CLINICAL PEDIATRIC ORTHOPEDICS

The Art of Diagnosis
and Principles of Management

CLINICAL PEDIATRIC ORTHOPEDICS

The Art of Diagnosis and Principles of Management

Mihran O. Tachdjian, MD
Professor of Orthopedic Surgery
Northwestern University Medical School
Chicago, Illinois

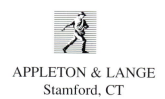

APPLETON & LANGE
Stamford, CT

Prentice Hall International (UK) Limited, *London*
Prentice Hall of Australia Pty. Limited, *Sydney*
Prentice Hall Canada, Inc., *Toronto*
Prentice Hall Hispanoamericana, S.A., *Mexico*
Prentice Hall of India Private Limited, *New Delhi*
Prentice Hall of Japan, Inc., *Tokyo*
Simon & Schuster Asia Pte. Ltd., *Singapore*
Editora Prentice Hall do Brasil Ltda., *Rio de Janiero*
Prentice Hall, *Upper Saddle River, New Jersey*

Tachdjian, Mihran O.
    Clinical pediatric orthopedics : the art of diagnosis and principles of management / Mihran O. Tachdjian.
        p.   cm.
    ISBN 0-8385-1106-6 (case : alk. paper)
    1. Pediatric orthopedics. I. Title.
    [DNLM: 1. Orthopedics—in infancy & childhood. 2. Musculoskeletal Diseases—diagnosis. 3. Muscholskeletal Diseases—therapy. WS 270 T117c 1996]
    RD732.3.C48T3283   1996
    617.3'0083—dc20
DNLM/DLC
for Library of Congress   96-8406
                                                                    CIP

Managing Editor Development: Kathleen McCullough
Production Editor: Sondra Greenfield
Designer: Libby Schmitz

PRINTED IN THE UNITED STATES OF AMERICA

ISBN 0-8385-1106-6

Dedicated to Sherman S. Coleman, MD,
A master clinician, teacher, and friend.

CONTENTS

PREFACE

Clinical Pediatric Orthopedics: The Art of Diagnosis and Principles of Management is a practical, concise, but thorough reference written for general orthopedic surgeons who treat children, orthopedic residents, pediatricians, primary care physicians, and allied health care personnel such as physical therapists, occupational therapists, and orthopedic nurses. I also hope the book is of value to radiologists who wish to refresh their recollection of the pathologic basis and clinical significance of imaging findings.

With changing patterns of health care, cost containment, and the demands for efficiency of utilization of time, the orthopedic resident-in-training often does not have the opportunity to be instructed in the art of history taking and physical examination. Often the key to diagnosis is a skillfully obtained clinical history and an examination performed with diligence. Many misdiagnoses are made because of incomplete histories and perfunctory, hurried examinations. Some so-called "modern" surgeons are treating radiograms, computed tomographic scans, and magnetic resonance images but not the child as a total person. The quest for a positive health care bottom line has sometimes depersonalized the physician-patient-parent relationship. The purpose of the book is to revive the art of medical diagnosis.

The book has six chapters. The first five chapters are regional in scope: Chapter 1, "Foot and Ankle"; Chapter 2, "Knee and Leg"; Chapter 3, "Hip and Thigh"; Chapter 4, "Neck and Upper Limb"; and Chapter 5, "Spine." Chapter 6 presents generalized conditions that involve the neuromusculoskeletal system. Only common and challenging orthopedic problems are presented because of space restrictions of the book. For the diagnosis of uncommon rare entities and the details of surgical management, the reader is referred to other voluminous works by this and other authors. This is a clinical rather than an operative textbook.

The format of the book is consistent from chapter to chapter. First, the presenting complaint or complaints of each orthopedic affection is given; next, each entity is defined with a brief statement of etiology, genetics, and pathology. This is followed by pertinent questions to ask during history taking. Then a step-by-step, orderly examination of the part and the entire child is described. To arrive at a clinical diagnosis, the orthopedic examination should follow a definite order: inspection (in stance and posture), gait, palpation, assessment of deformities, range of motion of joints, testing of motor power and muscle strength, and neurologic examination. The appropriate investigations by radiography, ultrasonography, computed tomography, magnetic resonance imaging, and various laboratory tests necessary to make a definitive diagnosis are discussed. Principles of management are presented.

The differential diagnosis of various conditions is presented by category of disease, system involved, and the age of the patient, as different deformities and affections of the neuromusculoskeletal system affect different age groups; also, some diseases affect children in all age groups.

It is hoped that the physician-surgeon will examine the child with concern, sympathy, kindness, and patience, combining his or her scientific knowledge with an understanding of the wants and needs of the child and its parents.

My thanks to Marguerite Aitken and Cindy Eller for their superb illustrations, all of which are original. I also would like to express my deep gratitude to Lynn Ridings for her expert editorial assistance.

Mihran O. Tachdjian

THE FOOT AND ANKLE

Anatomically the foot can be divided into three parts: (1) the forefoot, which consists of the metatarsals and the phalanges; (2) the midfoot, which is made up of the three cuneiforms and the cuboid bone (some surgeons include the navicular among the bones of the midfoot); and (3) the hindfoot, which consists of the calcaneus, talus, and navicular.

The ankle joint comprises the lower ends of the tibia and fibula and the dome of the talus. It is a true mortise joint. The axis of motion of the ankle is plantar flexion and dorsiflexion. The joint is stable and limited in all other planes of motion. The subtalar joint is a single-axis joint connecting the talus and calcaneus, allowing inversion and eversion. The transverse tarsal articulation consists of the calcaneocuboid and talonavicular joints. They allow adduction-inversion-plantar flexion and abduction-eversion-dorsiflexion. The tarsometatarsal, metatarsophalangeal, and interphalangeal joints allow flexion-extension.

Specific terms used to describe deformities of the ankle and foot depend upon the direction of joint motion. Neutral is the anatomic zero position. At the *ankle,* calcaneus denotes extension (dorsiflexion) deformity, whereas equinus describes flexion (plantar flexion) deformity; at the *subtalar* joint, inversion denotes heel varus and eversion heel valgus. At the midtarsal joint abductus denotes abduction; adductus adduction; cavus flexion; rocker-bottom extension (with the hindfoot-ankle in equinus); supination inversion-adduction; and pronation eversion-abduction. In the great and lesser toes flexion denotes flexion deformity and extension extension deformity. In motions of the great toe, the center of the foot is the reference point; that is, hallux valgus describes deviation of the great toe toward the center of the foot (away from the center of the body), whereas hallux varus describes deviation toward the center of the body away from the center of the foot. Joint deformity is due to contracture of the capsule, ligaments, and muscles. Table 1–1 summarizes the deformities of the foot and ankle.

GROWTH OF THE FOOT

The growth of the foot is very rapid during infancy and up to the age of 5 years. By 1 year in girls and 1.5 years in boys, the foot has reached one half of its adult size. After 5 years of age, the rate of growth of the foot decreases, reaching its mature length at the age of 12 years in girls and 16 years in boys. From a surgical standpoint, the skeleton of a foot is almost mature at 12 in girls and 14 in boys (Fig 1–1).

OSSIFICATION OF THE BONES OF THE FOOT AND ANKLE

In utero the tips of the distal phalanges in the foot are the first to ossify, followed by the metatarsals and later the proximal and middle phalanges.

In the newborn, the ossification centers of the calcaneus, talus, and cuboid are ordinarily present. However, it should be noted that cuboid bone ossification may be delayed until 3 weeks of age. Also, in the newborn, the metatarsals and the ossification centers of all of the metatarsals and phalanges are present. It should be noted that the growth plate of the first metatarsal is proximal and the growth plates of the second to fifth metatarsals are distal (Fig 1–2A, B and Fig 1–4).

The lateral cuneiform ossifies between the ages of 4 and 20 months, the medial cuneiform at around 2 years of age, the intermediate cuneiform at 3 years of age, and the navicular between the second and fifth years of age (Figs 1–3 and 1–4). The apophysis of the calcaneus ossifies between 4 and 6 years of age in girls and 5 and 7 years of age in boys (Fig 1–5). It fuses with the body of the calcaneus at 16 years of age in girls and 20 years of age in boys (Fig 1–6).

The ossification center of the distal tibial epiphysis is usually present at birth (Fig 1–7). The medial malleolus begins to ossify at 7 years of age in girls and 8 years of age in boys. The ossification center of the distal fibular epiphysis appears between postnatal months 11 and 18 (Fig 1–8).

ACCESSORY BONES OF THE FOOT

The foot is known for having numerous accessory bones. These should not be mistaken for fractures or osteochon-

TABLE 1–1. DEFORMITIES OF THE FOOT AND ANKLE ACCORDING TO RANGE OF MOTION OF JOINTS

Joint	Contracture	Deformity
Ankle	Extension (dorsiflexion)	Calcaneus
	Flexion (plantar flexion)	Equinus
Subtalar	Inversion	Heel varus
	Eversion	Heel valgus
Midtarsal	Adduction	Adductus
	Abduction	Abductus
	Flexion	Cavus
	Extension (with heel and ankle in equinus)	Rocker-bottom
	Inversion-adduction	Supination
	Eversion-abduction	Pronation
Lesser toes	Flexion	Flexion
	Extension	Extension
Great toe (hallux)	Deviation toward center of foot (away from the body)	Hallux valgus
Note: Reference point is center of foot, not center of body	Deviation away from center of foot toward center of body	Hallux varus
	Flexion	Flexion
	Extension	Extension

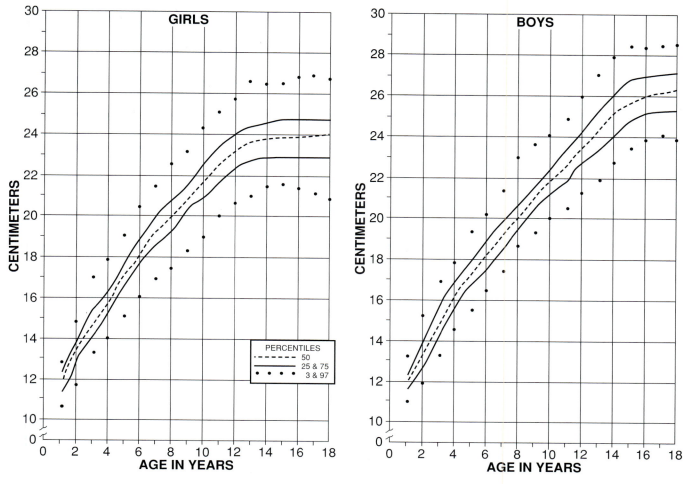

Figure 1-1. Length of normal foot derived from serial measurements of 512 children from 1 to 18 years of age. (From Blais MM, Green WT, Anderson M: Length of the growing foot. J Bone Joint Surg 38A:998, 1956. Reprinted by permission.)

dritis. In order of frequency these are os trigonum—13 percent, os fibulare—10 percent, os tibiale externum—10 percent, os intermetatarseum—9 percent, os sustentaculi I—5 percent, calcaneus secondarius—4 percent, os cuboideum secondarium—1 percent, talus secondarius—less than 1 percent, os vesalianum—less than 1 percent, os intercunei-forme—less than 1 percent, and pars fibularis ossis metatarsalis—seldom (Fig 1–9).

There may be separate ossification centers for the medial malleoli and distal end of the fibula. There may also be other abnormalities and variations that are not pathologic, such as a separate center of ossification for the head of the talus which develops on its dorsal aspect. An anomaly in which the head and neck of the talus are tilted dorsally is known as Africoid talus.

In 10 percent of children older than 7 years, a triangular or circular area of radiolucency may appear in the

inferior half of the body of the calcaneus, suggesting a pseudocyst, but it is a normal variation and not a deficiency of spongy bone. The calcaneus may have an enlarged trochlea that looks like an exostosis. Often a secondary center of ossification in the calcaneal apophysis develops in girls between 10.5 and 12 years and in boys between 11.5 and 13.5 years and quickly fuses with the body of the calcaneus. Occasionally two centers of ossification are present instead of one, and the cartilaginous junction between the two ossific nuclei suggests a fracture. Fragmentation and sclerosis of the apophysis of the calcaneus are normal.

A separate center of ossification of the tarsonavicular (os tibialis externus) is present in 10 percent of the population. It fuses to the tuberosity of the navicular in adolescence, but in 2 percent it persists as a separate bone.

The cuboid may have multiple, fine ossification centers. An accessory ossification center of the cuboid should not be

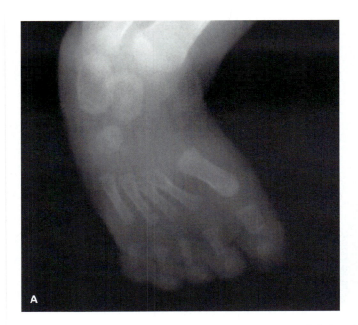

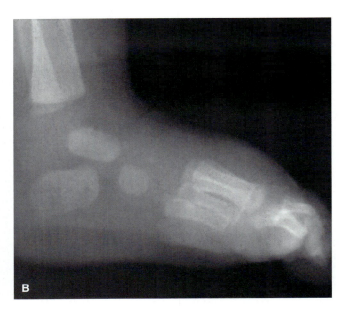

Figure 1-2. Ossification centers in a newborn. **A.** AP. **B.** Lateral. Note that the only ossification centers present are those of the calcaneus, talus, cuboid, metatarsals, and phalanges.

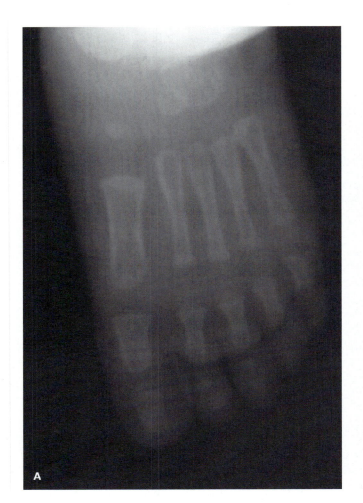

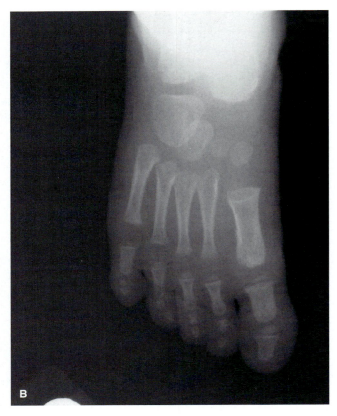

Figure 1-3. Ossification of cuneiform bones. **A.** AP radiogram of the foot in a 3-year-old child. Note the beginning of ossification of the medial cuneiform and intermediate cuneiforms. **B.** AP radiogram of the foot in a 4-year-old showing ossification of the intermediate, lateral, and medial cuneiforms.

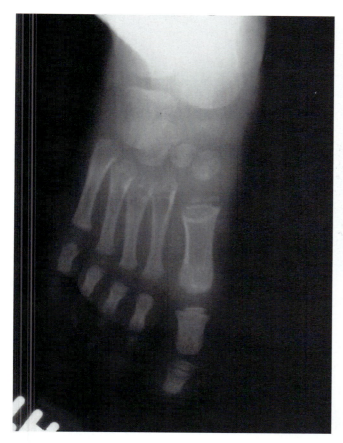

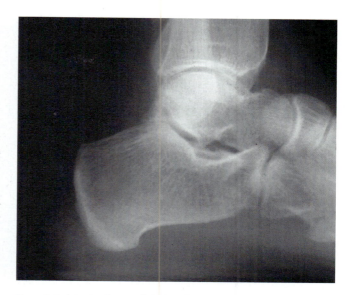

Figure 1–6. Lateral radiogram of the foot showing fusion of the apophysis of the calcaneus in a 16-year-old girl.

Figure 1–4. AP radiogram of the foot of a 4-year-old. Note the beginning of ossification of the navicular. The growth plate of the first metatarsal is proximal, whereas that of the second through fifth metatarsals is distal.

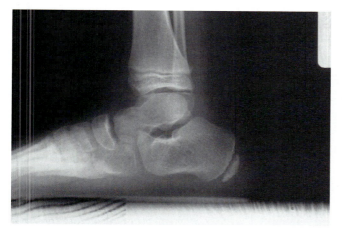

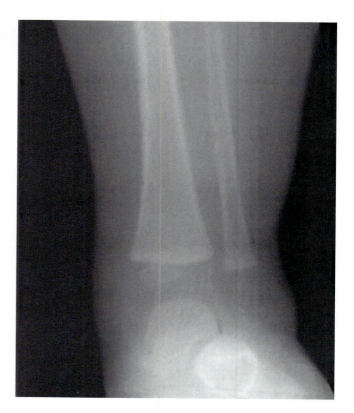

Figure 1–5. Lateral radiogram of the foot of a 6-year-old boy. Note the beginning of ossification of the apophysis of the calcaneus. This should not be mistaken for osteochondritis dissecans.

Figure 1–7. AP radiogram of the ankle in an 18-month-old girl showing the ossification centers of the distal tibial epiphysis and fibula.

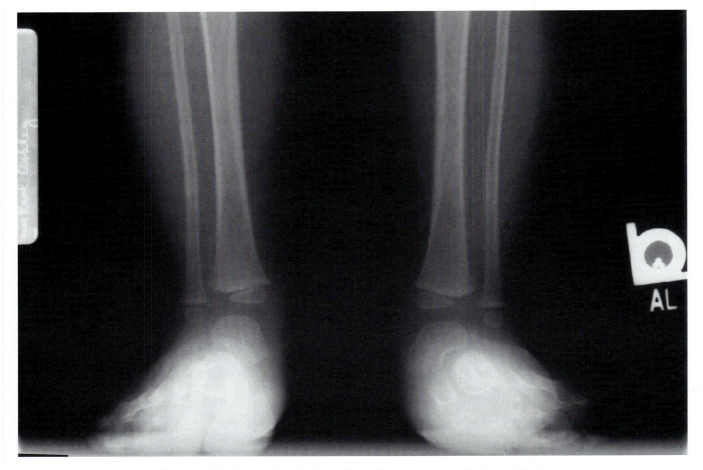

Figure 1–8. AP radiogram of the ankle showing the ossification center of the distal fibular epiphysis.

mistaken for a fracture; it is also referred to as os fibulare (Fig 1–10). In addition to an accessory navicular, there may be a small ossicle on the dorsum of the navicular known as os supranaviculare. The cuneiform edges may be irregular.

An accessory ossification center at the base of the fifth metatarsal (os vesalianum) runs parallel to the lateral cortex of the fifth metatarsal (Fig 1–11). It should not be mistaken for a fracture; the latter is transverse or oblique to the base of the fifth metatarsal.

The fifth toe may have two phalanges instead of three. Sclerosis of the epiphysis of the proximal phalanx is a normal variation. A pseudoepiphysis may be found at the base of the metatarsals.

■ POSTURAL AND CONGENITAL DEFORMITIES OF THE FOOT AND ANKLE

Deformities of the foot and ankle at birth may occur because of intrauterine malposture or congenital malfor-

mation, or they may be paralytic, as in myelomeningocele.

Normal posture of the newborn reflects intrauterine posture—the way the fetus was folded up and laid against the curvature of the wall of the uterus.

At birth the forefeet tend to be adducted with the soles facing each other in slight plantar flexion. The legs are medially rotated and bowed medially, and the knees are in 15 to 20 degrees of flexion. The hips are in 15 to 20 degrees of flexion (they cannot be extended fully) and are held in varying degrees of lateral rotation; the normal hip at birth, however, abducts fully. The spine has a long C curve—the round back resembling the curve of a banana, but it can be straightened fully on passive extension. The elbows and hands are postured in some flexion, and the fingers are clenched in the palm.

Abnormal posture at birth results in deformities that are not fixed; ordinarily they resolve and straighten fully once the baby is liberated from the tight intrauterine compartment. With skeletal growth secondary contractures occasionally develop, and active treatment is indicated. Pos-

A. Medial view

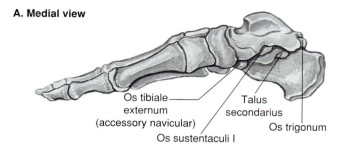

Os tibiale
externum
(accessory navicular)

Talus
secondarius

Os trigonum

Os sustentaculi I

B. Plantar view

Pars fibularis ossis metatarsalis I

Os tibiale externum

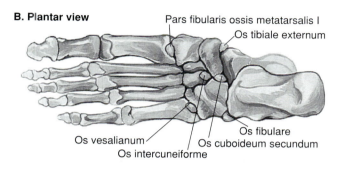

Os vesalianum

Os fibulare

Os cuboideum secundum

Os intercuneiforme

C. Lateral view

Os intercuneiforme

Os intermetatarseum

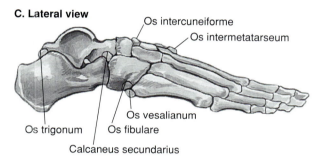

Os vesalianum

Os trigonum

Os fibulare

Calcaneus secundarius

Figure 1–9. Accessory bones of the foot.

tural deformation of the limbs, head, and neck is a packaging problem. Minimal deformities should be regarded as a variation of normal.

Postural deformities of the newborn in the foot and ankle are metatarsus adductus, metatarsus primus varus, postural clubfoot, calcaneovalgus, pes valgus, and equinus (Fig 1–12). The leg should be examined for medial and occasionally lateral tibiofibular torsion and the knee for genu recurvatum or hyperextension deformity. The hip is susceptible to lateral rotation contracture, pelvic obliquity with adduction contracture of one hip, and abduction contracture of the opposite hip. The spine is susceptible to positional infantile scoliosis and the head and neck to postural torticollis and plagiocephaly.

In this section only postural deformities of the foot and ankle are presented. However, it behooves the surgeon to examine the entire body to rule out associated postural deformities, as they often coexist.

The postural deformities in which the presenting complaint is turning-in of the foot are (1) metatarsus adductus, (2) metatarsus primus varus, (3) pes varus, and (4) pes equinovarus. Postural deformities in which the feet turn out are (1) calcaneovalgus and (2) pes valgus. Congenital deformities that cause turning-in of the foot are congenital metatarsus varus, congenital hallux varus, talipes equinovarus, and ankle varus due to congenital longitudinal deficiency of the tibia.

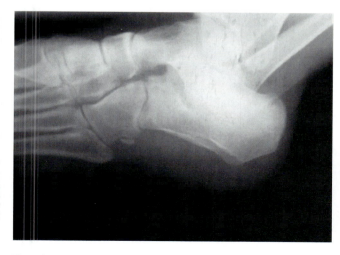

Figure 1–10. Radiogram of the foot showing an accessory bone of the cuboid which is referred to as os fibulare.

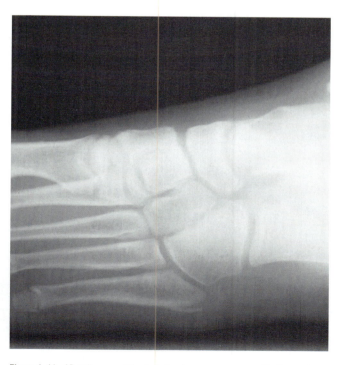

Figure 1–11. AP radiogram of the foot showing an accessory ossification center at the base of the fifth metatarsal, which is known as os vesalianum.

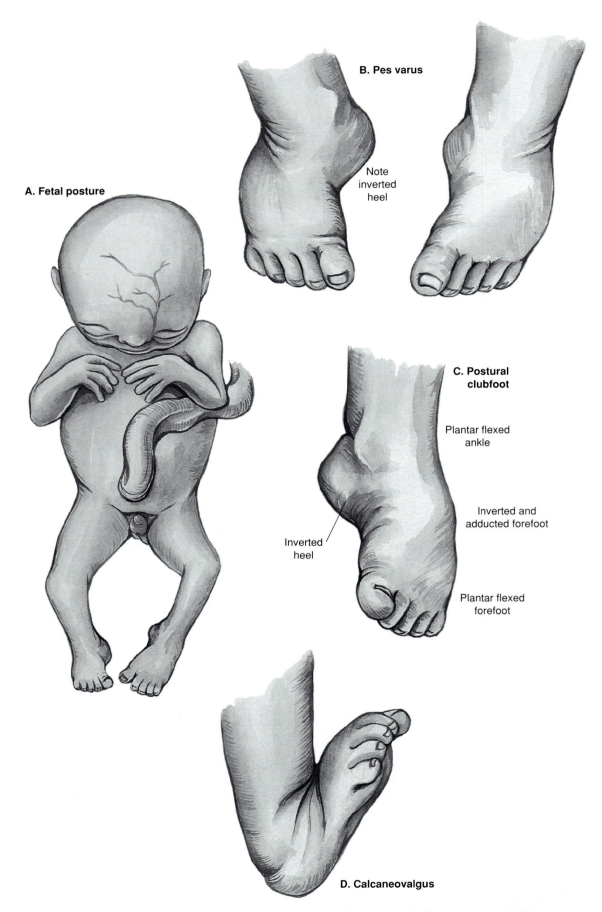

B. Pes varus

Note
inverted
heel

A. Fetal posture

**C. Postural
clubfoot**

Plantar flexed
ankle

Inverted and
adducted forefoot

Inverted
heel

Plantar flexed
forefoot

D. Calcaneovalgus

Figure 1–12. Normal fetal posture at birth and postural deformities of the feet and ankles. **A.** Normal fetal posture. **B.** Metatarsus adductus. **C.** Postural clubfoot. **D.** Calcaneovalgus. *(Continues)*

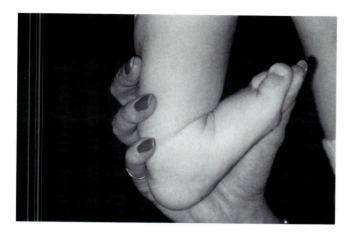

Figure 1–12 *(Continued).* **E.** Clinical appearance of calcaneovalgus of the foot.

TOEING-IN

Metatarsus Adductus

In this deformity the presenting complaint is that the foot turns in; the entire forefoot is adducted at the tarsometatarsal level. Usually the big toe is in more varus than the rest of the toes, with a wide gap between it and the second toe. The abductor hallucis muscle is taut. The hindfoot is in normal position. No crease is found on the medial plantar aspect of the foot. The deformity is not rigid; the forefoot can be passively manipulated into neutral position or slightly abducted (Fig 1–13). It should be distinguished from metatarsus primus varus, in which only the first metatarsal and the big toe are adducted.

Postural metatarsus adductus should be differentiated from congenital metatarsus varus; in the latter the deformity is rigid, it cannot be corrected by passive manipulation, and a crease is present on the medial plantar aspect of the foot at the tarsometatarsal joint level. It does not correct spontaneously.

Examine the hips to rule out developmental hip dysplasia. Infants with postural metatarsus adductus are at high risk for hip dislocation.

Treatment. In 90 percent of patients with metatarsus adductus, the feet tend to grow straight and correct spontaneously. They do not require active treatment. When the deformity is moderate or severe, however, it is best to perform passive stretching exercises. Only very occasionally does a metatarsus adductus foot develop fixed contractural deformity with skeletal growth and require serial casts or splinting.

Congenital Metatarsus Varus

The infant is presented with a chief complaint of the forefoot turning in. The forefoot is adducted and inverted at the tarsometatarsal joint, and a crease is present on the medial plantar aspect of the foot. The deformity is due to medial displacement (subluxation) of the tarsometatarsal joints. It occurs in about 1 in 1000 live births.[18] The deformity is evident at birth, and it increases in severity as the infant grows. The lateral border of the foot becomes convex, with the base of the fifth metatarsal prominent. On palpation the abductor hallucis muscle is taut, and on passive manipulation the varus deformity cannot be corrected (Fig 1–14).

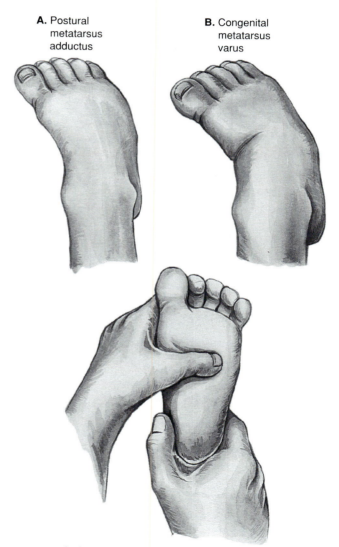

A. Postural metatarsus adductus

B. Congenital metatarsus varus

C. Correction with passive manipulation in postural metatarsus adductus

Figure 1–13. Metatarsus adductus. **A.** Postural. There is no crease on the medial plantar aspect of the foot. **B.** Congenital. Note the crease. **C.** Passive correction.

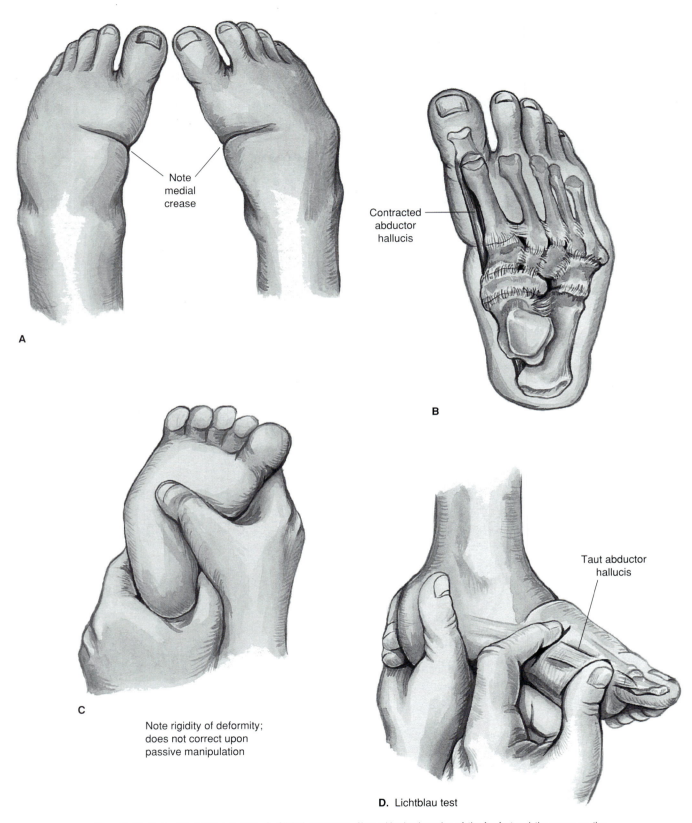

Figure 1–14. Congenital metatarsus varus. **A.** Clinical appearance. Note adduction-inversion of the forefoot and the crease on the medial plantar aspect at the level of the tarsometatarsal joint. **B.** The abductor hallucis is taut. **C.** Note the rigid deformity. It cannot be corrected on passive manipulation. **D.** Lichtblau test. On passive lateral deviation of the big toe, the taut tendon of the abductor hallucis is prominent.

Treatment. If mild, treatment consists of passive stretching exercises and splinting at night in an ankle-foot orthosis with the heel and the ankle in neutral position and the forefoot in maximal abduction. If moderate or severe, it is best corrected by serial stretching casts that are changed weekly. Within 2 to 3 weeks the deformity can be fully corrected. Following cast removal, passive stretching exercises are performed. Reverse-last shoes and splints should not be used when the deformity is severe and rigid, as they cause a skew or serpentine foot.

Serpentine or Skewfoot (Z Foot)

This complex deformity of the foot consists of a rigid metatarsus varus and hindfoot valgus with a flexible oblique talus and lateral subluxation of the talonavicular and calcaneocuboid joints. It is often due to inadequate treatment of congenital metatarsus varus in a child with ligamentous hyperlaxity. Weight-bearing radiograms of the foot depict the articular malalignment of the hindfoot, midfoot, and forefoot.

Treatment. In the young child an attempt should be made to correct the deformity by manipulation of the foot and serial casts—holding the heel in inversion and molding the longitudinal arch as you push the forefoot into valgus during application of the cast.

In the older child with fixed deformity and painful foot, surgical correction is indicated. It consists of osteotomy of the second through fourth metatarsals and capsulotomy of the first metatarsal–medial cuneiform joint or open-up wedge osteotomy of the medial cuneiform, correction of hindfoot valgus, and lateral subluxation of the talonavicular and calcaneocuboid joints by open-up osteotomy and bone graft of the anterior part of the calcaneus. Internal fixation is mandatory to maintain concentric reduction.

Metatarsus Primus Varus

In this deformity only the big toe and first metatarsal are deviated medially; the lesser toes and their metatarsals are aligned normally. The abductor hallucis is taut, pulling the hallux into varus and causing an abnormally wide gap between the big and second toes. It should be distinguished from congenital hallux varus, in which the deformity is rigid, the first metatarsal is short, and the first metatarsophalangeal joint is subluxated medially.

Radiograms are not ordinarily indicated in the infant and the young child. In standing AP radiograms of the feet, the angle between the first and second metatarsals is greater than 10 degrees.

Treatment. Treatment consists of passive stretching exercises and splinting at night. In the severe deformity, manipulation and cast application may be required, as it may take up to 1 year for complete correction. The parents become concerned by the persisting prehensile posture of the great toe and the toeing-in gait when the infant begins to ambulate.

Congenital Hallux Varus

In hallux varus the great toe is deviated medially at the metatarsophalangeal joint. Ordinarily the first metatarsal is short (Fig 1–15). It may be a primary deformity in which contracted fibrous tissues act as a tether, pulling the big toe into medial deviation, or it may be a varus deformity of the forefoot in which all of the metatarsals are deviated medially, the big toe more than the lesser toes. It may also be a part of a generalized bone dysplasia such as diastrophic dwarfism.

Treatment. Surgical correction is ordinarily carried out between the ages of 6 and 12 months. The technique depends upon the type. It is a more complex problem when the hallux is duplicated. Provide a skin flap on the medial aspect of the forefoot. Section all contracted soft tissues. A flap is taken from the plantar aspect of the foot and rotated to cover the defect on the medial side of the foot. The other sites of defect are covered with full-thickness skin grafts. When the hallux is duplicated, the extra big toe is excised.

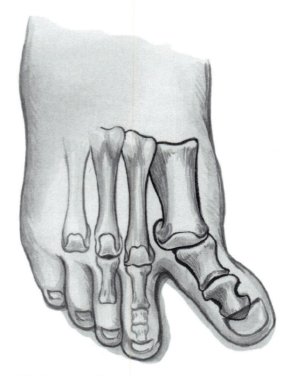

Figure 1–15. Congenital hallux varus. Note the medial subluxation of the first metatarsophalangeal joint and the short first metatarsal. The big toe is not duplicated in this form.

Postural Pes Varus

In this deformity, the forefoot is adducted and the hindfoot is in inversion. Range of dorsiflexion and plantar flexion is normal, and radiograms show normal talocalcaneonavicular and calcaneocuboid articular relationships. Treatment consists of passive stretching exercises. If the deformity is moderate to severe, splinting is used, and if it is very severe, manipulation and casts are employed to correct the deformity.

Postural Clubfoot

In this deformity the entire foot is plantar flexed at the ankle joint. The hindfoot is inverted and the forefoot is adducted and inverted. No abnormal skin crease is seen on the medial plantar aspect of the midfoot or the ankle (see Fig 1–12C).

On palpation, space is felt between the medial malleolus and the navicular, and the lateral malleolus and the calcaneus are not tethered. No atrophy of the calf is present, and the deformity of the foot is not rigid. On passive manipulation it can be partially or fully corrected.

The postural clubfoot should be distinguished from congenital talipes equinovarus, in which the deformity is rigid. Medial plantar and posterior ankle creases are present. The heel is drawn up with severe equinus deformity. The lateral malleolus and calcaneus are tethered, with limited range of plantar flexion and dorsiflexion of the ankle joint. The hallux appears shortened because of the proximal displacement of the medial column of the foot. The navicular abuts the medial malleolus. Moderate to severe calf atrophy is present.

Radiograms should be made to rule out congenital talipes equinovarus (clubfoot) (Fig 1–16A–D). In postural clubfoot the AP projection shows that the talar–first metatarsal angle is increased, but the talocalcaneal angle is normal (20 to 40 degrees) and no medial subluxation of the cuboid on the calcaneus is present. In the lateral projection, the talocalcaneal angle is normal (35 to 50 degrees). In intrinsic talipes equinovarus, the talocalcaneal angle in the AP view is less than 20 degrees and in the lateral projection less than 30 degrees.

Treatment. Treatment consists of passive stretching exercises and retention in cast followed by splinting. The prognosis is excellent, and the deformity can be corrected without any surgical measures within a few weeks. The importance of splinting the foot and ankle at night in slightly overcorrected posture cannot be overemphasized.

Congenital Talipes Equinovarus

Congenital talipes equinovarus is an in utero medial plantar displacement of the talocalcaneonavicular and calca-

neocuboid joints. The clinical appearance at birth is characteristic. The ankle is in fixed equinus with the heel drawn up and the calcaneus tethered to the fibula. Range of plantar flexion and dorsiflexion of the ankle is markedly restricted. The forefoot and midfoot are in fixed equinus and inversion. The navicular is displaced medially abutting the medial malleolus, and the calcaneocuboid joint is displaced medially. With medial angulation of the talar neck and head, the anterior part of the calcaneus follows the deformed anterior part of the talus and shifts medially, whereas the posterior part of the calcaneus shifts laterally. The calcaneus rotates medially in relation to the body of the talus, the interosseous ligament acting as a fulcrum. The subtalar joint has a medial spin. The talocalcaneonavicular and calcaneocuboid joints are displaced medially and plantarward under the tethering effect of contractures of the soft tissues, which are the triceps surae, posterior tibial, long toe flexors, calcaneofibular and talofibular ligaments, posterior capsule of the ankle and subtalar joints, anterior tibionavicular ligament, medial capsule of the subtalar joint, and short plantar muscles and ligaments (Fig 1–17).

Incidence. This congenital deformity is more common in males, with a male:female ratio of 2:1. The incidence in the male Caucasian is 1.6 per thousand and half that rate in the female Caucasian.[43,87] A definite racial predilection is seen: It is much more common in Hawaiians, with an incidence of 4.9 per thousand in mixed Hawaiians and 6.81 per thousand in full-blooded Hawaiians.[30,45] The incidence of talipes equinovarus is very low in Asians—0.57 per thousand. In about one of two clubfoot patients, both feet are affected.

Etiology. The condition is often referred to as idiopathic clubfoot because the exact cause is unknown. The deformity is multifactorial in its pathogenesis. It is important that one distinguish the various types of clubfoot.

Primary Germ Plasm Defect. Irani and Sherman[68] and Settle[75] have shown that the primary deformity of idiopathic talipes equinovarus is medial plantar tilting of the head and neck of the talus, with decrease of the declination angle of the talus (Fig 1–18). The normal declination angle of the talus is 150 to 160 degrees. In talipes equinovarus, it decreases to 115 degrees or less.

Arterial abnormalities have been demonstrated in talipes equinovarus, and arterial dysgenesis and disturbance of growth of the medial aspect of the talus may have a role in the pathogenesis of clubfoot.[80,81]

Neuromuscular Defect. Imbalance between the invertors and evertors and plantar flexors and dorsiflexors of the foot and ankle and fibrosis and contracture of the paralyzed

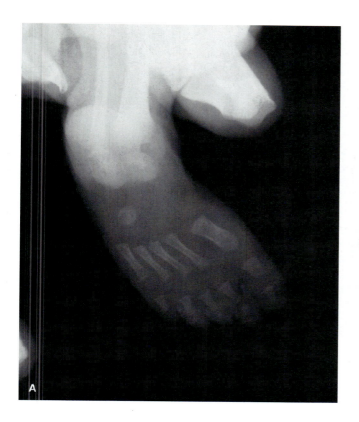

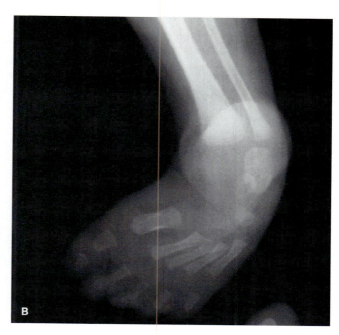

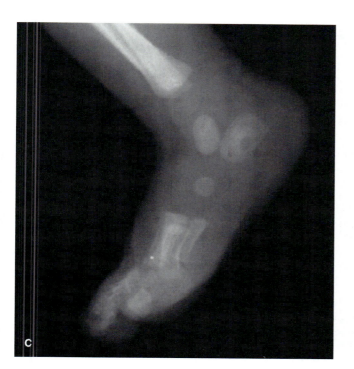

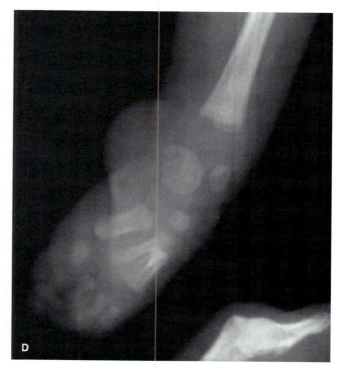

Figure 1–16. Radiograms of postural clubfoot and talipes equinovarus in the same child. **A.** AP radiogram of postural clubfoot. Note that the anterior ends of the talus and calcaneus are divergent. The hindfoot is inverted and the forefoot is adducted. **B.** AP radiogram of the left foot with talipes equinovarus. Note that the talocalcaneal angle is zero. The talo–first metatarsal angle is 50 degrees, and the cuboid is displaced medially. **C.** Lateral view of postural clubfoot. The lateral talocalcaneal angle is 45 degrees. The calcaneal pitch is 5 degrees of dorsiflexion, and the tibiocalcaneal angle is about 90 degrees. There is no forefoot equinus. **D.** Lateral radiogram of the foot in talipes equinovarus. Note that the lateral talocalcaneal angle is zero. Severe equinus of the ankle with a posterior crease at the ankle and severe cavus (forefoot equinus) with a crease on the plantar aspect of the foot are present.

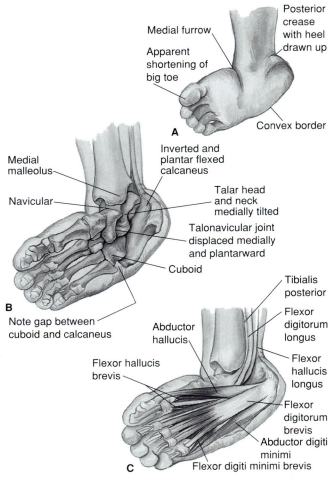

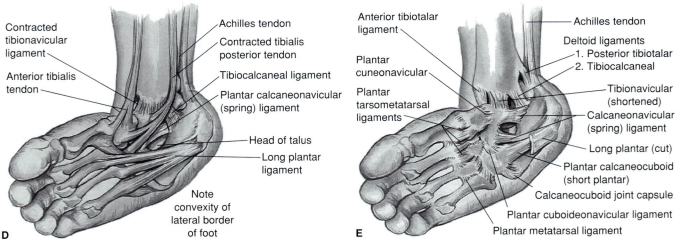

Figure 1–17. Pathologic findings in talipes equinovarus. **A–E.** Medial-plantar view. **A.** Clinical appearance. Note the inverted heel in marked equinus with a posterior crease at the ankle joint, the furrow on the medial plantar aspect of the midfoot with forefoot equinus, the apparent shortening of the hallux, the concave medial border of the foot with the forefoot adducted and inverted, and the convex lateral border of the foot. **B.** Articular and bony pathology. The talus is tilted and fixed in equinus with its head and neck tilted medially and plantarward. The calcaneus is in equinus and the heel is inverted. The talonavicular joint is displaced medially, with the navicular abutting the medial malleolus and displaced medially. The first ray appears shortened, and the calcaneocuboid joint is displaced medially. **C.** Muscle and tendon pathology. Posterior tibial, flexor digitorum longus, and flexor hallucis longus are contracted. The abductor hallucis is shortened. The plantar muscles are contracted, with an equinus and varus deformity of the forefoot and midfoot. **D, E.** Ligamentous and capsular pathology. Note the contractures of the following ligaments: tibionavicular, tibiocalcaneal, plantar calcaneonavicular (spring), and long plantar. It is imperative that these ligaments be released to obtain concentric alignment of the talocalcaneal navicular and calcaneocuboid joints. In **E**, note the contracture of the following capsules and ligaments: posterior tibiotalar, tibiocalcaneal, calcaneonavicular, plantar calcaneocuboid, calcaneocuboid joint capsule, plantar cuboideonavicular, plantar tarsometatarsal ligaments, and plantar cuneonavicular. *(Continues)*

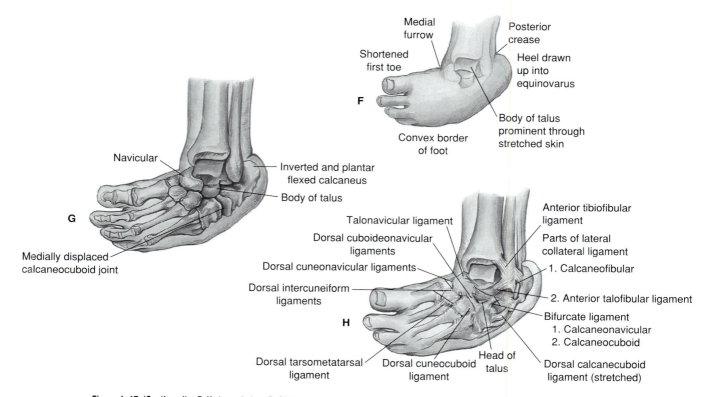

Medial
furrow

Posterior
crease

Shortened
first toe

Heel drawn
up into
equinovarus

F

Body of talus
prominent through
stretched skin

Convex border
of foot

Navicular

Inverted and plantar
flexed calcaneus

Body of talus

G

Medially displaced
calcaneocuboid joint

Talonavicular ligament

Anterior tibiofibular
ligament

Dorsal cuboideonavicular
ligaments

Parts of lateral
collateral ligament

Dorsal cuneonavicular ligaments

1. Calcaneofibular

Dorsal intercuneiform
ligaments

2. Anterior talofibular ligament

H

Bifurcate ligament
1. Calcaneonavicular
2. Calcaneocuboid

Head of
talus

Dorsal calcanecuboid
ligament (stretched)

Dorsal tarsometatarsal
ligament

Dorsal cuneocuboid
ligament

Figure 1–17 *(Continued).* **F–H.** Lateral view. **F.** Clinical appearance. Note the convex lateral border of the foot due to medial displacement of the calcaneocuboid joint, the shortened appearance of the hallux, and the prominent body of the talus on the dorsolateral aspect of the foot. **G.** Bony and articular pathology. Note the medially displaced calcaneocuboid joint and the prominent body of the talus. **H.** Ligamentous and capsular pathology. The calcaneus is tethered to the fibula by the contracted calcaneofibular ligament. *(Continues)*

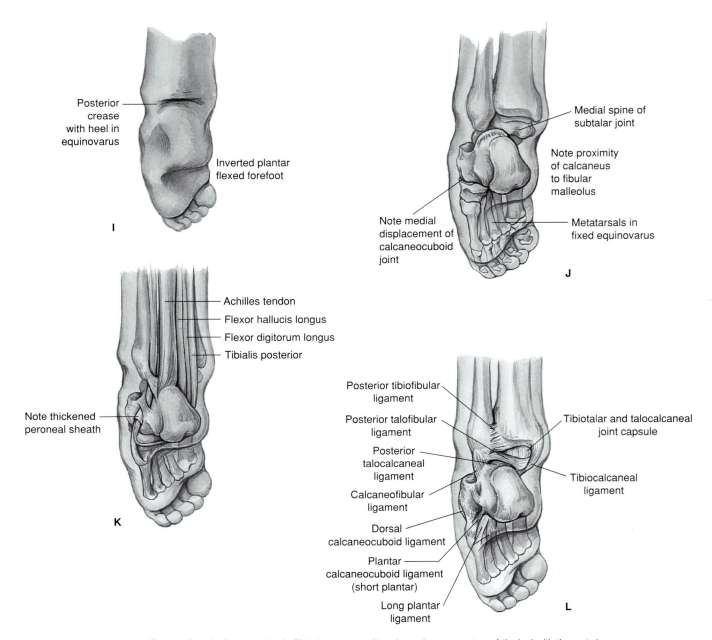

Figure 1–17 *(Continued).* **I–L.** Posterior view. **I.** Clinical appearance. Note the equinovarus posture of the heel with the posterior crease and the forefoot equinus. **J.** Bone and joint pathology. The calcaneus abuts the fibular malleolus, and the calcaneocuboid joint is displaced medially. The metatarsals are fixed in equinovarus. The calcaneus is rotated medially under the body of the talus. **K.** Muscle tendon pathology. Note the contractures of the Achilles tendon, flexor hallucis longus, flexor digitorum longus, and posterior tibial. The peroneal sheath is contracted and thickened. **L.** Ligamentous and capsular pathology. Note the contractures of the posterior tibiofibular, posterior talofibular, posterior talocalcaneal, calcaneofibular, plantar calcaneocuboid, and long plantar. The capsules of the tibiotalar and talocalcaneal joints are contracted posteriorly. *(Continues)*

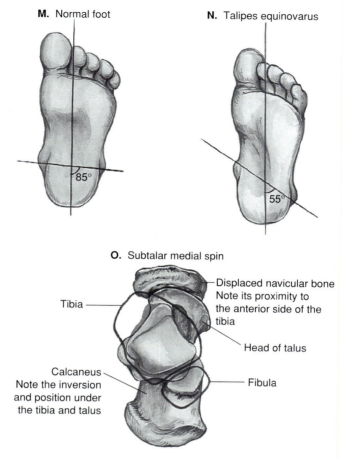

M. Normal foot

N. Talipes equinovarus

85°

55°

O. Subtalar medial spin

Displaced navicular bone
Note its proximity to
the anterior side of the
tibia

Tibia

Head of talus

Calcaneus
Note the inversion
and position under
the tibia and talus

Fibula

Figure 1–17 *(Continued).* M–O. The bimalleolar axis is decreased due to medial spin of the subtalar joint. **M.** Normal foot. Note the bimalleolar axis of 85 degrees. **N.** Talipes equinovarus. The bimalleolar axis is decreased to 55 degrees. **O.** Medial spin of the subtalar joint.

muscles are the causes of neuromuscular clubfoot. Evidence indicates an associated muscle paresis in idiopathic clubfoot. Whether this is primary or acquired is difficult to determine.

Connective Tissue Abnormalities. Deficiency of elastic tissues and an increased number of desmofibroblasts in clubfeet are pathogenic factors in contracture of ligamentous and capsular tissue. Idiopathic talipes equinovarus is not due to an arrest of fetal development.

Clinical Findings. The appearance of the foot is typical. It looks like a club—hence the name "clubfoot" (Fig 1–19A–E). The forefoot and midfoot are inverted and adducted. The big toe is relatively shortened. The lateral border of the foot is convex, and its medial border is concave with a furrow on the medial plantar aspect of the foot. The forefoot is in equinus. The heel is drawn up and inverted, and a deep skin crease is present on the posterior aspect of the ankle joint. The calf is atrophic. On manipulation, the foot is rigid; the forefoot cannot be abducted and everted, and the hindfoot cannot be everted out of varus. Range of motion of the ankle joint is limited. The foot cannot be dorsiflexed to neutral; attempting to do so causes a rocker-bottom deformity with the heel fixed in equinus and dorsiflexion at the tarsometatarsal joints. Range of the ankle is also restricted. The lateral malleolus is tethered to the calcaneus, and, on plantar flexion and dorsiflexion of the ankle, normal upward and downward movement of the lateral malleolus does not occur. The skin on the lateral aspect of the foot in front of the lateral malleolus is thin, with a prominent body of the talus under it. The cuboid is displaced medially in relation to the anterior end of the calcaneus. The navicular is displaced medially and plantar-

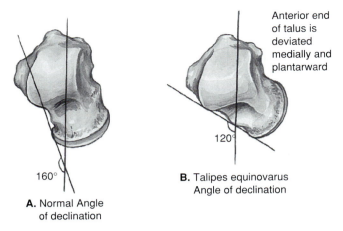

Anterior end of talus is deviated medially and plantarward

120°

B. Talipes equinovarus
Angle of declination

160°

A. Normal Angle
of declination

Figure 1–18. The angle between the head and neck and the body of the talus in the normal foot and in talipes equinovarus. **A.** Normal—the angle is 160 degrees. **B.** Talipes equinovarus—the angle is decreased to 120 degrees with medial tilting of the head and neck of the talus.

ward and tethered to the medial malleolus; the normal space between the medial malleolus and navicular is absent. The bimalleolar axis is decreased from a normal 85 degrees to 55 degrees in talipes equinovarus due to the subtalar medial spin. (see Fig 1–17, M–O)

Muscle testing for motor strength is difficult to perform in a newborn infant; however, by stimulation technique, one can determine whether or not muscles are functioning. The anterior and posterior tibial muscles are active and strong and contracted, whereas the peroneal muscles are weak and elongated. The toe extensors have normal motor strength; the toe flexors are shortened. The triceps surae muscle is strong. Because ruling out neuromuscular clubfoot is important, a muscle test should be performed, even though it is difficult to carry out.

Dorsalis pedis and tibial artery pulses are ordinarily present but vascular dysgenesis is possible, so it is important to assess circulation of the foot and ankle.

Next the spine of the infant should be examined to rule out spinal dysraphism and spina bifida. As a rule, I recommend AP and lateral radiography of the entire spine

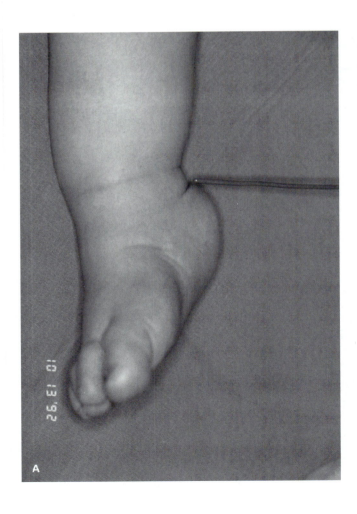

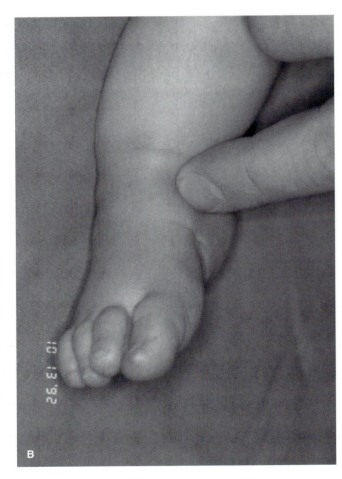

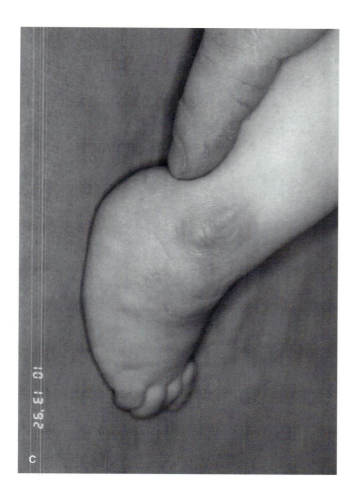

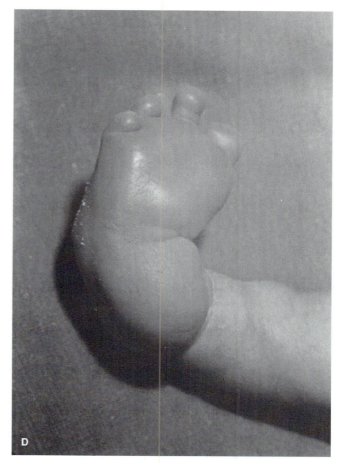

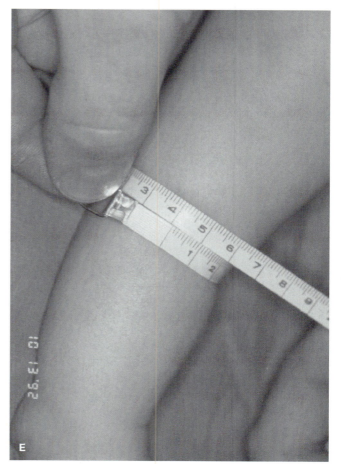

Figure 1–19. Clinical findings typical of talipes equinovarus. **A.** Severe rigid clubfoot with a crease over the midtarsal joints. The foot is in equinus and varus. **B.** Dorsal view showing palpation and absence of space between the medial malleolus and navicular, which abut. **C.** Lateral view showing the convexity of the lateral border of the foot due to medial displacement of the calcaneocuboid joint. **D.** Plantar view showing the medial posterior creases, apparent shortening of the hallux, and forefoot varus. **E.** Calf atrophy.

to rule out intraspinal pathology; in a child less than 4 to 6 months of age, ultrasonography of the spine should be performed when there is atrophy of the limb and a suggestion of neuromuscular deficit.

Other joints—the hips, knees, elbows, and shoulders—should be examined to rule out subluxation or dislocation. Hypoplasia of the tibia and medial subluxation of the ankle may be mistaken for clubfoot. Talipes equinovarus may be one of the manifestations of a generalized developmental syndrome.

The entire patient should be examined to rule out multiple malformations. Multiple congenital contractures (arthrogryposis multiplex congenita) manifest with decreasing muscle mass and fibrosis with rigidity of the joints. Streeter's dysplasia (congenital constriction bands) may be present. Clubfoot is one of the manifestations of diastrophic dysplasia, which is characterized by short first metacarpals and hitchhiker's thumb and by short first metatarsals with hallux varus; cauliflower ears and flexion deformity of the hips, knees, and elbows with webbing of the soft tissues are also evident. In Freeman-Sheldon syndrome (or craniocarpotarsal dysplasia) the face has a "whistling" appearance with a small mouth and protuberant lips; an H-shaped cutaneous crease pattern on the chin and ulnar deviation of the fingers and toes are also present. Larsen's syndrome is characterized by multiple dislocations of joints and a flat face with a widened nasal bridge and prominent forehead.

Imaging Findings. Radiographic assessment is indicated to determine the degree of displacement of the talocalcaneonavicular and calcaneocuboid joints and the severity of deformity prior to commencing treatment. During the course of treatment, radiograms are made to determine whether concentric reduction has been achieved and is being maintained. During a recurrence of deformity in follow-up, radiograms delineate pathologic anatomy and site and type of deformity, thereby assisting the surgeon in choosing appropriate treatment. As stated, radiograms of the spine and ultrasonography of the spine (in an infant less than 4 to 6 months of age) should be performed to rule out spinal pathology. In the older child with marked calf atrophy in whom neuromuscular clubfoot is suspected, magnetic resonance imaging (MRI) of the entire spinal cord is performed to rule out intraspinal pathology.

The feet should be positioned correctly and a standard technique of radiography should be used. The x-ray technician should be appropriately instructed.

For the *AP projection,* place the child in a sitting position with the hips and knees flexed 90 degrees and the feet bearing weight on the cassette with their medial borders touching and parallel. The ankles are in as much dorsiflexion as possible, and the forefeet are out of varus. The uncooperative infant requires gentle restraint by one or both parents. Shield the patient and parents to minimize radiation exposure. The x-ray tube is pointed to the hindfoot and directed 30 degrees cranial to the perpendicular. If the developed film shows the distal tibial shaft overlapping the hindfoot, when the distal ends of the talus and calcaneus are at different levels (greater than 2 mm) or when the metatarsals overlap, the radiographic technique is improper.

For the *lateral projection,* the hindfoot is placed parallel to the cassette, which is placed in a vertical cassette holder with the heel flat on the table and the x-ray tube centered on the hindfoot perpendicular to the cassette. In the developed film, the fibular malleolus displaced posterior to the tibia means that the hindfoot with the ankle mortise was in lateral rotation. The foot should be medially rotated so that the midfoot and forefoot are parallel to the cassette.

In the infant the navicular and cuneiform are not ossified; because they have the same density as surrounding soft tissues, they are radiologically "silent." The ossification centers of the calcaneus, talus, cuboid, metatarsals, and phalanges are present but delayed in skeletal maturation. To assess the articular relationships of the talus, calcaneus, navicular, and cuboid bones, longitudinal lines are drawn through the longitudinal axes of the talus, calcaneus, and shafts of the first and fifth metatarsals and the angles between these lines are measured.

In the AP projection the angle between the long axis of the talus and calcaneus (anteroposterior TC angle) in the normal foot measures 20 to 40 degrees (Fig 1–20A). In talipes equinovarus with inversion of the hindfoot, the anteroposterior TC angle is decreased from 20 to 40 degrees to 10 to 0 degrees, with the long axis of the talus and calcaneus becoming almost parallel to each other (Fig 1–20B).

The angle between the longitudinal axis of the first metatarsal and that of the talus (T-MT1) is measured to determine the articular relationship between the navicular and talus. In the normal foot the T-MT1 angle measures 0 to minus 15 degrees; in talipes equinovarus with medial displacement of the talonavicular joint and forefoot varus deviation, the T-MT1 angle becomes more negative—greater than minus 20 degrees (Fig 1–20A, B).

The relationship between the calcaneus and cuboid is assessed by measuring the angle between the long axis of the talus and that of the fifth metatarsal (T-MT5 angle). In the normal foot the T-MT5 angle measures 0; in talipes equinovarus with marked displacement of the calcaneocuboid joint, the T-MT5 angle diminishes to a negative value (Fig 1–20A, B).

In the normal foot, the TC angle in the lateral projection measures 35 to 50 degrees; in talipes equinovarus the lateral TC angle is decreased to 20 to −10 degrees (Fig 1–20C, D). If in doubt, make lateral radiograms of the foot in forced dorsiflexion at the ankle. This maneuver pulls the posterior apophysis of the calcaneus downward and its anterior end upward, thereby increasing the lateral TC angle. In talipes equinovarus the calcaneus is tethered into plantar

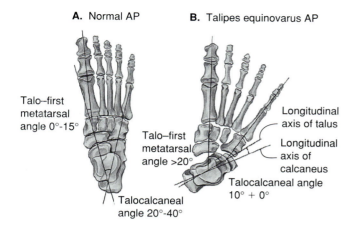

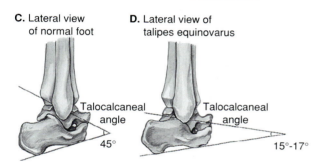

Figure 1–20. Diagram illustrating angles between the longitudinal axis of the talus, calcaneus, and first and fifth metatarsals in the normal foot and in talipes equinovarus. **A, C.** Normal. **B, D.** Talipes equinovarus.

flexion by the contracted Achilles tendon and posterior capsule; the calcaneus does not move and the talus tilts into slight dorsiflexion, thereby further decreasing the lateral TC angle. Also in the lateral projection, one can measure the tibiocalcaneal maximal dorsiflexion angle (normal is 40 ± 15 degrees) and the calcaneal pitch (15 degrees in the normal foot). The values of angular measurements in radiograms of normal feet and in talipes equinovarus are summarized in Table 1–2.

Recently ultrasonography of the foot has been used to show the articular relationship of the cartilaginous navicular to the medial malleolus and to the head of the talus. During the course of nonoperative treatment by manipulation and cast application, ultrasonography combined with clinical examination and radiography can demonstrate whether progress is being made toward achieving concentric reduction of the displaced talocalcaneonavicular joints.

Computed axial tomography (CT) determines whether subtalar medial spin is present and is a factor in persistent toeing-in during the postoperative period. MRI shows cartilaginous tarsal bones, but its application is in the investigative stage. The cost, the relative nonavailability of MRI,

and the fact that the child must be sedated make it impractical for routine use.

Treatment. Treatment of talipes equinovarus should begin immediately after birth. Following initial assessment of the deformity, the orthopedic surgeon should explain the goals, nature, and course of treatment to the parents.

The objectives of treatment are (1) to achieve and maintain a concentric, normal articular alignment of the displaced talocalcaneonavicular, calcaneocuboid, and ankle joints; (2) to establish a normal muscle balance between the evertors and invertors of the foot and the dorsiflexion and plantar flexion of the foot and ankle; and (3) to provide a mobile foot with normal weight-bearing and function.

At the outset, the parents must understand that nonsurgical methods of treatment often do not succeed and that open surgical reduction is required to achieve these goals. Conservative management of talipes equinovarus is open surgery. Just as the treatment for a ruptured appendix is surgery, the treatment for talipes equinovarus is operative.

A realistic approach is crucial. The family should understand that talipes equinovarus is an in utero deformation of the foot and that it can never be completely normal. Some residual atrophy of the calf will remain, the foot will be smaller than the opposite normal one, and normal range of motion will be somewhat restricted.

Treatment of talipes equinovarus may be divided into four sequential phases.

1. Manipulative stretching to elongate contracted soft tissues and skin and retention in cast. During this phase appropriate studies are performed to determine the type of clubfoot—idiopathic or neuromuscular—and to rule out other associated anomalies. Manipulative stretching and serial casts are usually applied for a period of 3 to 5 weeks. The correction is maintained by splinting at night and during part of the day.

TABLE 1–2. ANGLES BETWEEN LONGITUDINAL AXES OF THE TALUS, CALCANEUS, SHAFTS OF THE FIRST AND FIFTH METATARSALS AND BETWEEN THE LONGITUDINAL AXES OF THE TIBIA AND CALCANEUS IN RADIOGRAPHY OF THE FOOT

	Normal (degrees)	Talipes Equinovarus (degrees)
Anteroposterior Projection		
Talocalcaneal	20–50	15–0
Talo–first metatarsal	0 to −15	<−20
Talo–fifth metatarsal	0	<0
		−5 to −20
Lateral Projection		
Talocalcaneal	25–50	<20 to 0
Tibiocalcaneal	40 to −15	>70 degrees
Calcaneal pitch	15	0 to −15 to −20

2. Open reduction by posteromedial, lateral, plantar, and subtalar release.
3. Maintenance of reduction and restoration of mobility of the joints of the foot and ankle by splinting and active and passive exercises.
4. Management of problems such as recurrence of deformity, supination of the forefoot, and metatarsus varus.

Manipulative Stretching and Retention in Cast-Splint. The first step is passive stretching exercises to elongate contracted soft tissues and skin. The cardinal rule is to be gentle. The growth plates and articular cartilage are soft, in contrast to the contracted ligaments and capsule, which are rigid. Forceful manipulation should be avoided at all costs. A few days after discharge from the hospital, the foot is manipulated as follows: First, the triceps surae and posterior capsule of the ankle and subtalar joints and the calcaneofibular ligaments are elongated by pulling the heel down and pushing the midfoot up into dorsiflexion. Caution! Do not cause a rocker-bottom deformity. Count to five, let go, and repeat about 20 times.

The posterior tibial muscle and medial tibiocalcaneal ligaments are stretched by everting the hindfoot and midfoot.

Next, elongate the contracted plantar soft tissues by pushing the heel up and the forefoot up. Count to five and let go, and repeat 20 times. After the manipulation, the foot is painted with tincture of benzoin and an above-knee cast is applied to retain the elongation of the soft tissues. The cast is removed in 5 to 7 days, the manipulations are repeated, and another cast is applied.

Retention of Elongation of the Soft Tissues and Skin. Following removal of the final cast, a plastic splint is worn at night which consists of a posterior ankle-foot orthosis with the foot in neutral dorsiflexion, the heel in eversion, and the forefoot and midfoot in maximal abduction. The plastic splint is worn at night and during part of the day, and active and passive exercises are performed to develop muscle strength and maintain range of motion of the ankle, subtalar, and midtarsal joints.

Within 3 to 4 weeks, an attempt at closed reduction is made. With the foot and ankle in equinus position, distal traction is applied on the first ray and navicular and medial cuneiform. Attempt to bring the navicular bone distally and laterally over the anterior end of the talus. If the reduction is successful, the hallux appears longer, a palpable space opens between the medial malleolus and the navicular, and concavity on the medial column of the foot and convexity of the lateral column of the foot are eliminated. On palpation, the cuboid and the anterior end of the calcaneus are normally aligned. An above-knee cast is applied to maintain the reduction, and radiograms are made in AP and lateral projections to determine whether the articular relationships have been restored to normal. Do not be deceived by the external appearance of the foot. In the rigid true talipes equinovarus, concentric reduction by nonoperative means is very unlikely. The literature contains conflicting reports about the success of nonsurgical management of talipes equinovarus. Turco reported 30% success in correction of deformity.[84,85] In my experience, only occasionally can a moderately deformed foot be corrected nonsurgically.

In the rare case in which the deformity is minimal or moderate and one can obtain normal articular alignment as shown by radiography, the reduction must be maintained in an above-knee cast for 2 months, changing the cast every other week as the foot grows. Avoid prolonged immobilization (4 to 6 months) in a cast because it causes bone and muscle atrophy and stiffness of joints.

Open Reduction of the Talocalcaneonavicular and Calcaneocuboid Joints. Timing of open surgery is important. I follow the rule of four; that is, the child's foot should be 4 inches (10 cm) long, which is usually attained at approximately 4 to 6 months of age. Surgery is complex and very delicate and should be performed by an experienced pediatric orthopedic surgeon. At surgery, all elements of the deformity should be corrected. Concentric articular alignment should be obtained, and it should be maintained by internal fixation with pins across the talonavicular joint and, if necessary, across the calcaneocuboid and talocalcaneal joints. Overcorrection should be avoided.

Various surgical approaches are used—the Cincinnati incision, the posterior medial and lateral incision, and the Carroll technique of posterolateral and medial plantar incision. The choice of surgical approach is not critical. A word of caution, however: When the equinus deformity is very severe and rigid, the Cincinnati incision may result in skin slough posteriorly. The medial plantar technique as described by Carroll is technically demanding and should be performed only by a surgeon well trained in that technique.

It is beyond the scope of this book to describe surgical techniques, but the following structures are divided or elongated.

Posteriorly: Achilles tendon, posterior tibial muscle, toe flexors (if contracted), posterior capsule of the ankle and subtalar joints, calcaneofibular and posterior talofibular ligaments, and posterior part of the superficial deltoid ligament, but not the deep deltoid.

Medially: The tibionavicular capsule, anterior tibionavicular ligament, medial capsule of the subtalar joint, fibrous sheath of the knot of Henry, and abductor hallucis.

Plantarward: Plantar fascia, short toe flexor muscles, plantar calcaneonavicular and calcaneocuboid ligaments.

Laterally: The calcaneocuboid capsule. The calcaneocuboid joint should be normally aligned.

Subtalar: The talocalcaneal interosseous ligament is partially or totally sectioned if subtalar medial spin cannot be corrected.

Initially the foot is placed in equinus posture to allow skin healing; when the skin is healed—10 to 14 days after surgery—the foot is manipulated into dorsiflexion. The pins are removed 3 to 5 weeks postoperatively. Total immobilization in cast is about 6 to 8 weeks. Motion is life! Prolonged immobilization in cast and disuse atrophy should be avoided.

Maintenance of Reduction and Restoration of Motion of Joints and Muscle Strength. After removal of the cast, the infant is fitted with an ankle-foot orthosis with the heel in 5 degrees of eversion, the ankle in 5 degrees of dorsiflexion, and the forefoot and midfoot in 5 to 10 degrees of abduction and slight eversion. The chubby limb of an infant may require an above-knee splint with the knee in about 45 degrees of flexion to prevent the heel from sliding out of the splint. The splint is worn at night. Passive exercises are performed three to four times per day to develop range of dorsiflexion and plantar flexion of the foot and ankle, eversion and inversion of the subtalar joint and forefoot, and midfoot abduction and eversion. Active stimulation techniques are used to develop motor function of muscles controlling the foot and ankle. Ordinarily, shoe modifications or special shoes are not required.

Management of Problems and Complications. Talipes equinovarus deformity may recur for the following reasons. First, the primary pathology—medial plantar tilting of the head and neck of the talus—is not corrected by surgery because an osteotomy of the neck of the talus is not performed. It is expected to gradually correct with growth and remodeling of the foot in the corrected position. In severe deformities it may not, and the medial-plantar displacement of the talocalcaneonavicular joint may recur. The second cause of recurrence is fibrosis and contracture of the ligaments and capsule on the medial plantar aspect of the foot and the posterior aspect of the ankle. Collagen tissue in talipes equinovarus is abnormal and tends to scar. The third reason for recurrence of deformity is dynamic imbalance of muscles controlling the foot and ankle. Preoperatively, it should be explained to the parents that there is a likelihood of recurrence of deformity following surgical correction because of the preceding pathogenic factors.

The ankle joint is incongruous and limited in its range. The talus has forfeited its right of domicile in the ankle mortise. A problem often encountered is limitation of plantar flexion of the foot and ankle. This results in progressive atrophy of the calf and calcaneus deformity. Overlengthening of the Achilles tendon and weakness of the triceps surae muscle aggravate the problem. The importance of providing range of plantar flexion of the ankle as well as dorsiflexion cannot be overemphasized. Do not overlengthen the heel cord!

Equinus deformity often recurs because of scarring and contracture of the capsule and ligaments on the posterior aspect of the ankle and subtalar joint and of the triceps surae muscle. Splinting at night is important to prevent this problem, and one should not forget the value of intermittent stretching by means of walking casts. It is important to demonstrate radiographically that equinus deformity is corrected by restoration of normal tibiocalcaneal and talocalcaneal angles in the lateral projection.

In-toeing is commonly due to failure of correction of the medial spin of the subtalar joint. Other causes of in-toeing are forefoot supination, midfoot varus, and excessive medial tibial torsion.

Supination of the forefoot is due to dynamic imbalance between a strong anterior tibial muscle and weak peroneals. This is a progressive deformity that initially is managed by exercises and splinting, but not infrequently split anterior tibial tendon transfer—that is, transferring the lateral half of the anterior tibial tendon to the cuboid bone—is performed to provide dynamic balance of muscles acting on the foot.

Midfoot varus is due to failure of normal growth of the medial column of the foot as a result of dysplasia of the talus and a relative overgrowth of the lateral column of the foot. This is treated by a closing wedge osteotomy of the cuboid bone and opening wedge osteotomy of the medial cuneiform bone (the wedge of bone resected from the cuboid is inserted into the cuneiform). Lateral column stabilization in the form of a calcaneocuboid joint fusion (Evans' operation) should not be performed in the young child because it results in valgus deformity of the midfoot. The Evans operation is indicated in neuromuscular clubfoot or arthrogryposis, in which stabilization of the lateral column of the foot prevents recurrent varus of the midfoot.

Forefoot varus is due to contracture of the medial soft tissues. This is treated by manipulation and stretching casts in the young child, and in the older patient by osteotomy of the base of the metatarsals. The surgeon must remember that the growth plate of the first metatarsal is proximal and should not be disturbed by osteotomy. It is best to perform capsulotomy of the first metatarsal cuneiform joint.

The most common pitfall in clubfoot surgery is inadequate plantar release and failure to correct forefoot equinocavus deformity. This may be associated with *dorsal subluxation of the talonavicular joint.* This requires repeat surgical plantar release and, if the navicular is displaced dorsally more than 30 percent, open reduction of the talonavicular joint.

TOEING-OUT

Toeing-out caused by deformities of the foot may be due to calcaneovalgus, postural pes valgus, pes planovalgus with contracture of the triceps surae, flexible flatfoot with a short lateral column of the foot, congenital convex pes valgus (vertical talus), and tarsal coalition with ''spastic'' peroneal muscles. In this section, only calcaneovalgus and postural pes valgus are discussed.

Talipes Calcaneovalgus

This is the most common postural deformity of the foot. The presenting complaint by the parents is that the infant's feet are turned up and out. The foot is dorsiflexed at the ankle and everted and abducted at the midfoot; the hindfoot is in varying degrees of valgus (Fig 1–12D). The dorsiflexors of the ankle and the peroneus brevis muscles are contracted, restricting plantar flexion and inversion of the ankle and foot. The severity of the deformity varies. In mild cases the foot can be plantar flexed and inverted beyond neutral; in moderate cases, the foot passively plantar flexes only to neutral, whereas in severe cases the deformity is fixed with the ankle acutely dorsiflexed so that the toes almost touch the anterior aspect of the leg.

It is important to examine the hips of an infant with calcaneovalgus to rule out hip dysplasia and subluxation because of the high incidence of association between the two deformities. Examine the spine to rule out spina bifida or other defects in the vertebral column. Are there any external stigmata of spinal dysraphism such as a patch of hair or a hemangioma on the midline of the spine? Measure the circumference of the calves to rule out atrophy of the triceps surae muscle. Use stimulation techniques to assess motor function of the plantar flexors. Is there any sensory deficit? In boys test the cremasteric reflex, and in boys and girls check for the presence of the superficial abdominal umbilical reflex by stimulating the abdomen and inspecting the motion of the umbilicus. What is the Babinski response?

Rule out angular deformities of the tibia. Is there a dimple on the posterior aspect of the lower leg? Posterior medial angulation of the tibia and fibula are often associated with a moderate or severe calcaneal deformity of the foot.

Treatment. Treatment varies according to the severity of the deformity. Mild cases are simply observed or treated by gentle passive manipulation by the parent, consisting of bringing the foot into plantar flexion and inversion 15 to 20 times during several sessions each day. Moderate cases are treated by passive stretching exercises. In addition, if there is no response to exercises, a night splint with the foot and ankle held in plantar flexion and inversion is used. Severe cases require manipulation and retention in cast with the foot in plantar flexion and inversion.

The prognosis is good. Ordinarily the deformity can be fully corrected within several weeks. It is important to follow the infant until he or she begins to walk independently. An oblique talus and severe pes planovalgus deformity of the foot are common sequelae in the young child. These conditions require treatment in the form of support to the longitudinal arches of the feet such as UCBL (University of California Biomechanics Laboratory) orthoses.

Postural Pes Valgus

In this postural deformation, the midfoot and forefoot are abducted and everted with varying degrees of eversion of the hindfoot. The talus is plantar flexed and oblique to varying degrees. On plantar flexion of the ankle joint, the talonavicular relationship can be restored to normal; the deformity is flexible.

Differential Diagnosis. Postural pes valgus should be distinguished from three conditions. The first is *tarsal coalition,* in which the deformity is fixed. Check range of eversion and inversion of the hindfoot with the ankle in neutral dorsiflexion. Do not confuse range of ankle motion with that occurring at the subtalar joint. The second condition in the differential diagnosis is *congenital convex pes valgus,* in which there is rigid dorsolateral displacement of the talocalcaneal and calcaneocuboid joints. On plantar flexion of the ankle and inversion of the forefoot, the vertical position of the talus cannot be restored to normal. Stress radiograms of the foot may be indicated in borderline cases when the clinical diagnosis is uncertain. The third condition is acquired *peroneal spastic flatfoot,* an acquired valgus deformity of the foot due either to rheumatoid arthritis or another inflammatory condition affecting the talocalcaneal joint or to post-traumatic arthritis. Arthritis is characterized by synovial thickening of the sinus tarsi with increased local heat and pain upon inversion of the foot.

Treatment. Passive manipulation and splinting and, in severe cases, manipulation and retention in cast may be required to achieve correction. Prognosis is excellent, and the deformity can ordinarily be corrected within 3 to 4 weeks.

FLATFOOT (PES PLANUS)

A foot with absent or abnormally depressed longitudinal arch is referred to as flatfoot or pes planus; when the hindfoot is everted and the forefoot is abducted and everted, the term is further modified as pes planovalgus.

Flatfoot is subdivided into two general categories, depending upon the mobility of the tarsal joints—flexible and rigid. *Flexible flatfoot* may be *developmental* due to increased laxity of ligaments. It is physiologic and normal up to 4 to 6 years of age. The normal foot of infants and young children appears flat due to the presence of fat in the medial arch. Flexible flatfoot may be due to severe laxity of ligaments supporting the components of the longitudinal arch—talonavicular, talocalcaneal, and naviculocuneiform joints. This is referred to as *hypermobile flatfoot*. The ligamentous hyperlaxity is often familial, or it may be a part of a generalized syndrome such as Ehlers-Danlos, Marfan's, Down's, or osteogenesis imperfecta. A flexible flatfoot may be aggravated by contracture of the triceps surae and peroneal muscles. This is referred to as *hypermobile flatfoot with "tight heel cords."* The feet of infants with calcaneovalgus deformity due to intrauterine malposture are flat when the child starts standing and walking. A flexible flatfoot may also be due to *motor weakness and muscle imbalance,* as seen in hypotonia, muscular dystrophy, peripheral nerve lesions, spinal cord affections such as myelodysplasia and poliomyelitis, and cerebral palsy. It may also be due to *bony deformities* of the calcaneus such as hypoplasia of the sustentaculum tali or a short lateral column of the foot due to hypoplasia of the calcaneus.

Rigid flatfoot is very rare, comprising less than 0.1 percent of the cases. It may be *congenital,* such as in coalition of the tarsal bones (calcaneonavicular or talocalcaneal), or congenital, as in convex pes valgus (vertical talus). Congenital forms of rigid pes planus are often missed at birth. Rigid flatfoot may be due to *acquired causes*—inflammatory conditions involving subtalar and midtarsal joints such as rheumatoid arthritis, or traumatic arthritis following fractures involving the subtalar joint. Classification of flatfoot is given in Table 1–3.

History. When a child presents with flatfoot, the following questions should be asked of the family. Is there familial incidence of flatfeet and ligamentous hyperlaxity? If the parents or siblings had flatfeet, how was the condition treated? Did treatment succeed in restoring the longitudinal arch? Have they had other consultations with podiatrists or other physicians? What recommendations were given? Has any treatment been given in the form of special shoes or orthotics? Ask the parents if the child walks on his or her toes at times. Question the parents on birth history—especially hypoxia or prematurity. Inquire about whether developmental milestones were normal or delayed. Rule out cerebral palsy.

When flatfoot is noted in the newborn and young infant, the complaint is usually that the feet turn outward and are stiff. Often diagnosis of a *congenital convex pes valgus* is missed by the primary care physician, but its appearance is very characteristic. The forefoot and midfoot are ab-

TABLE 1–3. CLASSIFICATION OF FLATFOOT

Flexible
- A. Physiologic—due to ligamentous laxity in the infant and young child (this is normal)
- B. Excessive ligamentous laxity—hypermobile flatfoot
  1. Familial
  2. Part of generalized syndrome with severe ligamentous hyperlaxity such as Down's, Marfan's, Ehlers-Danlos, osteogenesis imperfecta
- C. Bony anomalies
  1. Hypoplasia of sustentaculum tali
  2. Short lateral column due to hypoplasia of the calcaneus
- D. Contractural—due to contracture of triceps surae or peroneals
- E. Motor weakness—muscle imbalance
  1. Tibialis posterior muscle with accessory tarso navicular
  2. Myopathic—as in muscular dystrophy
  3. Peripheral nerve lesions
  4. Spinal cord—myelodysplasia, poliomyelitis, Werdnig-Hoffmann disease
  5. Brain—cerebral palsy, hypotonic or spastic

Rigid
- A. Congenital
  1. Tarsal coalition—calcaneonavicular, talocalcaneal
  2. Congenital convex pes valgus (vertical talus)
- B. Acquired
  1. Inflammatory lesions involving the subtalar and midtarsal joints such as in rheumatoid arthritis
  2. Traumatic arthritis due to fractures involving subtalar joints

ducted, the head of the talus is plantar flexed, and the heel is pulled up into equinus.

Tarsal coalition often is not detected until the juvenile or early adolescent period, when pain and peroneal muscle spasm develop.

If the parents noted the child's flatfeet when he or she began to stand and walk, it is most often flexible, which is normal and physiologic due to the fact that the longitudinal arch of the foot has not fully developed yet and a large fat pad is present in the hollow of the foot. Under body weight the talus drops into plantar flexion, the calcaneus everts, and the midfoot and forefoot abduct. The severity of flatfoot in the toddler varies. The normal foot does not cause a problem with shoe wear, but a moderate flexible pes planus with ligamentous hyperlaxity and an oblique talus and hindfoot valgus may cause abnormal shoe wear—a rapid wearing away of the medial sole and counter. The parents often bring old shoes along to document their concern. The grandparents often accompany the child and not infrequently display their own "painful" flatfeet and state that they do not want their grandchildren's feet to be like theirs.

An older child or young adolescent with flatfeet usually presents with foot pain, often due to contracture of the triceps surae or to tarsal coalition that was not diagnosed earlier. Has the patient noted any fatigue, foot and leg cramps, or inability to keep up with peers? Is there family history of myopathy such as muscular dystrophy? Does anything in the past history indicate minimal cerebral palsy or other paralytic conditions such as peripheral nerve affections?

B. Non–weight-bearing

A. Weight-bearing

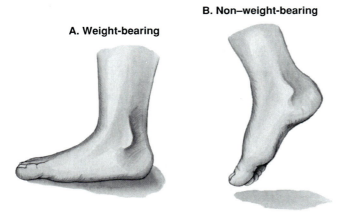

Figure 1–21. Flexible flatfoot. **A.** The medial longitudinal arch is depressed and absent on weight-bearing. **B.** When weight-bearing is removed, the longitudinal arch is restored to normal.

Flexible Flatfoot Due to Ligamentous Hyperlaxity (Hypermobile Flatfoot). *Pathoanatomy.*

The joints that constitute the longitudinal arch of the foot are the talonavicular, talocalcaneal, and naviculocuneiform. The stability of the longitudinal arch is provided by the plantar calcaneonavicular (spring), interosseus, talocalcaneal, plantar naviculocuneiform capsule and ligaments, and calcaneocuboid bifurcate ligaments. The configuration of the tarsal bones provides further integrity to the longitudinal arch. Active contraction of the muscles of the foot and leg does not maintain the medial longitudinal arch.[90]

When the ligaments supporting the longitudinal arch are lax and elongated and the foot is loaded under body weight, the head of the talus moves medially and plantar-ward and the anterior end of the calcaneus moves laterally and dorsally and the heel everts. Horizontal motion occurs at the talonavicular joint (the navicular moves laterally in relation to the head of the talus) and at the calcaneocuboid joint. Mechanical axis deviation occurs.

Assessment of Deformity. In the flexible flatfoot the longitudinal arch is depressed or absent on weight-bearing, but the longitudinal arch returns to normal when weight is removed (Fig 1–21). Determine the severity of the flatfoot by inspecting the medial border of the weight-bearing foot (Fig 1–22). In the *mild or first-degree* flatfoot, the longitudinal arch is depressed but still present (Fig 1–22B). On the medial view, rule out the presence of an accessory navicular, which may be associated with insufficiency of the posterior tibial muscle. In the *moderate or second-degree* flatfoot, the longitudinal arch is absent (Fig 1–22C). In the *severe or third-degree* form, the longitudinal arch is absent and the medial border of the foot is convex due to plantar flexion of the head of the talus (Fig 1–22D).

Next inspect the foot posteriorly and determine whether the heel is in neutral position or in valgus and establish the degree of obliquity of the talus (Fig 1–23). Is the head of the talus prominent on the sole? Clinically try to estimate the *calcaneal pitch.* Is it neutral, dorsiflexed 15 to 20 degrees, or in equinus? In flatfoot due to myostatic contracture of the triceps surae—"tight heel cords"—the calcaneal pitch is zero, whereas in congenital convex pes valgus the heel is in varying degrees of equinus.

Ask the child to stand on *tiptoe* and see whether the heel inverts to neutral or some varus (Fig 1–24). If the position of the heel does not change on tiptoe rising (it

A. Normal   **B. Mild flatfoot**   **C. Moderate flatfoot**   **D. Severe flatfoot**

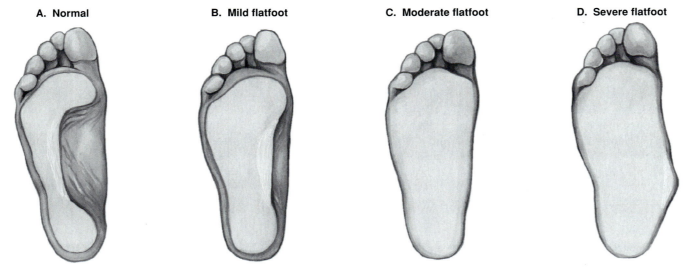

Figure 1–22. Footprints of a normal foot and varying degrees of flatfoot. **A.** Normal. Note the normal longitudinal arch. **B.** Mild. Note the minimal longitudinal arch. **C.** Moderate. The longitudinal arch is completely obliterated. **D.** Severe. Note the convex medial border of the foot.

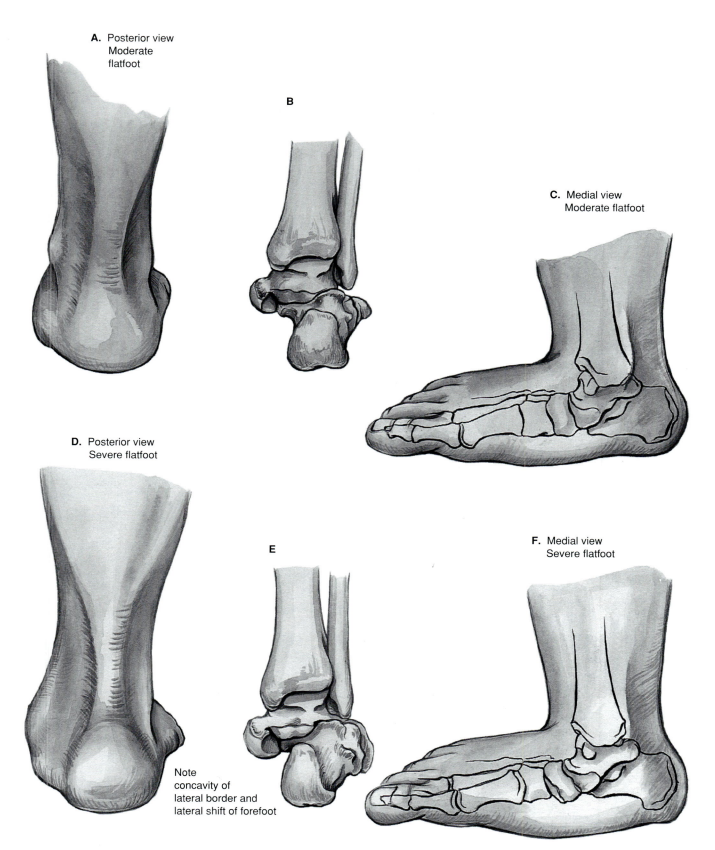

A. Posterior view
Moderate
flatfoot

B

C. Medial view
Moderate flatfoot

D. Posterior view
Severe flatfoot

E

F. Medial view
Severe flatfoot

Note
concavity of
lateral border and
lateral shift of forefoot

Figure 1–23. Assessment of severity of deformity of hindfoot in pes planovalgus. **A–C.** Moderate degree of flatfoot. Note that the heel is in 15 degrees of valgus and the talus is oblique but not vertical. Also note the sagging of both the talonavicular and naviculocuneiform joints. **D–F.** Severe pes planovalgum. Note that the head of the talus is prominent on the plantar aspect of the foot and the talus has dropped into almost vertical position. The lateral border of the foot is concave and the medial border is convex.

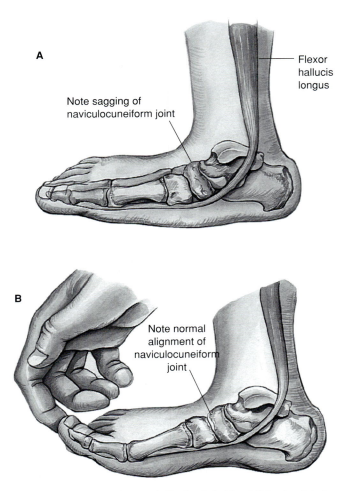

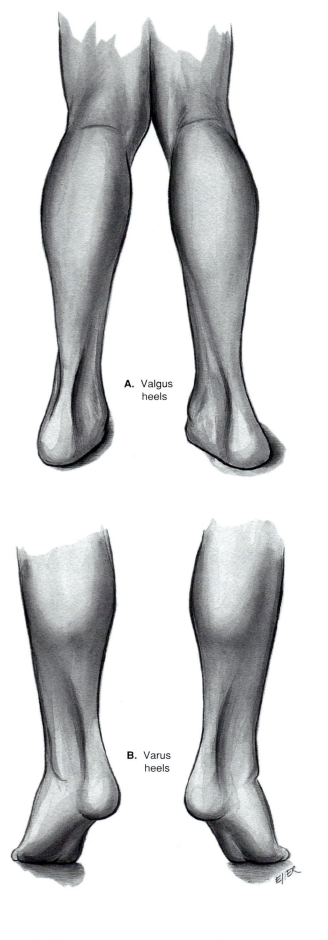

A. Valgus
heels

B. Varus
heels

Note sagging of
naviculocuneiform joint

Flexor
hallucis
longus

Note normal
alignment of
naviculocuneiform
joint

Figure 1–25. Jack toe-raising test. **A.** The foot is in full weight-bearing. Note the sagging of the naviculocuneiform joint. **B.** The big toe is raised into hyperextension. The longitudinal arch is restored by the tautness of the flexor hallucis longus tendon on the plantar aspect of the naviculocuneiform joint.

remains in valgus), a rigid flatfoot is present. Also from the posterior view see if the heel touches the floor or there is equinus of the hindfoot.

Inspect the *lateral border of the foot* and see if it is concave and whether abduction of the midfoot and a short lateral column are present. From the *medial view*, determine the *site of sagging* of the longitudinal arch—the talonavicular joint, the naviculocuneiform joint, or both. The *Jack toe-raising* test is of some value in clinical determination of maximal site of sagging of the longitudinal arch.[109] With the patient bearing full weight on the floor, passively raise the big toe into hyperextension (Fig 1–25). When the sag is at the talonavicular joint due to plantar flexion of the talus, the longitudinal arch is not restored because the flexor

Figure 1–24. Tiptoe rising test in pes planovalgus. **A.** In stance the heels are in 15 degrees of valgus. **B.** On tiptoe rising, the heels invert.

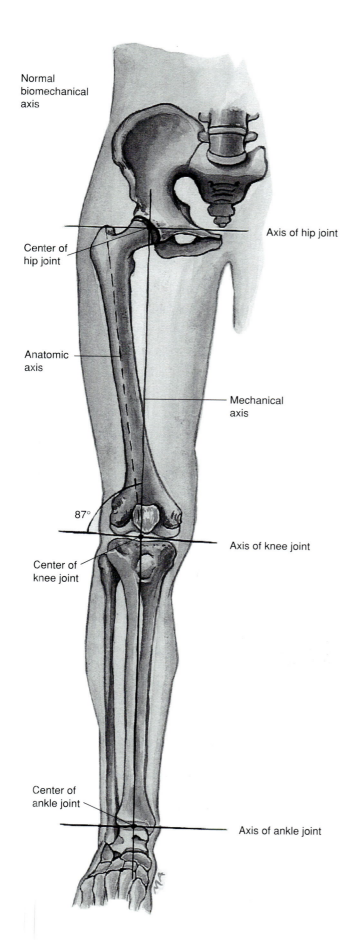

Normal
biomechanical
axis

Center of
hip joint

Axis of hip joint

Anatomic
axis

Mechanical
axis

87°

Axis of knee joint

Center of
knee joint

Center of
ankle joint

Axis of ankle joint

Figure 1–26. Normal mechanical axis of the lower limb. Note that the plumb line from the center of the hip joint falls between the first and second metatarsals. It is important in assessment of flatfoot to rule out associated genu valgum and lateral tibiofibular torsion, which increase weight-bearing stresses on the foot.

A

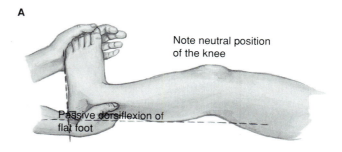

Note neutral position
of the knee

Passive dorsiflexion of
flat foot

B

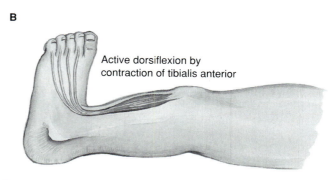

Active dorsiflexion by
contraction of tibialis anterior

Figure 1–27. Passive range of dorsiflexion of the ankle. **A, B.** With the knee in extension and the heel inverted, dorsiflex the foot and ankle. Be sure that the anterior tibialis muscle is not contracted because if it contracts, the triceps surae relaxes and more range of dorsiflexion is obtained.

hallucis longus tendon does not have adequate leverage to translate the navicular under the head of the talus. When the sag is at the naviculocuneiform joint, the longitudinal arch elevates on passive hyperextension of the big toe. In the presence of a triceps surae contracture, the Jack toe-raising test is not reliable because the flexor hallucis longus is inefficient.

From the front, determine the mechanical axis of the lower limb—whether the plumb line from the anterosuperior iliac spine falls between the first and second toe on weight-bearing (Fig 1–26). Rule out associated rotational and angular deformities of the lower limbs, specifically genu valgum and excessive lateral tibiofibular torsion.

Next, determine the *range of motion of the ankle and tarsal joints*. Passively dorsiflex the ankle with the knee in extension and flexion. Be sure that the patient is not actively dorsiflexing the foot because when the anterior tibial contracts, the triceps surae relaxes because of reciprocal innervation of agonist-antagonist muscles (Fig 1–27). Determine subtalar joint motion by inverting and everting the hindfoot. Be sure to hold the distal tibia and fibula steady

A. Normal

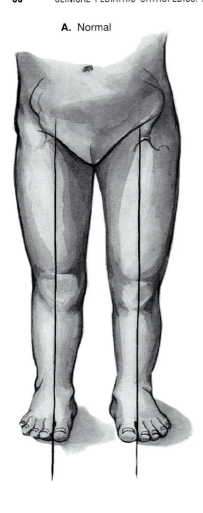

B. Moderate flexible flatfoot

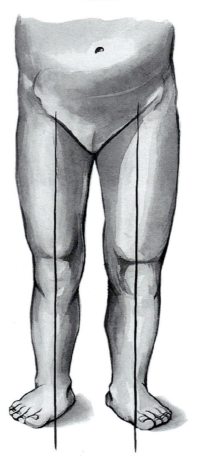

C. Overcorrection during walking

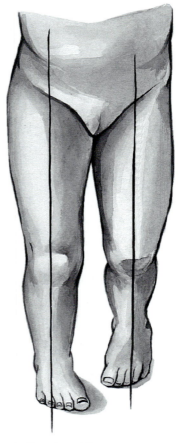

Note that plumb line falls medial to first metatarsal

Figure 1–28. Protective toeing-in in flexible flatfoot. **A.** In the normal foot the plumb line from the anterosuperior iliac spine and the center of the hip joint falls between the first and second metatarsals. **B.** In moderate or severe pes planovalgum the plumb line falls medial to the first metatarsal. **C.** In order to prevent stresses on the foot, the child toes in by medial rotation at the hip and forefoot adduction when walking.

and invert and evert the hindfoot with the other hand holding the ankle in neutral dorsiflexion. Also determine range of motion of the talonavicular and calcaneocuboid joints by abducting and adducting the midfoot and forefoot.

Ask the patient to walk. Is the foot progression angle normal or is the child toeing-out or toeing-in? In protective toeing-in, the foot shifts medially so that the body weight in the stance phase of gait falls on the center of the foot (Fig 1–28).

Next, determine motor strength of muscles controlling the foot, ankle, and lower limb. Rule out myopathy and hypotonia. Perform the *slip-through test*. Lift the child by holding him under the arm pits. When hypotonia is present, the child slips through (Fig 1–29A, B). Is there any pseudohypertrophy of the gastrocnemius soleus muscles? (Fig 1–29E). Perform a Gower's test (Fig 1–29C). Ask the patient to lie or sit on the floor and to stand unassisted without his hands climbing up his thighs for support. Note the posture in stance—is there hyperlordosis of the lumbar spine? (Fig 1–29D). Is the gait pattern normal heel-toe, or is it toe-heel or toe-toe? If there is any suspicion of central nervous system disorder, ask the patient to walk in tandem and to hop on one foot. Inspect the shoes for any abnormal wear.

Imaging. Routine radiography of flexible flatfoot should not be performed. Make radiograms when the child has painful feet with restricted motion or when the deformity is so severe that treatment by orthosis or surgery is being considered. Radiograms show the site of the sagging in the longitudinal arch and the severity of the deformity of the joints. The degree of valgus of the hindfoot is reflected by the talocalcaneal angle in the AP projection of the hindfoot and the posteroplantar projection of the hindfoot and ankle (Bush-Poznanski view). In the AP view any lateral displacement of the talonavicular and calcaneocuboid joints is noted. Is the lateral column of the foot short? Note the length of the calcaneus in relation to the talus. The alignment of the forefeet is determined—is there any forefoot varus indicating a serpentine or Z foot?

Radiograms of the feet are made with the patient standing in full weight-bearing and the muscles controlling the foot and ankle completely relaxed. Instruct the x-ray technician to position the feet correctly and use the correct technique of radiography.

Draw a longitudinal line through the center of the bodies of the talus, navicular, medial cuneiform, and shaft of the first metatarsal. Also draw a vertical line through the center of the navicular parallel to its proximal articular surface. In the normal foot the longitudinal line forms a straight line and is perpendicular to the vertical line drawn through the body of the navicular (Fig 1–30A, B). When the *sagging is at the talonavicular joint,* the longitudinal line through the center of the body of the talus is tilted into plantar flexion and forms an angle of varying degrees with the longitudinal line drawn through the naviculocuneiform–first metatarsal (Fig 1–30C, D). When the *sagging is at the naviculocuneiform joint,* the longitudinal axis through the talus and navicular forms a straight line and bisects a vertical line through the body of the navicular at a right angle and exits on the plantar aspect of the medial cuneiform joint (Fig 1–30E). When the *sagging is at both the talonavicular and naviculocuneiform joints,* a line is drawn through the longitudinal axis of the navicular and extended proximally and distally. The line is plantar to the talus and the first metatarsal segments (Fig 1–30F). In the AP projection, the talocalcaneal angle is increased, with varying degrees of lateral displacement of the talonavicular and calcaneocuboid joints.

The *calcaneal pitch* is determined on a standing lateral radiogram of the foot. Draw a line along the plantar aspect of the calcaneus between the anterior and posterior tuberosities and a horizontal line between the posterior tuberosity of the calcaneus and the first metatarsal head. The angle formed between these two lines is the calcaneal pitch; nor-

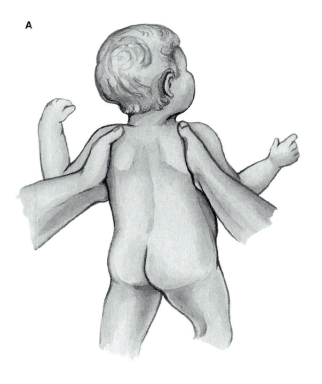

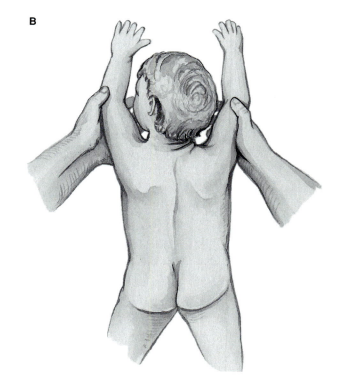

Figure 1–29. Slip-through test to rule out hypotonia. **A.** Hold the child under the arm pits and lift him up. **B.** When marked shoulder weakness is present, as in Werdnig-Hoffmann disease, the child slips through your hands. *(Continues)*

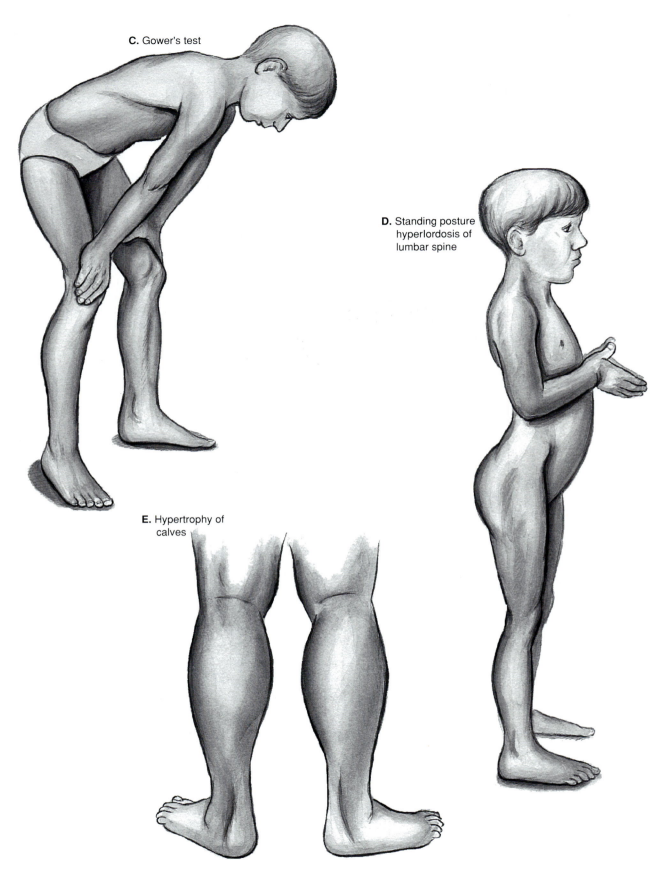

C. Gower's test

D. Standing posture hyperlordosis of lumbar spine

E. Hypertrophy of calves

Figure 1–29 *(Continued).* **C–E.** Gower's test and other signs of muscular dystrophy.

mally it measures 15 degrees (see Fig 1–30A). In pes plano-valgus it is decreased, and with a contracture of the triceps surae it may be as low as zero or even a negative angle (see Fig 1–30C).

Treatment. *Physiologic (or Developmental) Flatfoot.* Physiologic flexible flatfoot in the infant and young child is physiologic and normal. The plantar surface of the foot of an infant and a young child appears flat for two reasons: (1) the area of the longitudinal arch of the foot has abundant subcutaneous fat, and (2) the joints of infants and children are lax, and when the child stands the ligaments elongate under stress loading of the body weight and the longitudinal arch flattens. As the child gets older the fat pad shrinks, the ligaments become taut, and the longitudinal arch spontaneously develops up to 6 years of age. The clinical studies of Asher[89] and the radiographic studies of Staheli et al[118,119] and Wenger et al[120,121] have well documented this fact.

Physiologic flexible flatfeet—that is, full range of subtalar, midtarsal, and ankle joints—are asymptomatic. They do not cause pain and disability. Radiograms of the feet are not indicated, and treatment is not required. With growth, normal longitudinal arches develop. No scientific evidence indicates that shoe modifications or shoe inserts or orthotics alter the outcome. Even though they appear flat, the feet of these infants and young children are normal and should be left alone. By age 4 to 6 years, the ligaments become taut, the fat pad shrinks, and a normal longitudinal arch develops. Mild or moderate flexible flatfeet do not become painful. Parents should be educated as to the innocuous nature of physiologic, flexible flatfeet.

When a flexible flatfoot in a child is painful, other pathologic conditions should be explored.

Factors That Complicate Management. One or more of five conditions may complicate management of flexible flatfoot.

1. The 2- to 4-year-old child with *moderate* flexible flatfeet who *toes-in* (see Fig 1–28C). Parents or grandparents are very concerned. Sometimes well-meaning friends harass the parents—"You should take your poor child to a foot doctor!" Some children have had shoe inserts or orthotics which, according to the parents, have aggravated the toeing-in.

   Examine the hips and the legs to rule out femoral antetorsion or excessive medial tibiofibular torsion. Often no rotational malalignment of the lower limb is present. In the child with moderate or severe flexible flatfoot, the center of gravity of the body falls medial to the first metatarsal on weight-bearing. The child toes in with active contraction of the anterior and posterior tibial muscles and toe flexors so that the body weight is shifted laterally toward the center of the foot, thereby protecting the child

   from foot strain. Explain to the parents that toeing-in is good for the child's foot and should not be discouraged or prevented by special shoe modifications. Previous foot orthotics or shoe inserts should be discarded. Reassure the parents and practice the art of doing nothing.

2. The child with *moderate* flexible flatfoot who *toes out.* Examine the passive range of dorsiflexion of the ankle with the knee in extension and the rotational and angular alignment of the entire lower limb. The toeing-out may be due to myostatic contracture of the triceps surae, excessive lateral tibiofibular torsion with or without associated genu valgum, or contracture of soft tissues on the lateral aspect of the hip or diminished femoral antetorsion or femoral retrotorsion.

   When flexible flatfoot is associated with myostatic contracture of the triceps surae, the child complains of pain in the calf. Mild equinovalgus deformity is treated by elongation of the contracted triceps surae by passive stretching exercises, manual or against the wall (Fig 1–31). Moderate or severe contracture of the triceps surae often requires serial stretching cast application.

   When excessive lateral tibiofibular torsion and genu valgum are associated with moderate or severe flexible pes planovalgus, the mechanical axis deviation—that is, medial shift of the weight-bearing forces of the body—causes foot strain and pain. In such cases more definitive therapy is indicated by supporting the feet in good shoes with longitudinal arch supports or, in severe pes planovalgus, in UCBL foot orthoses. Excessive lateral tibiofibular torsion does not correct spontaneously. Perform Ober's test to rule out contracture of the iliotibial band; if present, it should be stretched out by passive manual exercises (see Fig 3–33). When lateral tibiofibular torsion exceeds 30 degrees, it is best for the child to wear a Fillauer bar at night (no greater than 4 to 6 inches [12 to 15 cm] wide) with the feet turned in 30 to 45 degrees by the medially rotated shoes. In a young child (3 to 5 years of age) such an external device, in the experience of this author, assists in correcting excessive lateral tibiofibular torsion within 3 to 6 months. The obese child should lose weight.

   When medial rotation of the hips is restricted, the lateral rotators of hip should be stretched by passive stretching exercises (see Fig 3–33).

3. The child 3 to 4 years of age who has *marked ligamentous hyperlaxity* and severe flexible flatfoot. The wear of the shoes is definitely abnormal: The medial upper of the shoes is caved in and the medial part of the heel is worn away. Some parents bring a batch of shoes and line them up on the

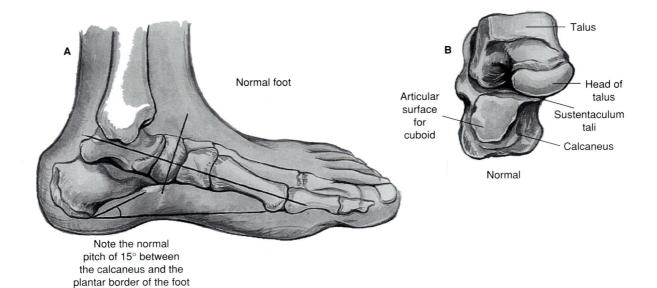

A

Normal foot

Note the normal
pitch of 15° between
the calcaneus and the
plantar border of the foot

B

Talus

Articular
surface
for
cuboid

Head of
talus

Sustentaculum
tali

Calcaneus

Normal

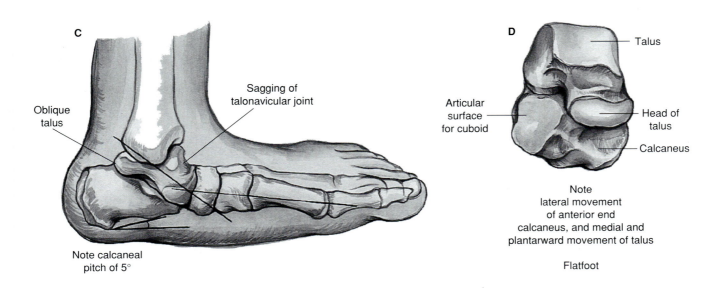

C

Oblique
talus

Sagging of
talonavicular joint

Note calcaneal
pitch of 5°

D

Talus

Articular
surface
for cuboid

Head of
talus

Calcaneus

Note
lateral movement
of anterior end
calcaneus, and medial and
plantarward movement of talus

Flatfoot

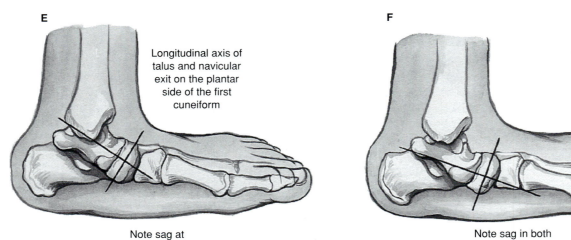

E

Longitudinal axis of
talus and navicular
exit on the plantar
side of the first
cuneiform

Note sag at
naviculocuneiform joint

F

Note sag in both
talonavicular and
naviculocuneiform joints

tudinal arch is being restored by the orthosis by making standing radiograms of the feet with the UCBL foot orthoses in the shoes (Fig 1–32).[107,111]

Explain to the parents that such orthotic support does not tighten the loose ligaments and restore the longitudinal arch to normal permanently. In these cases, UCBL foot orthoses relieve foot strain and pain, improve gait pattern, make shoe wear more even, and, if worn faithfully, prevent structural deformation of the tarsal bones.[92]

4. *Pes planovalgus with short lateral column of the foot.* The heels are markedly everted (20 degrees or more), the talus is plantar flexed 60 degrees or more, the calcaneus is short in relation to the talus, and the calcaneocuboid and talonavicular joints are displaced laterally. Some of these problems are the residual deformity of severe calcaneovalgus feet in infancy (note: in such feet the obliquity of the talus is minimal); others are a developmental growth abnormality of the calcaneus. These patients usually present in the office at 6 to 8 years of age. The parents have noted that the flatfeet are becoming worse, and the child is complaining of foot strain and is toeing out in gait. Manage such feet by support in UCBL orthoses during the juvenile period. After 10 to 12 years of age, lengthening of the lateral column of the foot (reverse Evans procedure) is performed by inserting a wedge of bone in the anterior part of the calcaneus. The results of surgery are very satisfactory.[88,96,113]

5. *Congenital or developmental hypoplasia of the sustentaculum tali of the calcaneus.* This rare deformity is readily documented by CT or MRI. These children have severe flexible flatfoot with severe obliquity of the talus. These feet are supported in UCBL foot orthoses during childhood, and after 10 years of age a Grice extra-articular subtalar arthrodesis is performed.[100,101]

Surgical Treatment. Surgery is rarely indicated, and should not be performed in children under 10 years of age. Indications are pain and marked deformation of the shoes because of the foot deformity. If the triceps surae is contracted and does not elongate with stretching exercises and casts, a heel cord lengthening is performed and the Achilles ten-

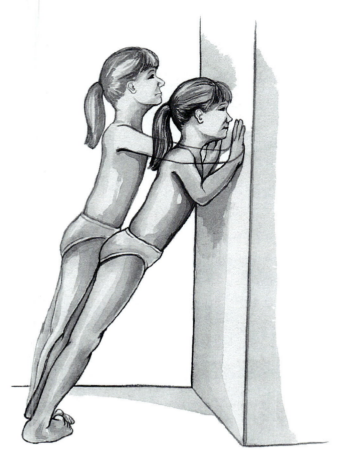

Figure 1–31. Passive stretching exercises for contracted triceps surae.

examining table to document the problem. There is a strong family history of ligamentous hyperlaxity. A parent or grandparent takes off his shoes and shows the severe flatfoot and severe loose-jointedness. Their feet hurt, and they don't want their child's feet to be painful and have a deformity like theirs. They demand treatment. How is one to manage these children and their parents?

Make standing radiograms of the feet and ankles in the AP and lateral projections and determine the degree and site of sagging of the longitudinal arch. The feet of these children are best supported by UCBL foot orthoses. Document that the longi-

Figure 1–30. Assessment of deformity of flatfoot, medial view. **A, B.** Normal. No sagging of the talonavicular or naviculocuneiform joints is present. The calcaneal pitch is normal at 15 degrees. **C, D.** Oblique talus with sagging at the talonavicular joint. Note that the longitudinal line through the center of the body of the talus is tilted plantarward, forming an angle with the longitudinal line drawn through the naviculocuneiform–first metatarsal. **E.** The sagging is at the naviculocuneiform joint. Note that the longitudinal line drawn through the talus and navicular is straight and bisects the vertical line through the body of the talus at right angles but exits on the plantar aspect of the medial cuneiform. It is continuous with a longitudinal line drawn through the navicular and first metatarsal. **F.** Sagging at both the talonavicular and naviculocuneiform joints. Note that the line drawn through the longitudinal axis of the navicular and extended proximally and distally is plantar to the talus and first metatarsal segments.

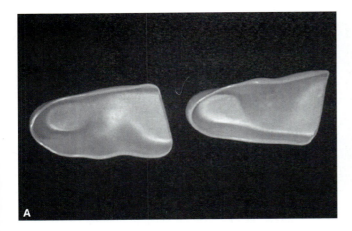

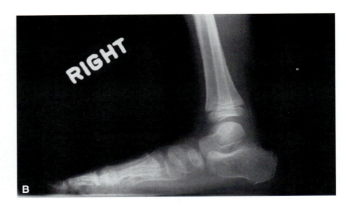

Figure 1–32. A. University of California Biomechanics Laboratory (UCBL) foot orthoses. **A.** Photographs of the brace. **B.** Standing lateral radiogram of the foot without the brace. **C.** Standing lateral of the right foot with the brace. Note the restoration of the longitudinal arch.

don is divided laterally in its distal part and medially in its proximal part.

When the heel is in marked valgus, medial displacement osteotomy of the calcaneus is performed. This is a very satisfactory procedure to restore mechanical axis deviation to normal. If the lateral column of the foot is short with a valgus deformity at the calcaneocuboid joint, a reverse Evans procedure to lengthen the lateral column of the foot with autogenous bone graft from the ilium is performed.

If the sag is at the naviculocuneiform joint, a naviculocuneiform fusion with transfer of the anterior tibial tendon and tightening of the plantar calcaneonavicular (spring) ligament and posterior tibial tendon is performed (Giannestras operation).[97,98]

Paralytic pes planovalgus deformity usually requires stabilization of the subtalar joint with restoration of dynamic balance of muscles acting on the foot. In the skeletally immature foot in the cerebral palsy child, oblique or flexible vertical talus is best corrected by subtalar arthroereisis (Crawford staple fixation).[94] It is combined with appropriate lengthening of the heel cord or contracted peroneal muscles if indicated. The Grice extra-articular arthrodesis is a more definitive procedure in the older child. Use autogenous bone graft from the ilium and not the fibula in order to avoid the problem of ankle valgus due to shortening of the fibula and a high-riding lateral malleolus. In paralytic, severe flexible pes planovalgus, triple arthrodesis by inlay bone graft (Williams-Menelaus technique) is indicated.[122a]

Congenital Convex Pes Valgus (Congenital Vertical Talus)

This rigid, rocker-bottom flatfoot deformity is present at birth and can be detected by the astute clinician. Often,

→

Figure 1–33. Congenital convex pes valgus. **A.** Clinical appearance. Child presents with rigid flatfoot and the foot and leg pointing outward. **B.** Medial view of the foot. Note the vertical talus and dorsal displacement of the navicular on the neck of the talus. **C.** Dorsal view showing lateral subluxation of the calcaneocuboid and talonavicular joints. **D.** Ligamentous and muscle pathology. The triceps surae is contracted, pulling the calcaneus into equinus. The long toe extensors and peroneals are contracted. The capsule and spring ligament (calcaneonavicular ligament) on the medial plantar aspect of the talonavicular joint are stretched out.

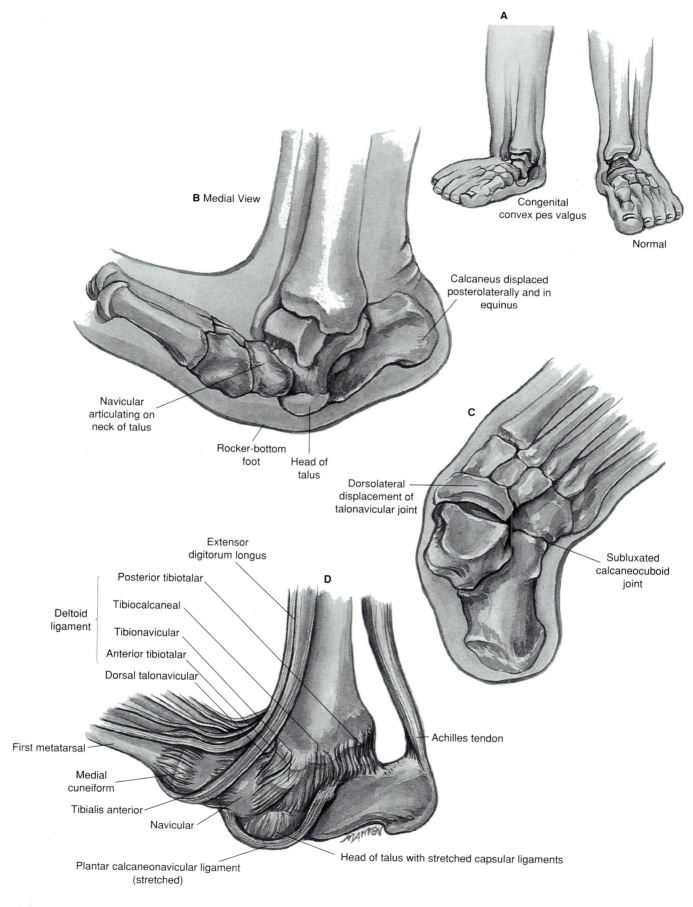

A

Congenital convex pes valgus

Normal

B Medial View

Calcaneus displaced posterolaterally and in equinus

Navicular articulating on neck of talus

Rocker-bottom foot

Head of talus

C

Dorsolateral displacement of talonavicular joint

Subluxated calcaneocuboid joint

Extensor digitorum longus

D

Deltoid ligament
- Posterior tibiotalar
- Tibiocalcaneal
- Tibionavicular
- Anterior tibiotalar

Dorsal talonavicular

Achilles tendon

First metatarsal

Medial cuneiform

Tibialis anterior

Navicular

Head of talus with stretched capsular ligaments

Plantar calcaneonavicular ligament (stretched)

however, it is not diagnosed until later in infancy or when the child begins to stand and walk. The parents bring the child to the doctor with the complaint that the foot is very flat, turns out, and appears strange with its convex sole and the bony prominence (the head of the talus) on the plantar aspect of the foot (Fig 1–33A). The child toes out when walking, and fitting shoes is difficult.

Fortunately it is a rare deformity. The talus is fixed in 90 degrees plantar flexion (vertical), with its head projecting into the plantar surface of the foot. The sole of the foot is convex; the heel is drawn up into equinus and the forefoot-midfoot are everted and abducted. Congenital convex pes valgus is due to in utero dorsolateral displacement of the talocalcaneonavicular and calcaneocuboid joints. The talus is locked in 90 degrees of plantar flexion, and the navicular is displaced on the dorsolateral aspect of the neck of the talus; the calcaneus is fixed in equinus and the forefoot is dorsiflexed and everted, giving the sole of the foot a rocker-bottom convex shape (Fig 1–33B, C).

The capsules and ligaments on the dorsolateral aspect of the talonavicular and calcaneocuboid joints are contracted, tethering the tarsal bones in the displaced position. The deformity cannot be corrected by plantar flexion and inversion of the foot and ankle. The medial plantar capsule of the talonavicular joints and the plantar calcaneonavicular ligaments are stretched out and thin. The triceps surae, extensor hallucis longus, extensor digitorum longus, peroneus brevis and tertius, and anterior tibial muscles are contracted, whereas the posterior tibial muscle is stretched out (Fig 1–33D).

Etiology. The exact cause of this prenatal deformity is unknown. It has been proposed to be due to arrest of prenatal development of the foot.[126] Paralysis and contracture of soft tissues have been implicated in its pathogenesis. Experimentally in rabbits, Ritsila[151] has produced vertical talus deformity by shortening of the triceps surae and dorsiflexion of the foot and ankle, fixing the hindfoot in equinus and the forefoot in dorsiflexion-eversion, and by sectioning of the ligamentum transversus cruris.

The deformity is rare. Its exact incidence is unknown. Although familial cases have been reported, no definite hereditary pattern has been identified.

Classification. Congenital convex pes valgus may be *primary,* occurring as an isolated deformity or in association with other musculoskeletal deformities or part of a syndrome, or it may be *secondary* to neuromuscular disorders such as myelomeningocele, sacral or lumbosacral agenesis, caudal regression syndrome, or arthrogryposis multiplex congenita. Associated musculoskeletal deformities include dislocation of the hip, congenital dislocation of the knee, talipes equinovarus or calcaneovalgus deformity of the contralateral foot, ischiocalcaneal band, and pollex varus. In autosomal trisomy 13-15 and trisomy 18, congenital convex

TABLE 1–4. CLASSIFICATION OF CONGENITAL CONVEX PES VALGUS

Primary
  A. Isolateral
  B. In association with other musculoskeletal deformities
    1. Ischiocalcaneal band
    2. Congenital dislocation of hip
    3. Congenital dislocation of knee
    4. Talipes equinovarus or calcaneovalgus deformity of opposite foot and ankle
    5. Pollex varus
  C. Part of trisomy 13-15 or 18

Secondary—Neuromuscular
  A. Myelomeningocele
  B. Lumbosacral or sacral agenesis
  C. Caudal regression syndrome
  D. Arthrogryposis multiplex congenita

pes valgus is present as one of numerous anomalies (Table 1–4).

Clinical Picture. The rocker-bottom appearance of the foot is typical (Fig 1–34). The heel is drawn up and is in valgus; the forefoot and midfoot are dorsiflexed, everted, and abducted. The head of the talus is prominent and fixed in its position on the medial plantar aspect of the sole. The contracted muscles and tendons can be readily palpated. The deformity is rigid; it cannot be corrected by simple plantar flexion and inversion of the foot. Walking is delayed and the gait is awkward. Shoe wear is abnormal. Feet with congenital convex valgus deformity are ordinarily not painful until later in adult life.

Imaging Findings. Radiographic investigations of congenital convex pes valgus should consist of the following: stress, weight-bearing, AP and lateral projections of the foot centered on the hindfoot, and a lateral view of the foot and ankle in maximal plantar flexion–inversion (Fig 1–35). All patients with congenital convex pes valgus should also have thorough investigation of the spine to rule out anomalies of the vertebral column such as sacral agenesis, diastematomyelia, spina bifida, and intraspinal pathology such as lipoma or hydromyelia. Make AP and lateral radiograms of the entire spine and, in infants up to 4 to 6 months of age, perform ultrasonography of the entire spine.

Normally in the newborn only the talus, calcaneus, and metatarsals are ossified. The ossification center of the cuboid may be present or delayed in appearance until the third week of life. The cuneiform bones ossify between 1 and 2 years of age, and the navicular begins to ossify at about 3 years of age. As the navicular is cartilaginous during the first 3 years of life and not visible in the radiogram, the articular relationship of the talus and navicular bones is delineated by drawing lines through the longitudinal axis of the talus and first metatarsal.

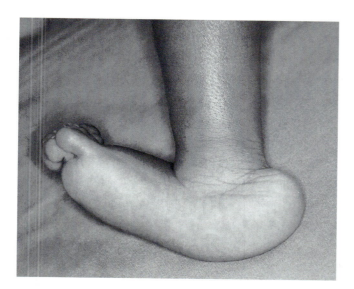

Figure 1–34. Clinical appearance of congenital convex pes valgus. Note the rocker-bottom deformity with hindfoot equinus and forefoot dorsiflexion.

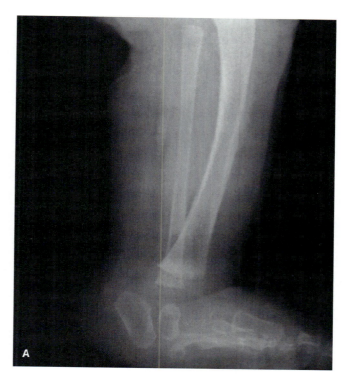

Take a ruler and marking pen and draw lines through the longitudinal axis of the talus, calcaneus, and tibia in the lateral projection and through the longitudinal axis of the calcaneus and talus in the AP projection.

In congenital convex pes valgus in the lateral projection of the foot and ankle, the longitudinal axis of the talus is vertical, almost parallel to the longitudinal axis of the tibia. Also, the longitudinal axis of the talus passes through the anterior end of the calcaneus, posterior to the cuboid. In a normal foot the longitudinal axis of the talus is oblique, passing through the plantar half of the cuboid. In maximal flexion in congenital convex pes valgus, the vertical position of the talus is fixed—it does not change.

Draw the longitudinal axis of the first metatarsal and note its relationship to the head of the talus. In congenital convex pes valgus the longitudinal axis of the first metatarsal points dorsal to the head of the talus, indicating that the navicular is displaced dorsal to the head of the talus. The talo–first metatarsal relationship does not alter in maximal plantar flexion of the foot. In the oblique talus and in the normal foot, the long axis of the talus and the long axis of the first metatarsal line up with the foot in extreme plantar flexion. Next, draw the longitudinal axis of the calcaneus. In congenital convex pes valgus it is tilted into plantar flexion and it passes plantar to the cuboid. In the normal

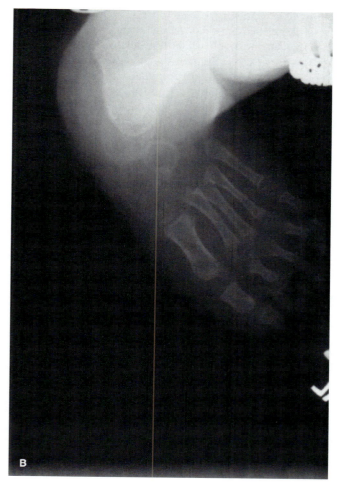

Figure 1–35. Radiographic appearance of congenital convex pes valgus. **A.** In the lateral projection note the 90 degree plantarflexed (vertical) talus with hindfoot equinus and dorsolateral displacement of the midfoot and forefoot. A line drawn through the longitudinal axis of the first metatarsal passes dorsal to the head and neck of the talus. **B.** In the AP projection note the marked increase of the talocalcaneal angle and the lateral subluxation of the midfoot and forefoot.

foot the long axis of the calcaneus cuts through the upper half of the cuboid. The lateral talocalcaneal angle in congenital convex pes valgus is 85 to 90 degrees, whereas in the normal foot it is 35 to 50 degrees.

In the AP projection of the foot, the talocalcaneal angle is measured. In the normal foot it measures 20 to 40 degrees, whereas in congenital convex pes valgus it is markedly increased. Also, note the relationship of the lateral border of the ossific centers of the cuboid and calcaneus. In the normal foot they form a continuous line, whereas in congenital convex pes valgus, the calcaneocuboid joint is displaced laterally and the calcaneocuboid line is broken. In the child older than 3 years of age, the ossific centers of the navicular appear and the dorsal subluxation of the talonavicular joint is evident.

The lateral radiogram of the foot with the ankle in maximal plantar flexion is the important radiographic examination. In oblique talus due to ligamentous hyperlaxity and in paralytic pes planovalgus with contraction of the triceps surae in which the ankle is plantar flexed, the position of the talus changes and the long axis of the talus lines up normally with that of the calcaneus and the first metatarsal (Fig 1–36).

Differential Diagnosis. The following conditions should be distinguished from congenital convex pes valgus: (1) oblique talus in flexible pes planovalgus due to ligamentous hyperlaxity and (2) paralytic pes planovalgus due to myostatic contracture of the triceps surae. In these two conditions the talus is oblique or vertical in position, but the dorsolateral displacement of the talonavicular joint is flexible and reducible when the ankle and foot are maximally plantar flexed and the foot is inverted. In congenital convex pes valgus the rocker-bottom flatfoot deformity is fixed and the vertical position of the talus and dorsolateral displacement of the talonavicular joint are irreducible. The importance of making lateral radiograms of the foot in maximal plantar flexion cannot be overemphasized.

Ordinarily peroneal spastic flatfoot due to tarsal coalition or irritable lesions of the subtalar joint such as rheumatoid arthritis may be mistaken for congenital convex pes valgus. Radiograms of the foot depict the pathology and allow one to make an accurate diagnosis. CT scanning or MRI of the foot may be indicated in the skeletally immature foot of the infant. Prominence of an accessory navicular on the medial aspect of the foot should not be mistaken for the head of the talus.

Treatment. In the neonate and young infant, treatment consists of passive stretching exercises to stretch skin and elongate contracted soft tissues followed by retention in cast. The casts are changed at weekly intervals for 3 to 4 weeks. Then splints are worn at night. These closed methods of management are unsuccessful in achieving concentric reduction of the dorsolaterally displaced talocalcaneonavicular and calcaneocuboid joints.

Open reduction by soft tissue release and internal fixation with a pin across the talonavicular joint are carried out at 4 to 8 months of age. Ordinarily the Cincinnati incision is used for surgical approach. The following ligaments on the dorsolateral aspect of the foot are sectioned: (1) the dorsal and lateral parts of the talonavicular capsule, (2) the tibionavicular ligament, (3) the lateral and dorsal capsule of the calcaneocuboid joint, (4) the bifurcated or Y ligament, that is, the calcaneonavicular and calcaneocuboid limbs, (5) the calcaneofibular ligament, and (6) the talocalcaneal interosseous ligament (if necessary). Posteriorly the Achilles tendon is lengthened, and often posterior capsulectomy of the ankle and subtalar joints is performed. Ordinarily musculotendinous fractional lengthening of the peroneus longus and brevis and long toe extensors is required in severe rigid cases.

On the medial plantar aspect of the foot, the stretched-out capsule of the talonavicular joint is tautened by capsular plication, and the posterior tibial tendon and the spring (calcaneonavicular) ligament are transferred distally to support the longitudinal arch of the foot. The anterior tibial tendon is split into halves and one half of the tendon is transferred to the head of the talus for dynamic support. The talonavicular joint is fixed internally with a pin, which is removed 4 to 6 weeks postoperatively. After removal of the pin, the foot and ankle are immobilized in a below-knee cast for an additional 3 weeks. It is vital to support the foot in an ankle-foot orthosis or UCBL foot orthosis for a prolonged period to prevent recurrence of deformity.

In the older child with rigid deformity, partial or complete excision of the tarsal navicular may be required to shorten the medial column of the foot. The medial cuneiform articulates with the head of the talus. Subtalar stabilization, either by stapling or Grice extra-articular arthrodesis, may be necessary.

The results of surgery in idiopathic congenital convex valgus are usually satisfactory if surgical correction is carried out at 6 to 12 months of age. Paralytic cases require continued support of the feet in an ankle-foot orthosis. Recurrence of deformity is a problem. Avascular necrosis of the talus is a potential complication, particularly after extensive surgery! Untreated or failed surgical cases develop callosities and pain over the convex rocker-bottom sole of the foot; they are managed by triple arthrodesis for relief of symptoms and facilitation of shoe-fitting.

Tarsal Coalition

The child with tarsal coalition presents with the chief complaint of *rigid flatfoot*. On non–weight-bearing the longitudinal arch is not restored, and on passive manipulation no motion occurs between the affected tarsal bones.

A history of repeated *ankle sprains* and *pain* in the ankle and foot is not uncommon; with rigidity of the subtalar joint compensatory stress is exerted on the ankle and talonavicular and calcaneonavicular joints, causing the

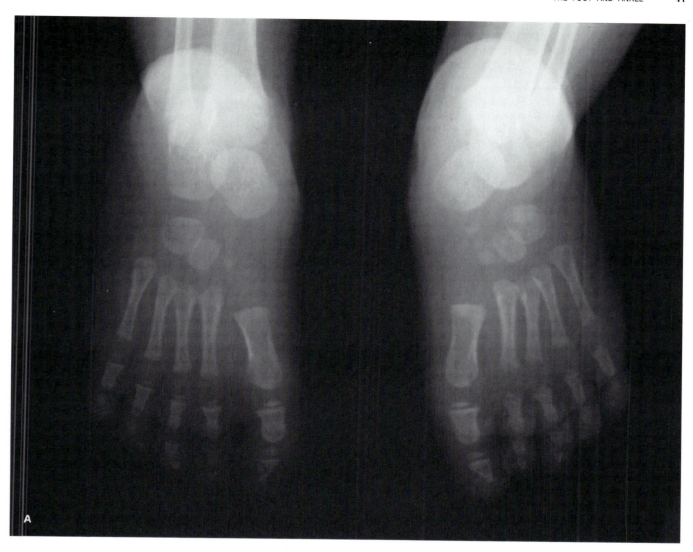

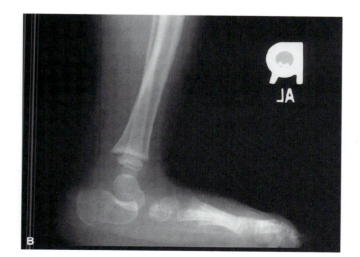

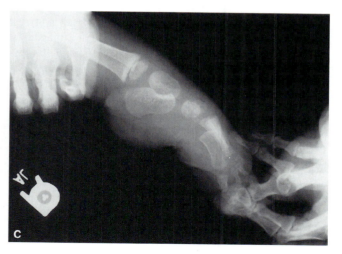

Figure 1–36. Radiograms of oblique talus in flexible pes planovalgum. Do not misdiagnose as vertical talus. **A, B.** AP and lateral projections. Note in the AP view the increased talocalcaneal angle and in the lateral view, the almost 90 degree vertical position of the talus. The calcaneal pitch is zero. **C.** In maximal plantar flexion, the talus assumes a normal inclination.

capsule and ligaments to stretch. Peroneal muscle spasm and occasionally anterior and/or posterior tibial muscle spasm may be other presenting complaints.

Etiology. The union between the tarsal bones may be completely osseous (synostosis), cartilaginous (synchondrosis), or fibrous (syndesmosis). This congenital anomaly is present in the fetus and is due to failure of differentiation and segmentation of the primitive mesenchyme forming the tarsal bones and the consequent lack of joint formation.[173]

It is a genetic disorder; its inheritance pattern is autosomal dominant.[177] Often tarsal coalition is an isolated anomaly, but it can occur in association with coalition between carpal bones or phalanges or with other major lower limb anomalies such as congenital longitudinal deficiency of the fibula or proximal femoral focal deficiency. Occasionally it is part of a syndrome such as the Nievergelt-Perlman syndrome, in which tarsal synostosis is associated with clubfeet, dysplasia of the elbows with radioulnar synostosis, and dysplasia of the tibia and fibula, or Apert's syndrome, in which coalition of the tarsal bones is associated with craniosynostosis, midfacial hypoplasia, syndactyly of fingers and toes, and a broad distal phalanx of the thumb and great toe.[179] Massive coalition of the tarsal bones can occur but is rare.

In the tarsus, the most common and clinically significant coalitions are between the talus and calcaneus and between the calcaneus and navicular. They may cause painful flatfeet and impede ambulation. One or both feet may be involved; 60 percent of the calcaneonavicular coalitions and 50 percent of the talocalcaneal coalitions are bilateral. Ordinarily both feet are affected in talonavicular coalitions.

Clinical Picture. Lack of motion between the affected tarsal bones is usually missed in infancy and childhood because it is not painful and because the coalition between the two bones is fibrous or cartilaginous and not apparent on routine radiograms. It should also be noted that tarsal coalition in the adult may be totally asymptomatic and discovered incidentally on a radiogram made for some other reason.

Symptoms develop when ossification of the coalition takes place and excessive stress and strain are exerted on the foot with increasing body weight and participation in strenuous physical activity and sports. Ordinarily calcaneonavicular coalition becomes symptomatic between 8 and 12 years of age and talocalcaneal coalitions between 12 and 14 years of age. Talonavicular coalitions are usually silent clinically; in the rare symptomatic case, pain may develop as early as 2 years of age.

Physical Examination. The salient physical finding in talocalcaneal and calcaneonavicular coalition is restriction and loss of motion at the subtalar or calcaneonavicular joints. In testing range of subtalar motion, the ankle should be in neutral dorsiflexion and not in plantar flexion (Fig 1–37). When the foot is in neutral position, the talus is locked in the ankle mortise, and no motion occurs at the ankle joint on inversion-eversion of the hindfoot. When the foot is in equinus and the talus is not locked in the ankle mortise, motion does occur at the ankle joint which can be mistaken for motion at the subtalar joint.

With the patient sitting and relaxed and the ankle and foot in neutral position, ask him or her to invert and evert the foot; in calcaneonavicular or talocalcaneal coalition with loss of motion in the subtalar joint, the child is unable to do so. Hold the heel between the fingers and thumb of one hand, and with the other hand hold the medial and lateral malleoli steady. With the ankle in neutral position, passively attempt to invert and evert the hindfoot. In the normal foot in neutral position, there should be 15 degrees of inversion and 10 to 15 degrees of eversion, whereas in talocalcaneal or calcaneonavicular coalition, there is no motion.

Ask the patient to stand on tiptoe and note the position of his heels. In the normal foot, the heels invert 15 degrees,

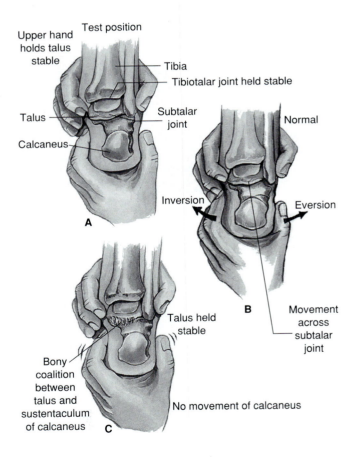

Figure 1–37. Method of testing range of subtalar motion. **A.** The ankle should be in neutral position. With one hand, steady the medial and lateral malleolus between your thumb and fingers. With the other hand, hold the heel with the patient in prone position and totally relaxed. **B.** In a normal foot, on inversion-eversion there are 10 to 15 degrees of motion in each direction. **C.** In calcaneonavicular or talocalcaneal coalition, there is no motion.

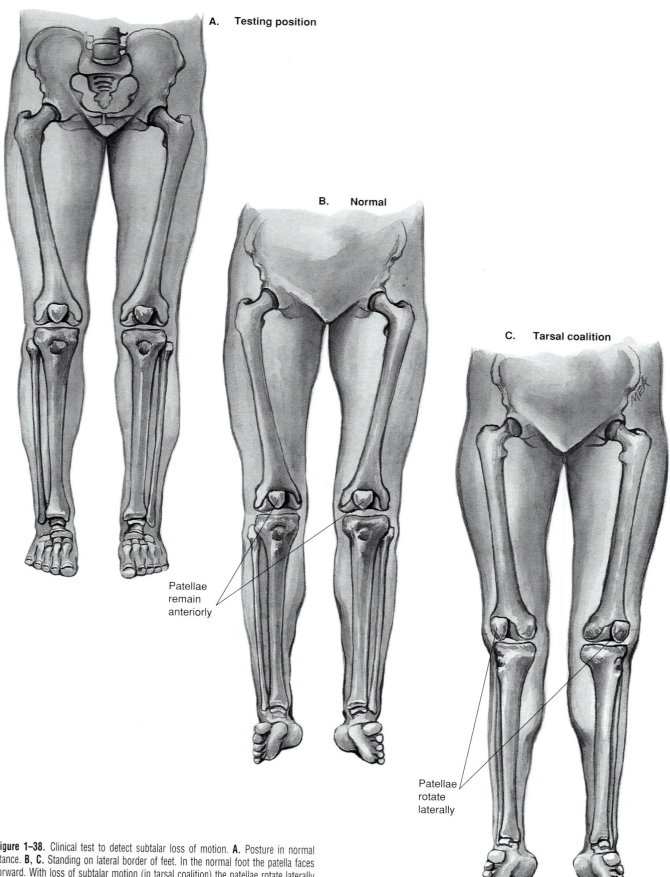

A.   Testing position

B.   Normal

C.   Tarsal coalition

Patellae
remain
anteriorly

Patellae
rotate
laterally

Figure 1–38. Clinical test to detect subtalar loss of motion. **A.** Posture in normal stance. **B, C.** Standing on lateral border of feet. In the normal foot the patella faces forward. With loss of subtalar motion (in tarsal coalition) the patellae rotate laterally by lateral rotation of the hip as a compensatory mechanism.

whereas in tarsal coalition, range of heel inversion is restricted, there is no change in position of the heels. In equinus, the talus moves forward and is not locked in the ankle mortise, allowing some degree of eversion-inversion to take place in the ankle mortise. This should not be mistaken for subtalar motion. With the patient facing you, ask him to stand on the outer borders of his feet. In the normal foot the patellae point forward on this maneuver, whereas in tarsal coalition with loss of subtalar motion, compensatory lateral rotation takes place at the hip and the patellae rotate laterally (Fig 1–38).

Inspect the child from the front, back, and side. Look at the position of the feet. Are they flat? Are the heels everted, neutral, or inverted? If the hindfeet are in valgus, note the degree of heel eversion.

Viewing the child from the side, inspect the peroneal tendons. Are they taut? Do they stand out? Peroneal "spastic" flatfoot is a common physical finding in tarsal coalition. The peroneal tendons are short, but true spasticity is absent. On passive inversion, the spasm of the tendons increases. Occasionally the anterior and posterior tibialis muscles are in spasm and the midfoot and the forefoot are in varus.

Inspect the child's gait. In the normal gait cycle, the tibiae rotate medially 15 to 20 degrees during the swing phase of gait and the first one-eighth of the stance phase. Then the tibiae rotate laterally, reaching their peak of lateral rotation at toe-off. These rotatory motions of the tibiae are translocated to the talus and then via the subtalar joint to the calcaneus. Medial rotation of the tibiae causes inversion of the calcaneus, whereas lateral rotation of the tibiae causes the calcaneus to evert. With loss of subtalar motion, this normal inversion-eversion of the calcaneus in the gait cycle is lost. An astute observer detects this abnormality of gait.

In the normal foot during eversion, the talus moves forward on the calcaneus, and during inversion it moves posteriorly. When the navicular is fused to the calcaneus, this movement is blocked and the talus cannot move forward. It moves plantarward, pulling the capsule and causing a traction spur (beak) on the head of the talus. This should not be mistaken for arthritis of the talonavicular joint. No narrowing of the articular cartilage space exists (Fig 1–39).

On palpation, there may be tenderness of the talonavicular joint or at the ankle joint over the deltoid or calcaneofibular ligaments. No synovial thickening or effusion or increased heat of the subtalar joint is present to suggest arthritis. Nor are areas of tenderness present over the body of the talus or calcaneus to indicate the presence of a painful lesion such as osteoid osteoma, infection or osteomyelitis, or traumatic arthritis due to fracture.

Imaging. When tarsal coalition is suspected, initial radiographic views of the foot should consist of an AP, lateral, and 45-degree oblique view made with the patient standing on the film and the x-ray beam projected from the lateral to the medial side and a 45-degree axial (Harris) view of the calcaneus to show the subtalar joint.

Calcaneonavicular coalitions are visualized in the 45-degree oblique view of the foot (Fig 1–40). When the coalition is bony, it is clearly depicted in the radiogram. When it is cartilaginous or fibrous, detection is not that simple. One should suspect such syndesmosis or synchondrosis when the anterior end of the calcaneus and navicular abut each other, with flattening of their opposing cortical surfaces. In the lateral projection, a tubular prolongation anteriorly over the superior calcaneus approaching or overlapping the midportion of the navicular may be present, which has been termed "anteater nose" (Fig 1–41).[180] When clinical findings warrant, MRI shows the cartilaginous union between the calcaneus and navicular. However, such an indication is rare.

In time, secondary changes develop in calcaneonavicular coalition: (1) beaking on the dorsal and lateral aspect of the navicular next to the talonavicular joint, (2) broadening of the lateral part of the talus, and (3) narrowing of the cartilaginous space of the posterior subtalar joint (Fig 1–42).

Talocalcaneal coalition is difficult to visualize on routine radiograms. Its presence should be suspected when blurring of the joint is seen in the lateral projection. Also, before a Harris view is taken, it is best to determine the angle of the sustentaculum tali in the lateral projection; it may vary from 30 to 45 degrees. The axial Harris view should be directed accordingly (Fig 1–43). At present the best way to demonstrate subtalar coalition is by CT scan, which shows whether it is partial, medial, or complete (Fig 1–44). If cartilaginous coalition is suspected, MRI is indicated. Talonavicular and calcaneocuboid coalitions are clearly visualized in the AP and lateral radiograms. A radiogram of the ankle in the AP and oblique projection should always be made to rule out ball-and-socket ankle joint or, in the painful ankle, osteochondritis dissecans in the dome of the talus.

Treatment. The presence of a bar is not necessarily an indication for surgical excision. When pain and deformity are present, definitive treatment should be carried out. A peroneal spastic flatfoot that is painful and of recent onset after strenuous physical activity is best managed by immobilization in a below-knee cast for 3 to 4 weeks. During this period the patient and parents are educated about the nature of this congenital failure of segmentation, its natural history and indications for surgical excision of the bar, results and problems, and complications of treatment. In general, calcaneonavicular bar excision and fat interposition to prevent recurrence of bony union are very successful and should be recommended (Fig 1–45).[187]

In the older adolescent and adult patient with pain in the talonavicular and subtalar joints and fixed valgus

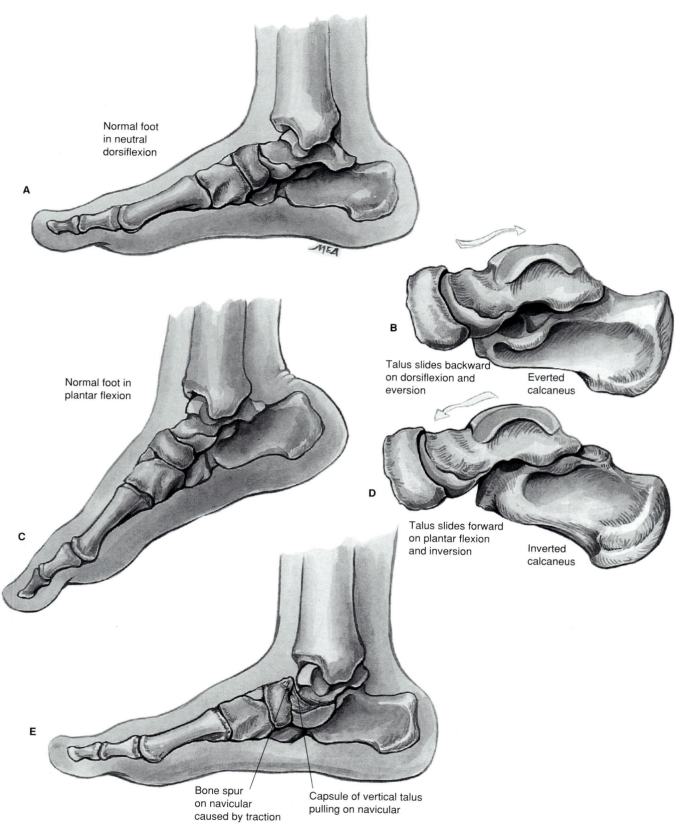

Normal foot in neutral dorsiflexion

A

Talus slides backward on dorsiflexion and eversion

Everted calcaneus

B

Normal foot in plantar flexion

C

Talus slides forward on plantar flexion and inversion

Inverted calcaneus

D

E

Bone spur on navicular caused by traction

Capsule of vertical talus pulling on navicular

Figure 1–39. Pathomechanics of the foot in calcaneonavicular coalition. **A.** Normal foot with the talus in normal position. **B.** During dorsiflexion and eversion, the talus moves backward on the calcaneus. **C, D.** During plantar flexion and inversion, the talus moves forward. **E.** In the infant and young child, the bar of calcaneonavicular coalition between the talocalcaneonavicular joints is cartilaginous. In the older patient, when the bar ossifies, the navicular cannot be pushed forward. Therefore, the talus tilts into plantar flexion, stretches the talonavicular capsule, and causes a traction "beaking" on the navicular bone. This should not be mistaken for degenerative arthritis.

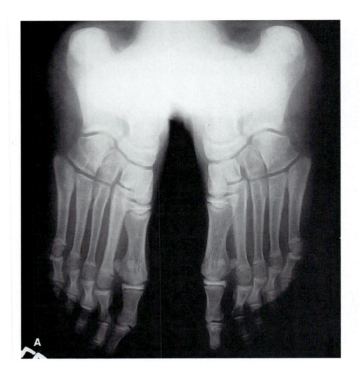 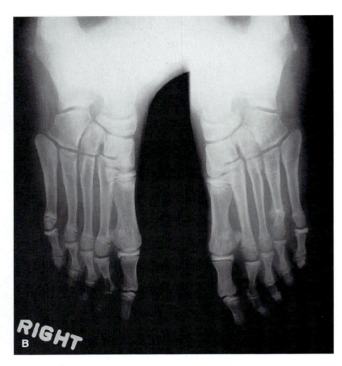

Figure 1–40. Bilateral calcaneonavicular coalition. **A.** On the left the bar is bony. **B.** On the right it is cartilaginous.

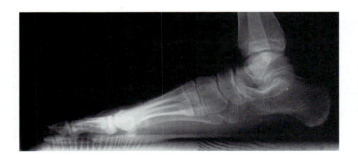

Figure 1–41. "Anteater nose" appearance in a lateral projection of a foot with calcaneonavicular coalition.

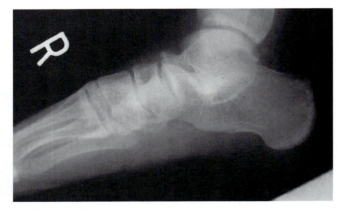

Figure 1–42. "Beaking" of the dorsolateral aspect of the navicular next to the talonavicular joint. This is a traction spur and not a sign of degenerative arthritis. Note the broadening of the lateral part of the talus and narrowing of the cartilage space of the posterior subtalar joint.

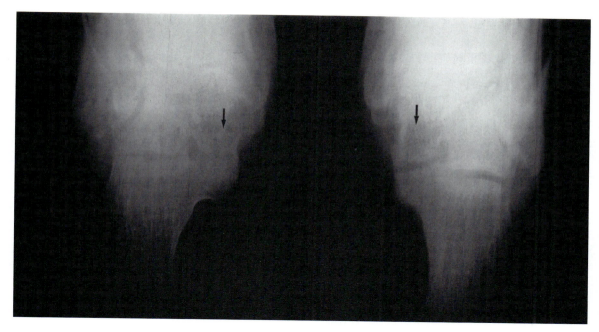

Figure 1–43. Harris view showing talocalcaneal coalition.

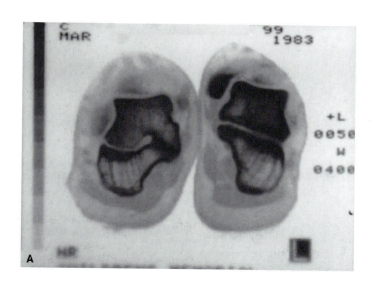

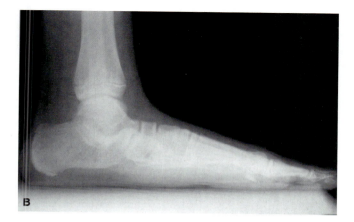

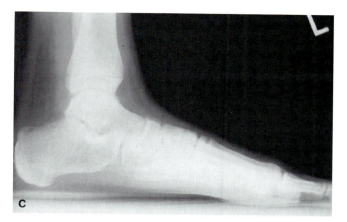

Figure 1–44. Talocalcaneal coalition. **A.** Computed tomography scan of both feet showing talocalcaneal coalition of the right foot. **B.** Lateral projection of the involved right foot. Note the narrowing of the posterior talocalcaneal facet joint space and the broadening of the lateral process of the talus, which shows a rounded appearance. **C.** Lateral projection of normal left foot.

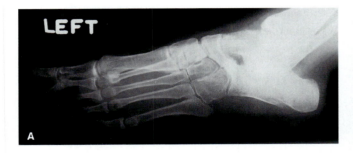

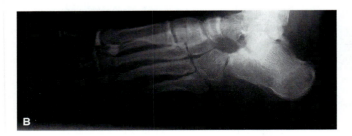

Figure 1–45. Oblique view of the left foot with calcaneonavicular coalition. **A.** Preoperative radiogram showing the bar. **B.** Postoperative radiogram following excision of the bar with fat interposition.

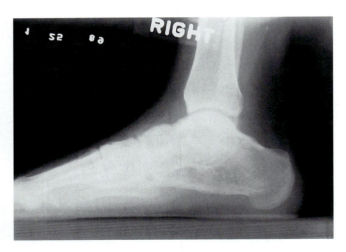

Figure 1–46. A painful talocalcaneal coalition treated by triple arthrodesis.

deformity, triple arthrodesis should be considered. It corrects the deformity and relieves the symptoms. It behooves the surgeon to assess the ankle joint and rule out ankle instability by making stress radiograms.

Treatment of talocalcaneal coalition should be individualized. Resection and fat interposition of the symptomatic medial facet coalition are recommended. Results have been reported to be satisfactory in about 80 percent of cases. Failed resections and painful feet are treated by triple arthrodesis (Fig 1–46). Complete talocalcaneal coalitions cannot be excised successfully; they are best treated by correction of the deformity and fusion of the subtalar joint if no degenerative changes are present in the talonavicular joint. If the latter are present, it is best to perform triple arthrodesis.

PES CAVUS

The patient with pes cavus presents with the chief complaint of high arch of the foot; that is, the longitudinal arch of the foot is abnormally elevated due to fixed equinus deformity of the forefoot on the hindfoot. The age of presentation is between 8 and 12 years. Occasionally pes cavus is present at birth with clawing of the great toe.

With drop of the forefoot the extremities of the tripod that support the foot—the heel and the heads of the first and fifth metatarsals—approximate and the longitudinal arch is raised. In the beginning the deformity is flexible; that is, it can be corrected by simple elevation of the forefoot. Later on it becomes fixed, first with shortening and

contracture of soft tissues—muscles, fasciae, ligaments, and capsules—on the plantar and medial aspect of the foot and later with deformation of the bones and joints of the metatarsals and tarsus. The toes may be normal; often, however, with progression of the deformity, the toes become retracted and clawed.

TABLE 1–5. CAUSES OF PES CAVUS

Neuromuscular
  Peripheral and spinal nerve root level
    1. Charcot-Marie-Tooth disease
    2. Déjérine-Sottas interstitial hypertrophic neuritis
    3. Polyneuritis
    4. Traumatic lesions
  Spinal cord level
    5. Spinocerebellar tract, Friedreich's ataxia, Roussy-Levy syndrome
    6. Spinal muscular atrophy
    7. Myelomeningocele
    8. Poliomyelitis
    9. Syringomyelia
    10. Spinal cord tumors
    11. Diastematomyelia
    12. Spinal dysraphism—tethered cord
    13. Arthrogryposis multiplex congenita
  Muscular level
    14. Muscular dystrophy—distal type
    15. Overlengthened triceps surae—calcaneocavus
  Cerebral and cerebellar level
    16. Spastic or athetoid cerebral palsy
    17. Primary cerebellar disease

Old treated or untreated talipes equinovarus

Traumatic
    18. Compartment syndrome
    19. Severe burns
    20. Crush injury

Idiopathic

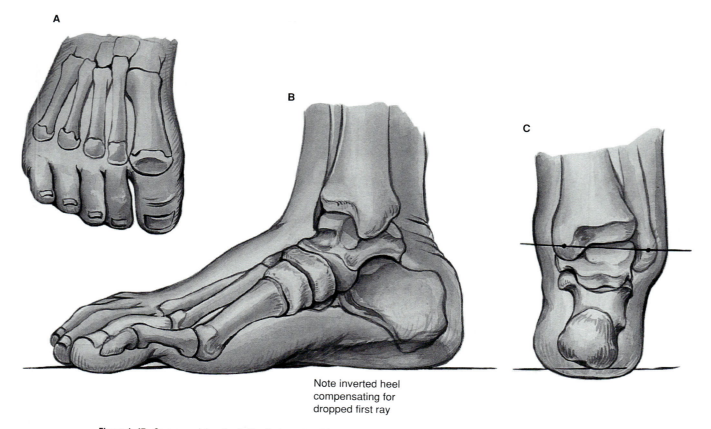

Note inverted heel
compensating for
dropped first ray

Figure 1–47. Cavovarus deformity. **A.** The first metatarsal has dropped into equinus and eversion (pronation). **B, C.** In order to get the first and fifth metatarsal heads even on the ground, the first metatarsal supinates and the hindfoot follows into inversion when there is normal mobility between the forefoot and hindfoot.

Clinical Features. In addition to the *high arch* of the foot, other associated complaints are (1) difficulty with shoe fit with pain on the dorsum of the midfoot due to rubbing by the shoe, (2) abnormal shoe wear because excessive loading is exerted over a smaller area of the forefoot and heel, (3) plantar callosities over the metatarsal heads, (4) pain and callosity at the posterior tuberosity of the heel as it moves up and down and rubs on the counter of the heel of the shoe, (5) clawing of the toes, (6) inversion instability of the ankle due to hindfoot varus, and (7) rigidity and pain in the midfoot at the apex of the high arch. In contrast to flatfoot, cavus foot often becomes symptomatic and progresses in the severity of deformity.

Diagnosis. Pes cavus is a manifestation of a neuromuscular disease with dynamic muscle imbalance unless proven otherwise. The various causes of pes cavus are listed in Table 1–5. In examination and assessment of the cavus deformity, the following steps are carried out.

First, determine the *type* of pes cavus. Is it simple cavus (plantaris), cavovarus, calcaneocavus, or equinocavus? In *simple cavus* both the first and fifth metatarsals are in fixed equinus with even distribution of weight on their heads, and the heel is in neutral or slight valgus. In *cavo-*

varus the first metatarsal is in *fixed equinus* and the fifth metatarsal is in normal longitudinal alignment; therefore the medial limb of the tripod of the foot is longer than the lateral limb. The medial ray of the foot is pronated (Fig 1–47A). On weight-bearing the fifth metatarsal head and the heel cannot touch the floor. The forefoot and heel invert so that the three points of the tripod touch the floor (Fig 1–47B, C). Initially the varus deformity of the heel is flexible; that is, when the fixed equinus and pronation deformity of the first metatarsal are corrected, the varus deviation of the heel disappears. In time, however, the hindfoot inversion becomes fixed. In *pes calcaneocavus* the hindfoot is in fixed calcaneus and the forefoot in fixed equinus. It is encountered in myelomeningocele and other flaccid paralytic conditions such as poliomyelitis. It also develops as a secondary deformity when the Achilles tendon is overlengthened and the triceps surae is markedly weakened. In *pes equinocavus* the ankle, hindfoot, and forefoot are in fixed equinus; it is seen in congenital clubfoot. *Congenital pes cavus* (or talipes cavus) is present at birth; it is a rare deformity in an otherwise normal infant. Often it is associated with clawing of the great toe.

Second, *assess the deformity.* Examine the feet in stance from the front, medial (one foot in front of the other), lateral, and posterior views. In pes cavus, the longitudinal arch is abnormally elevated. Determine the apex of the high arch. Is it anterior, at the tarsometatarsal and naviculocuneiform joints (as in pes cavovarus), or posterior, at the talonavicular and calcaneocuboid joints (as in calcaneocavus). Is it global; that is, does the equinus occur at both tarsometatarsal and calcaneocuboid and talonavicular joints (as in simple cavus and often in equinocavus)?

Inspect the position of the hindfoot from the rear. Is the heel in varus, neutral, or eversion? Assess the pitch of the calcaneus. Is it normal (10 to 30 degrees of dorsiflexion), is it in excessive dorsiflexion (more than 40 degrees, indicating calcaneus deformity of the hindfoot), or is it in plantar flexion as seen in equinocavus deformity?

Note the position of the toes. Are they normal or are they clawed with hyperextension of the metatarsophalangeal joints and flexion of the interphalangeal joints (Fig 1–48)? Do the tips of the toes touch the floor? On passive manipulation, can the claw deformity be corrected (flexible) or is it rigid? Inspect the dorsum of the interphalangeal joints. Is there adventitious bursitis (because of pressure and rubbing from shoes) or keratoses over the dorsum of the interphalangeal joints?

Next ask the patient to walk. Is any abnormality of gait present? Have the patient walk in tandem, on his or her toes, heels, and inner and outer borders of his or her feet. Observe balance and assess motor function of muscles controlling the foot and ankle.

Next have the patient sit with his or her feet dangling over the edge of the table. Feel the soft tissues of the plantar aspect of the foot. When the metatarsal heads are pushed into maximal dorsiflexion, are the plantar soft tissues taut and contracted, pulling and fixing the forefoot in equinus (Fig 1–49)? Is there pronation—that is, plantar flexion and eversion of the medial rays of the foot (first and second metatarsals)? Test the range of motion of the ankle, subtalar, midtarsal, tarsometatarsal, metatarsophalangeal, and interphalangeal joints. In equinocavus deformity, the range of ankle dorsiflexion is limited, whereas in calcaneocavus deformity, the range of ankle plantar flexion is restricted. In idiopathic cavovarus deformity, ordinarily the ankle has normal range of motion. Manually test the passive range of eversion and inversion of the subtalar joint. Is the hindfoot varus fixed or flexible?

An important determination is the mobility of the hindfoot on the forefoot. This can be determined in two ways: The first method is the Coleman standing lateral block test—the cavovarus test. Ask the patient to stand on a 1- to 1.5-inch thick wooden block bearing weight on the heel with the lateral border of the foot and the first through third metatarsals hanging freely into plantar flexion and pronation. If the heel varus returns to normal heel eversion, the mobility between the hindfoot and forefoot is normal; if the hindfoot remains in varus, the deformity is rigid (Fig 1–50A–D). The second method is the Carroll test. Have the

patient stand on a 2- to 3-inch wooden block, bearing weight on his hindfoot with the forefoot dangling over the edge. When there is mobility between the hindfoot and the forefoot, the heel varus corrects to normal position (Fig 1–50E, F).

Next, check mobility of the first metatarsal medial cuneiform joint. Hold the heel with one hand and raise the first metatarsal head into maximal dorsiflexion. Can you correct the equinus deformity of the first metatarsal, or is it fixed? The flexibility of the metarsophalangeal and interphalangeal joints is tested by the Kelikian "push-up" test. Passively dorsiflex the metatarsal heads. If mobility is normal, the hyperextended metatarsophalangeal joints extend to neutral position and the flexed interphalangeal joints extend fully.

Next examine the plantar aspect of the foot for abnormal pressure areas and painful callosities and ulcerations under the metatarsal heads.

Perform manual muscle testing for strength of the muscles controlling the foot and ankle. Is there any invertor-evertor dynamic muscle imbalance? Is the anterior tibial muscle weak and the peroneus longus strong? Is the peroneus brevis weak? Examine the shoes for abnormal wear.

The third step is to determine the *cause* of the cavus. Although the exact cause of pes cavus is unknown, it can be classified into two general categories: paralytic and idiopathic. In the latter a neuromuscular deficit or other specific cause cannot be demonstrated. A positive family history of cavus makes the probability of an underlying neuromuscular affection as the cause of pes cavus more likely. Neuromuscular causes of pes cavus are Charcot-Marie-Tooth disease, Déjérine-Sottas interstitial hypertrophic neuritis, polyneuritis, Friedreich's ataxia, Roussy-Levy syndrome, spinal cord tumors, tethered cord and spinal dysrhaphism, myelomeningocele, poliomyelitis, dystonia

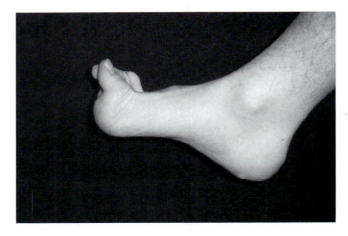

Figure 1–48. Pes cavus with hyperextension deformity of the metatarsophalangeal joints and flexion deformity of the interphalangeal joints of the big toe and lesser toes.

musculorum deformans, spinal muscular atrophy, spastic or extrapyramidal type of cerebral palsy, and distal type of muscular dystrophy (see Table 1–5).

Carry out the following investigations to determine the cause:

1. Perform *muscle testing* to rule out paralysis and dynamic imbalance of muscles acting on the foot. The peroneus longus depresses the first metatarsal, whereas the anterior tibial elevates the first metatarsal. A weak anterior tibial and a strong peroneus longus cause equinus and pronation of the medial ray of the foot. The extensor digitorum longus is overactive to compensate for the loss of motor strength of the weak anterior tibialis and aggravates the eversion of the forefoot.[202,210] Triceps surae muscle weakness causes a calcaneal deformity of the hindfoot and results in a calcaneocavus defor-

mity. Intrinsic muscles of the foot, lumbricals, interossei, and short toe flexors and extensors should be carefully assessed as well as the function of extensor digitorum longus and flexor digitorum longus.[203] The posterior tibialis muscle is usually normal in motor strength and the last to lose its function in Charcot-Marie-Tooth disease and other hereditary and sensory neuropathies. This is a factor in varus deformation of the hindfoot and midfoot in paralytic cavovarus deformity. Is there atrophy and inverted champagne bottle appearance of the legs (seen in Friedreich's ataxia and Charcot-Marie-Tooth disease)?

2. *Sensory testing.* Besides testing touch and sensory pin prick function, determine position sense and vibratory sensation with a tuning fork. This is important to detect hereditary motor and sensory neuropathies.

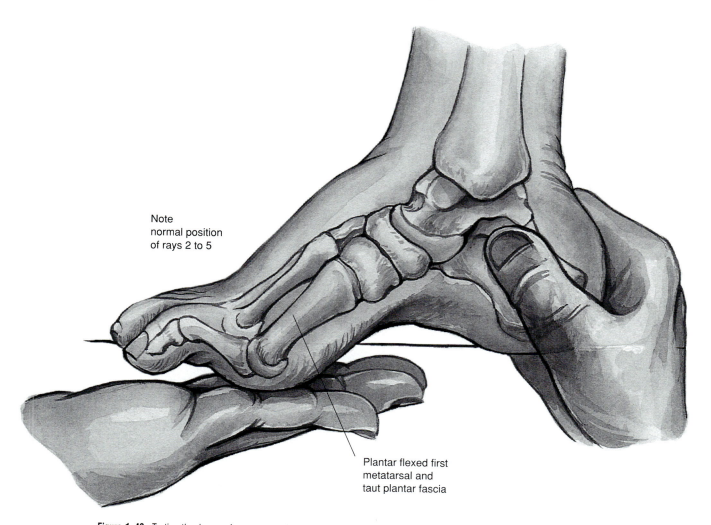

Note
normal position
of rays 2 to 5

Plantar flexed first
metatarsal and
taut plantar fascia

Figure 1–49. Testing the degree of contracture of the plantar soft tissues and flexibility of the equinus deformity of the forefoot. Hold the hindfoot with one hand and with the other, push the metatarsal heads into maximal dorsiflexion. Feel the tautness of the plantar soft tissues. Passive dorsiflexion of the metatarsal heads also determines the flexibility of the MP and IP joints. If they are mobile, the toes will straighten (Kelikian push-up test).

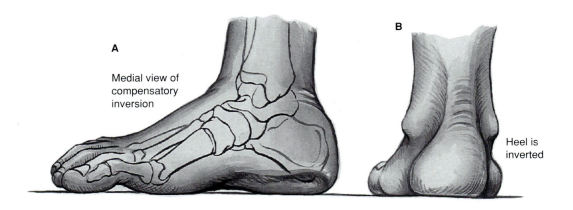

A

Medial view of compensatory inversion

B

Heel is inverted

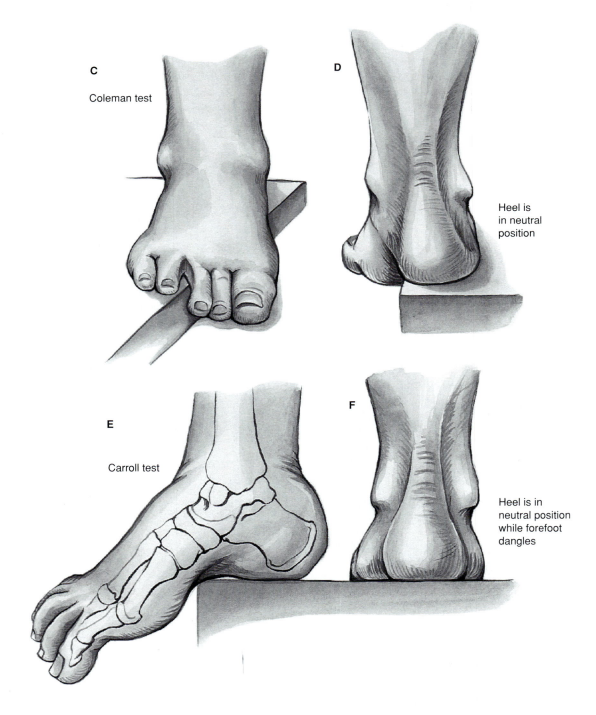

C

Coleman test

D

Heel is in neutral position

E

Carroll test

F

Heel is in neutral position while forefoot dangles

Figure 1–50. Methods of testing mobility between the hindfoot and the forefoot in pes cavovarus. **A, B.** Note the interdependence between the hindfoot and the forefoot. The heel, first metatarsal head, and fifth metatarsal head have a tripod relationship. When the first metatarsal is pronated, the forefoot supinates to get the first and fifth metatarsal heads flat on the floor and the hindfoot inverts. **C, D.** In the Coleman standing lateral block test, the heel and lateral border of the foot are on a 1.5-inch block, and the first and second metatarsals dangle at the edge of the block into pronation. When mobility is present between the hindfoot and the forefoot, the heel moves to its normal position of 5 degrees eversion. **E, F.** In the Carroll test, the patient stands with his hindfoot on a 2- or 3-inch wooden block (or a hard book) and the forefoot dangles free at the edge of the block. When flexibility between the hindfoot and forefoot is normal, the heel everts to normal position.

←

3. Have the child walk in tandem and also perform a finger-to-nose and Romberg test.

4. Inquire about urinary incontinence and anal sphincter control. Do not forget to test for the presence of the cremasteric reflex in boys and the umbilical abdominal skin reflex for upward or lateral excursion of the umbilicus in girls and boys to rule out spinal cord pathology. Deep tendon reflexes should be tested and the presence of a positive Babinski sign ruled out.

Examine the upper limbs, especially the hand. Are the metatarsophalangeal joints in hyperextension and the interphalangeal joints in flexion due to intrinsic muscle paralysis? Is the thumb lying flat to the side of the index finger with flatness of the thenar eminence due to paralysis of the thenar muscles? Check for opposition between the pulps of the thumb and index fingers? In Charcot-Marie-Tooth disease and Friedreich's ataxia, progressive paralysis of these muscles may occur.

Examine the child's spine. Is a hairy patch present, indicating spinal dysrhaphism? Is there scoliosis or kyphosis? What is the flexibility of the spine? Ask the patient to bend laterally to each side and then to hyperextend and flex the lumbosacral spine. Can he touch his toes? Are the hamstring muscles taut and spastic? In the presence of a progressive intraspinal cord lesion, paraspinal muscular rigidity is evident.

Imaging Findings. Make AP and lateral weight-bearing radiograms of the foot. Determine the apex of the deformity and its severity. Draw a longitudinal line through the center of the body of the talus, navicular, medial cuneiform, and first metatarsal shaft. Next, draw a vertical line through the center of the body of the navicular. In the normal foot this longitudinal line is straight and bisects the vertical line through the navicular at a right angle (Fig 1–51). In pes cavus the forefoot is in fixed equinus. Draw a line through the center of the longitudinal axis of the first metatarsal and another longitudinal line through the center of the calcaneus and measure the angle between the two lines on the plantar aspect of the foot (Hibbs angle) (Fig 1–52).

When the equinus deformity is in the forefoot or midfoot, it is best measured by the Meary method. Draw a longitudinal line through the center of the talus and another longitudinal line through the center of the first metatarsal

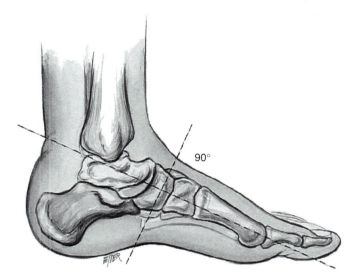

Figure 1–51. Drawing of a lateral view of a normal foot. Draw a longitudinal line through the center of the body of the talus, navicular, medial cuneiform, and first metatarsal shaft. Draw a vertical line through the center of the body of the navicular. In the normal foot this longitudinal line is straight and bisects the vertical line through the navicular at a right angle.

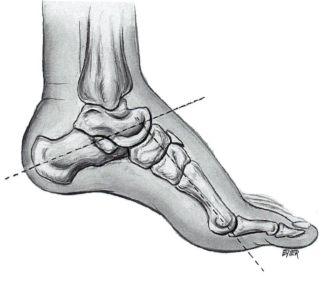

Figure 1–52. Hibbs angle in pes cavus. Draw a line through the center of the longitudinal axis of the first metatarsal and another longitudinal line through the center of the calcaneus. Measure the angle between these two lines on the plantar aspect of the foot.

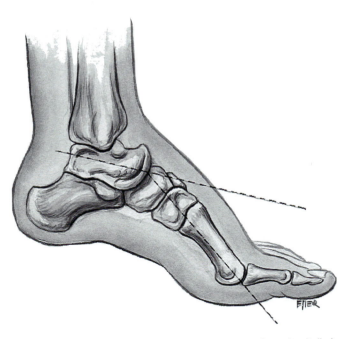

Figure 1–53. Meary angle to determine the degree of pes cavus. Draw a longitudinal line through the center of the talus and another longitudinal line through the center of the first metatarsal. The angle formed determines the degree of pes cavus.

(Fig 1–53). The angle formed by these lines determines the degree of cavus.[211]

AP and lateral radiograms of the entire spine should be made. Diastematomyelia is suggested by widening of the interpediculate distance and a radiopaque central bone spike. In slowly growing intraspinal tumors such as astrocytomas, the spinal canal is widened. Other congenital deformities of the vertebral column such as congenital scoliosis or kyphosis should be ruled out.

Nerve conduction velocity and electromyographic studies are performed to rule out hereditary motor and sensory neuropathies. In Charcot-Marie-Tooth disease the nerve conduction is slowed and electromyography shows evidence of muscle atrophy. If neurologic findings indicate spinal or brain pathology, an MRI of the entire spinal cord and brain is performed. Creatine phosphokinase and aldolase blood levels are determined to rule out myopathy. It is always wise to obtain a neurologic consultation with a competent pediatric neurologist.

Treatment. Asymptomatic cavus feet do not require treatment because a painless foot may become painful after surgery. Simple observation is in order. Document the severity and flexibility of the deformity. Passive stretching exercises are performed several times a day to elongate the contracted plantar fascia and short plantar muscles. Hold the heel steady with one hand and with the other hand push the metatarsal heads into dorsiflexion. In time the cavus may increase in the degree of deformity and a flexible foot may become rigid.

Treatment is indicated when painful calluses develop under the metatarsal heads and over the claw toes and when the patient complains of difficulty in fitting shoes, abnormal excessive shoe wear, and pain and inversion instability of the ankle due to heel varus.

When the deformity is *mild,* symptomatic relief may be provided by (1) special shoes with a wide toe portion and thin padding on the tongue of the shoe, (2) supportive soft molded insoles to relieve pressure from the metatarsal heads and increase the weight-bearing area of the foot to relieve discomfort. When the heel is in varus, it has been customary to give a 1/8- to 3/16-inch wedge in the lateral side of the shoe. An ankle-foot orthosis that holds the heel out of varus and the metatarsal heads in dorsiflexion may be worn at night. These measures, however, do not correct the cavus deformity, and it is questionable whether they are of any value in preventing progression of the severity of the cavus.

Surgery is indicated when the deformity is *moderate* or *severe* and symptoms are disabling. Prior to any surgical procedure it is vital to rule out progressive neuromuscular deficit by thorough serial examinations. The neuromuscular picture should be stable.

It is best to release contractural deformities of plantar soft tissues and provide dynamic balance of muscles acting on the foot before rigid bony deformity develops. Proper timing is crucial. Test mobility of the hindfoot on the forefoot and that of the first metatarsal medial cuneiform joint. If both are flexible, then perform a plantar soft tissue release. Subcutaneous section of the plantar fascia is ordinarily not sufficient to provide full correction, and it may result in a painful fibrositis of the plantar fascia. It is best to perform an open release of the plantar fascia and short plantar muscles and calcaneonavicular ligament at their origin from the tuberosity of the calcaneus and calcaneocuboid ligaments.[191,221,222]

A capsulotomy and plantar release of the naviculocuneiform and first metatarsal medial cuneiform joint are carried out if equinus deformity of the first metatarsal cannot be corrected by release of the plantar soft tissues from the origin. If the first metatarsal cuneiform joint is rigid, a dorsiflexion osteotomy is performed at its base. Avoid injury to the growth plate of the first metatarsal in the skeletally immature child. Do not combine osteotomy with capsulotomy because the unstable proximal segment may cause fixation problems. The anterior tibial tendon can be hemisectioned near its insertion and one half of it transferred dorsally to enhance its dorsiflexion power on the first metatarsal. Following surgery, below-knee walking casts are changed every 2 weeks for a total period of 6 weeks.

Extensor digitorum longus and extensor hallucis longus muscles are transferred to the metatarsal heads when, upon active dorsiflexion of the foot, the toes hyperextend and the metatarsal heads do not elevate. The metatarsal heads elevate upon transfer of the long toe extensors to the metatarsal heads and prevent recurrence of deformity.

When the varus deformity of the heel is fixed, a lateral closing wedge and lateral displacement osteotomy of the calcaneus are performed simultaneously with open plantar release. Because of the extensive nature of surgery and problems of vascular compromise, one should not combine plantar release and calcaneal osteotomy with long toe extensor transfer to the metatarsal heads. When the toes are clawed, the interphalangeal joint fusion can be simultaneously performed with long toe extensor transfer to the metatarsal heads. If the metatarsophalangeal joints are still subluxated dorsally, a dorsal capsulotomy of the metatarsophalangeal joints is performed and temporarily fixed internally with a Steinmann pin for 3 to 4 weeks to prevent rotatory and angular malalignment of the metatarsophalangeal joints.

In Charcot-Marie-Tooth disease or Friedreich's ataxia with progressive paralysis of the anterior tibial and toe extensors, the posterior tibial tendon is transferred by the interosseous route through the dorsum of the foot. When midfoot deformity is rigid and osseous, dorsal wedge osteotomy of the midtarsus is performed.[195,207]

When calcaneocavus deformity is present, plantar soft tissue release is combined with a posterior displacement osteotomy of the calcaneus.[213,217,218] In the paralytic foot, a triple arthrodesis provides stability of the joints, corrects deformity, and enhances action of the weakened muscles controlling the foot.

In equinocavus deformity, usually seen as a residual of clubfoot, the medial plantar release is combined with a posterior capsular–ligamentous release and Achilles tendon lengthening. Indications for the various surgical procedures are summarized in Table 1–6.

ADOLESCENT OR JUVENILE HALLUX VALGUS (BUNION) AND METATARSUS PRIMUS VARUS

The presenting complaint is the bunion. It is a rather common familial developmental deformity that is more frequent in girls. About 40 to 50 percent of bunions in the adult have their onset in the juvenile or adolescent age period. The deformity is typical: The big toe is deviated into valgus in varying degrees, and the first metatarsal is angled medially with its head prominent—the bunion. An adventitious bursa develops from pressure and friction against the shoe. The bursa may become inflamed and painful.

Etiology. The following factors have been implicated in the pathogenesis of hallux valgus:

1. Ligamentous hyperlaxity causes flattening of the metatarsal arch and splaying of the forefoot.
2. On pronation of the foot, the axis of the first ray is rotated so that the metatarsophalangeal joint of the big toe assumes an oblique orientation. Normally, the abductor hallucis provides medial and plantar stability of the metatarsophalangeal joint and the adductor hallucis provides support to the lateral aspect of the joint. The dorsal aspect of the metatarsophalangeal joint of the big toe is covered by an extensor hood, which is rather thin and stretchable. With medial rotation of the axis of the first ray, the abductor hallucis shifts plantar ward and the extensor hood assumes a medial position, thereby weakening the ligamentous support on the medial side of the metatarsophalangeal joint. The pull of the abductor hallucis deviates the big toe into valgus.
3. Dynamic imbalance is present between the adduc-

TABLE 1–6. INDICATIONS AND SURGICAL PROCEDURES TO CORRECT PES CAVUS

Indications	Operative Procedure
Fixed cavovarus deformity with mobility of hindfoot on the forefoot and over the first metatarsal medial cuneiform joint.	Medial plantar release of contracted plantar fascia, short plantar muscles, and calcaneonavicular and calcaneocuboid ligaments. Split anterior tibial tendon transfer near its insertion to dorsum of first metatarsal.
As above but with rigid equinus-pronation deformity of first metatarsal cuneiform joint	As above with dorsiflexion-inversion osteotomy of the base of first metatarsal. Caution! Do not injure growth plate at base of first metatarsal.
Following correction of cavovarus deformity when toes hyperextend but metatarsal heads do not elevate	Transfer long toe extensors and extensor hallucis longus to metatarsal heads.
Cavovarus deformity with stiff subtalar joint. No mobility between fixed equinus forefoot and varus hindfoot	Medial plantar release and lateral closing wedge osteotomy of calcaneus. Caution! Do not combine it with long toe extensor transfer to metatarsal heads to avoid vascular compromise.
Rigid equinus deformity at the midfoot (anterior cavus)	Medial plantar release, dorsal wedge osteotomy of midtarsus and first metatarsal
Rigid calcaneocavus deformity	Medial plantar release, posterior and lateral displacement osteotomy of calcaneus
Equinocavus deformity (ordinarily residual of clubfoot)	Medial plantar release and posterior release and Achilles tendon lengthening
Paralytic cavovarus or calcaneocavus with weak muscles controlling foot and ankle	Triple arthrodesis
Paralytic cavovarus as in severe Charcot-Marie-Tooth disease	Medial plantar release, arthrodesis and anterior transfer of posterior tibial tendon through interosseous route

tor hallucis and abductor hallucis, and contracture of the capsule and ligamentous tissues occurs on the lateral side of the metatarsophalangeal joint and ligamentous and capsular insufficiency on its medial side.

4. The first metatarsal and hallux are long (Roman foot). Pointed shoes worn by females deviate the big toe into valgus.

History.   The following questions are asked of the patient and parents: Do any other family members have bunions? Is there "loose jointedness" or flatfeet in the family? Was surgery required on the family members with bunions? How did the foot of the patient appear at birth? Was there metatarsus varus? Did it require treatment in the form of passive stretching exercises, splints, or casts? When was the deformity of the hallux and the bunion noted? Is it increasing in severity and becoming more and more painful? Are the feet flat? What types of shoes does the patient wear?

Do wide soft shoes relieve the symptoms? Has any orthotic device been used to try to correct the deformity? Are there painful keratoses under the second, third, or fourth metatarsal heads? Is there a hammer-toe deformity? Is there a bunionette?

Assessment of the Deformity.   This is carried out by clinical examination and by true AP standing radiograms of the feet.

1. Determine the angle between the longitudinal axis of the first and second metatarsals. When the *intermetatarsal angle* is greater than 9 degrees, it is abnormal (see Fig 1–54A).
2. Assess the degree of hallux valgus by measuring the angle between the longitudinal axis of the proximal phalanx of the great toe and the first metatarsal. If the hallux valgus is greater than 16 degrees, it is abnormal (see Fig 1–54A).

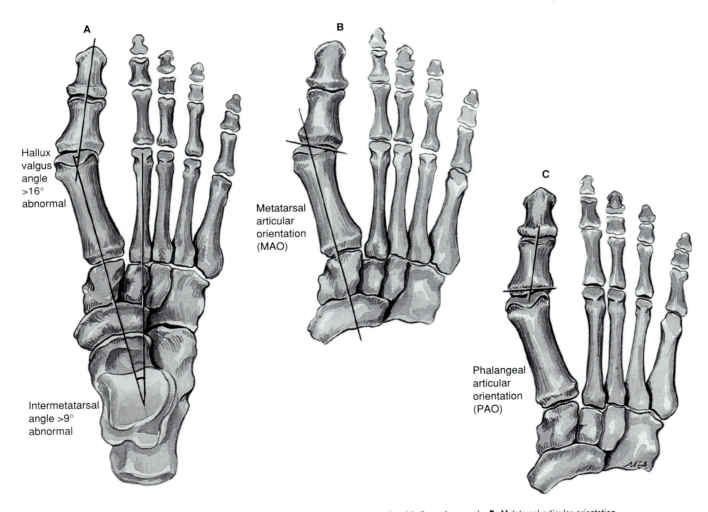

Figure 1–54. Radiographic assessment of hallux valgus. **A.** Intermetatarsal and hallux valgus angle. **B.** Metatarsal articular orientation (MAO). **C.** Phalangeal articular orientation (PAO). *(Continues)*

Hallux valgus angle >16° abnormal

Intermetatarsal angle >9° abnormal

Metatarsal articular orientation (MAO)

Phalangeal articular orientation (PAO)

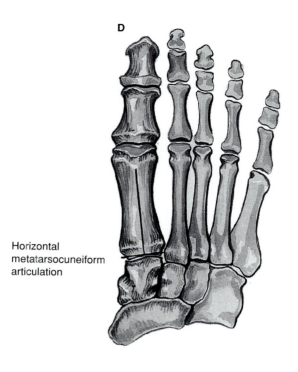

Horizontal
metatarsocuneiform
articulation

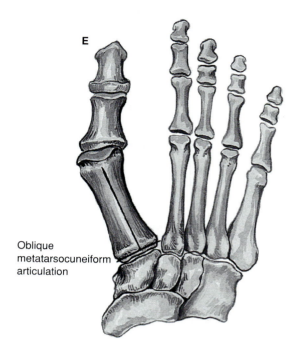

Oblique
metatarsocuneiform
articulation

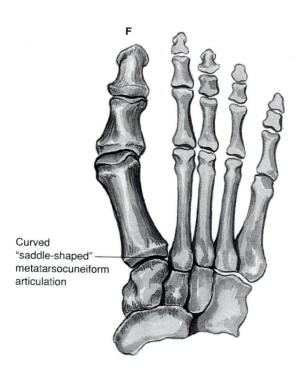

Curved
"saddle-shaped"
metatarsocuneiform
articulation

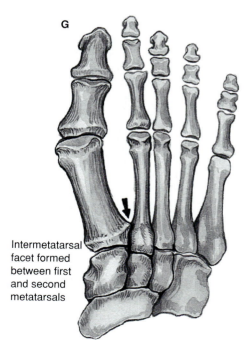

Intermetatarsal
facet formed
between first
and second
metatarsals

Figure 1–54 *(Continued).* **D, E.** Horizontal and oblique metatarsal cuneiform articulation. The horizontal is stable; the oblique is unstable. **F.** Curved "saddle-shaped" metatarsocuneiform articulation. **G.** Intermetatarsal facet between first and second metatarsal base. *(Continues)*

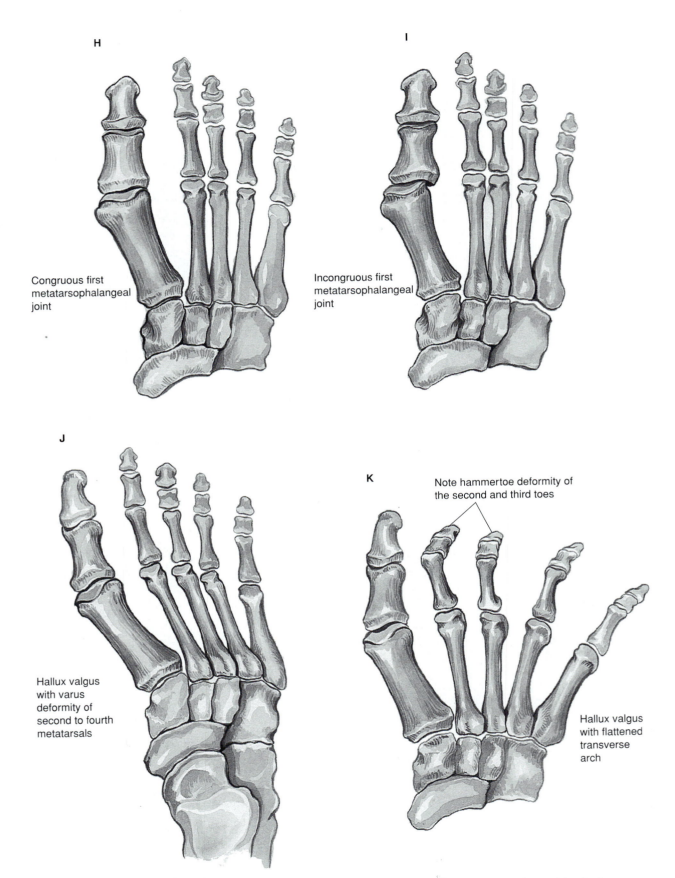

H

Congruous first
metatarsophalangeal
joint

I

Incongruous first
metatarsophalangeal
joint

J

Hallux valgus
with varus
deformity of
second to fourth
metatarsals

K

Note hammertoe deformity of
the second and third toes

Hallux valgus
with flattened
transverse
arch

Figure 1–54 *(Continued)*. **H, I.** Congruous and incongruous first metatarsophalangeal joint. **J.** Hallux valgus with varus deformity of second, third, and fourth metatarsals. **K.** Hallux valgus with splaying of the forefoot and flattening of the transverse arch.

3. Determine the orientation of the articular surface of the first metatarsal head and the base of the proximal phalanx of the great toe. The metatarsal articular orientation (MAO) is determined by measuring the angle between a line drawn parallel to the articular surface of the distal metatarsal articular surface and the longitudinal axis of the first metatarsal (Fig 1–54B). The phalangeal articular orientation (PAO) is measured by drawing a line parallel to the proximal articular surface of the proximal phalanx and the longitudinal axis of the proximal phalanx of the great toe (Fig 1–54C). The hallux valgus deformity tends to progressively increase when the MAO, PAO, or both angles are abnormally high, indicating increased lateral tilt of the distal metatarsal articular surface.

4. Determine the orientation of the metatarsal cuneiform joint. Is it horizontal or oblique? A horizontal orientation is stable, whereas an oblique orientation tends to increase the first–second intermetatarsal angle (Fig 1–54D, E). A curved metatarsal cuneiform articulation also tends to be unstable and causes medial deviation of the first ray (Fig 1–54F).

5. Is a facet present between the bases of the first and second metatarsals (Fig 1–54G)? If so, it restricts correction of the intermetatarsal angle at surgery.

6. Assess the configuration of the first metatarsal head. Is it round and smooth or is it enlarged and irregular with degenerative changes and a sagittal sulcus?

7. Determine whether the metatarsophalangeal joint is congruent (no lateral subluxation) or incongruent (presence of lateral subluxation). A congruous metatarsophalangeal joint is stable and ordinarily the degree of hallux valgus does not increase, whereas an incongruous joint is at risk for progressive hallux valgus deformity (Fig 1–54H, I).

8. The physis of the first metatarsal is near its base; when it is open, recurrence rate is high.

9. Assess the degree of any varus deformity of the second, third, and fourth metatarsals and splaying and flattening of the transverse metatarsal arch due to ligamentous hyperlaxity (Fig 1–54J, K).

10. Is there any deformity of the lesser toes?

Treatment. An asymptomatic bunion should be left alone unless it is so severe that it causes difficulty in shoe fitting and wear. When an associated flexible pes planus is present, a longitudinal arch support is provided to correct the pronation and lateral rotation of the first ray. A wide soft shoe relieves pressure on the bony prominence of the first metatarsal head. Bunion splints are of questionable value.

Surgical treatment is indicated when the bunion is symptomatic and the deformity is severe. The patient should demand correction of the deformity for pain but not necessarily for cosmesis. In general, the results of bunion surgery are very satisfactory; however, problems and complications can develop and the foot may become more painful and cause great disability. Varus orientation of the first metatarsal is corrected by osteotomy of the metatarsal at its base, either by a closing wedge osteotomy if the first metatarsal is long, opening wedge osteotomy if the first metatarsal is short, or crescentic wedge osteotomy if the first metatarsal is normal in length. If the metatarsal cuneiform joint is oblique, an open-up osteotomy of the medial cuneiform with a wedge of bone graft is performed to convert the varus orientation of the metatarsal cuneiform joint to horizontal. All of these osteotomies are fixed with threaded pins or screws (Fig 1–55).

Hallux valgus deformity is corrected by tenotomy of the adductor hallucis and capsulotomy on the lateral side of the first metatarsophalangeal joint. On the medial side of the metatarsophalangeal joint, the capsule is tightened and the abductor hallucis shifted medially from its plantar displaced position. Capsular stability and dynamic balance of muscle forces should be provided. Avoid overcorrection.

HALLUX VALGUS INTERPHALANGEUS

In this deformity varying degrees of valgus deviation of the big toe are present at the interphalangeal joint (Fig 1–56). In the severe case, in which blisters and a painful adventitious bursa develop over the prominent interphalangeal joint, surgical correction is indicated. In the adult arthrodesis of the interphalangeal joint of the hallux in normal alignment is carried out. In the skeletally immature foot the growth plate of the distal phalanx (which is proximal) should not be disturbed; the deformity is corrected by cuneiform osteotomy of the proximal phalanx near the interphalangeal joint with resection of a wedge of bone based medially.

BUNIONETTE (TAILOR'S BUNION)

Prominence of the fifth metatarsal head with or without lateral deviation of its neck and shaft cause abnormal increased pressure from tight shoes and result in a painful adventitious, swollen bursa over the bone (Fig 1–57A).

Treatment. Mild or moderate symptoms are relieved by wearing a wide-toed shoe with appropriate padding. Severe cases are treated surgically by sliding osteotomy of the fifth metatarsal neck (Fig 1–57B).[233,234]

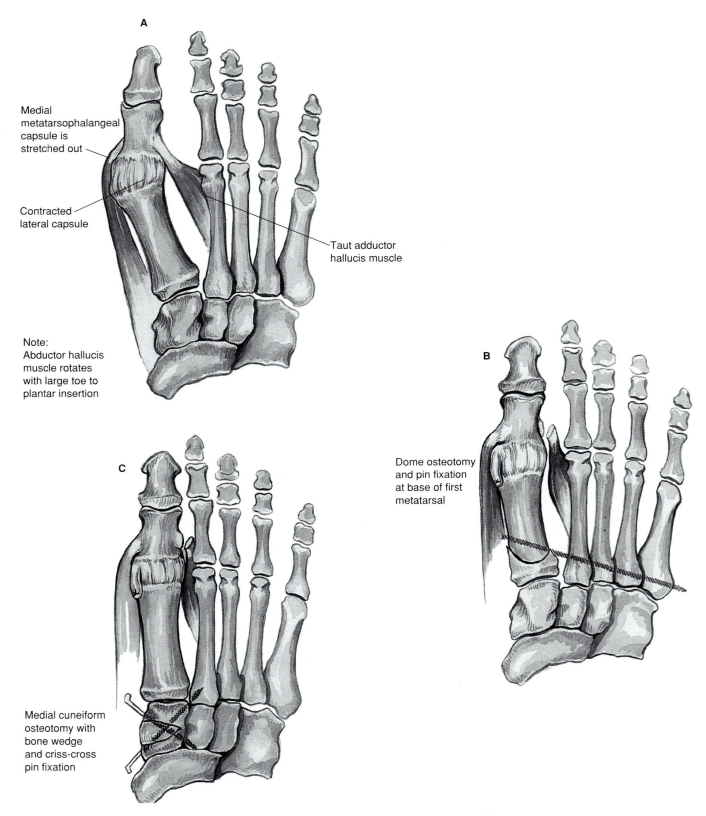

A

Medial metatarsophalangeal capsule is stretched out

Contracted lateral capsule

Taut adductor hallucis muscle

Note: Abductor hallucis muscle rotates with large toe to plantar insertion

B

Dome osteotomy and pin fixation at base of first metatarsal

C

Medial cuneiform osteotomy with bone wedge and criss-cross pin fixation

Figure 1–55. Surgical treatment of hallux valgus. **A.** The pathologic anatomy. **B.** Adductor myotomy and medial capsular plication of the metatarsal cuneiform joint and dome osteotomy of the base of the first metatarsal and intermetatarsal fixation with one threaded Steinmann pin. **C.** Open-up osteotomy of medial cuneiform with wedge bone graft to correct varus orientation of the first metatarsal cuneiform joint.

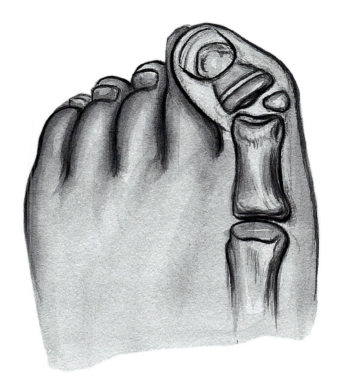

Figure 1–56. Hallux valgus interphalangeus. Note the valgus deformity at the interphalangeal joint of the great toe. The metatarsophalangeal joint is normal.

SPLAYFOOT

The presenting complaint is a broad forefoot due to increased intermetatarsal angles caused by hyperlaxity of the ligaments. Involvement is bilateral and is seen more frequently in the female and adolescent with generalized ligamentous hyperlaxity or as a part of a syndrome such as Marfan's or Down's.

Often the problem is one of fitting shoes and eventually pain over the fifth and first metatarsal heads, with flattening of the transverse metatarsal arch. These patients develop pain under the second, third, and fourth metatarsal heads.

Treatment. Soft shoe inserts with a metatarsal pad to relieve the symptoms should be prescribed. In severe cases with pain and difficulty in ambulation, proximal osteotomies of the first and fifth metatarsals can narrow the foot. Reinforcement by tendon graft to tighten the stretched intermetatarsal ligaments has not been successful.

LOBSTER CLAW OR CLEFT FOOT DEFORMITY

This rare malformation presents with absence of the central two or three rays of the foot (Fig 1–58). Often it is inherited

as an autosomal dominant trait with bilateral involvement and sometimes in conjunction with lobster clawing of the hands. In the rare form, involvement is unilateral and not hereditary. Associated deformities such as cleft lip and palate may be present.

Treatment. Treatment consists of osteotomy of the lateral and medial metatarsals at their bases, approximation of their spread distal ends, and partial surgical syndactyly.

SYNDACTYLY

Fusion of the toes is a congenital deformity representing failure of separation of parts which may be partial or complete (Fig 1–59). It does not cause any symptoms and should be left alone. Do not separate the toes. The postsurgical scar may form a keloid that can become painful from irritation by the shoes.

MICRODACTYLY

Congenital hypoplastic toes may occur as an isolated deformity or in association with congenital constriction band syndrome (Streeter's dysplasia). Acquired microdactyly may result from vascular insufficiency in thromboembolic or vascular diseases. Surgical treatment is not necessary because hypoplasia of the toes does not cause any functional deficiency. If shoe size is a problem, a soft shoe insert with appropriate padding may be used.

MACRODACTYLY

Gigantism of the toes is rare; it may involve one or more rays of the foot. The corresponding digital nerves are enlarged, and varying degrees of hyperplasia of adipose and lymphatic tissue are present. It may be primary and idiopathic or secondary to neurofibromatosis or hemihypertrophy. In true gigantism, all tissue elements are affected. It should be distinguished from false gigantism, in which one tissue is primarily involved, such as bone in Ollier's disease or melorheostosis, vascular as in Klippel-Trenaunay syndrome, hemangiomatosis as in atrioventricular fistula, neural as in neurofibromatosis, fat as in lipomatous macrodactyly, or lymph as in congenital lymphedema.

Macrodactyly may be one of the many manifestations of Proteus syndrome—a congenital hamartomatous condition of overgrowth of various parts of the body, hemihypertrophy, macrodactyly of digits, and various deformities of the limbs such as valgus deformity of the knees, ankles, and hips and muscle hemangiomas and dislocations of joints.

The gigantic toe often has a grotesque appearance and interferes with shoe-fitting and weight-bearing, requiring surgical treatment.

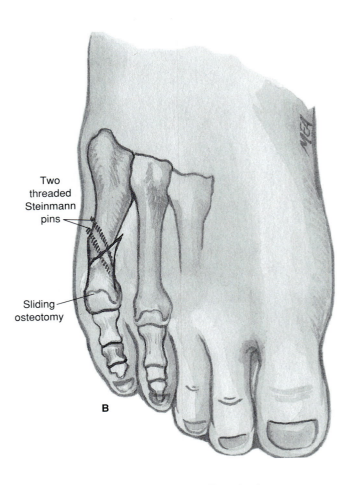

Two
threaded
Steinmann
pins

Sliding
osteotomy

Figure 1–57. Bunionette. **A.** Deformity of bunionette. Note fibular angulation of the fifth metatarsal, prominence of the fifth metatarsal head, and tibial angulation of the little toe. **B.** Surgical correction by sliding osteotomy of the neck and distal shaft of the fifth metatarsal and internal fixation with two threaded Steinmann pins.

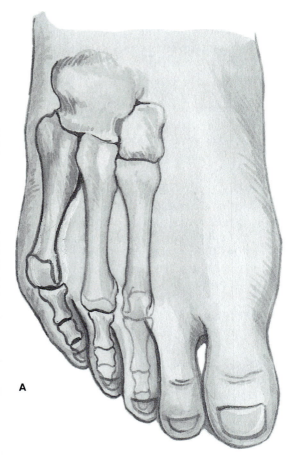

Figure 1–58. Bilateral lobster claw feet.

Treatment. The severely involved gigantic toe is best treated by ablation and partial or complete resection of the corresponding metatarsal. The remaining adjacent digits are partially syndactylized.

Moderate or minimally enlarged toes are treated by growth arrest of the metatarsal and phalanges and partial to complete debulking of the hypertrophied soft tissues. Vascular impairment is a definite complication. Perform the surgery in two or three stages.

POLYDACTYLY OR SUPERNUMERARY DIGITS

Supernumerary digits may be preaxial, on the medial side of the big toe, or postaxial, on the lateral side of the little toe; occasionally they are central. Polydactyly is more common in the female and in blacks. Often it is transmitted as an autosomal dominant trait. There may be associated polydactyly of the hand.

Examine the whole child for other associated anomalies such as Ellis–van Creveld chondroectodermal dysplasia

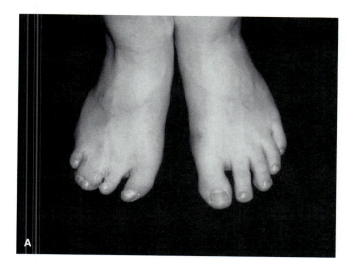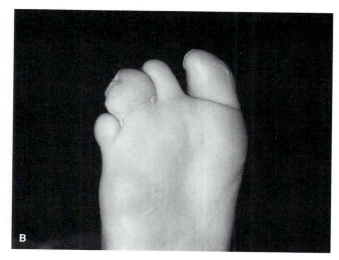

Figure 1–59. Syndactyly of the third and fourth toes of the right foot. **A.** Dorsal view of both feet. **B.** Plantar view of the right foot.

or Jeune's infantile thoracic dystrophy. An associated longitudinal deficiency of the tibia may also be present.

Treatment. Ablation of the extra toe is usually carried out before the first year of life when the infant begins to stand and take steps and the foot is large enough. Do not disturb growth! Repair the capsule to prevent subluxation of the metatarsophalangeal joints. Ordinarily when the little toe is duplicated the extra digit on the fibular side is removed and when the big toe is duplicated, the one on the tibial side is excised. The incisions should be placed in such a way that the operative scars are not irritated by the shoe, and the width and normal contour of the foot should be restored.

SYMPHALANGISM

Symphalangism, a term coined by Harvey Cushing, is characterized by fusion of two or three phalanges of a digit due to failure of separation of the parts. It is a hereditary malformation that is inherited as an autosomal dominant trait. There is a definite racial predilection for Caucasians; it occurs occasionally in Asians and hardly ever in Blacks.

Symphalangism may occur as an isolated malformation, ordinarily affecting more than one finger. Any of the interphalageal joints may be fused. It may be associated with other malformations of the hands and feet such as a short or absent middle phalanx of the involved digit or may be associated with syndactylism, as in Apert's syndrome.

Clinically the affected joint of the finger or toe is stiff, with no motion on passive manipulation of the articulation. The transverse creases overlying the fused interphalangeal joint are absent; the skin is smooth. Periarticular soft tissues

are atrophic. The affected digit is usually stiff in extension, especially when the proximal interphalangeal joint is fused. In the foot, there is no functional impairment. In the hand, when the long finger is involved, the appearance of the hand can be cosmetically and socially objectionable when the child attempts to make a fist. Symphalangism interferes with fine motor activities such as picking up small objects.

The stiff joint can be detected at birth; the radiograms appear normal, however, because the cartilaginous components at the articulation have the same density as the surrounding soft tissues. With skeletal maturation and growth in adolescence the bony fusion becomes evident.

Treatment. Flexion osteotomy of the digit fused in extension may provide some improvement of function. Arthroplasty to restore motion should not be performed because it does not succeed. In symbrachydactyly the digit is short due to hypoplasia or aplasia of the middle phalanx. When the thumb, index, or long finger is involved, lengthening of the fused phalanges by either the Ilizarov or callotasis orthofix technique may be indicated. Such surgical procedures should be delayed until adolescence.

HAMMER TOE

This common deformity is a flexion contracture of the proximal interphalangeal joint; the distal interphalangeal joint and the metatarsophalangeal joints are in neutral extension (Fig 1–60A). Involvement is usually bilateral. Often the second toe is affected; the adjacent third or fourth toe may also be involved. The congenital form has a high familial incidence. Hammer-toe deformity may develop when an abnormally long toe is forced into flexion in a small shoe.

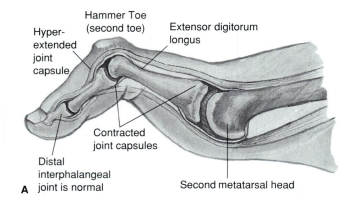

A Hyper-extended joint capsule

Hammer Toe (second toe)

Extensor digitorum longus

Contracted joint capsules

Distal interphalangeal joint is normal

Second metatarsal head

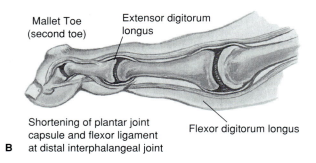

B Mallet Toe (second toe)

Extensor digitorum longus

Shortening of plantar joint capsule and flexor ligament at distal interphalangeal joint

Flexor digitorum longus

Figure 1–60. Hammer toe and mallet toe. **A.** Hammer toe (second toe). Note that the proximal interphalangeal joint is in flexion and the distal interphalangeal and metatarsophalangeal joints are in neutral position. **B.** Mallet toe (second toe). Note that the distal interphalangeal joint is in flexion, whereas the proximal interphalangeal and metatarsophalangeal joints are in neutral position.

Painful calluses and an adventitious bursa may develop over the prominent interphalangeal joint and the depressed metatarsal head.

Treatment. In infants and children the deformity is asymptomatic and ordinarily not corrected. Ignore a minor degree of hammer toe. When it is moderate or severe, manage it by passive stretching of the interphalangeal joint into complete extension and by providing shoes with adequate room.

In the moderate deformity in the older child, when one plantar flexes the metatarsophalangeal joint and the interphalangeal joint becomes fully extended, simple division of the long flexor tendon of the affected toe corrects the hammer-toe deformity.

In the adolescent and adult when the deformity is fixed and severe, causing pain and problems with shoe fitting, it is treated by a wedge resection of the proximal interphalangeal joint with its base dorsal and with fusion of the interphalangeal joint in neutral extension. When the metatarsophalangeal joint is hyperextended and the metatarsal

head is depressed with a painful callus under the metatarsal head, the long toe extensor is transferred to the metatarsal neck.

MALLET TOE (CONGENITAL FLEXED TOE)

In mallet toe the flexion deformity is at the distal interphalangeal joint, in contrast to hammer toe, in which the flexion deformity is at the proximal interphalangeal joint (Fig 1–60B). Ordinarily a single toe or two adjacent toes are affected. It is asymptomatic in childhood, but in the adolescent or adult a painful corn may develop on the tip of the flexed toe.

Treatment. Treatment is conservative in the growing child, whereas in the adolescent the long toe flexor is divided and the distal interphalangeal joint is fused in extension.

CLAW TOE

In this deformity the proximal and distal interphalangeal joints are flexed, whereas the metatarsophalangeal joint is hyperextended and subluxated dorsally (Figs 1–61A, B and 1–62). The condition is often associated with pes cavus; it is severe in paralytic and progressive disorders such as myelomeningocele. Occasionally it presents as an isolated congenital deformity in the infant.

Initially it is flexible, but later it may become fixed. Flexibility of claw toe is determined by the push-up test (Fig 1–63). On dorsiflexion of the metatarsal head, if the joint is flexible, the metatarsophalangeal joint extends to neutral position and the interphalangeal flexed joint extends fully. The great toe is usually more severely affected than the lesser toes. Pressure keratoses develop under the metatarsal heads and over the flexed proximal interphalangeal joints.

Treatment. If the deformity is moderate or severe and symptomatic, transfer the long toe extensors to the metatarsal neck and the short toe extensor to the stump of the long toe extensor and fuse the interphalangeal joint in neutral position. Occasionally when contracture of the dorsal capsule of the dorsally subluxated metatarsophalangeal joint is very severe, a dome capsulotomy of the metatarsophalangeal joint may be required.

CURLY TOE (CONGENITAL VARUS TOE)

In this common congenital deformity the affected toe is flexed, rotated laterally, and deviated at the proximal interphalangeal or at both the proximal and distal interphalangeal joints (Fig 1–64). The curled toe lies underneath the

A. Claw great toe

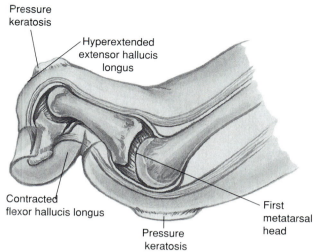

Pressure keratosis

Hyperextended extensor hallucis longus

Contracted flexor hallucis longus

Pressure keratosis

First metatarsal head

B. Claw second toe

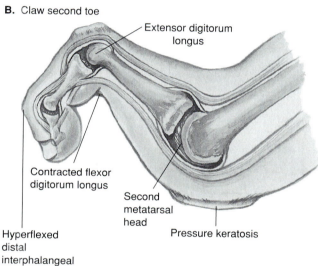

Extensor digitorum longus

Contracted flexor digitorum longus

Second metatarsal head

Pressure keratosis

Hyperflexed distal interphalangeal joint

Figure 1–61. Diagram illustrating claw toe deformity of the big and second toe. The metatarsophalangeal joint is hyperextended and subluxated dorsally. **A.** In the big toe the proximal interphalangeal joint is flexed, whereas in the second toe (**B**) both the proximal and distal interphalangeal joints are flexed.

adjacent toe. Involvement is usually bilateral, often affecting the second or third toe. It is believed to be caused by hypoplasia of the intrinsic muscles of the affected toe. Curly toe has a high familial incidence. It tends to increase with growth and does not correct spontaneously. The underriding toe tends to become uncomfortable in the shoe and causes pain and limping when walking.

Treatment. Ignore the deformity when it is mild and asymptomatic. Strapping the toes with adhesive tape does not correct the deformity. When the deformity is moderate and can be fully corrected by flexion of the toe and passive manipulation, a tenotomy of the flexor tendon through a

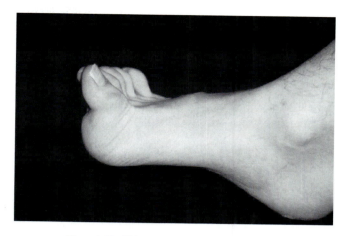

Figure 1–62. Clinical appearance of claw toe deformity.

transverse plantar incision straightens the toe. When curling of the toe is severe, section and transfer the long toe flexor tendon of the affected toe to its dorsolateral aspect.

CONGENITAL DIGITUS MINIMUS VARUS

In this common deformity the fifth toe is deviated dorsally and medially at its metatarsophalangeal joint, overriding the base of the fourth toe (Fig 1–65A). No flexion deformity of the interphalangeal joints is present. The long extensor tendon of the fifth toe, the dorsomedial aspect of the capsule of the fifth metatarsophalangeal joint, and the skin on the dorsum between the fourth and fifth toes become contracted. In children the deformity is asymptomatic. In the adolescent and adult, irritation by the shoe causes a painful, hard callus over the dorsum of the fifth toe. The condition is usually familial and involvement often bilateral.

Treatment. Passive stretching exercises of the little toe into plantar flexion and abduction and strapping of the little toe in normal position can be performed on the infant, but the strapping is cumbersome. Surgical correction is indicated in the adolescent or adult when a painful callus develops on the dorsum of the fifth toe. Two techniques are effective. In the Butler operation, recommended for children and adolescents, the little toe and the end of the fifth metatarsal are exposed through a racquet-shaped dorsal skin incision, with a second handle of the racquet on the plantar aspect. The long extensor tendon of the fifth toe and the dorsomedial capsule of the metatarsophalangeal joint are divided and plantar capsule adhesions are released. The toe is manipulated into normal position in the plantar handle of the racquet incision, and the subcutaneous tissue and skin are closed. A simple dressing and Ace bandage are applied.

In the adolescent with severe deformity and in the adult, the McFarland-Kelikian operation is recommended.

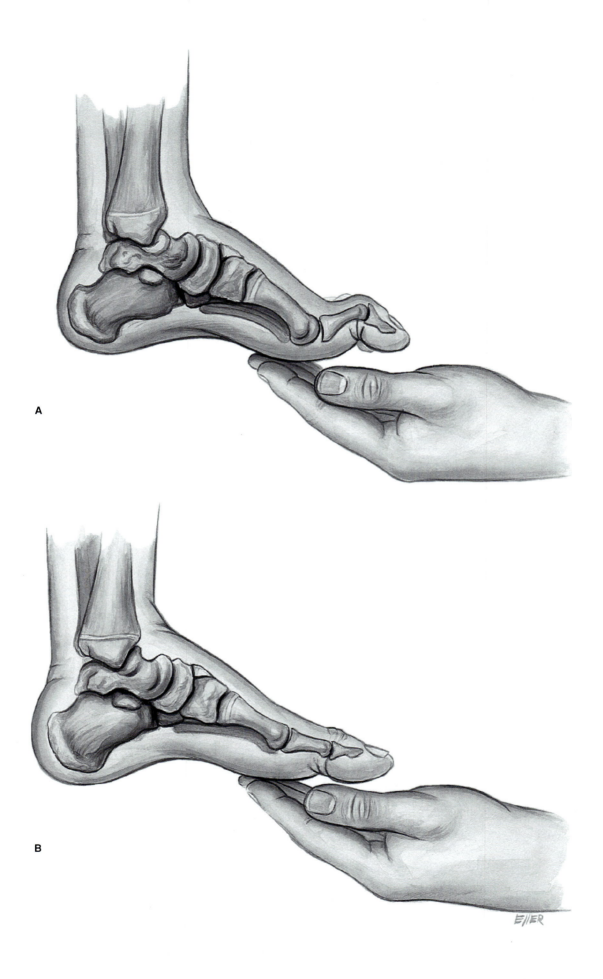

Figure 1–63. The "push-up" test to determine the flexibility of claw toe. **A.** The deformity with hyperextension of the metatarsophalangeal joint and flexion of the interphalangeal joint. **B.** On pushing the first metatarsal out of equinus, the metatarsophalangeal and interphalangeal joints straighten out, indicating that the deformity is flexible.

In this technique, the long extensor tendon of the little toe and the dorsomedial capsule of the metatarsophalangeal joint are divided, the proximal phalanx of the little toe is excised, and a surgical syndactyly of the fourth and fifth toes is performed (Fig 1–65B).

NAIL DEFORMITIES

Congenital Onychogryposis

A very rare growth deformity of the nail in children, congenital onychogryposis usually affects the great toe and presents as a thick, irregular corrugated nail. It may cause difficulty with wearing of socks and shoes and may become painful. Treatment consists of removal of the nail and excision of the nail bed.

Absence or Hypoplasia of Nails

Dystrophy of nails is more common in the hand than in the foot. Examine the knees and pelvis, as the nail dystrophy may be part of the nail-patella syndrome—hereditary onycho-osteodysplasia—which is characterized by absence or hypoplasia of the patellas and iliac horns. There is no specific treatment.

■ THE PAINFUL FOOT AND ANKLE

Pain in the foot and ankle is a common complaint. Its cause varies in different age groups. A diagnosis is readily made by careful physical examination to determine the site of local tenderness, swelling, increased heat, restriction of range of motion, and aggravation with stress (Fig 1–66).

KOHLER'S DISEASE

When pain is over the apex of the medial longitudinal arch, avascular necrosis of the tarsonavicular joint (Kohler's disease) should be suspected. In its acute phase, the child walks with an antalgic limp, supinating the foot and bearing weight on the lateral border of the foot. Palpation demonstrates local tenderness over the body of the tarsonavicular, with minimal swelling of the posterior tibial tendon near its insertion. No increased heat or fluid is present, and the range of motion of the midtarsal and subtalar joints is normal. Examine the opposite foot for any local tenderness over the tarsonavicular. Bilateral involvement is not uncommon. Ask for a history of acute injury or excessive stress on the foot due to overzealous physical activity. The age of a child with Kohler's disease is usually 5 years in boys and 4 years in girls. The condition is four times more common in boys than in girls. The cause of Kohler's disease is repetitive compression forces resulting in avascular necrosis of the tarsonavicular. Histologic examination of the involved navicular has shown evidence of aseptic necrosis, resorption of dead bone, and formation of new bone.

Imaging Findings. Make radiograms of both feet in AP, lateral, and oblique projections. The tarsonavicular begins

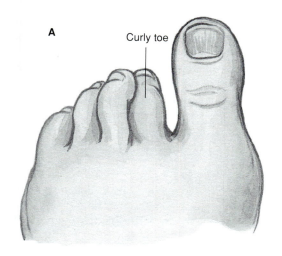

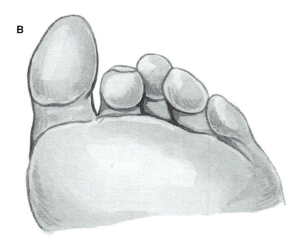

Figure 1–64. Congenital curly second toe. **A.** Dorsal view. **B.** Plantar view.

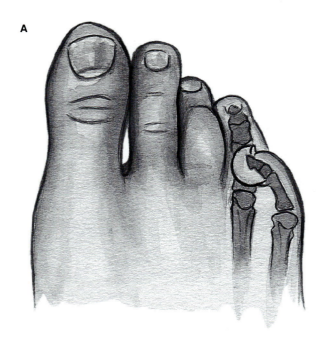

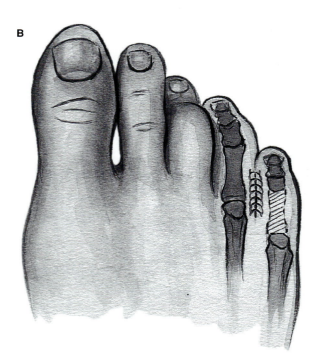

Figure 1–65. Congenital digitus minimus varus. **A.** Clinical appearance. **B.** Postoperative view of correction by the McFarland-Kelikian technique.

to ossify at around 2 years of age in girls and 2 1/2 years in boys. Irregularity of ossification of the tarsonavicular is a common, normal finding and should not be mistaken for Kohler's disease. Diagnostic findings are flattening of the tarsonavicular, as evidenced in the lateral projection by decrease of its AP diameter (Fig 1–67). Follow-up serial radiograms show rarefaction, sclerosis, and irregular ossification.

Bone imaging with technetium-99m is ordinarily not indicated unless there is a question about diagnosis. Imaging shows decreased uptake of radionuclides during its early stages, followed by increased uptake during revascularization.

Treatment. Treatment should be individualized according to the severity of symptoms. If moderate to severe, causing the child to limp, a below-knee walking cast is applied for 3 to 6 weeks, followed by support with a 3/8-inch longitudinal arch support or UCBL foot orthosis and avoidance of strenuous physical activities such as running, jumping from heights, and contact sports. When the pain is minimal (which is often the finding with the contralateral foot), a simple longitudinal arch support is all that is necessary. The prognosis is excellent. Within 1 year, the radiographic appearance of the navicular is restored to normal; long-term results have shown no evidence of arthritis of the talonavicular or naviculocuneiform joints.

FREIBERG'S INFRACTION

When pain occurs over the second or third metatarsal head, Freiberg's infraction should be suspected. This is a disease of the adolescent which occurs after 13 years of age. In one of 10, involvement is bilateral. In contrast to Kohler's disease, which is more common in boys, Freiberg's infraction is more common in girls, occurring in females in 75 percent of cases. The second metatarsal head is the most common site. The cause of Freiberg's infraction is repetitive trauma, compression, and aseptic necrosis of the affected metatarsal head.

Physical findings are quite typical—local tenderness and swelling of the affected metatarsal head, usually the second. The range of motion of the metatarsophalangeal joint is restricted.

Imaging Findings. Radiograms show flattening of the metatarsal head (Fig 1–68). However, bony and articular pathology is best depicted by MRI. The flattening, rarefaction, and irregular sclerosis of the metatarsal head are clearly demonstrated on CT scan. A bone scan with tech-

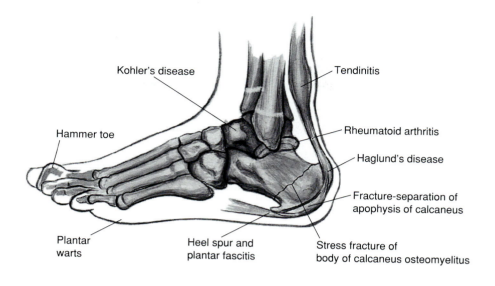

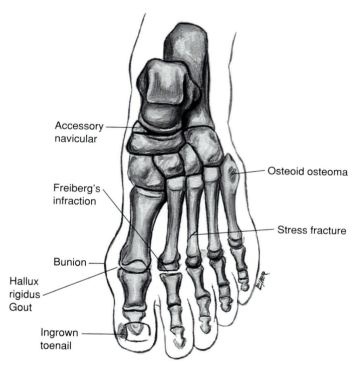

Figure 1–66. Differential diagnosis of foot pain according to its anatomic site.

netium-99m shows increased uptake due to healing of a stress fracture.

Treatment. Early diagnosis and treatment are crucial to prevent permanent structural deformation of the affected metatarsal head. In its acute painful stage when radiograms show simple flattening of the metatarsal head with minimal sclerosis, the foot is protected in a below-knee walking cast for 3 to 4 weeks, followed by a foot orthosis that extends to the toes and does not allow flexion-extension of the metatarsophalangeal joints. Strenuous physical activities such as running, jumping from heights, and contact sports are avoided. If symptoms persist and do not respond to the above measures or if the patient is seen late with flattening of the affected metatarsal head and sclerosis and irregularity of the bone, I recommend curettage and removal of the

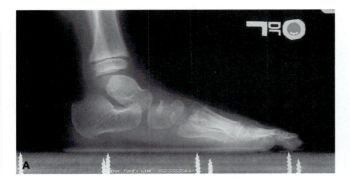 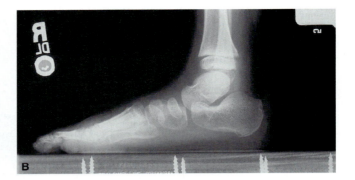

Figure 1–67. Radiogram of Kohler's disease (avascular necrosis of navicular bone) of left foot. **A.** Lateral view of the left foot showing compression and flattening of the tarsonavicular. **B.** Lateral view of right foot showing normal configuration of the tarsonavicular.

dead bone, grafting with cancellous bone, and protection in a cast for 6 weeks. Resection of the metatarsal head is reserved for cases diagnosed late, in which the head is markedly flattened and degenerative arthritis of the metatarsophalangeal joint is present. Resection is a salvage procedure. When the metatarsal head is resected, the toe of the affected ray is syndactylized to the adjacent toe to maintain its stability and length. The importance of early diagnosis and prevention of arthritis and preservation of the metatarsal head cannot be overemphasized. Silicone prosthetic implants to replace the resected metatarsal head are not recommended.

ACCESSORY NAVICULAR[267–271]

An accessory tarsal navicular may cause pain over the bony prominence due to formation and inflammation over an adventitious bursa. Often associated, nonspecific tenosynovitis of the posterior tibial tendon occurs near its insertion. The longitudinal arch is flattened. Fracture-separation of the cartilaginous synchondrosis of an accessory navicular is acutely painful.

Three types of accessory navicular have been identified based upon the size and location of the ossicle and the presence or absence of a synchondrosis between the accessory bone and the navicular. Type I is a sesamoid bone in the substance of the posterior tibial tendon. In type II the accessory bone is connected to the navicular by a cartilaginous synchondrosis, and in type III the accessory navicular is connected to the navicular by an osseous bridge. It is referred to as a cornuate navicular.[270]

Radiograms show the separate center of ossification to be proximal and somewhat plantar to the medial tip of the body of the navicular. The interval between the two may be fibrous connective tissue or fibrocartilage. In the radiogram it appears smooth and rounded, distinguishing it from traumatic fracture (Fig 1–69). In adolescence the fibrocartilaginous connection between the accessory navicular and the navicular bone may ossify; however, it persists in 2 percent of the adult population. Involvement is often bilateral.

Treatment. Treatment should be conservative, supporting the longitudinal arch in mild cases and applying a below-knee walking cast for 3 to 4 weeks when the pain is mod-

Figure 1–68. Freiberg's infraction of the second metatarsal head of the right foot. Note the flattening of the articular surface and sclerosis of the metatarsal head.

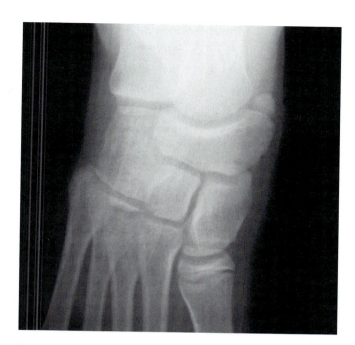

Figure 1–69. Accessory navicular. Note the separate center of ossification of the navicular.

erate or severe. Often symptoms subside with these measures. Only very occasionally do local swelling and pain persist. In such instances, excision of the accessory tarsal navicular is appropriate. It is combined with distal and plantar transfer of the posterior tibial tendon. However, it is crucial that the surgeon explain to the patient and family that this surgical procedure does not correct the planovalgus deformity.

HEEL PAIN

Tendinitis of the Heel Cord

When pain is in the heel at the insertion of the Achilles tendon, nonspecific tendinitis of the heel cord is the most common cause. Symptoms usually begin following strenuous physical activity such as running track. Achilles tendinitis is caused by repeated stretching of a contracted triceps surae due to overuse. On examination, the Achilles tendon is swollen and tender near its insertion. Dorsiflexion of the ankle and stretching of the triceps surae aggravate the pain. The bone is not tender on gentle palpation of the calcaneus, and the subtalar joint has normal range of motion. Radiograms in the AP, lateral, and os calcis views show fragmentation and irregular radiopacity of the calcaneal apophysis; these are normal findings, and an erroneous diagnosis of calcaneal apophysitis or Sever's disease should not be made. The radiographic appearance of the posterior surface of the calcaneus is smooth in the infant and young child. The calcaneal apophysis ossifies from several centers of ossification which appear between 4 and 7 years of age in girls and 7 and 10 years in boys. These ossification centers coalesce, forming an irregular outline, and the calcaneal apophysis fuses with the body of the calcaneus between 12 and 15 years of age, at which time it has the same density as the rest of the bone. An irregular sclerotic apophysis is normal, and "Sever's disease" does not exist.

Treatment. If pain and swelling are moderate or severe, a heel lift is given (3/8 inch tapered to the front to 1/8 inch). A nonsteroidal anti-inflammatory drug such as ibuprofen can be given orally. If the pain is very severe and does not respond to the above measures, a well-padded below-knee cast may be applied with the ankle and foot in slight equinus for a period of 3 weeks. Ordinarily the tendinitis subsides. Injection of corticosteroids into the inflamed tendon is not recommended because of the potential for rupture of the tendon.

Osteomyelitis of the Bones of the Foot[272–275]

The child with osteomyelitis of the foot presents with antalgic limp and pain, local tenderness, and soft tissue swelling over the site of the affected bone. The calcaneus is the most common site. Often the infection is caused by external inoculation of the pathogen through a puncture wound sustained by stepping on a nail, thorn, or sharp piece of glass. In the nursery the heel may be infected by puncture from a contaminated needle. *Pseudomonas* osteomyelitis is the most common. Infection is indolent, with paucity of systemic manifestations of fever, leukocytosis, and elevation of erythrocyte sedimentation rate.

Early radiographic changes are distortion and loss of trabecular bone structure; later on (within 10 to 21 days) bone destruction and periosteal new bone formation develop. Bone imaging with radionuclides detects osteomyelitis before radiographic changes are evident.

Treatment. The site of maximum tenderness is aspirated to isolate the pathogenic organism. A smear and Gram's stain and cultures are made. Appropriate antibiotics are administered according to sensitivity test results. If the response to antibiotic therapy is inadequate, surgical incision and drainage are indicated. *Pseudomonas* osteomyelitis is a difficult problem requiring immediate operative intervention.

Haglund's Disease[276–280]

Haglund's disease is an abnormal protuberance of the posterosuperior calcaneal tuberosity which causes retrocalcaneal adventitious bursitis, often referred to by laymen as a pump bump (Fig 1–70). The bony enlargement is a developmental anomaly. The pressure of the rigid counter of the shoe against the bony protuberance of the calcaneus irritates the Achilles tendon and causes progressive swelling of the retrocalcaneal bursa. In contrast to Achilles tendinitis, the local tenderness and swelling are above the insertion of the Achilles tendon.

The radiographic appearance in the lateral projection of the prominent posterosuperior tuberosity of the calcaneus is characteristic.

Treatment. Treatment should be conservative initially in the form of relieving the pressure from the shoe. The counter of the heel is softened, and wearing of a stiff heel counter is avoided. If symptoms persist, cause disability, and interfere with shoe wear, surgical excision of the prominent posterosuperior tuberosity of the calcaneus is indi-

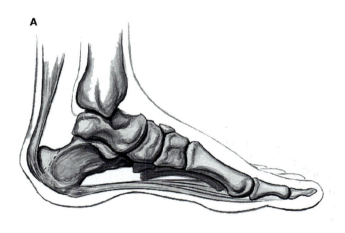

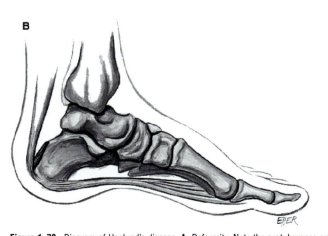

Figure 1–70. Diagram of Haglund's disease. **A.** Deformity. Note the protuberance on the posterosuperior calcaneal tuberosity and the thickened, inflamed Achilles tendon with retrocalcaneal bursitis. **B.** Treatment by excision of the abnormal bony protuberance.

cated. Use a horizontal incision in line with the skin creases; it is more aesthetic and the scar is not irritated by the shoe.

Heel Spurs

Heel spurs are not common in children and adolescents but can occur and cause pain. They are managed by appropriate padding to relieve heel pressure, a longitudinal arch support, and on occasion elevation of the heel.

STRESS FRACTURES

Calcaneus. When a child or adolescent complains of generalized heel pain after running track or other strenuous athletic activity, stress fracture of the calcaneus should be suspected. The condition is quite disabling. The child walks with an antalgic limp. On palpation, the tenderness is diffuse. Initial radiograms may appear normal. Bone imaging with technetium-99m shows increased uptake of the radionuclide at the fracture site. Follow-up radiograms show the healing fracture. Treatment consists of a below-knee walking cast for about 3 to 4 weeks.

Metatarsals. The presenting complaint is an antalgic limp after a child has participated in strenuous sports such as running and jumping. There is no history of acute trauma. On palpation the fractured metatarsal is tender, with some localized swelling. The initial radiograms may be negative, but follow-up radiograms show the subperiosteal callus and the fracture line.

Sesamoid Bones. Fractures of the sesamoid bone are rare except in dancers. The pain and tenderness are localized over the affected sesamoid bones under the first metatarsal head.

Treatment of stress fractures of the metatarsals and sesamoid bones consists of protection of the foot in a below-knee cast for 3 weeks.

PLANTAR FASCITIS

Plantar fascitis is rare in the pediatric population. The pain is localized near the origin of the plantar aponeurosis and is aggravated by standing and walking for prolonged periods (Fig 1–71).

On examination, the pain can be elicited by dorsiflexion of the metatarsophalangeal joints. This stretches the plantar aponeurosis. Radiograms may show a calcaneal spur.

Treatment consists of the use of soft shoes and oral intake of nonsteroidal anti-inflammatory medication. When symptoms are not relieved, local injection of corticosteroids is performed. Occasionally in the severe and recalcitrant case, excision of the heel spur is indicated.

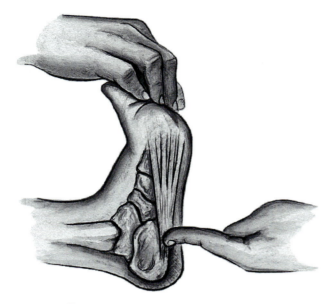

Figure 1–71. Plantar fascitis. Point of tenderness.

Tarsal tunnel syndrome and nerve entrapment are extremely rare in children and adolescents.

RHEUMATOID ARTHRITIS (PAUCIARTICULAR TYPE)

Rheumatoid arthritis may have its onset in the subtalar or midtarsal joint, which are restricted in range of motion, painful, with local soft tissue swelling and increased local heat. Radiograms are nonspecific and show the localized osteoporosis and soft tissue thickening. Imaging with technetium-99m shows increased local uptake. Laboratory tests for rheumatoid factors may be positive.

Treatment. Treatment consists of protection of the part and medicinal management with nonsteroidal anti-inflammatory drugs such as naproxen or tolmetin sodium. Only very rarely is surgical synovectomy indicated.

HALLUX RIGIDUS[281–283]

Hallux rigidus is multifactorial in its pathogenesis and presents as pain and stiffness in the metatarsophalangeal joint of the great toe. A rare lesion in the child and uncommon in the adolescent, it is familial in incidence and more common in the female. It may be caused by inflammatory disorders of the metatarsophalangeal joint such as arthritis or osteochondritis dissecans of the first metatarsal head.

Often mechanical factors such as dorsal elevation of the first metatarsal and a longer first metatarsal than second metatarsal are the cause of hallux rigidus. The weight is borne by the big toe rather than the first metatarsal head.

Imaging Findings. Radiographic features are normal in the beginning, but later dorsal elevation of the first metatarsal head becomes apparent. Subsequently the cartilage space of the metatarsophalangeal joint narrows, the first metatarsal head flattens, and osteophyte formation occurs.

In the differential diagnosis one should consider gout, which is rare in the adolescent but can occur. Determination of uric acid blood level helps make the diagnosis. Rheumatoid arthritis of the metatarsophalangeal joint of the great toe can occur and should be considered in the differential diagnosis.

Treatment. Nonsurgical measures should always be tried first in the form of stiffening the sole of the shoe between the shank and the big toe and purchase of larger shoes. If symptoms persist and protracted pain causes disability and abnormality in gait, surgical correction of the deformity is indicated.

A dorsiflexion osteotomy of the base of the proximal phalanx is performed in the skeletally mature foot. In children it is imperative that the growth plate at the base of the proximal phalanx not be disturbed. Waterman's cuneiform osteotomy of the first metatarsal is the procedure of choice. Only rarely is fusion of the metatarsophalangeal joint of the great toe required to relieve symptoms permanently.

PLANTAR WARTS

These cauliflower-like warts are clearly delineated from the surrounding normal skin and have a punctate appearance due to minute hemorrhages in the papillae. When compressed by weight-bearing or pressure from shoes, they are painful. They are viral in origin and highly contagious.

Treatment. Ignore plantar warts if they do not cause pain; they disappear spontaneously. If they are painful and large, causing difficulty with walking, chemical destruction by application of salicylic acid or liquid nitrogen is the best method of treatment. Refrain from surgical excision or cauterization, especially if the warts are in the weight-bearing area on the plantar aspect of the foot because the resulting scars may cause more discomfort and difficulty with walking.

INGROWING TOENAIL

A rather common problem in the adolescent with large feet who wears tight socks and shoes and sweats excessively is the ingrowing toenail. The big toe is almost always affected, and the cause of ingrowth of the nail is the external pressure of tight shoes and socks. Curvilinear trimming of the toenail and poor foot hygiene aggravate and perpetuate the problem. The edge of the curved nail digs into the nail fold and causes formation of granuloma, which may become infected. One or both sides of the nail may be affected.

Treatment. Conservative measures should be taken initially. The toenail is cut transversely and pledgets of sterile cotton are inserted under the nail edge. Several times a day the feet are immersed in lukewarm water to decrease the inflammation, and antibiotics are given if suppuration is present. Sandals are worn, and tight socks and shoes are avoided.

When the granulation-infected toenail fails to respond to the above measures, surgery is indicated. Under anesthesia the nail is excised, infected granulation soft tissue is debrided, and a wedge of the nail bed is destroyed with a curette.

TUMORS OF THE FOOT AND ANKLE

The presenting complaint with a tumor is a swelling or mass, which may be asymptomatic or may be painful and cause an antalgic limp. If the lump is large or in the weight-bearing portion of the foot, there may be some difficulty in fitting shoes.

The origin of the tumor may be in the *soft tissues*—skin, subcutaneous tissue, fascia, tendon or tendon sheath, muscle, nerve, or vessels—or it may originate in bone or in the joint (Table 1–7).

First, locate the exact *site* of the tumor. Ask the parents to identify and show you the suspected swelling. Compare the involved foot with the contralateral normal limb with the patient weight-bearing and then sitting with the feet dangling.

Next, determine the *consistency* of the mass: Is it soft and cystic or firm, hard, and bony? What is its *size*? Measure its transverse and longitudinal diameter, if possible. Delineate the *boundaries* of the tumor: Is it well defined or is it irregular and infiltrating adjacent tissues? What is its *mobility*—freely movable or fixed to subjacent structures? Inspect the color and consistency of the overlying *skin:* Are the superficial veins dilated? Feel the temperature of the swelling with the dorsum of the proximal phalanx of your fingers: Is there increased local heat? Does the swelling pulsate, suggesting a vascular lesion? If an aneurysm or blood vessel lesion is suspected, apply a tourniquet on the

TABLE 1–7. TUMORS AND TUMOROUS CONDITIONS OF THE FOOT AND ANKLE

Origin	Tumor
Skin	Plantar warts
Subcutaneous tissue	Lipoma
Fascia	Fibromatosis
	Fibrosarcoma
Tendon–tendon sheath	Ganglion
	Xanthomatosis of tendon sheath
Muscle	Rhabdomyosarcoma
Nerve	Neuroma
	Neurofibroma
	Neurofibrosarcoma
Vessels	Hemangioma
	Hemangiopericytoma
	Hemangiosarcoma
Joint	Synovial hemangioma
	Synovial sarcoma
	Pigmented villonodular synovitis
Bone	*Painful*
	Osteoma—subungual exostosis
	Osteoid osteoma
	Osteoblastoma
	Aneurysmal bone cyst
	Unicameral bone cyst–fracture
	Asymptomatic
	Intraosseous lipoma

proximal limb and determine if the swelling decreases in size under tourniquet ischemia. Does the mass transilluminate, suggesting a ganglion? Palpate the regional lymph nodes: Are they enlarged, firm or soft, or tender?

Imaging studies are made to depict the soft tissues and bony changes; they consist of radiography, ultrasonography, and MRI.

Some of the common *soft tissue* tumors are as follows:

1. *Lipoma.* This presents as a soft tissue mass, usually on the instep of the foot, often in the subcutaneous tissue and occasionally deep to the plantar fascia. On palpation the mass feels soft, lobulated, and flabby but contained in a capsule. It does not transilluminate. Radiograms depict a soft tissue mass of fatty consistency. MRI is not indicated unless liposarcoma is suspected. Surgical treatment is rarely indicated except when the lipoma is large and interferes with gait and shoe fitting. Then the lipoma should be completely excised; if not, it will recur.

2. *Ganglion.* This may occur anywhere on the dorsal, medial, or lateral aspect of the foot. It may originate from the tendon sheath or the synovium of a joint. The mass transilluminates. Radiograms are made to rule out a spur, which may irritate the tendon and require removal. If the mass is large, tense, and firm, ultrasonography shows its fluid consistency. Treatment should be nonsurgical in the beginning.

However, if the ganglion enlarges and causes pain and difficulty in wearing shoes, it is surgically excised.

3. *Hemangioma.* Blood vessel tumors in the foot are usually the cavernous type, or they may be deep and involve the muscles and tendons. The lesion is usually tender and interferes with gait. It may bleed and become infected. Treatment by embolization may be attempted. If embolization is unsuccessful, the lesion is excised surgically. A preoperative angiogram should be obtained to delineate the extent of the lesion and the adequacy of circulation.

4. *Neurofibroma.* This can occur in the foot. If painful, it is excised.

5. *Fibrosarcoma, rhabdosarcoma,* and *synovial sarcoma.* These are very rare. Treatment consists of staging of the lesion, biopsy, and radical excision.

Bone tumors are infrequent in the foot. Exostosis, intraosseous lipoma, unicameral bone cysts, aneurysmal bone cysts, and enchondromas are some of the lesions encountered. When painful, osteoid osteoma or osteoblastoma should be suspected. A *subungual exostosis* presents as a bony mass under the nail of the distal phalanx of the toe, usually the hallux. The nail becomes deformed and elevated. The tumor is painful on pressure of the nail. Radiographic features are typical. Treatment consists of surgical excision through a transverse incision at the distal end of the toe.

OSTEOCHONDRITIS DISSECANS OF THE DOME OF THE TALUS[286-299]

The presenting complaint is pain, clicking, stiffness, and swelling of the ankle joint. When the osteochondral fragment is completely detached and loose in the joint, the ankle may lock.

In osteochondritis dissecans, a part of the articular cartilage with its underlying subchondral bone separates (''cuts out''—*dissecare*) from the surrounding osteocartilaginous tissue. In the ankle the osteochondral fragment is in either the superolateral or superomedial corner of the dome of the talus. The *lateral* lesions are usually caused by trauma: Upon forced inversion of the foot, the superolateral aspect of the talus is compressed against the fibular malleolus. Initially the fibular collateral ligament is intact (Fig 1–72A). Following further inversion of the foot, the fibular ligament ruptures, the dome of the talus tilts, and a segment of the transchondral bone chips (Fig 1–72B). This osteochondral segment may be partially or completely detached; it may remain in place or float loose in the ankle and cause locking of the joint (Fig 1–72C).

Osteochondritis dissecans of the *medial* dome of the talus may be post-traumatic, but often a history of specific injury cannot be obtained. Postinjury compression on the medial upper border of the dome of the talus is caused by lateral rotation of the tibia with the foot and ankle in plantar flexion and inversion (Fig 1–72D). With further lateral rotation of the tibia the compressed medial dome of the talus chips and becomes a loose fragment in the ankle (Fig 1–72E). In the nontraumatic lesions, heredity and constitutional features play an etiologic role.

The salient physical finding is localized tenderness over the lesional area. Plantar flex the foot and with the tip of the index finger compress the medial and lateral dome of the talus. Simulate the mechanism of injury—for lateral dome lesions forcefully invert the foot, and for medial lesions invert the foot and laterally rotate the tibia—to see if you can elicit pain. Always compare the symptomatic ankle with the contralateral normal one.

Imaging.   Radiographic findings are typical. In either the lateral or medial dome of the talus a circumscribed fragment of subchondral bone is partially or completely demarcated from the surrounding osteochondral tissue. The fragment may be crescent or saucer shaped (Fig 1–73). Make oblique-lateral radiograms. CT scanning is indicated when diagnosis is suggested clinically and not clearly depicted in routine radiography or when one cannot determine whether the fragment is partially or completely detached. Occasionally MRI is performed. Although it is an expensive study, it clearly demonstrates the cartilaginous break in continuity of the osteochondral fragment and extent of the lesion; it is indicated when surgical intervention is contemplated.

Treatment.   In children less than 12 years of age, treatment should always be nonsurgical initially when the fragment is not completely detached. A below-knee cast is applied and weight-bearing is not allowed for 6 to 8 weeks. Ordinarily the lesion heals.

In the adolescent (13 years of age or older), particularly when the fragment is beginning to separate, arthroscopy and multiple drilling of the fragment to increase its blood supply are carried out. A below-knee cast is applied and the dome of the talus is protected from weight-bearing as described above. When the fragment is completely detached, it is removed through the arthroscope. In the dome of the talus the fragment is usually small, and replacement and pinning of the fragment are not indicated.

ANKLE INSTABILITY

Ankle instability may be post-traumatic (due to ligamentous sprain), it may be due to a congenital deformity of the foot and ankle such as tarsal coalition or ball-and-socket ankle joint, or it may be due to an acquired varus deformity of the hindfoot such as in pes cavovarus or following varus

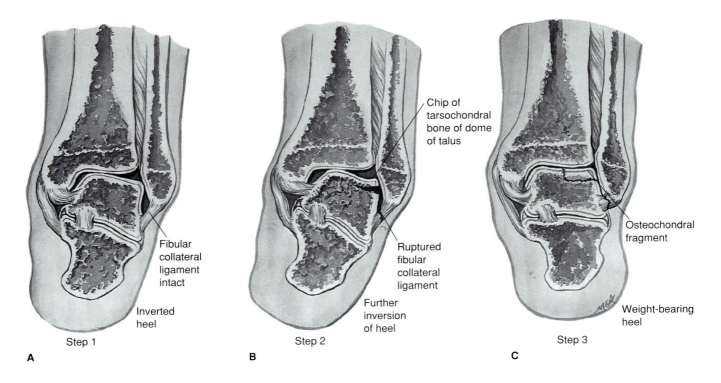

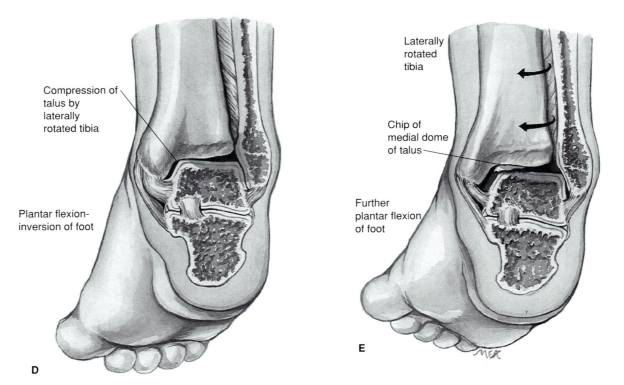

Figure 1–72. Osteochondritis of the dome of the talus. **A.** In the lateral region it is caused by forced inversion of the foot. The superolateral corner of the talus is compressed against the fibular melleolus, and the fibular collateral ligament is intact. **B.** Further inversion of the heel causes rupture of the fibular collateral ligament and fracture of a segment of transchondral bone of the lateral dome of the talus. **C.** Osteochondral fragment completely detached but in situ. **D.** Osteochondritis dissecans of the medial dome of the talus. It is caused by lateral rotation of the tibia with the foot and ankle in plantar flexion and inversion. **E.** Note a chip of osteochondral fragment caused by further lateral rotation of the tibia.

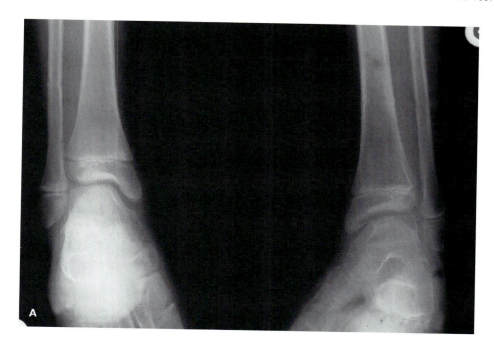

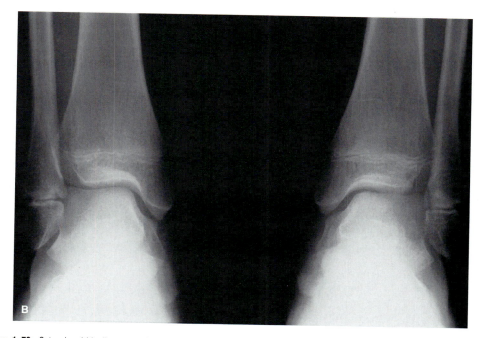

Figure 1–73. Osteochondritis dissecans of the lateral dome of the talus. **A.** AP view of the ankle at initial presentation. Note the clearly demarcated osteochondral fragment; it is not detached or loose. **B.** Three months following treatment with non–weight-bearing cast. Note the healing osteochondral fragment.

ankle due to asymmetric growth arrest of the distal tibial physis due to ankle fracture. When an adolescent presents with a history of recurrent sprain of the ankle joint, always rule out *talocalcaneal or talonavicular coalition.* Make oblique radiograms and Harris views of the foot in addition to the AP, lateral, and oblique views of the ankle. If the subtalar joint is rigid and routine radiograms are not conclusive, a CT scan of the hindfoot and midfoot should be performed to rule out tarsal coalition.

Ball-and-socket ankle joint is a rare congenital deformity, and sometimes it is acquired secondary to subtalar fusion. It is characterized by a dome shape of the upper end of the talus in both the AP and lateral radiographic projections, with a corresponding hemispheric articulation of the lower end of the tibia. The congenital form may occur as an isolated deformity or be associated with major congenital malformations of the lower limb such as congenital longitudinal deficiency of the fibula and talocalcaneal coalition. Congenital ball-and-socket ankle joint does not usually cause any problem in childhood, but in the adolescent who is obese or heavily involved in sports, it may cause repeated ankle sprain and pain.

The *varus hindfoot* causes repeated ankle sprain because of mechanical axis deviation.

Post-traumatic ankle instability is often caused by severe ligamentous sprain of the ankle, either medial or lateral, which was inadequately treated by a simple Ace bandage and the patient was allowed to participate in sports and strenuous physical activity prior to adequate healing of the sprain. Prevention is the best treatment for these cases. Severe sprain of the ankle should be managed by a below-knee walking cast for 3 weeks. Make stress AP sagittal radiograms in eversion and inversion to document the degree of instability of the ankle and the subtalar joint.

An attempt should be made to stabilize the ankle by an ankle orthosis. If the orthosis is unsuccessful and the disability is severe, operative treatment should be undertaken to shorten the anterior talofibular and calcaneofibular ligaments (modified Brostrom procedure) or to reconstruct the tendon to restore normal ligamentous restraints of the ankle and subtalar joint.[300–304]

REFERENCES

1. Blais MM, Green WT, Anderson M: Length of the growing foot. *J Bone Joint Surg* 38A:998, 1956
2. McDougall A: The os trigonum. *J Bone Joint Surg* 37B:257, 1955
3. Powell HDW: Extra centre of ossification for the medial malleolus in children. Incidence and significance. *J Bone Joint Surg* 43B:107, 1961
4. Roches AF, Sunderland S: Multiple ossification centers in the epiphyses of the long bones of the human hand and foot. *J Bone Joint Surg* 41B:375, 1959
5. Shands AR Jr: The accessory bones of the foot. *South Med Surg* 93:326, 1931
6. Sirry A: The pseudocystic triangle in the normal os calcis. *Acta Radiol* 36:516, 1951
7. Templeton AW, McAlister WH, and Zim ID: Standardization of terminology and evaluation of osseous relationships in congenitally abnormal feet. *Amer J Roentgen,* 93:374, 1965
8. Trolle D: *Accessory Bones of the Human Foot.* Copenhagen, Munksgaard, 1948
9. von Lanz T, Wachsmuth W: *Praktische Anatomie.* Berlin, Julius Springer, 1938
10. Zeide MS, and Robbins H: Glossary of eponyms: Orthopaedic signs, lines, and tests. *Bull Hosp Joint Dis* 36:177, 1975

Congenital Metatarsus Varus

11. Bleck EE: Metatarsus adductus: Classification and relationship to outcomes of treatment. *J Pediatr Orthop* 3:2, 1983
12. Kite JH: Congenital metatarsus varus. Report of 300 cases. *J Bone Joint Surg* 32A:500, 1950
13. Kite JH: Congenital metatarsus varus. *J Bone Joint Surg* 46A:525, 1964
14. Lichtblau S: Section of the abductor hallucis tendon for correction of metatarsus varus deformity. *Clin Orthop* 110:227, 1975
15. Mitchell GP: Abductor hallucis release in congenital metatarsus varus. *Int Orthop* 3:299, 1980
16. Reimann I, Werner HH: Congenital metatarsus varus. A suggestion for possible mechanism and relation to other foot deformities. *Clin Orthop* 110:223, 1975
17. Reimann I, Werner HH: Congenital metatarsus varus. On the advantages of early treatment. *Acta Orthop Scand* 46:857, 1975
18. Wynne-Davies R: Family studies and the cause of congenital clubfoot—talipes equinovarus, talipes calcaneovalgus and metatarsus varus. *J Bone Joint Surg* 46B:445, 1964

Serpentine or Skewfoot (Z Foot)

19. Berg EE: A reappraisal of metatarsus adductus and skewfoot. *J Bone Joint Surg* 68A:1185, 1986
20. McCormick DW, Blount WP: Metatarsus adductovarus: "Skewfoot." *JAMA* 141:449, 1949
21. Mosca VS: Skewfoot deformity in children: Correction by calcaneal neck lengthening and medial cuneiform open wedge osteotomies. *J Pediatr Orthop* 13:807, 1993
22. Peabody CW, Murrow F: Congenital metatarsus varus. *J Bone Joint Surg* 15A:171, 1933
23. Peterson HA: Skewfoot (forefoot adduction with heel valgus). *J Pediatr Orthop* 6:24, 1986
24. Scully SP, Ferguson R: Association of metatarsus adductovarus (skewfoot) with Angelman's (happy puppet) syndrome. *Orthopedics* 16:1270, 1993

Congenital Hallux Varus

25. Farmer AW: Congenital hallux varus. *Am J Surg* 95:274, 1958

Congenital Talipes Equinovarus

26. Adams W: *Club Foot, Its Causes, Pathology and Treatment.* London, J & A Churchill, 1866
27. Altar D, Lehman WB, Grant AD: Complications in clubfoot surgery. *Orthop Rev* 20:233, 1991
28. Aronson J, Puskarich CL: Deformity and disability from treated clubfoot. *J Pediatr Orthop* 10:109, 1990
29. Attenborough CG: Severe congenital talipes equinovarus. *J Bone Joint Surg* 48B:31, 1966
30. Beals RK: Clubfoot in the Maori: A genetic study of 50 kindreds. *NZ Med J* 88:144, 1978
31. Beatson RR, Pearson JR: A method assessing correction in club feet. *J Bone Joint Surg* 48B:40, 1966
32. Ben-Menachem Y, Butler JE: Arteriography of the foot in congenital deformities. *J Bone Joint Surg* 56:1625, 1974

33. Bensahel H, Guillaume A, Czukonyi Z, Desgrippes Y: Results of physical therapy for idiopathic clubfoot: A long-term follow-up study. *J Pediatr Orthop* 10:189, 1990

34. Bensahel H, Huguenin P, Themar-Noel C: The functional anatomy of clubfoot. *J Pediatr Orthop* 3:191, 1983

35. Bensahel H, Csukonyi Z, Desgrippes Y, Chaumien JP: Surgery in residual clubfoot: One-stage medioposterior release "a la carte." *J Pediatr Orthop* 7:145, 1987

36. Bohm M: Zur Pathologie und Rontgenologie des angeborenen Klumfusses. *Munchen Med Wochenschr* 55:1492, 1928

37. Bohm M: The embryologic origin of clubfoot. *J Bone Joint Surg* 11:229, 1929

38. Brockman EP: *Congenital Clubfoot (Talipes Equinovarus).* New York, William Wood & Co, 1930

39. Brougham DI, Nicol RO: Use of the Cincinnati incision in congenital talipes equinovarus. *J Pediatr Orthop* 8:696, 1988

40. Campos da Paz A Jr, DeSouza V: Talipes equinovarus: Pathmechanical basis of treatment. *Orthop Clin North Am* 9:171, 1978

41. Carroll NC: Congenital clubfoot: Pathoanatomy and treatment. *AAOS Instr Course Lect* 36:117, 1987

42. Carroll NC: Clubfoot, in Morrissy RT (ed): *Lovell and Winter's Pediatric Orthopaedics.* Philadelphia, JB Lippincott, 1990, pp 92–96

43. Carter CO, Fairbank JJ: Talipes equinovarus, in *The Genetics of Locomotor Disorder.* London, Oxford University Press, 1974, pp 100–102

44. Catterall A: A method of assessment of the clubfoot deformity. *Clin Orthop* 264:48, 1991

45. Chung CS, Nemechek RW, Larsen IJ, Ching GHS: Genetic and epidemiological studies of clubfoot in Hawaii: General and medical considerations. *Hum Hered* 19:321, 1969

46. Crawford AH, Marxsen JL, Osterfeld DL: The Cincinnati incision: A comprehensive approach for surgical procedures for the foot and ankle in childhood. *J Bone Joint Surg* 64A:1355, 1982

47. Downey DJ, Drennan JC, Garcia JF: Magnetic resonance image findings in congenital talipes equinovarus. *J Pediatr Orthop* 12:224, 1992

48. Edelson JG, Husseini N: The pulseless club foot. *J Bone Joint Surg* 66B:700, 1984

49. Elmslie RC: The principles of treatment of congenital talipes equinovarus. *J Orthop Surg* 2:669, 1920

50. Evans D: Treatment of cavovarus foot and clubfoot. *J Bone Joint Surg* 39B:789, 1957

51. Evans D: Relapsed club foot. *J Bone Joint Surg* 43B:722, 1961

52. Fahrenbach G, Kuehn D, Tachdjian MO: The use of computerized tomography in assessing residual deformities in talipes equinovarus. *J Pediatr Orthop* 6:334, 1986

53. Farrill J: Tibioperoneal tenoplasty for congenital clubfoot with peroneal insufficiency. *J Bone Joint Surg* 38A:329, 1956

54. Freeman EA, Sheldon JH: Cranio-carpal-tarsal dystrophy. An undescribed congenital malformation. *Arch Dis Child* 13:277, 1938

55. Fripp AT, Shaw NE: *Club-foot.* Edinburgh, E & S Livingstone, 1967

56. Garceau GJ: Anterior tibial transposition in recurrent congenital clubfoot. *J Bone Joint Surg* 22:932, 1940

57. Garceau GJ, Palmer RM: Transfer of the anterior tibial tendon for recurrent clubfoot. A long-term follow-up. *J Bone Joint Surg* 49A:207, 1967

58. Goldner JL: Congenital talipes equinovarus—fifteen years of surgical treatment. *Curr Pract Orthop Surg* 4:61, 1969

59. Green ADL, Lloyd-Roberts GC: The results of early posterior release in resistant club feet. A long-term review. *J Bone Joint Surg* 67B:588, 1985

60. Greider TD, Siff SJ, Gerson P, Donovan MM: Arteriography in clubfoot. *J Bone Joint Surg* 64A:837, 1982

61. Grill F, Franke J: The Ilizarov distractor for the correction of relapsed or neglected clubfoot. *J Bone Joint Surg* 69B:593, 1987

62. Handelsman JE, Badalamente MA: Club foot: A neuromuscular disease. *Dev Med Child Neurol* 24:3, 1973

63. Harrold AJ, Walker CJ: Treatment and prognosis in congenital clubfoot. *J Bone Joint Surg* 65B:8, 1983

64. Herzenberg JE, Carroll NC, Christofferson MR, Lee EH, White S, Muroe R: Clubfoot analysis with three-dimensional computer modeling. *J Pediatr Orthop* 8:257, 1988

65. Hjelmstedt A, Sahlstedt B: Talar deformity in congenital clubfeet. An anatomical and functional study with special reference to the ankle joint mobility. *Acta Orthop Scand* 45:628, 1974

66. Hootnick DR, Levinsohn EM, Randall PA, Packard DS Jr: Vascular dysgenesis associated with skeletal dysplasia of the lower limb. *J Bone Joint Surg* 62:1123, 1980

67. Hutchins PM, Foster BK, Paterson DC, Cole EA: Long-term results of early surgical release in clubfeet. *J Bone Joint Surg* 67B:791, 1985

68. Irani RN, Sherman MS: The pathological anatomy of clubfoot. *J Bone Joint Surg* 45A:45, 1963

69. Laaveg SJ, Ponseti IV: Long-term results of treatment of congenital clubfoot. *J Bone Joint Surg* 62A:23, 1980

70. Magone JB, Torch MA, Clark RN, Kean JR: Comparative review of surgical treatment of idiopathic clubfoot by three different procedures at Columbus Children's Hospital. *J Pediatr Orthop* 9:49, 1989

71. McKay DW: New concept of approach to clubfoot treatment: Section II—Correction of the clubfoot. *J Pediatr Orthop* 3:10, 1983

72. McKay DW: New concept of and approach to clubfoot treatment: Section III—Evaluation and results. *J Pediatr Orthop* 3:141, 1983

73. Nather A, Bose K: Conservative and surgical treatment of clubfoot. *J Pediatr Orthop* 7:42, 1987

74. Porter RW, Youle K: Factors that affect surgical correction in congenital talipes equinovarus. *Foot Ankle* 14:23, 1993

75. Settle GW: The anatomy of congenital talipes equinovarus: Sixteen dissected specimens. *J Bone Joint Surg* 45A:1341, 1963

76. Simons GW (ed): *The Clubfoot. The Present and a View of the Future.* New York, Springer Verlag, 1994

77. Simons GW: Complete subtalar release in clubfeet: Part I—A preliminary report. *J Bone Joint Surg* 67A:1044, 1985

78. Simons GW: Complete subtalar release in clubfeet: Part II—Comparison with less extensive procedures. *J Bone Joint Surg* 67A:1056, 1985

79. Simons GW: Analytical radiography of clubfeet. *J Bone Joint Surg* 59B:485, 1977

80. Sodre H, Bruschini S, Mestriner LA, Miranda F Jr, Levinsohn EM, Packard DS Jr, Crider RJ Jr, Schwartz R, Hootnick DR: Arterial abnormalities in talipes equinovarus as assessed by angiography and the Doppler technique. *J Pediatr Orthop* 10:101, 1990

81. Stanitski CL, Ward WT, Grossman W: Noninvasive vascular studies in clubfoot. *J Pediatr Orthop* 12:514, 1992

82. Tachdjian MO: *Atlas of Pediatric Orthopedic Surgery.* Philadelphia, WB Saunders Co, 1994

83. Thometz JG, Simons GW: Deformity of the calcaneocuboid joint in patients who have talipes equinovarus. *J Bone Joint Surg* 75:190, 1993

84. Turco VJ: Resistant congenital clubfoot—one-stage posteromedial release with internal fixation. *J Bone Joint Surg* 61A:805, 1978

85. Turco VJ: Resistant congenital clubfoot—one-stage posteromedial release with internal fixation. A follow-up report of a fifteen-year experience. *J Bone Joint Surg* 61A: 805, 1979

86. Wijesinha SS, Menelaus MB: Operation for calcaneus deformity after surgery for clubfoot. *J Bone Joint Surg* 71B: 234, 1989

87. Wynne-Davies R: Family studies and cause of congenital clubfoot. *J Bone Joint Surg* 46B:445, 1964

Flatfoot (Pes Planus)

88. Armstrong AF, Fowler SB: Anterior calcaneal osteotomy for symptomatic juvenile pes planus. *Foot Ankle* 4:274, 1984

89. Asher C: Flatfoot and valgus heel, in *Postural Variations in Childhood.* London, Butterworth & Co, 1974, pp 76–101

90. Basmajian JR, Bentzon JW: An electromyographic study of certain muscles of the leg and foot in the standing position. *Surg Gynecol Obstet* 98:662, 1954

91. Bleck EE: The shoeing of children: Sham or science? *Dev Med Child Neurol* 13:188, 1971

92. Bleck EE, Berzins UJ: Conservative management of pes valgus with plantar flexed talus, flexible. *Clin Orthop* 122:85, 1977

93. Bordelon RL: Correction of hypermobile flatfoot in children by molded insert. *Foot Ankle* 1:132, 1980

94. Crawford AH, Kucharzyk D, Roy DR, Bilbo J: Subtalar stabilization of the planovalgus foot by staple arthroereisis in young children who have neuromuscular problems. *J Bone Joint Surg* 72A:840, 1990

95. Engel GM, Staheli LT: The natural history of torsion and other factors influencing gait in childhood. A study of the angle of gait, tibial torsion, knee angle, hip rotation, and development of the arch in normal children. *Clin Orthop* 99: 12, 1974

96. Evans DC: Calcaneovalgus deformity. *J Bone Joint Surg* 57B:270, 1975

97. Giannestras NJ: Static foot problems in the pre-adolescent and adolescent stages, in *Foot Disorders. Medical and Surgical Management.* Philadelphia, Lea & Febiger, 1967, pp 119–155

98. Giannestras NJ: Flexible valgus flatfoot resulting from naviculocuneiform and talonavicular sag. Surgical correction in the adolescent, in Bateman JE (ed): *Foot Science.* Philadelphia, WB Saunders Co, 1976, pp 67–105

99. Gould N, Moreland M, Alvary R, Trevino S, Fenwick J: Development of the child's arch. *Foot Ankle* 9:241, 1989

100. Grice DS: An extra-articular arthrodesis of the subastragalar joint for correction of paralytic flat feet in children. *J Bone Joint Surg* 34A:246, 1955

101. Grice DS: Further experience with extra-articular arthrodesis of the subtalar joint. *J Bone Joint Surg* 37A:246, 1955

102. Harris RI, Beath T: Hypermobile flatfoot with short tendo-Achillis. *J Bone Joint Surg* 30A:116, 1948

103. Henderson WH, Campbell JW: UCBL shoe insert: Casting and fabrication. The Biomechanics Laboratory. University of California at San Francisco and Berkeley. *Technical Report 53,* August 1967

104. Hicks JH: The mechanics of the foot. I. The joints. *J Anat* 87:343, 1953

105. Hicks JH: The mechanics of the foot. II. The joints. *J Anat* 88:25, 1954

106. Hoke M: An operation for the correction of extremely relaxed flat feet. *J Bone Joint Surg* 13:773, 1931

107. Inman VT: UCBL dual axis control system and UCBL shoe insert. *Bull Prosthet Res* 10:11, 1969

108. Inman VT: *The Joints of the Ankle.* Baltimore, Williams & Wilkins, 1976

109. Jack EA: Naviculocuneiform fusion in the treatment of flatfoot. *J Bone Joint Surg* 35B:279, 1953

110. Koutsogiannis E: Treatment of mobile flatfoot by displacement osteotomy of a calcaneus. *J Bone Joint Surg* 53B:96, 1971

111. Mereday C, Dolan CME, Lusskin R: Evaluation of the University of California Biomechanics Laboratory shoe insert in "flexible" pes planus. *Clin Orthop* 82:45, 1972

112. Penneau K, Lutter LD, Winter RB: Pes planus: Radiographic changes with foot orthoses and shoes. *Foot Ankle* 2:299, 1982

113. Phillips GE: A review of elongation of os calcis for flat feet. *J Bone Joint Surg* 65B:15, 1983

114. Rose GK, Welton EA, Marshall T: The diagnosis of flat foot in the child. *J Bone Joint Surg* 67B:71, 1985

115. Schede F: Die Operation des Platfusses. *Z Orthop Chir* 50: 528, 1929

116. Seymour N: The late results of naviculo-cuneiform fusion. *J Bone Joint Surg* 49B:558, 1967

117. Smith SD, Millar EA: Arthrosis by means of a subtalar polyethylene peg implant for correction of hindfoot pronation in children. *Clin Orthop* 181:15, 1983

118. Staheli LT, Griffin L: Corrective shoes for children: A survey of current practice. *Pediatrics* 65:13, 1980

119. Staheli LT, Chew DE, Corbett M: The longitudinal arch. A survey of 882 feet in normal children and adults. *J Bone Joint Surg* 69A:426, 1987

120. Wenger DR, Mauldin D, Morgan D, Sobol MG, Pennebaker M, Thaler R: Foot growth rate in children age one to six years. *Foot Ankle* 3:207, 1983

121. Wenger DR, Mauldin D, Speck C, Morgan D, Lieber RL: Corrective shoes and inserts as treatment for flexible flatfoot in infants and children. *J Bone Joint Surg* 71A:800, 1989

122. Wetzenstein H: The significance of congenital pes calcaneovalgus in the origin of pes planovalgus in children. *Acta Orthop Scand* 30:64, 1960

122a. Williams PF, Menelaus MB: Triple arthrodesis by inlay grafting—a method suitable for the undeformed or valgus foot. J Bone Joint Surg 59B:333, 1977

Congenital Convex Pes Valgus (Vertical Talus)

123. Adelaar RS, Williams RM, Gould JS: Congenital convex pes valgus: Results of an early comprehensive release and a review of congenital vertical talus at Richmond Crippled Children's Hospital and the University of Alabama in Birmingham. *Foot Ankle* 1:62, 1980
124. Badelon O, Rigault P, Pouliquen JC, Padovani JP, Guyonvarch J: Congenital vertical talus. A diagnostic and therapeutic study of 71 cases. *Int Orthop* 8:211, 1984
125. Becker-Andersen H, Reimann I: Congenital vertical talus. *Acta Orthop Scand* 45:130, 1974
126. Campos da Paz Jr, De Souza V, De Souza DC: Congenital convex pes valgus. *Orthop Clin North Am* 9:207, 1978
127. Clark MW, D'Ambrosia RD, Ferguson AB Jr: Congenital vertical talus. *J Bone Joint Surg* 59A:816, 1977
128. Coleman SS, Martin AF, Jarrett J: Congenital vertical talus: Pathogenesis and treatment. *J Bone Joint Surg* 48A:1442, 1966
129. Colton CL: The surgical management of congenital vertical talus. *J Bone Joint Surg* 55B:566, 1973
130. Connolly JF, Dornenburg P, Holmes CD: Congenital convex pes valgus deformities, in Bateman JE (ed): *Foot Science*. A selection of papers from the Proceedings of the American Orthopaedic Foot Society, Inc., 1974 and 1975. Philadelphia, WB Saunders Co, 1976, pp 47–66
131. Drennan JC, Sharrard WJW: The pathological anatomy of convex pes valgus. *J Bone Joint Surg* 53B:455, 1971
132. Duckworth T, Smith TW: The treatment of paralytic convex pes valgus. *J Bone Joint Surg* 56B:305, 1974
133. Eyre-Brook A: Congenital vertical talus. *J Bone Joint Surg* 49B:618, 1967
134. Fitton JM, Nevelos AB: The treatment of congenital vertical talus. *J Bone Joint Surg* 61B:481, 1979
135. Grice DS: The role of subtalar fusion in the treatment of valgus deformities of the feet. *AAOS Instr Course Lect* 16:127, 1959
136. Hamanishi C: Congenital vertical talus: Classification with 69 cases and new measurement system. *J Pediatr Orthop* 4:318, 1984
137. Hark FW: Rocker-foot due to congenital subluxation of the talus. *J Bone Joint Surg* 32A:344, 1950
138. Harrold AJ: Congenital vertical talus in infancy. *J Bone Joint Surg* 49B:634, 1967
139. Henken R: Contribution a l'étude des formes osseuses du pied valgus congénital. Thèse de Lyon, 1914
140. Herndon CH, Heyman CH: Problems in the recognition and treatment of congenital convex pes valgus. *J Bone Joint Surg* 45A:413, 1963
141. Heyman CH: The diagnosis and treatment of congenital convex pes valgus or vertical talus. *AAOS Instr Course Lect* 16:117, 1959
142. Hughes JR: Congenital vertical talus. *J Bone Joint Surg* 39B:580, 1957
143. Jackson D: Acquired vertical talus due to burn contractures. *J Bone Joint Surg* 60:215, 1978
144. Jacobsen ST, Crawford AH: Congenital vertical talus. *J Pediatr Orthop* 3:306, 1983
145. Lamy L, Weissman L: Congenital convex pes valgus. *J Bone Joint Surg* 21:79, 1939
146. Lichtblau S: Congenital vertical talus. *Bull Hosp Joint Dis* 39:165, 1978
147. Lloyd-Roberts GC, Spence AJ: Congenital vertical talus. *J Bone Joint Surg* 40B:33, 1958
148. Osmond-Clarke H: Congenital vertical talus. *J Bone Joint Surg* 38B:334, 1956
149. Patterson WR, Fitz DA, Smith WS: The pathologic anatomy of congenital convex pes valgus. *J Bone Joint Surg* 50A:458, 1968
150. Pouliquen JC: Pied convexe congénital. *Rev Chir Orthop* 2(suppl):370, 1974
151. Ritsila VA: Talipes equinovarus and vertical talus produced experimentally in newborn rabbits. *Acta Orthop Scand* Suppl 121, 1969
152. Robbins H: Naviculectomy for congenital vertical talus. *Bull Hosp Joint Dis* 37:77, 1976
153. Schlesinger AE, Deeney VF, Caskey PF: Sonography of the nonossified tarsal navicular cartilage in an infant with congenital vertical talus. *Pediatr Radiol* 20:134, 1989
154. Seimon LP: Surgical correction of congenital vertical talus under the age of 2 years. *J Pediatr Orthop* 7:405, 1987
155. Sharrard WJW, Grosfield I: The management of deformity and paralysis of the foot in myelomeningocele. *J Bone Joint Surg* 50B:456, 1968
156. Specht EE: Congenital paralytic vertical talus. *J Bone Joint Surg* 57A:842, 1975
157. Stern HJ, Clark RD, Stroberg AJ, Shohat M: Autosomal dominant transmission of isolated congenital vertical talus. *Clin Genetics* 36:427, 1989
158. Stone KH, Lloyd-Roberts GC: Congenital vertical talus: A new operation. *Proc R Soc Med* 56:1, 1963
159. Storen H: On the closed and open correction of congenital convex pes valgus with a vertical astragalus. *Acta Orthop Scand* 36:352, 1965
160. Tachdjian MO: Congenital convex pes valgus. *Orthop Clin North Am* 3:131, 1972
161. Towns PL, Dettart GK, Hecht F, Manning JA: Trisomy 13-15 in a male infant. *J Pediatr* 60:528, 1962
162. Uchida IA, Lewis AJ, Bowman JM, Wang HC: A case of double trisomy: No. 18 and triple-X. *J Pediatr* 60:498, 1962
163. Wainwright D: Congenital vertical talus in infancy. *J Bone Joint Surg* 48B:588, 1966
164. Walker AP, Ghali NN, Silk FF: Congenital vertical talus. *J Bone Joint Surg* 67B:117, 1985

Tarsal Coalition

165. Braddock GTF: A prolonged follow-up of peroneal spastic flatfoot. *J Bone Joint Surg* 43B:734, 1961
166. Chambers RB, Cook TM, Cowell HR: Surgical reconstruction for calcaneonavicular coalition. *J Bone Joint Surg* 64A:829, 1982
167. Conway JJ, Cowell HR: Tarsal coalition: Clinical significance and roentgenographic demonstration. *Radiology* 92:799, 1969

168. Cowell HR: Extensor brevis arthroplasty. *J Bone Joint Surg* 52A:820, 1970

169. Cowell HR: Talocalcaneal coalition and new causes of peroneal spastic flatfoot. *Clin Orthop* 85:16, 1972

170. Cowell HR: Diagnosis and management of peroneal spastic flatfoot. *AAOS Instr Course Lect* 24:94, 1975

171. Cowell HR, Elener V: Rigid painful flatfoot secondary to tarsal coalition. *Clin Orthop* 177:54, 1983

172. Gonzalez P, Kumar SJ: Calcaneonavicular coalition treated by resection and interposition of the extensor digitorum brevis muscle. *J Bone Joint Surg* 72A:71, 1990

173. Harris BJ: Anomalous structures in the developing human foot, abstracted. *Anat Rec* 121:399, 1955

174. Harris RI: Rigid valgus foot due to talocalcaneal bridge. *J Bone Joint Surg* 37A:169, 1955

175. Harris RI: Retrospect: Peroneal spastic flatfoot (rigid valgus foot). *J Bone Joint Surg* 47A:1657, 1965

176. Inglis G, Buxton RA, Macnicol MF: Symptomatic calcaneonavicular bars. The results 20 years after surgical excision. *J Bone Joint Surg* 68B:128, 1986

177. Leonard MA: The inheritance of tarsal coalition and its relationship to spastic flatfoot. *J Bone Joint Surg* 55B:881, 1973

178. Mosier KM, Asher M: Tarsal coalitions and peroneal spastic flatfoot. *J Bone Joint Surg* 66A:976, 1984

179. Nievergelt K: Positiver Vaterschaftsnachweis auf Grand erblicher Missbildungen der Extremitaten. *Arch Klaus Stift Vererbungforsch* 19:157, 1944

180. Oestreich AE, Mize WA, Crawford AH, Morgan RC Jr: The "anteater nose": A direct sign of calcaneonavicular coalition on the lateral radiograph. *J Pediatr Orthop* 7:709, 1987

181. Olney BW, Asher MA: Excision of symptomatic coalition of the middle facet of the talocalcaneal joint. *J Bone Joint Surg* 69A:539, 1987

182. Pearlman HS, Edkin RE, Warren RF: Familial tarsal and carpal synostosis with radial head subluxation. *J Bone Joint Surg* 46A:585, 1964

183. Scranton PE: Treatment of symptomatic talocalcaneal coalition. *J Bone Joint Surg* 69A:533, 1987

184. Slomann HC: On coalition calcaneo-navicularis. *J Orthop Surg* 3:586, 1921

185. Slomann HC: On demonstration and analysis of calcaneonavicular coalition by roentgen examination. *Acta Radiol* 5:304, 1926

186. Snyder RB, Lipscomb AB, Johnston RK: The relationship of tarsal coalitions to ankle sprains in athletes. *Am J Sports Med* 9:313, 1981

187. Swiontkowski MF, Scranton PE, Hansen S: Tarsal coalitions: Long-term results of surgical treatment. *J Pediatr Orthop* 3:287, 1983

Pes Cavus

188. Alvik I: Operative treatment of pes cavus. *Acta Orthop Scand* 23:137, 1953

189. Barenfeld PA, Weseley MS, Shea JM: The congenital cavus foot. *Clin Orthop* 79:119, 1971

190. Bentzon PGK: Pes cavus and the m. peroneus longus. *Acta Orthop Scand* 4:50, 1933

191. Bost FC, Schottstaedt ER, Larsen LJ: Plantar dissection. An operation to release the soft tissues in recurrent or recalcitrant talipes equinovarus. *J Bone Joint Surg* 42A:151, 1960

192. Bradley GW, Coleman SS: Treatment of the calcaneo-cavus foot deformity. *J Bone Joint Surg* 63A:1159, 1981

193. Brewerton DA, Sandifer PH, Sweetman DR: "Idiopathic" pes cavus, an investigation of its etiology. *Br Med J* 358:659, 1963

194. Chuinard EG, Baskin M: Clawfoot deformity. Treatment by transferring the long extensors into the metatarsals and fusion of the interphalangeal joints. *J Bone Joint Surg* 55A:351, 1973

195. Cole WH: The treatment of clawfoot. *J Bone Joint Surg* 22:895, 1940

196. Coleman SS: *Complex Foot Deformities in Children.* Philadelphia, Lea & Febiger, 1983

197. Coleman SS, Chesnut WJ: A simple test for hindfoot flexibility in the cavovarus foot. *Clin Orthop* 123:60, 1977

198. Dekel S, Weissman SL: Osteotomy of the calcaneus and concomitant plantar stripping in children with talipes cavovarus. *J Bone Joint Surg* 55B:802, 1973

199. Duchenne BG: *Physiology of Motion.* (Translated and edited by EB Kaplan.) Philadelphia, WB Saunders Co, 1959, p 384

200. Dwyer FC: Osteotomy of the calcaneum for pes cavus. *J Bone Joint Surg* 41B:80, 1959

201. Dwyer FC: The present status of the problem of pes cavus. *Clin Orthop* 106:254, 1975

202. Fowler B, Brooks AL, Parrish TF: The cavo-varus foot. *J Bone Joint Surg* 41A:757, 1959

203. Garceau GJ: Pes cavus. *AAOS Instr Course Lect* 18:184, 1961

204. Giriat A, Taussig G, Masse P: Plantar release in the treatment of pes cavus in childhood. Technique and indications. (Author's transl.) *Rev Chir Orthop* 65:77, 1979

205. Gould N: Surgery in advanced Charcot-Marie-Tooth disease. *J Foot Ankle* 4:267, 1984

206. Jahss MH: Tarsometatarsal truncated-wedge arthrodesis for pes cavus and equinovarus deformity of the forepart of the foot. *J Bone Joint Surg* 62A:713, 1980

207. Japas LM: Surgical treatment of pes cavus by tarsal V-osteotomy. Preliminary report. *J Bone Joint Surg* 50A:927, 1968

208. Kelikian HA: *Hallux Valgus, Allied Deformities of the Forefoot, and Metatarsalgia.* Philadelphia, WB Saunders Co, 1965, p 305

209. Mann R, Inman VT: Phasic activity of intrinsic muscles of the foot. *J Bone Joint Surg* 46A:469, 1964

210. Mann RA, Missirian J: Pathophysiology of Charcot-Marie-Tooth disease. *Clin Orthop* 234:221, 1988

211. Meary R: Le pied creux essentiel. Symposium. *Rev Chir Orthop* 53:389, 1967

212. Meary R, Mattei CR, Tomeno B: Tarsectomie anterieure pour pied creux. Indications et résultats lointains. *Rev Chir Orthop* 62:231, 1976

213. Mitchell GP: Posterior displacement osteotomy of the calcaneus. *J Bone Joint Surg* 59B:233, 1977

214. Paulos CE, Coleman SS, Samuelson KM: Pes cavovarus: Review of a surgical approach using soft tissue procedures. *J Bone Joint Surg* 62A:942, 1980

215. Price AE, Maisel R, Drennan JC: Computed tomographic analysis of pes cavus. *J Pediatr Orthop* 13:646, 1993

216. Sabir M, Lyttie D: Pathogenesis of pes cavus in Charcot-Marie-Tooth disease. *Clin Orthop* 175:173, 1983

217. Samilson RL: Calcaneocavus feet—a plan of management in children. *Orthop Rev* 10:121, 1981

218. Samilson RL, Dillin W: Cavus, cavovarus and calcaneocavus. An update. *Clin Orthop* 177:125, 1983

219. Sherman FC, Westin GW: Plantar release in the correction of deformities of the foot in childhood. *J Bone Joint Surg* 63A:1382, 1981

220. Siffert RS, Forster RI, Nachamie B: "Beak" triple arthrodesis for correction of severe cavus deformity. *Clin Orthop* 45:101, 1966

221. Steindler A: Operative treatment of pes cavus. *Surg Gynecol Obstet* 24:612, 1917

222. Steindler A: Stripping of the os calcis. *J Orthop Surg* 2:8, 1920

223. Watanabe RS: Metatarsal osteotomy for the cavus foot. *Clin Orthop* 252:217, 1988

224. Yale AC, Hugar DW: Pes cavus: The deformity and its etiology. *J Foot Surg* 20:159, 1981

Adolescent or Juvenile Hallux Valgus (Bunion) and Metatarsus Primus Varus

225. Coughlin MJ, Mann RA: The pathophysiology of the juvenile bunion. *AAOS Instr Course Lect* 36:123, 1987

226. Helal B, Gupta S, Gojaseni P: Surgery for adolescent hallux valgus. *Acta Orthop Scand* 45:271, 1974

227. Houghton G, Dickson R: Hallux valgus in the younger patient: The structural abnormality. *J Bone Joint Surg* 61B:176, 1979

228. Piggott H: The natural history of hallux valgus in adolescence and early adult life. *J Bone Joint Surg* 42B:749, 1960

229. Scranton P, Zuckerman J: Bunion surgery in adolescents: Results of surgical treatment. *J Pediatr Orthop* 4:39, 1984

230. Simmonds F, Menelaus M: Hallux valgus in adolescents. *J Bone Joint Surg* 42B:761, 1960

231. Young JD: A new operation for adolescent hallux valgus. *Univ PA Med Bull* 23:459, 1910

Hallux Valgus

232. Coughlin MJ, Bordelon RL, Johnson K, Mann RA: Symposium-Presidents' forum—evaluation and treatment of juvenile hallux valgus. *Contemp Orthop* 21:169, 1990

Bunionette (Tailor's Bunion)

233. Hansson G: Sliding osteotomy for tailor's bunion. Brief report. *J Bone Joint Surg* 71B:324, 1989

234. Sponsel KH: Bunionette correction by metatarsal osteotomy. *Orthop Clin North Am* 7:809, 1976

Macrodactyly

235. Ackland MK, Uhthoff HK: Idiopathic localized gigantism: A 26-year follow-up. *J Pediatr Orthop* 6:618, 1986

236. Demetriades MD, Hager J, Nikolaides N, Malamitsi-Puchner A, Bartsocas CS: Proteus syndrome: Musculoskeletal manifestations and management: A report of two cases. *J Pediatr Orthop* 12:106, 1992

237. Dennyson WG, Bear JN, Bhoola KD: Macrodactyly in the foot. *J Bone Joint Surg* 59B:355, 1977

238. Kumar K, Kumar D, Gadegone WM, Kapahtia NK: Macrodactyly of the hand and foot. *Int Orthop* 9:259, 1985

239. Wiedemann HR, Burgio GR, Adenhoff P, Kunze J, Kaufmann HJ, Schirg E: The Proteus syndrome. *Eur J Pediatr* 140:5, 1983

Hammer Toe

240. Jones R: *Notes on Military Orthopaedics.* New York, PB Hoeber, 1917, pp 38–57

241. Ross ERS, Menelaus MB: Open flexor tenotomy for hammer toes and curly toes in childhood. *J Bone Joint Surg* 66B:770, 1984

242. Soule RE: Operation for the cure of hammertoe. *NY Med J* 91:649, 1910

Claw Toe

243. Dickson FD, Dively RL: Operation for correction of mild claw foot, the result of infantile paralysis. *JAMA* 87:1275, 1926

244. Forrester-Brown MF: Tendon transplantation for clawing of the great toe. *J Bone Joint Surg* 20:57, 1938

245. Heyman CH: Operative treatment of claw foot. *J Bone Joint Surg* 14:335, 1932

246. Hibbs RA: An operation for "claw foot." *JAMA* 73:1583, 1919

247. Taylor TG: The treatment of claw toes by multiple transfers of flexor into extensor tendons. *J Bone Joint Surg* 33B:539, 1951

Curly Toe (Congenital Varus Toe)

248. Biyani A, Jones DA, Murray JM: Flexor to extensor tendon transfer for curly toes. 43 children reviewed after 8 (1–25) years. *Acta Orthop Scand* 63:451, 1992

249. Pollard JP, Morrison PJM: Flexor tenotomy in the treatment of curly toes. *Proc R Soc Med* 68:480, 1975

250. Ross ER, Menelaus MB: Open flexor tenotomy for hammer toes and curly toes in childhood. *J Bone Joint Surg* 66B:770, 1984

251. Sharrard WJW: Congenital varus (curly) toes, in *Paediatric Orthopaedics and Fractures and Developmental Abnormalities of the Foot and Toes.* Oxford, Blackwell, 1971, pp 295–299

252. Sweetnam R: Congenital curly toes. An investigation into the value of treatment. *Lancet* 2:398, 1958

Congenital Digitus Minimus Varus

253. Biyani A, Jones DA, Murray JM: Flexor to extensor tendon transfer for curly toes. 43 children reviewed after 8 (1–25) years. *Acta Orthop Scand* 63:451, 1992

254. Cockin J: Butler's operation for an overriding fifth toe. *J Bone Joint Surg* 50B:78, 1968

255. Kelikian H: *Hallux Valgus, Allied Deformities of the Forefoot, and Metatarsalgia.* Philadelphia, WB Saunders Co, 1965

256. McFarland B: Congenital deformities of the spine and limbs, in Platt H (ed): *Modern Trends in Orthopedics*. New York, PB Hoeber, 1950, p 107

Kohler's Disease

257. Ippolito E, Pollini PTR, Falez F: Kohler's disease of the tarsal navicular. Long-term follow-up of 12 cases. *J Pediatr Orthop* 4:416, 1984
258. Karp M: Kohler's disease of the tarsal scaphoid. *J Bone Joint Surg* 19:84, 1937
259. Kohler A: Eine typische Erkrankung des 2. Metatarsophalangealgelenkes. *Munch Med Wochenschr* 67:1289, 1920
260. Waugh W: The ossification and vascularization of the tarsal navicular and their relation to Kohler's disease. *J Bone Joint Surg* 40B:765, 1958
261. Williams GA, Cowell HR: Kohler's disease of the tarsal navicular. *Clin Orthop* 158:53, 1981

Freiberg's Infraction

262. Braddock GTF: Experimental epiphysial injury and Freiberg's disease. *J Bone Joint Surg* 41:154, 1959
263. Freiberg AH: Infraction of the second metatarsal bone; a typical injury. *Surg Gynecol Obstet* 19:191, 1914
264. Freiberg AH: The so-called infraction of the second metatarsal bone. *J Bone Joint Surg* 8:257, 1926
265. Hoskinson J: Freiberg's disease: A review of the long-term results. *Proc R Soc Med* 67:106, 1974
266. Jewett EL: A case of Freiberg's disease treated by a walking cast. *J Bone Joint Surg* 21:778, 1939

Accessory Navicular

267. Bennett GL, Weiner DS, Leighley B: Surgical treatment of symptomatic accessory tarsal navicular. *J Pediatr Orthop* 10:445, 1990
268. Grogan DP, Gasser SI, Ogden JA: The painful accessory navicular: A clinical and histopathological study. *Foot Ankle* 10:164, 1989
269. Macnicol MF, Voutsinas S: Surgical treatment of the symptomatic accessory navicular. *J Bone Joint Surg* 66B:218, 1984
270. Sella EG, Lawson JP, Ogden JA: The accessory navicular synchondrosis. *Clin Orthop* 209:280, 1986
271. Sullivan JA, Miller WA: The relationship of the accessory navicular to the development of the flat foot. *Clin Orthop* 144:233, 1979

Osteomyelitis of the Bones of the Foot

272. Borris LC, Helleland H: Growth disturbance of the hind part of the foot following osteomyelitis of the calcaneus in the newborn. *J Bone Joint Surg* 68A:302, 1986
273. Canale ST, Manugian AH: Neonatal osteomyelitis of os calcis. A complication of repeated heel punctures. *Clin Orthop* 156:178, 1981
274. Feigin RD, McAlister WH, San Joaquin V, Middlekamp JN: Osteomyelitis of the calcaneus. *Am J Dis Child* 119:61, 1970
275. Lilien LD, Harris VJ, Ramamurthy RS, Pildes RS: Neonatal osteomyelitis of the calcaneus: Complication of heel puncture. *J Pediatr* 88:478, 1976

Haglund's Disease

276. Dickinson PH, Coutts MB, Woodward EP, Handler D: Tendo Achilles bursitis. *J Bone Joint Surg* 48A:77, 1966
277. Haglund P: Beitrag Zur Uliwik der Achillesse Have. *Z Orthop Chir* 49:49, 1928
278. Heneghan MA, Pavlov H: The Haglund painful heel syndrome. *Clin Orthop* 187:228, 1984
279. Jones DC, James SL: Partial calcaneal osteotomy for retrocalcaneal bursitis. *Am J Sports Med* 12:72, 1984
280. Keck SW, Kelly PJ: Bursitis of the posterior part of the heel. *J Bone Joint Surg* 47A:267, 1965

Hallux Rigidus

281. Kelikian H: *Hallux Valgus, Allied Deformities of the Forefoot, and Metatarsalgia*. Philadelphia, WB Saunders Co, 1965, p 273
282. Kessel L, Bonney G: Hallux rigidus in the adolescent. *J Bone Joint Surg* 40B:668, 1958
283. Watermann H: Die Arthritis deformans Grosszehengrundgelenkes. *Z Orthop Chir* 48:346, 1927

Ingrowing Toenail

284. Ceh SE, Pettine KA: Treatment of ingrown toenail. *J Musculoskel Med* 7:62, 1990
285. Zadek FR: Obliteration of the nail bed of the great toe without shortening the terminal phalanx. *J Bone Joint Surg* 32B:66, 1950

Osteochondritis Dissecans of the Dome of the Talus

286. Anderson DV, Lyne ED: Osteochondritis dissecans of the talus: Case report on two family members. *J Pediatr Orthop* 4:356, 1984
287. Anderson IF, Crichton KJ, Gratton-Smith T, Cooper RA, Brazier D: Osteochondral fracture of the dome of the talus. *J Bone Joint Surg* 71A:1143, 1989
288. Bauer M, Jonsson K, Linden B: Osteochondritis dissecans of the ankle: A 20-year follow-up study. *J Bone Joint Surg* 69B:93, 1987
289. Berndt AL, Harty M: Transchondral fractures (osteochondritis dissecans) of the talus. *J Bone Joint Surg* 41A:988, 1959
290. Bourrel P, Maistre B, Palinacci JC, Gourul JC, Jardin M: Osteochondrite de l'astragale. A propos de 9 observations. *Rev Chir Orthop* 58:609, 1972
291. Canale ST, Belding RH: Osteochondral lesions of the talus. *J Bone Joint Surg* 62A:97, 1980
292. David MW: Bilateral talar osteochondritis dissecans with lax ankle ligaments. *J Bone Joint Surg* 52A:168, 1970
293. DeGinder WL: Osteochondritis dissecans of the talus. *Radiology* 65:590, 1955
294. DeSmet AA, Fisher DR, Burnstein MI: Value of MR imaging in staging osteochondral lesions of the talus (osteochondritis dissecans): Results in 14 patients. *AJR* 154:555, 1990
295. Heare MM, Gillespy T III, Bittar ES: Direct coronal computed tomography arthrography of osteochondritis dissecans of the talus. *Skeletal Radiol* 17:187, 1988

296. Mukherjee SK, Young AB: Dome fracture of the talus: A report of ten cases. *J Bone Joint Surg* 55B:319, 1973

297. Scharling M: Osteochondritis dissecans of the talus. *Acta Orthop Scand* 49:89, 1978

298. Smith GR, Winquist RA, Allan TNK, Northrop CH: Subtle transchondral fractures of the talar dome: A radiological perspective. *Radiology* 124:667, 1977

299. Zinman C, Reis ND: Osteochondritis dissecans of the talus: Use of high resolution computed tomography scanner. *Acta Orthop Scand* 53:697, 1982

Ankle Instability

300. Brostrom L: Sprained ankles. I. Anatomic lesions in recent sprains. *Acta Chir Scand* 128:483, 1964

301. Brostrom L: Sprained ankles. III. Clinical observations in recent ligament ruptures. *Acta Chir Scand* 130:560, 1965

302. Brostrom L: Sprained ankles. V. Treatment and prognosis in recent ligament ruptures. *Acta Chir Scand* 130:560, 1965

303. Brostrom L: Sprained ankles. VI. Surgical treatment of "chronic" ligament ruptures. *Acta Chir Scand* 132:551, 1966

304. Brostrom L, Liljedahl SO, Lindvall N: Sprained ankles. II. Arthrographic diagnosis of recent ligament ruptures. *Acta Chir Scand* 129:485, 1965

THE KNEE AND LEG

Knee and leg deformities and complaints are quite common in infants and children. The underlying problem may be a simple developmental variation or more serious pathology. The disease entity varies in different age groups. The cause may be congenital malformation, developmental abnormality, postural deformation, trauma, rotational or angular malalignment, infection, arthritis, or tumor.

■ CONGENITAL DISLOCATION AND SUBLUXATION OF THE KNEE

In this very rare congenital deformity (1.7 per 100,000 births), the newborn exits the birth canal with an alarming appearance: One or both knees are severely hyperextended and the hips are in hyperflexion with the toes touching the upper chest, shoulders, or chin (Fig 2–1A, B).

History. Inquire as to the presentation of the fetus at birth. Often babies with congenital dislocation of the knee are the product of a breech presentation and not infrequently were delivered by cesarean section to prevent fetal distress. Ask about familial incidence of dislocation of joints—knee, hip, or elbow. Inspect the facies of the parents and siblings. In some syndromes such as Larsen's, the facies is distinctive—hypertelorism and prominent forehead.

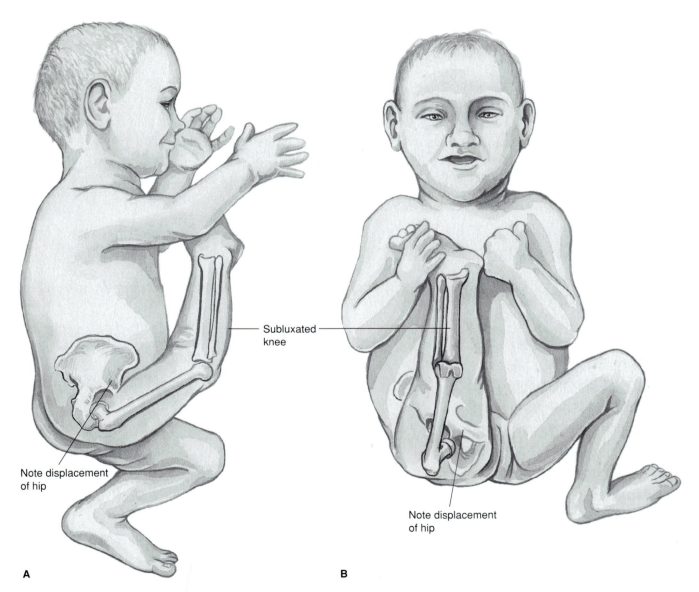

Subluxated knee

Note displacement of hip

Note displacement of hip

A

B

Figure 2–1. Congenital dislocation of the knee in a newborn. **A.** Lateral view. **B.** Posterior view of the affected lower limb. Note the severe hyperextension deformity of the knee, with the femoral condyles prominent in the popliteal region. The ipsilateral hip is dislocated. Don't miss it!

Examination. On inspection the femoral condyles are prominent in the popliteal region, and transverse creases or folds are present in the front of the knee. On passive manipulation, knee flexion is markedly restricted; on releasing the flexion force, the knee bounces back into hyperextension. Hyperextension of the knee is associated with varying degrees of genu valgum with contracture of the lateral intermuscular septum and iliotibial band. In severe dislocation of the knee, the hamstrings, particularly the medial, are displaced anteriorly and act as knee extensors. The quadriceps muscle is contracted and the patellar tendon is shortened. The patella is hypoplastic. In severe cases massive fibrous tissue proliferation and adhesions in the suprapatellar pouch tether the quadriceps mechanism. The cruciate ligaments of the knee may be absent.

Determine the severity of anterior displacement of the knee. Leveuf and Pais subdivide it into three progressive grades. In *grade I* the knee can be passively flexed beyond neutral to 45 to 60 degrees, but on release of flexion force it bounces up to 10 to 20 degrees of hyperextension. The anterior displacement of the tibia is minimal (Fig 2–2A). In *grade II* the anterior subluxation is moderate, with some contact remaining between the articular surfaces of the femur and tibia. On passive manipulation the knee can be flexed only to neutral, and the knee is postured in 20 to 40 degrees of hyperextension (Fig 2–2B). *Grade III* involves complete anterior dislocation with total loss of contact between the articular surfaces of the distal femur and the proximal tibia (Fig 2–2C). Leveuf and Pais' classification was based on arthrographic studies in five cases of congenital dislocation of the knee. Parsch and Schulz confirmed Leveuf and Pais' classification by ultrasonography of 10 congenitally hyperextended knees in 10 patients; they found

two simple knee hyperextensions, five knee subluxations, and three total dislocations.[12,17]

It is vital to examine the entire child and rule out associated deformities. About 50 percent of dislocated-subluxated knees have associated hip dislocation. Rule out elbow dislocation, which occurs in 10 percent of the cases. Foot deformities—talipes equinovarus, pes calcaneus, convex pes valgus—are present in about one third of the cases.

Is the dislocation of the knee part of a syndrome such as Down's or Ehlers-Danlos syndrome? Is there hypermobility of all of the joints and severe ligamentous hyperlaxity? In Larsen's syndrome the facies is distinctive and dislocation of the knee is accompanied by multiple dislocations of the hips, feet, ankles, and elbows.[11,21] Arthrogryposis multiplex congenita is characterized by rigidity of multiple joints. The hip and knee may be dislocated and the feet deformed into talipes equinovarus or convex pes valgus, and the upper limbs may be involved.

Other associated anomalies may be imperforate anus, cryptorchidism, spina bifida, hydrocephalus, cleft palate, facial paralysis, and camptodactyly of the little fingers.

Imaging. Initially routine radiography in the anteroposterior (AP) and *true* lateral projection is done. The ossification centers of the distal femur and proximal tibia are delayed; however, the plain radiograms clearly depict the varying degrees of anterior displacement of the tibia over the femur.

The problem is distinguishing simple knee hyperextension (genu recurvatum) deformity from true anterior subluxation-dislocation. Ultrasonography is performed to differentiate the two. Anterior, lateral, and popliteal scanning approaches are used. Ultrasonographic images clearly depict the cartilaginous relationship of the distal femur and proximal tibia; a computed sonography machine should be used.[17] Ultrasonography is also used during the course of treatment to determine the success or failure of conservative treatment and to decide on the timing of open surgical reduction of the dislocated knee.

Arthrography to depict the intra-articular pathology is not recommended because it is invasive. It is best to perform magnetic resonance imaging (MRI); it depicts articular cartilage, menisci, cruciate ligaments, and the presence or absence of the suprapatellar pouch and the soft tissue pathology.

Treatment. Management depends upon the severity of the deformity. Grade I is best managed by serial splinting of the knee into progressive flexion following gentle passive manipulation. Once 90-degree knee flexion is obtained, a Pavlik harness is used for dynamic retention of knee flexion.[7]

Grade II is treated by serial cast application followed by a period of dynamic splinting. Use ultrasonography to confirm reduction of the subluxation. Do not use the Pavlik harness when rotatory lateral subluxation is present. Resis-

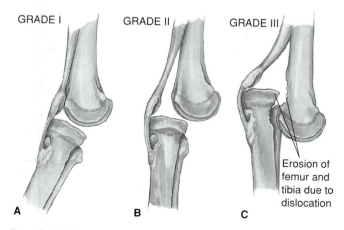

Figure 2–2. Grades of congenital subluxation and dislocation of the knee. **A.** Grade I—Note the minimal anterior displacement of the tibia and the degree of hyperextension of the knee of 10 to 20 degrees. **B.** Grade II—The anterior subluxation is moderate. Note that there is still some contact between the articular surfaces of the distal femur and proximal tibia. The degree of hyperextension deformity is 20 to 40 degrees. **C.** Grade III—Note the complete anterior dislocation. There is no contact between the articular surfaces of the distal femur and proximal tibia.

tant rigid extension contracture of the knee and failure of reduction by manipulation and cast application require simple quadriceps lengthening. Traction—skin or skeletal—is an alternative method; I do not recommend it because it is cumbersome, is not well tolerated by an infant (not to mention the parents), and introduces a risk of skin slough and vascular complications.

Grade III requires major open reduction. The results of surgery are good. The natural history of untreated dislocation or subluxation of the knee is joint instability, pain, degenerative arthritis, and severe disability in adulthood requiring total joint replacement.

■ KNEE HYPEREXTENSION (GENU RECURVATUM) AND FLEXION DEFORMITY

In utero the fetus is in a confined compartment with knees and hips flexed. The knees and hips of the normal neonate have flexion contractures, and following delivery they gradually stretch out. Broughton et al studied the range of knee motion and the degree of hip flexion contracture in 57 normal neonates; the mean degree of knee flexion contracture was 21.4 degrees at birth, and decreased to 10.7 degrees at 3 months and 3.3 degrees at 6 months. The mean range of knee flexion was 154.4 degrees at birth, diminishing to 145.5 degrees at 3 months and 141.7 degrees at 6 months of age. The mean range of hip flexion contracture was 34.1 degrees at birth, diminishing to 18.9 degrees at 3 months and 7.5 degrees at 6 months. Hip flexion contracture and range of knee motion do not correlate clinically.[22]

GENU RECURVATUM

In genu recurvatum the knee extends beyond 2.5 SD of the mean, but the proximal articular surface of the tibia has contact with the distal articular surface of the femur. Distinguish genu recurvatum from congenital subluxation of the knee—the latter demonstrates a varying degree of loss of contact between the proximal end of the tibia and the distal end of the femur.

Imaging.   Radiograms in the AP and true lateral projection in maximal hyperextension are made to rule out associated bony pathology. Ultrasonography depicts the articular relationships of the cartilaginous knee.

Management.   No active treatment is indicated. Occasionally there is extensor contracture of the knee. If it is present, passive stretching exercises to obtain normal range of knee flexion are performed several times a day. Splints and orthotic devices are not necessary because the knees stabilize with tautening of the ligaments. In very severe knee hyperextension deformity, use of the Pavlik harness for a period of 4 to 6 weeks is appropriate. When associated de-

TABLE 2–1. CONDITIONS THAT CAUSE KNEE FLEXION DEFORMITY

Spasticity of hamstrings: upper motor neuron lesion—cerebral palsy, spinal cord tumor, tethered cord, etc
Congenital dislocation of the patella (tibia is rotated laterally)
Cartilaginous bony deformity of the upper tibia–lower femur: bone dysplasia, multiple hereditary exostosis, tarsoepiphyseal dysplasia
Arthrogryposis multiplex congenita
Internal derangement of knee: torn meniscus, loose body
Inflammatory lesions of the synovium: rheumatoid arthritis, pigmented villonodular synovitis
Hemarthrosis in bleeding disorders
Pterygium syndromes: ischiocalcaneal band

velopmental hip dysplasia with dislocation is present, it is treated accordingly.

KNEE FLEXION DEFORMITY

The presenting complaint is that the infant's knees do not straighten—he is "walking with his knees and hips bent." As stated above, knee flexion contracture is normal in the newborn, decreasing gradually up to 6 months of age. When the degree of knee flexion contracture exceeds 2 SD for the age of the patient, it is regarded as a deformity.

When knee flexion contracture persists and is very marked, examine the hamstrings. Are they taut and spastic, indicating an upper motor neuron lesion such as cerebral palsy or tethered spinal cord? With the hip in 90 degrees of flexion, extend the knee and determine the popliteal thigh–leg angle. Rule out hip flexion deformity or ankle equinus. In these conditions knee flexion posture is secondary and compensatory. In congenital dislocation of the patella, the knee has a flexion deformity and the leg is rotated laterally.

Bone dysplasia and intra-articular bony-cartilaginous deformity of the upper tibia and/or the lower femur cause loss of knee extension. Check the elbows—do they extend fully? Imaging studies, routine radiography, ultrasonography, and sometimes MRI establish the diagnosis.

Rule out arthrogryposis multiplex congenita. Is there a popliteal pterygium or ischiocalcaneal band? Inflammatory conditions of the knee—rheumatoid arthritis, pigmented villonodular synovitis, synovial chondromatosis, or hemarthrosis in bleeding disorders such as hemophilia—result in knee flexion deformity. Treatment of this condition depends upon the diagnosis. Common causes of knee flexion deformity are listed in Table 2–1.

■ CONGENITAL ABSENCE OF THE PATELLA

The child presents with flattening of the anterior aspect of the knee which is accentuated when the knee is bent. When the quadriceps muscle is intact, no functional deficit exists.

However, when it is associated with deficiency of the quadriceps mechanism, progressive weakness of the knee extensors and knee flexion deformity are present. On palpation, absence of the patella can be detected.

Examine the entire child to rule out associated syndromes such as nail-patella and arthrogryposis multiplex congenita. Involvement is often bilateral.

Imaging. The patella ossifies between 3 and 4 years of age. In the older child, radiograms show absence of the patella. In the infant and young child, ultrasonography demonstrates absence of the cartilaginous patella.

Management. Treatment is not necessary if no flexion deformity or quadriceps weakness is present. If the quadriceps is absent or hypoplastic, first correct the knee flexion deformity and then transfer the medial and lateral hamstrings anteriorly to provide active knee extension. Neglected, late cases with fixed knee flexion deformity are best treated by the Ilizarov technique.

■ CONGENITAL DISLOCATION OF THE PATELLA[28–32]

In this very rare derangement of the knee extensor mechanism, the patella is displaced laterally on the lateral femoral condyle. The dislocation takes place in utero as a result of failure of normal medial rotation of the myotome containing the quadriceps femoris and the patella. Involvement may be bilateral or unilateral. It may be an isolated anomaly or part of a genetic chromosomal abnormality, Larsen's syndrome, or arthrogryposis multiplex congenita.

The dislocation is present at birth but is often missed. The infant presents with fixed flexion deformity of the knee and excessive lateral rotation of the tibia. All newborns have flexion deformity of the knees due to the flexed posture of the knees and hips in utero. In fact, when you can extend the knee of a newborn fully, you should suspect developmental dislocation of the hip. In the normal lower limb of the newborn, the leg is medially rotated. Suspect congenital dislocation of the patella when fixed flexion of the knee is combined with lateral rotation deformity of the tibia.

On palpation the patella is found to lie on the lateral aspect of the knee above the fibular head and not in its normal location on the anterior aspect of the knee. The dislocated patella is tethered and fixed by contracted fascial bands and is irreducible by passive manipulation. The entire quadriceps mechanism is displaced and rotated laterally, pulling the tibia into valgus and lateral rotation. With delayed diagnosis and treatment, flexion and valgus deformities of the knee increase and the motor strength of the quadriceps femoris weakens. There is 20 to 30 degrees of extensor lag of the knee.

Independent ambulation is slightly delayed; the child walks with an out-toeing gait in spite of the knee flexion deformity and inability to extend the knee fully. In childhood, pain and discomfort are not complaints.

Imaging Findings. The patella ossifies between 3 and 4 years of age; therefore, prior to the appearance of the ossific center of the patella, routine radiograms do not show the patellar dislocation. In the AP projection of the thigh and knee, the soft tissue shadow of the quadriceps femoris is displaced laterally from its normal anterior position.

Ultrasonograms show the laterally dislocated patella.[32] MRI also depicts both the nonossified patella, the muscle–soft tissue pathology and hypoplasia of the lateral femoral condyle and trochlear sulcus. In spite of its cost and the necessity of sedation, this author recommends preoperative MRI, not for diagnostic purposes but for its value in surgical planning.

Treatment. Closed manipulative reduction of the patella is not successful. Treatment is by open surgery. It should be performed early—between 6 and 12 months of age. The quadriceps mechanism is realigned by mobilization of the vastus lateralis, sectioning of the contracted lateral patellar retinaculum and fibrous bands tethering the dislocated patella, medial capsular plication-imbrication, transfer of the semitendinosus tendon to the patella (Galeazzi-Dewar procedure), and hemisection of the patellar tendon and transfer of the lateral half medially. Postoperative habilitation and splinting are crucial for success. Results of surgery are good if open reduction is carried out prior to development of bony deformity.

Untreated patients develop progressive genu valgum, lateral rotation and displacement of the tibia, and knee flexion deformity and pain due to patellofemoral arthritis. The importance of early realignment of the quadriceps and reduction of the patella cannot be overemphasized.

■ BIPARTITE PATELLA[33–37]

The presenting complaint is pain on the superolateral pole or lateral border of the patella during or following vigorous exercise or after a direct blow to the knee. Some patients present with swelling at the site of the accessory ossicle or with catching of the knee. Acute flexion of the knee, pressure from kneeling, or forceful contraction of the quadriceps aggravates the pain. Most cases of bipartite patella, however, are detected incidentally in radiograms of the knee made for other reasons.

Normally the cartilaginous anlage of the patella ossifies from one center of ossification. In 0.4 percent of the population, the patella ossifies from two ossification centers.[35] The junction between the separate ossicle and the

A. Superlateral

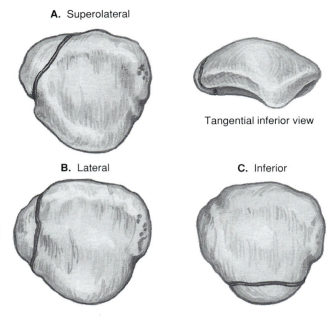

Tangential inferior view

B. Lateral   **C.** Inferior

Figure 2–3. Anatomic sites of accessory ossification centers of the patella. **A.** Superolateral pole. **B.** Lateral part. **C.** Inferior pole.

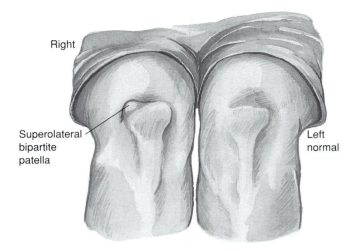

Right

Superolateral
bipartite
patella

Left
normal

Figure 2–4. Clinical appearance of bipartite patella. Note the prominence and swelling of the superolateral pole of the right knee.

body of the patella may be fibrous or cartilaginous. Trauma may disrupt the union between the patellar fragments. Painful bipartite patellae are more common in males.[34] The main body of the patella begins ossification at 3 to 4 years of age; the accessory center of ossification, however, appears later, between 8 and 12 years of age.

The most common site of an accessory ossification center of the patella is the superolateral corner of the patella (about 75 percent); next in frequency is the lateral margin of the patella (20 percent). The inferior pole of the patella is involved in 5 percent of the cases (Fig 2–3).

Clinical Examination. Inspection of the knees in 90 degrees of flexion may reveal a prominence on the superolateral pole or lateral border of the patella (Fig 2–4). The patella feels wider than usual on palpation. Local tenderness may occur at the junction of the displaced accessory ossification center and the body of the patella. Manipulation of the patella ordinarily elicits no abnormal mobility of the displaced ossicle.

Imaging. Routine radiograms in the AP, lateral, and infrapatellar tangential views demonstrate the accessory ossification center of the patella (Fig 2–5). Sometimes it is difficult to distinguish between a stress fracture of the patella and an acutely separated accessory ossification center, particularly when the ossification center is at the inferior pole of the patella. Involvement is unilateral in about 60 percent of cases.

Treatment. Acute painful separated bipartite patellae are treated in an above-knee cast with the knee in extension for

a period of 3 to 4 weeks. Most cases heal with complete relief of symptoms. Treat the patient and not the radiogram—ignore the persistence of a radiolucent line between the accessory ossicle and the body of the patella.

When diagnosis and treatment are delayed, healing may not take place, and with persistent forceful repeated knee flexion fibrous non-union may develop. When painful fibrous non-union is present, treat the patient initially with immobilization in an above-knee cylinder cast for 6 weeks. Do not inject steroids into the site of painful non-union in

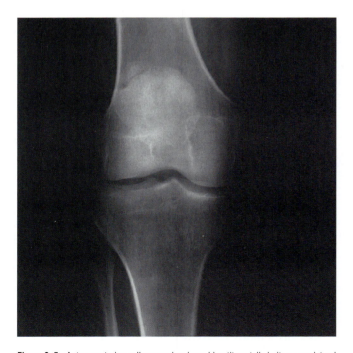

Figure 2–5. Anteroposterior radiogram showing a bipartite patella in its superolateral corner.

an effort to provide symptomatic relief, as pain will recur. Skin slough following cortisone injection is a problem.

Chronically painful accessory ossification of the patella, when disabling, is excised surgically. The result is good, with complete relief of symptoms and no interference with function. Only very occasionally is a traumatically separated large patellar fragment openly reduced and fixed internally with screws; those cases are managed as fracture-separations.

■ PATELLOFEMORAL JOINT

Anterior knee pain and instability of the knee are very common complaints in the adolescent, particularly in those who are active in sports and overuse the extensor mechanism of the knee or in those with angular or torsional malalignment of their lower limbs. Careful inquiry and physical examination to determine the location of the pain often make the diagnosis (Fig 2–6).

Patellofemoral disorders are very common problems in the obese adolescent female with a wide pelvis and knock knees. Clinically a pragmatic classification of patellofemoral disorders is (1) those causing primarily *pain,* (2) those causing primarily *instability,* and (3) those causing both *pain and instability.*[61]

History. Involvement—is it bilateral or unilateral? If involvement is bilateral, does one knee hurt more than the other?

Determine the location of pain—where is the pain and where does it hurt most? Is it at the medial patellar region (indicating recurrent lateral subluxation of the patellofemoral joint), or is it at the inferior pole of the patella (Sinding-Larsen-Johansson disease), superior pole of the patella (extensor tendinitis), diffuse peripatellar region (chondromalacia of the patella), medial joint line (meniscal pathology), or over the collateral ligaments (ligamentous strain or bursitis)? Often in patellofemoral malalignment syndrome, the pain is diffuse in its topography.

Onset. How did the pain begin? Was it gradual or spontaneous in onset, did it follow an acute injury such as a direct blow on the patella resulting from a fall on the knee, or did it ensue after overuse or repetitive trauma during sports such as playing hockey or basketball?

Duration and Relation to Level of Activity. How long have the knees been bothering the patient? Does the pain increase with activity and decrease with rest? Ordinarily patellofemoral pain is aggravated by going up and down stairs or sitting for prolonged periods with the knees flexed such as in a movie theater or a small car. Rest and curtailment from sports ameliorate the symptoms.

Is there any history of swelling; if present, where is the *swelling?* In patellofemoral disorders, acute or chronic effusion of the knee is usually not present. Sometimes, however, there may be recurrent minimal, diffuse puffiness, especially after strenuous physical activity such as running or a sports activity. Is there any *increased local heat*—does the involved knee feel warmer than the other knee?

Does the patient feel any *"grinding"* sensations in the patellofemoral joint when he or she bends and straightens the knee? Is there any history of *locking* of the knee? For example, when he or she stands up from sitting with the legs crossed or from the tailor's position, is he or she unable to straighten the knee? A history of locking of the knee indicates a torn meniscus or the presence of a loose body in the knee joint. Ordinarily it is not a symptom of patellofemoral joint malalignment syndrome. A *"popping"* sound when the knee is straightened from a bent position indicates the presence of a medial synovial plica.

Is there any complaint of *giving way* of the knee, as if the leg is about to collapse under the body weight? Did the patella jump out of place, a feeling of the patella displacing laterally—a subluxation? Did the patient have to push the patella into place manually?

Question the patient as to previous treatment—medication (what type?), splinting, exercises, physical therapy—and the response to such measures.

Is the pain increasing in severity over time, staying the same, or decreasing in intensity? What is the degree of disability? What does the patient desire to do that the pain in the knee is preventing?

Other painful joints—such as the elbows, wrists, ankles—or diffuse muscular pains may indicate a generalized systemic disorder such as rheumatoid disease or lupus erythromatosus. Does the patient have any skin rashes? Any history of tick bite? Always consider Lyme disease. Does the patient have any allergies?

Inquire in detail as to the family history of orthopedic afflictions and the past history of the patient. Table 2–2 lists

---

TABLE 2–2. QUESTIONS TO ELICIT THE CAUSE OF PATELLOFEMORAL JOINT PAIN

1. Involvement—unilateral or bilateral?
2. Site—peripatellar, superior or inferior pole of patella, medial or lateral patellar region, joint line?
3. Onset—spontaneous, gradual, acute following trauma or repetitive trauma or overuse?
4. Duration?
5. Relation to level and type of activity?
6. Swelling—local increased temperature or inflammation?
7. Crepitation—popping, locking?
8. Giving way—quadriceps insufficiency?
9. Instability—subluxation, dislocation?
10. Course—getting worse, static, improving?
11. Previous treatment—rest, brace, medication, response to previous management?
12. Any other peripheral joint pains?
13. Family history, past history of patient?

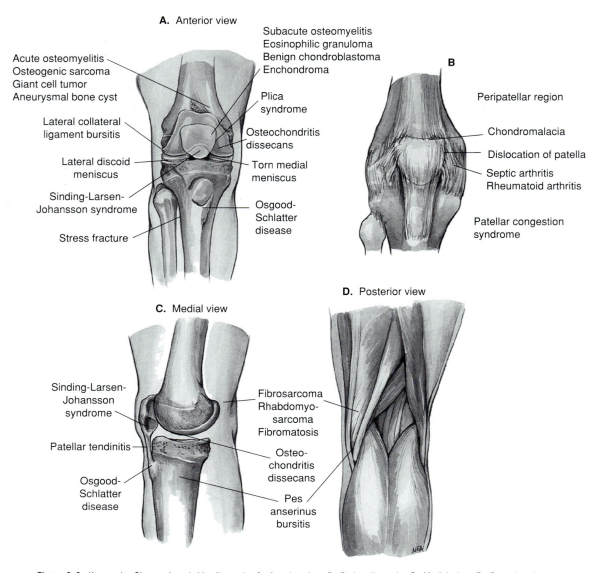

Figure 2–6. Knee pain. Sites and probable diagnosis. **A.** Anterior view. **B.** Peripatellar pain. **C.** Medial view. **D.** Posterior view. *(Continues)*

the questions to ask in order to elicit the cause of the patellofemoral joint pain.

Examination. It is vital to examine the bones, joints, muscles, and entire lower limb from the hip to the foot. Assess the lower limb as a whole and then each individual segment. Rule out causes of "knee pains" referred from the hip, such as Legg-Calvé-Perthes disease or slipped capital femoral epiphysis. First examine the normal or less involved limb and then the symptomatic affected knee. Patellofemoral malalignment is often bilateral. A thorough physical examination ensures that you do not miss unusual causes of knee pain.

An adolescent girl or boy is frequently shy and self-conscious and hesitant to take off jeans or trousers. Insist that the patient be properly attired in a gown or shorts. Respect the privacy of the adolescent, but don't be Victorian and examine her through her clothes or with her jeans rolled up.

First, *inspect* the patient *standing* from the front, back, and side. Is there any angular malalignment of the lower limbs? Is the *mechanical axis* normal, or is it deviated into valgus or varus? *Genu valgum* is often associated with patellofemoral joint malalignment (Fig 2–7A, B). Another common finding in patellofemoral joint disorders is apparent *genu varum*. When the patient stands with the knees in full extension with the feet facing straight for-

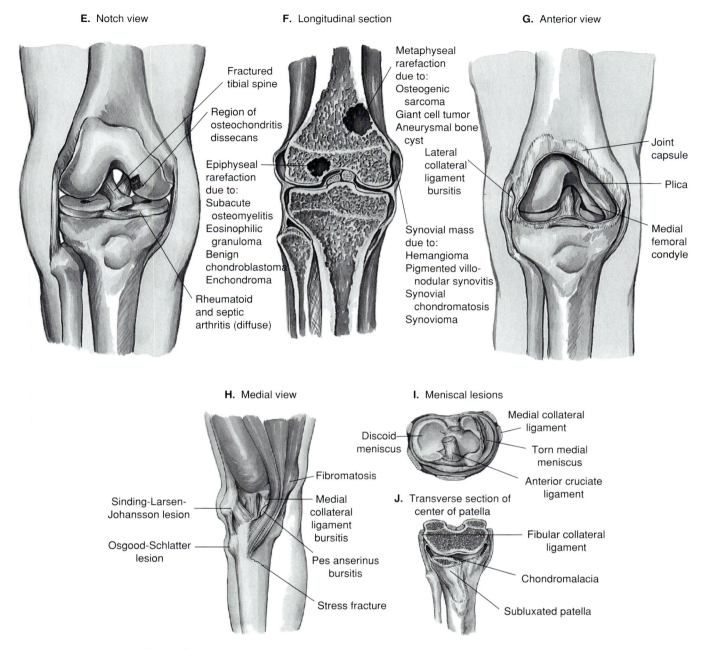

E. Notch view

Fractured tibial spine

Region of osteochondritis dissecans

Epiphyseal rarefaction due to:
Subacute osteomyelitis
Eosinophilic granuloma
Benign chondroblastoma
Enchondroma

Rheumatoid and septic arthritis (diffuse)

F. Longitudinal section

Metaphyseal rarefaction due to:
Osteogenic sarcoma
Giant cell tumor
Aneurysmal bone cyst

Lateral collateral ligament bursitis

Synovial mass due to:
Hemangioma
Pigmented villo-nodular synovitis
Synovial chondromatosis
Synovioma

G. Anterior view

Joint capsule

Plica

Medial femoral condyle

H. Medial view

Sinding-Larsen-Johansson lesion

Osgood-Schlatter lesion

Fibromatosis

Medial collateral ligament bursitis

Pes anserinus bursitis

Stress fracture

I. Meniscal lesions

Medial collateral ligament

Discoid meniscus

Torn medial meniscus

Anterior cruciate ligament

J. Transverse section of center of patella

Fibular collateral ligament

Chondromalacia

Subluxated patella

Figure 2–6 *(Continued).* E. Notch view. F. Longitudinal section. G. Anterior view showing medial plica. H. Medial view. I. Superior view of meniscal lesions. J. Transverse section of center of patella.

ward and the ankles touching each other, the knees are held apart; they do not touch each other (apparent varus) and the patellae are twisted inward facing each other (the "cross-eyed" patellae) (Fig 2–8A). There is rotatory malalignment at the knee. Because of excessive femoral antetorsion, the femora are rotated medially so that the femoral heads are concentrically centered in the acetabulae and the tibiae are rotated laterally to compensate for the medial rotation (antetorsion) deformity of the femurs. The feet appear to be in valgus with the heels everted. When the pa-

tellae face straight forward, the bowlegged appearance disappears (Fig 2–8B).

Next determine the position of the patellae in stance—are they normally located or displaced laterally or superiorly? What is the Q (quadriceps) angle in stance (Fig 2–9)?

Inspect the patient from the side and from behind to rule out genu recurvatum and popliteal masses. Are the iliac crests level? Is there any lower limb length disparity or scoliosis? Ask the patient to walk and determine his or her

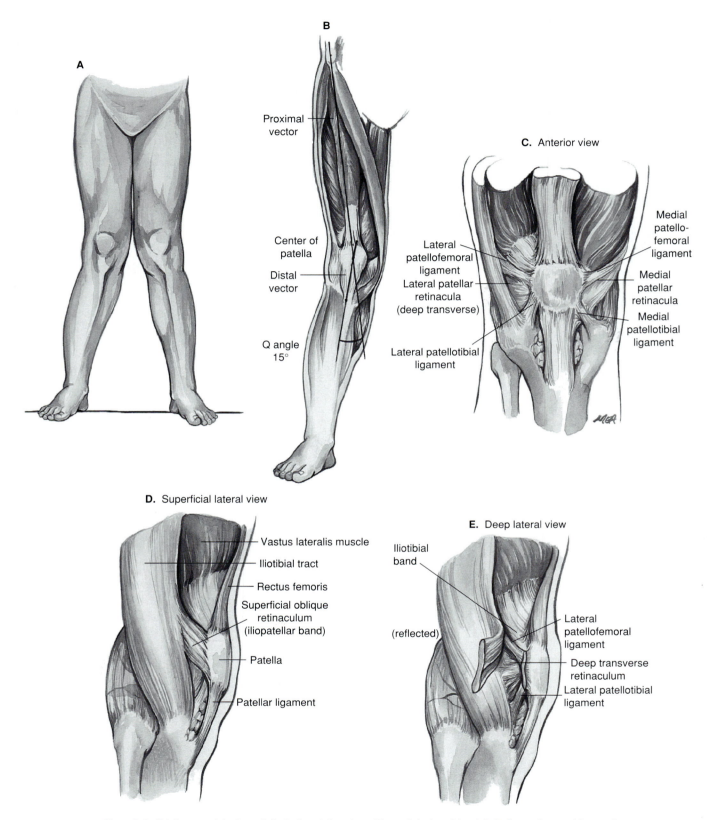

Figure 2–7. Malalignment of the lower limb. Static and dynamic stabilizers of the knee joint. **A & B.** Genu valgum and increased quadriceps (Q) angle. **C.** Anterior view showing the dynamic and static stabilizers of the knee. **D.** Superficial lateral view showing the iliotibial band and its attachment to the patella. **E.** Deep lateral view showing the lateral patellotibial and patellofemoral ligaments and the deep transverse retinaculum.

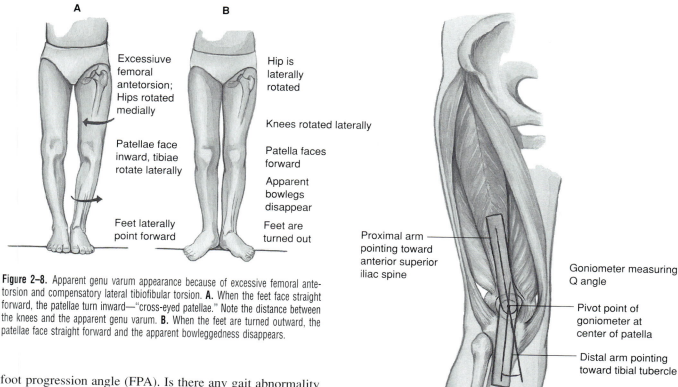

A. Excessiuve femoral antetorsion; Hips rotated medially

Patellae face inward, tibiae rotate laterally

Feet laterally point forward

B. Hip is laterally rotated

Knees rotated laterally

Patella faces forward

Apparent bowlegs disappear

Feet are turned out

Figure 2–8. Apparent genu varum appearance because of excessive femoral ante-torsion and compensatory lateral tibiofibular torsion. **A.** When the feet face straight forward, the patellae turn inward—"cross-eyed patellae." Note the distance between the knees and the apparent genu varum. **B.** When the feet are turned outward, the patellae face straight forward and the apparent bowleggedness disappears.

Proximal arm pointing toward anterior superior iliac spine

Goniometer measuring Q angle

Pivot point of goniometer at center of patella

Distal arm pointing toward tibial tubercle

Figure 2–9. Quadriceps or Q angle. It is measured with the patient supine, the knee in full extension, and the quadriceps isometrically contracted. Note the pivot point of the goniometer at the center of the patella with its upper arm directed toward the anterosuperior iliac spine and the lower arm pointing toward the tibial tubercle.

foot progression angle (FPA). Is there any gait abnormality such as short leg or antalgic limp, or quadriceps weakness (the patient leans forward in the stance phase of gait)? Have the patient step up and step down the examining stool to exaggerate any quadriceps weakness; he or she steadies the lower thigh with the hand and/or leans forward further if the quadriceps is weak. Ask the patient to squat on both legs and then on one leg at a time. Observe the patient for any abnormal lateral shift of the patella as it engages and disengages the trochlea. Can he or she duck walk? Is it painful? Have him or her squat on one leg holding the examination table and then get up while rotating the hip—this is a combination of the McMurray and Apley tests. When meniscal tears are present, the patient complains of pain.

Completely assess the *rotation (torsion) profile* by having the patient lie prone on the examination table and determine hip rotation in extension (HR), thigh-foot angle (TFA), and transmalleolar axis (TMA) and the presence or absence of any foot deformity (see Fig 2–68) pp. 154 and 155. (FPA has already been observed in gait.) Is there any metatarsus varus with a convex lateral border of the foot or pes valgus with a concave lateral border of the foot? In pes calcaneus there is abnormal wear of the foot—callosity of the heel with limitation of plantar flexion range of the ankle-foot, whereas in equinus the metatarsal head region is more worn with restriction of range of ankle dorsiflexion. Inspect the skin of the sole for abnormal callosities on the lateral or medial border of the foot.

Next have the patient seated in a relaxed position on the examination table with knees bent at right angles and legs dangling free over the edge of the table. Determine the

position of the patellae—are they normally located facing straight forward (Fig 2–10A) or are they tilted laterally and riding high, indicating patellofemoral lateral malalignment (Fig 2–10B)?

The superoinferior position of the patella is best assessed from the lateral view. In the normal knee (flexed 90 degrees), the patella faces straight forward with its superior pole aligned to the longitudinal axis of the anterior cortex of the femur (Fig 2–11A). When the patella is riding high (patella alta), it faces toward the ceiling (Fig 2–11B).

A practical clinical method of determining the superoinferior position of the patella is measuring the ratio of the greatest longitudinal length of the patella (LP) to the length of the patellar tendon (LT) from its origin at the inferior pole of the patella to its insertion into the tibial tubercle. The patient's knee is flexed 30 degrees. Determine the ratio or simply use your fingers to measure the lengths of the patella and patellar tendon. Normally the LP:LT ratio is 1:1. When the patellar tendon is stretched and elongated, the LP:LT ratio decreases. A ratio of less than 0.8 indicates a high-riding patella (Fig 2–12).[46]

A. Normal anterior view

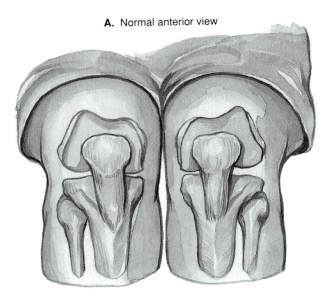

B. Patella alta

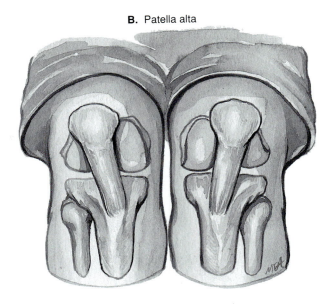

Figure 2–10. Position of the patella as seen from the anterior view. **A.** Normal. The patellae are facing straight forward centered in the trochlea of the femur and soft tissue outline of the knee. **B.** Abnormal, seen in lateral patellofemoral malalignment. The patellae are riding high and tilted laterally. Some surgeons refer to this as the appearance of grasshopper eyes.

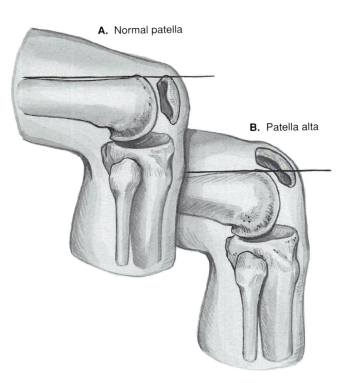

Figure 2–11. Superoinferior position of the patella as viewed from the lateral projection. **A.** Normal. The patella faces straight forward, with its superior pole aligned with the anterior cortex of the femoral shaft. **B.** In patella alta, the patella faces toward the ceiling.

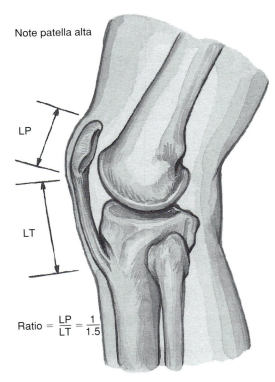

$$\text{Ratio} = \frac{LP}{LT} = \frac{1}{1.5}$$

Figure 2–12. Clinical determination of the superoinferior position of the patella by measuring the greatest longitudinal length of the patella (LP) and that of the patellar tendon (LT) with the knee flexed 30 degrees. Use a tape or finger-breadths for mensuration. In the normal knee, the LP : LT ratio is 1 : 1, whereas in high-riding patella (patella alta) it is decreased to less than 0.8.

Is the tibial tubercle prominent and enlarged, indicating chronic or healed Osgood-Schlatter lesion as the cause of patella alta? Palpate the patellar tendon and tibial tubercle—are they tender? Flex the knee acutely—is the pain increased? These findings indicate acute Osgood-Schlatter lesion. Inspect and palpate to rule out effusion or synovial thickening in the knee.

Next determine the Q angle—the relationship of the distal restraint vector (patellar tendon–center of patella to tibial tubercle) to the proximal vector (the line of pull of the quadriceps from the pelvis to the patella) (see Fig 2–9). With the patient in the supine position, ask him or her to isometrically contract the quadriceps and determine the angle formed between the line drawn from the antero-superior iliac spine to the center of the patella and the line drawn from the center of the patella to the center of the tibial tubercle. A simple and practical method of measuring the Q angle is to place the pivot point of the goniometer at the center of the patella with its upper arm pointing to the anterosuperior iliac spine and its distal arm to the tibial tubercle and measuring the angle. The average normal Q angle is 14 degrees; however, it varies with gender, being greater in females because of their greater genu valgum due to their wider pelvis. A Q angle of up to 10 degrees in the male and up to 15 degrees in the female is normal. A Q angle of more than 20 degrees is definitely abnormal. The Q angle is increased in lateral patellar subluxation, excessive genu valgum, and excessive femoral antetorsion and compensatory lateral tibial torsion.

Next determine the 90-degree tubercle sulcus angle, which more accurately determines the malalignment of the distal vector alone (Fig 2–13). (1) Ask the patient to sit with the knees flexed 90 degrees. (2) Palpate and determine the transepicondylar axis of the femur. Then (3) draw a line from the center of the patella to the tuberosity of the tibia. An angle of 0 degrees is normal, whereas an angle of 10 degrees or more is abnormal. It should be noted, however, that when there is fixed lateral displacement of the patella (subluxation), the tubercle sulcus angle may decrease.

In patellofemoral joint malalignment with recurrent lateral subluxation of the patella, there is definite muscle imbalance between a dysplastic, weak vastus medialis obliquus (VMO) and a strong vastus lateralis muscle. Inspection and palpation reveal depression and atrophy of the muscle in the medial and superomedial region of the patella. Measure the distal thigh circumference at a set distance proximal to the knee joint line, but do not use the superior border of the patella as a reference point because in patella alta it may vary between the right and left sides. With the knees flexed 45 degrees there will be a distinct *lateral tilt* of the patella in patellofemoral joint lateral subluxation and malalignment.

Flex and extend the knee and observe the tracking of the patella. The course of excursion of the patella is deter-

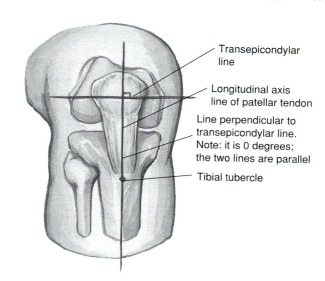

Figure 2–13. Tubercle sulcus angle, the angle formed between the axis of the patellar tendon and a line drawn perpendicular to the transepicondylar axis of the femur with the knee flexed 90 degrees. Normally it is 0 degrees; a value greater than 10 degrees is abnormal.

mined by bony and soft tissue constraints. When there is a dynamic imbalance between a weak vastus medialis obliquus and a strong vastus lateralis and/or the patella is riding high and the buttress of the lateral femoral condyle is lost, the patella displaces laterally when the knee begins to extend fully. The "screw home mechanism" by rotation of the tibia on the femur causes a sudden lateral shift of the patella (Fig 2–14).

Observe the position of the patella with the knee in full extension and the quadriceps muscle relaxed. In the normal knee the patella is located in the midline between the two femoral condyles (Fig 2–15A). Ask the patient to actively contract the quadriceps; normally the patella moves straight upward or in an equal ratio of superior and lateral excursions (Fig 2–15B). Some degree of lateral glide of the patella is present in most patients and is not clinically significant. Movement of the patella straight laterally or more laterally than proximally on quadriceps contracture indicates the presence of a pathologic vector force due to dynamic imbalance between the weak vastus medialis obliquus and strong vastus lateralis or contracture of lateral patellar retinaculum (Fig 2–15C). This is referred to as the *lateral pull sign*.

Patellar Tilt. Mediolateral tilt occurs when the lateral patellar retinaculum, especially the deep portion, is contracted. To detect patellar tilt, observe the patient from the foot of the examining table with the knee in full extension and the quadriceps relaxed. Determine the horizontal axis of the patella in relation to the plane of the floor; when the two axes are parallel the patellar tilt angle is neutral.

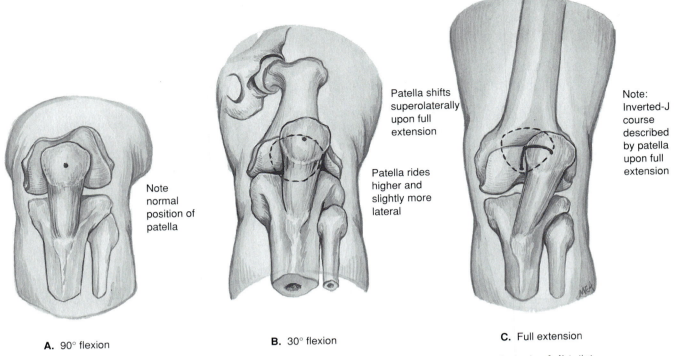

Patella shifts superolaterally upon full extension

Patella rides higher and slightly more lateral

Note normal position of patella

Note: Inverted-J course described by patella upon full extension

A. 90° flexion   **B.** 30° flexion   **C.** Full extension

Figure 2–14. Patellar tracking, the excursion of the course of the patella from 90 degrees of flexion to neutral extension. **A.** Note that at 90 degrees of knee flexion the patella faces straight forward. **B.** At 30 degrees of flexion the patella is beginning to ride high and slightly laterally. **C.** Near or at full extension the patella suddenly shifts laterally. This is abnormal and is referred to as inverted-J sign of the patella. It is observed when there is a dynamic imbalance between a weak vastus medialis obliquus and a strong vastus lateralis. It is also abnormal when the patella is riding high and the lateral buttress of the patella is lost.

Next, perform the *patellar tilt test* (Fig 2–16A, B).[48] Press the medial edge of the patella posteriorly and measure the degree of elevation of the lateral edge of the patella from the lateral femoral condyle. When the lateral patellar retinaculum is contracted (taut) the lateral edge of the patella is below the neutral position (negative patellar tilt angle), and on the passive patellar tilt test the lateral border of the patella does not elevate to neutral. When comparing the levels of medial and lateral patellar borders, it is crucial that the patella is in its normal position in the trochlea and not displaced laterally or medially.

Next, inspect the relationship of the inferior and superior poles of the patella as to rotation of the patella in its longitudinal axis in relation to the longitudinal axis of the femur and the relationship of the patellar poles to the AP plane.

Then test mobility of the patella—is it hypermobile, decreased, or normal? The best way to test this is to have the patient supine with the knee in 30 degrees of flexion and resting on folded sheets with the quadriceps completely relaxed. First, with your thumbs on the medial side of the patella, push the patella laterally and second with your index fingers on the lateral side of the patella, push the patella medially (Fig 2–17A, B). Visually divide the width of the patella into four longitudinal quadrants. Normally the me-

dial or lateral displacement of the patella should not exceed one half of its width (Fig 2–17C). When the lateral patellar retinaculum is taut, medial displacement of the patella is restricted. When the vastus medialis obliquus is dysplastic and the medial patellar retinaculum is stretched out (inadequate medial dynamic and static restraint), the patella displaces laterally more than one half of its width. The patella may be passively dislocated laterally. A global hypermobile patella is displaced medially and laterally three or four quadrants. When there is a history of previous painful dislocation of the patella, the patient becomes fearful when testing for hypermobility of the patella, especially when the patella is about to dislocate laterally. The patient is apprehensive of acute pain; he or she reaches over and seizes the examiner's hand and straightens the knee in order to prevent dislocation or pain (Fig 2–18). (Fairbanks apprehension test.)

Methodically palpate the anterior, medial, lateral, and posterior aspects of the knee for the site of maximum local tenderness. Is it in the patella, peripatellar soft tissues, inferior or superior poles of the patella, patellar tendon, or tibial tubercle? Carefully palpate the joint line anteromedially and anterolaterally and also the medial and collateral ligaments. Turn the patient to the prone position and, with the knee in maximal extension, palpate the posterior aspect

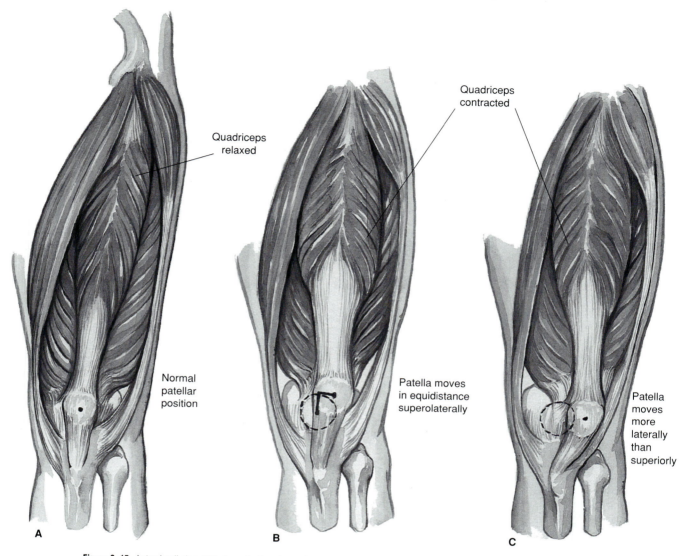

Quadriceps
relaxed

Quadriceps
contracted

Normal
patellar
position

Patella moves
in equidistance
superolaterally

Patella
moves
more
laterally
than
superiorly

A

B

C

Figure 2–15. Lateral pull sign. With the patient supine and the knee fully extended, note the position of the patella with the quadriceps relaxed and on active muscle contraction of the quadriceps. **A.** Quadriceps relaxed—normal knee. Note that the patella is in the midline between the femoral condyles. **B.** Upon contraction of the quadriceps, normally the patella moves straight upward or an equal distance superiorly and laterally. **C.** In the abnormal knee the patella moves more laterally than superiorly.

of the knee for any sites of acute tenderness. A common pitfall is to forget to examine the posterior aspect of the knee.

Next, examine the range of motion of the foot and ankle, knee, and hip to rule out contractural deformity of the hamstrings (limited straight-leg raising), quadriceps (prone Ely test), and triceps surae (restricted range of ankle dorsiflexion).

Imaging Findings. When a patient presents with patellofemoral joint pain and instability, the following radiographic studies are ordinarily made: (1) AP, (2) lateral, (3) notch, and (4) tangential or axial views. Proper posi-

tioning of the knee and centering of the x-ray beam are crucial.

An AP projection is made with the knee in complete extension. If any significant mechanical axis deviation is present clinically, long standing films are made including the hips, knees, and ankles.

Rule out osteochondritis dissecans of the femoral condyles or of the patella or traction changes such as an Osgood-Schlatter lesion of the tibial tubercle or a Sinding-Larsen-Johansson lesion of the inferior pole of the patella. Loose bodies are best detected in the tunnel-notch view. First, diligently inspect for other causes of knee pain, such as tumors (osteoid osteoma, osteoblastoma, osteogenic sar-

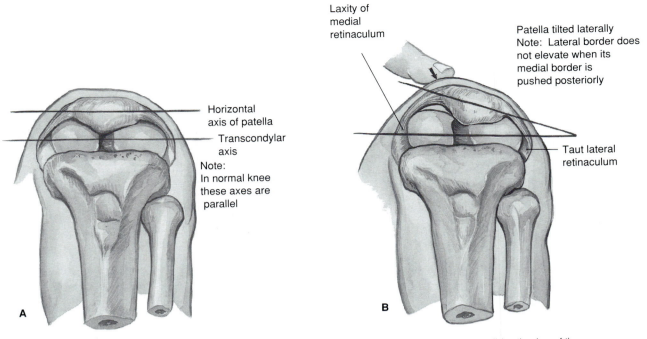

Figure 2–16. Passive patellar tilt test (Kolowich). **A.** In the normal knee the horizontal axis of the patella is parallel to the plane of the floor—the patellar tilt angle is neutral. **B.** When the lateral patellar retinaculum is taut, the lateral border of the patella is tilted posteriorly and the medial border of the patella anteriorly (patellar tilt angle is abnormal). On pressing the medial border of the patella posteriorly, the lateral border of the patella cannot be elevated anteriorly to neutral position.

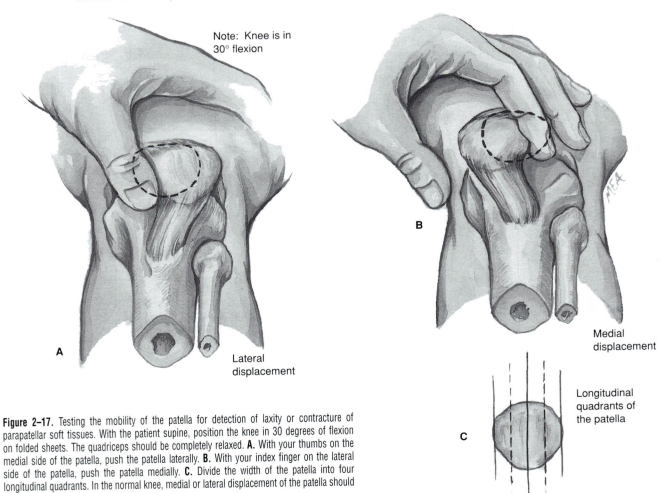

Figure 2–17. Testing the mobility of the patella for detection of laxity or contracture of parapatellar soft tissues. With the patient supine, position the knee in 30 degrees of flexion on folded sheets. The quadriceps should be completely relaxed. **A.** With your thumbs on the medial side of the patella, push the patella laterally. **B.** With your index finger on the lateral side of the patella, push the patella medially. **C.** Divide the width of the patella into four longitudinal quadrants. In the normal knee, medial or lateral displacement of the patella should not exceed one half of its width.

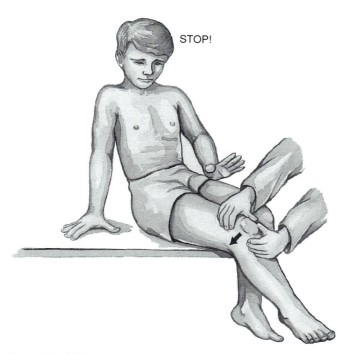

Figure 2–18. Fairbank's apprehension test. With the patient's knee in 30 to 40 degrees of flexion and the quadriceps relaxed, place both of your thumbs on the medial side of the patella and push the patella laterally over the lateral femoral condyle. When there is a history of previous painful acute patellofemoral dislocation, the patient straightens the knee and asks you to stop. The fear of pain and resistance by the patient are referred to as a positive apprehension test.

STOP!

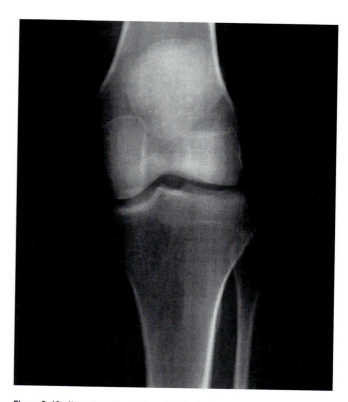

Figure 2–19. Normal position of the patella in the AP projection of the knee, made with the knee in full extension and the x-ray beam centered at the femoral notch. Note that the inferior pole of the patella is in line with the superior margin of the femoral notch.

coma, eosinophilic granuloma, enchondroma) or infection such as subacute osteomyelitis or synovial lesions such as chondromatosis or loose bodies in the knee joint. Are there accessory ossification centers of the patella? Is there hypoplasia of the femoral condyles? Is there degenerative joint disease? What is the degree of genu valgum or varum?

Next, determine the position of the patella. In the AP projection made with the knee in neutral extension and the x-ray beam correctly centered in the femoral notch, the inferior pole of the patella is in line with the superior margin of the intercondylar notch shadow (Fig 2–19).

In the lateral projection made with the knee in 90 degrees of flexion, a line drawn along the anterior cortex of the distal femoral diaphysis normally passes above the superior pole of the patella. When the patella is high-riding, the superior pole of the patella is above the projected line. Also in the lateral projection measure the greatest vertical length of the patella and the length of the patellar tendon. The ratio between the two is 1.0 ± 20 percent.

$$\frac{PL}{PT} = 1.0 \pm 20\%$$

A ratio of 0.8 or less indicates patella alta, and a ratio above 1.2 indicates patella baja. The problem with the technique is the difficulty of accurately determining the lower point of the patellar tendon.

In the axial view of Merchant, determine the *congruence angle* (Fig 2–20).[55] The radiograph is made with the cassette held between the ankles and the x-ray taken above the knee with the knee flexed 45 degrees and the quadriceps relaxed. First locate the lowest point of the intercondylar sulcus (R) and the highest points of the medial (B) and lateral (C) condyles of the femur. Draw the *sulcus angle* by bisecting these points. Second, locate the lowest point of the articular median ridge of the patella (D). Third, bisect the sulcus angle by drawing the reference line RO. Fourth, draw a line from the lowest point of the articular ridge of the patella to the apex of the sulcus angle (line RD). The angle formed between the lines RO and RD is the congruence angle. If the apex of the articular ridge of the patella (line RD) falls medial to the reference line RO, the congruence is expressed in negative degrees; if it falls lateral to the RO reference line, it is expressed in positive degrees. In the normal patellofemoral joint, the congruence angle is −6 degrees with a standard deviation of 11 degrees; an angle greater than 16 degrees is abnormal.

The lateral patellofemoral angle of Laurin is measured by the angle formed between the horizontal line drawn between the anterior highest points of the medial and lateral femoral condyles and the line between the limb of the slope

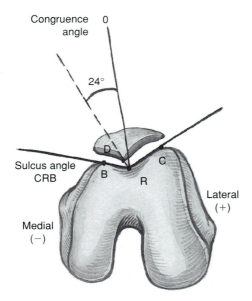

Figure 2–20. Patellofemoral congruence angle of Merchant. (See text for technique of determination.) Normal value is −6 degrees with 11 degrees standard deviation. A value greater than 16 degrees is abnormal.

of the lateral facet of the patella. In the normal knee the lateral patellofemoral angle is open laterally, whereas in lateral subluxation of the patella it is parallel or open medially (Fig 2–21).[52]

Computed tomography (CT) clearly demonstrates the congruence angle, lateral tilt, and degree of subluxation of the patellofemoral joint.[43,44] It is made with the knee in full extension, at 10 degrees of flexion, and at 30 degrees of flexion, the arc of knee motion at which much of the maltracking and abnormal position of the patella takes place. The congruence angle is measured similarly to that of the conventional axial x-ray. The normal value is greater than 0 degrees at 10 degrees of knee flexion. The patellar tilt angle is that formed between a line parallel to the posterior femoral condyles and the line drawn between the limbs of the lateral facet of the patella. In the normal knee it measures greater than 8 degrees in 10 degrees of knee flexion (Fig 2–22). The drawbacks of CT are the ionizing radiation and cost.

Abnormal findings in a CT study of the patellofemoral joint can be subgrouped into three types. Type I is lateral subluxation without patellar tilt, type II is lateral subluxation with a lateral patellar tilt, and type III is lateral tilt without subluxation (Fig 2–23).[57]

Magnetic resonance imaging demonstrates the same patellofemoral articular relationships as the CT scan and also depicts meniscal, ligamentous, cartilaginous, and other soft tissue pathology. It is performed when muscle and other soft tissue or cartilage pathology is suspected. Although availability and cost are problems, a definite advantage of MRI is the lack of radiation.[49,58]

A bone scan with technetium-99m with blood flow studies is performed when a bone lesion is suspected or when the diagnosis of reflex sympathetic dystrophy is entertained.

Patellofemoral Joint Instability in Recurrent Lateral Subluxation. The presenting complaint is peripatellar pain following physical activities that involve repetitive knee flexion-extension movements during which the patella impinges on the lateral femoral condyle. Giving way of the

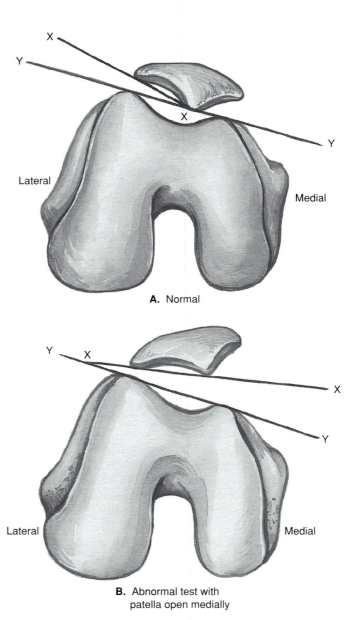

A. Normal

B. Abnormal test with patella open medially

Figure 2–21. The lateral patellofemoral angle of Laurin, the angle formed between the line YY drawn between the anterior summits of the lateral and medial femoral condyles and the line XX drawn between the limbs of the lateral part of the patella. **A.** In the normal knee it is open laterally. **B.** In lateral subluxation of the patella it is open medially or the lines are parallel.

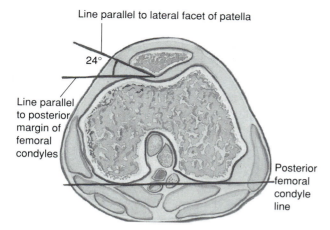

Figure 2–22. Computed tomography determination of patellofemoral joint orientation and congruence. Lateral patellar tilt, the angle formed between a line drawn parallel to the posterior femoral condyles and a line between the end points of the lateral patellar facet. In the normal knee it is greater than 8 degrees at 10 degrees of knee flexion.

knee, locking and popping with minimal swelling, and crepitation are other complaints. Some teenagers are more explicit, "My knee cap slips out of place and my knee gives way."

Physical examination discloses malalignment of the knee extensor mechanism, a taut lateral patellar retinaculum, a dysplastic and weak vastus medialis obliquus, lateral hypermobility of the patella, and a positive apprehension test. On performing the Ober test, the iliotibial band may be contracted. It is important to determine when the patella subluxates. When the iliotibial band is contracted, the patella displaces laterally on knee flexion. These cases are treated by release of the contracted iliotibial band, either by closed arthroscope or by open surgery.[62] In the presence of patella alta with elongation of the patellar tendon, ligamentous hyperlaxity, or contracture of the vastus lateralis with dysplasia of the vastus medialis, the patella displaces laterally on knee extension. These cases are treated by semitendinosus tenodesis to the patella and quadricepsplasty. The treatment modality used depends on whether the patella subluxates in flexion or extension.

Lateral Patellar Retinacular Release. This is indicated when (1) the patient complains of chronic intermittent anterior knee pain, aggravated by flexion-extension of the knee, (2) physical examination shows a contracted lateral patellar retinaculum and soft tissues, (3) imaging documents lateral patellar subluxation or tilt or both, (4) the patient fails to respond to nonsurgical measures of management, or (5) arthroscopy demonstrates lateral tracking of the patella.

Lateral patellar release is best performed through the arthroscope. Results of lateral patellar retinacular release are not satisfactory when ligamentous hyperlaxity is severe

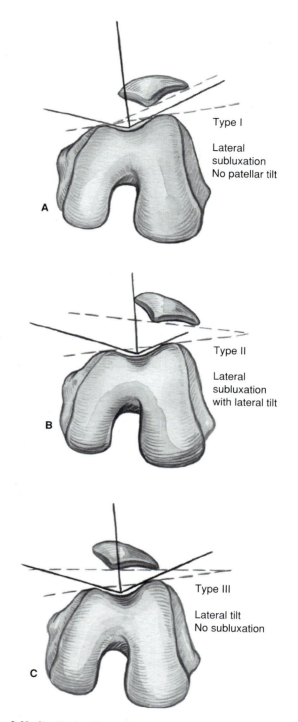

Figure 2–23. Classification of abnormal findings in a CT study of the patellofemoral joint. **A.** Type I—lateral subluxation without lateral tilt. **B.** Type II—lateral subluxation with lateral tilt. **C.** Type III—lateral tilt without lateral subluxation.

or a high-riding patella with recurrent subluxation and dislocation and a Q angle of greater than 20 degrees indicates a severe malalignment of the quadriceps mechanism. These patients require proximal and/or distal realignment of the quadriceps mechanism.

Complications of lateral release are (1) medial patellar subluxation (this is seen with hyperlaxity of ligaments and extensive lateral release), (2) hemarthrosis, (3) electrocautery burns of the skin when coagulation is used through the arthroscope, and (4) reflex sympathetic dystrophy.

Semitendinosus tenodesis to the patella (Galeazzi-Dewar operation) is performed when the patella is riding high, it is dislocating laterally, and/or there is ligamentous hyperlaxity such as in Down's syndrome. *Quadricepsplasty* with release and realignment of the vastus lateralis and distal and lateral transfer of the vastus medialis with release of the contracted lateral patellar retinaculum and plication of the medial patellar retinaculum is indicated when malalignment of the quadriceps mechanism is severe and accompanied by a dysplastic vastus medialis obliquus and a strong contracted vastus lateralis. It is important not only to transfer the vastus medialis distally and laterally but also to change its direction of pull from oblique to transverse to counteract the lateral pull of the vastus lateralis.

The *Goldthwaite-Hauser procedure* (distal and medial transfer of the tibial tubercle) is not indicated in the growing skeleton because of problems of growth arrest, genu recurvatum, and excessive lateral torsion of the tibia.

Post-traumatic Recurrent Lateral Subluxation.

This is encountered in inadequately treated acute lateral dislocations of the patella in which the medial parapatellar soft tissues (capsule, patellar retinaculum, and vastus medialis) are torn, stretched out, and weak. An osteochondral fracture and a loose body may be associated findings in the post-traumatic lateral subluxation of the patella. Adequate treatment of acute lateral dislocation of the patella would have prevented recurrent subluxation. These cases are treated by reefing of the medial capsule and medial patellar retinaculum and distal lateral transfer of the vastus medialis and release of the vastus lateralis if contracted.

Lateral Patellar Compression Syndrome.

The presenting complaint is dull, aching anterior knee pain aggravated by prolonged sitting, ascending or descending stairs, or jogging or running. This condition shows no lateral subluxation, but there is lateral patellar tilt with compression of the lateral facet of the patella on the lateral femoral condyle. The cause of pain is synovial irritation or abnormal increase of subchondral bone pressure. On examination, the apprehension test is negative, and the patella is not dislocatable or subluxatable. Lateral parapatellar tissues are taut, and local palpation reveals lateral retinacular and lateral patellar facet tenderness.

Axial radiograms and CT scan show the lateral tilt of the patella with no subluxation.

Treatment consists of lateral patellar retinacular release.

Recurrent Dislocation of the Patella.

This is usually seen in patients with severe ligamentous hyperlaxity such as in Down's or Marfan's syndromes or familial ligamentous hyperlaxity, Ehlers-Danlos syndrome, or arthrochalasis multiplex congenita or patella alta with marked deficiency of the lateral condyle. The knee gives way and locks. The Q angle is markedly increased, patella alta is present, and the apprehension test is positive. The lateral condyle may be dysplastic. This complex problem is difficult to treat: Ligamentous tissues are tightened, and semitendinosus and, if necessary, semimembranosus tenodesis to the patella is performed. Any mechanical axis deviation is corrected. Prognosis is guarded.

Principles of Management.

The following general principles of management should be followed in patellofemoral joint instability. *Nonsurgical measures* should always be tried initially, even when operative intervention is planned in the future. It consists of the following: (1) Active exercises to strengthen the quadriceps, particularly the vastus medialis, are performed with the knee in extension (not flexion-extension). Quadriceps setting, straight leg-raising, and eccentric isokinetic exercises are performed several times a day, always stopping short of pain. The iliotibial band, hamstrings, and triceps surae are passively stretched. (2) If the pain is severe and disabling a static patellar immobilizer with a buttress to checkrein lateral displacement of the patella or dynamic patellofemoral braces with an elastic strap pulling the patella medially are commonly used. (3) Nonsteroidal anti-inflammatory medications such as naproxen (Naprosyn) or tolmetin sodium (Tolectin) are administered as necessary to provide symptomatic relief. (4) Curtailment of strenuous physical activities such as contact sports, hockey, basketball, volleyball, bicycle riding, and descending and ascending stairs is appropriate. (5) The obese teenager should be on a weight-reduction program, and valgus flat feet should be supported by longitudinal arch supports.[42]

Operative measures are indicated when conservative management fails to relieve symptoms and the patient is disabled.

Prior to undertaking surgical treatment, carefully reassess the cause of pain. Examine the knee objectively by appropriate imaging—radiography and CT scan for patellar tilting, subluxation, and patellofemoral joint incongruity. MRI is performed as necessary. Bone scan with technetium-99m with regional blood flow studies is carried out when reflex sympathetic dystrophy or tumorous lesions such as osteoid osteoma are suspected. Contraindications to surgery are (1) a psychologically unstable teenager, (2) patients who are noncompliant and have demonstrated no interest or cooperation in a physical therapy and rehabilitation program, and (3) reflex sympathetic dystrophy.

The type of operative procedure used depends upon the following factors: (1) degree of lateral displacement, whether it is moderate or severe or complete dislocation, (2) whether it is a lateral subluxation due to a contracted lateral patellar retinaculum and iliotibial band and insufficiency of the vastus medialis obliquus, (3) proximal malalignment of the entire quadriceps mechanism with a Q angle greater than 20 degrees, (4) whether the patella is riding high with an elongated patellar tendon and no lateral bony buttress to prevent lateral displacement of the patella, and (5) the psychological profile of the teenager.

■ OSGOOD-SCHLATTER LESION

The presenting complaint is pain in the anterior aspect of the knee in the region of the proximal tubercle, which is swollen, prominent, and tender. Onset of symptoms is vague and intermittent. The degree of discomfort is mild, enabling the patient to participate in sports and play activities. Running, jumping (such as in volleyball and basketball), squatting, kneeling, and ascending and descending stairs aggravate the severity of pain, whereas rest relieves the symptoms. The incidence is definitely higher in adolescents who engage in rigorous athletic activities. The age of onset of symptoms is 9 to 14 years—the prepubescent period and the midst of the adolescent growth spurt.

The tibial tubercle is cartilaginous up to 11 years of age in girls and 13 years in boys (Fig 2–24A). The secondary ossification center of the tibial tubercle (an apophysis) appears between 8 and 12 years in the female and 9 and 14 years in the male (Fig 2–24B). During this apophyseal stage of development of the tibial tubercle the Osgood-Schlatter lesion occurs. With further ossification the tibial tubercle forms a tongue-shaped bone that fuses with the primary center of ossification of the proximal tibial epiphysis between 10 and 15 years of age in the female and 11 and 17 years of age in the male; this is the epiphyseal stage of development of the tibial tubercle (Fig 2–24C). Finally, the growth plates of the proximal tibia close on the average at 14 to 15 years in girls and 15 to 16 years in boys. This is the bony stage of development (Fig 2–24D).[63,70,71]

Etiology. The lesion is an extra-articular osteochondral stress fracture of the apophysis caused by repeated strong contractions of the quadriceps mechanism. Tension forces produce avulsion fracture-separation of an osteochondral fragment that includes a segment of the secondary ossification center of the tibial tubercle and the cartilage anterior to it (Fig 2–25A). With healing of the fracture, new bone forms in the gap between the separated osteochondral frag-

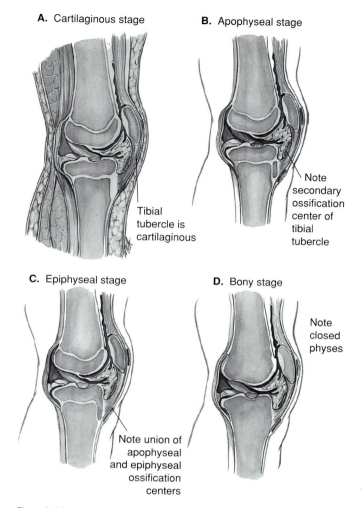

Figure 2–24. Development of tibial tubercle. **A.** Cartilaginous stage. **B.** Apophyseal stage. Note the appearance of the secondary ossification center of the tibial tubercle. **C.** Epiphyseal stage. The epiphyseal and apophyseal ossification centers unite. **D.** Bony stage.

ment and the tibial tubercle, which is deviated and prominent. The patella rides high (Fig 2–25B). Repetitive trauma and stress fracture are the causes of the Osgood-Schlatter lesion.

Contributing factors are contracture of muscles around the knee: The quadriceps (particularly rectus femoris) is taut, hamstrings are shortened as demonstrated by a positive Ely test and by limitation of straight-leg raising, and the triceps surae is contracted as shown by restriction of range of ankle dorsiflexion. The Q angle is increased and gradually the patella rides high.

Imaging Findings. Routine radiographic findings are nonspecific in Osgood-Schlatter lesion. They are made to rule out other pathologic lesions such as subacute osteomyelitis of the proximal tibial apophysis or tumors such as osteo-

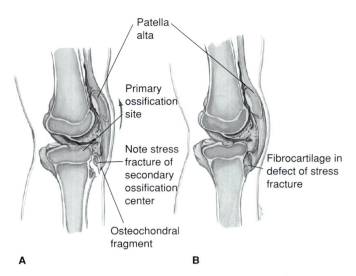

Figure 2–25. Pathogenesis of the Osgood-Schlatter lesion. **A.** Stress fracture of the secondary ossification center of the apophysis of the tibial tubercle. Note the fracture-separation and elevation of the tibial tubercle. **B.** Healing of the fracture with fibrocartilaginous filling-in of the defect. Note the high-riding patella.

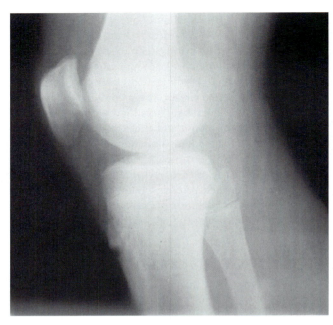

Figure 2–26. Lateral radiogram of the knee showing fragmentation and elevation of the tibial tubercle.

blastoma, osteoid osteotoma, eosinophilic granuloma, and enchondroma.

The tibial tubercle is best depicted in the lateral projection made with the knee in slight medial rotation. The acute stage is marked by soft tissue swelling of the patellar ligament with blurring of its margins and a convex posterior border.

The tibial tubercle is prominent and elevated, with soft tissue swelling anterior to it. Variation in the ossification of the tibial tubercle is great; irregularity, fragmentation, and increased density of its ossification center are common (Fig 2–26). These findings are normal and not diagnostic of Osgood-Schlatter lesion. With healing of the stress fracture sometimes the osteochondral fragments fail to unite with the ossifying tibial tubercle and persist as ossicles that may become painful.

Treatment. The modality of treatment depends upon the severity of symptoms. In the mild or moderate case, symptoms subside following restriction of sports and strenuous physical activities such as running and jumping. Contracted muscles, such as quadriceps, hamstrings, and triceps surae, are stretched. In severe cases in noncompliant adolescents with persisting symptoms the knee is immobilized in an above-knee cylinder cast for a period of 3 to 4 weeks.

An ununited ossicle that is painful requires simple surgical excision; results are excellent.[66] Do not inject cortisone.[73]

A bony prominence of the tibial tubercle may be cosmetically objectionable in the female. Patella alta may pre-dispose to recurrent subluxation of the patella.[75,76] Avulsion fractures of the tibial tubercle are more common in the vigorous athletic adolescent with Osgood-Schlatter lesion. Very occasionally a recurvatum deformity of the tibia may develop because of premature fusion of the proximal tubercle.[68]

■ KNEE EXTENSOR TENDINITIS

Knee extensor tendinitis includes patellar tendinitis, Sinding-Larsen-Johansson disease, and quadriceps tendinitis. The presenting complaint is chronic anterior knee pain of insidious onset in adolescents or children who engage in running or jumping sports such as basketball and volleyball. Some patients experience discomfort following ascending or descending stairs or prolonged sitting. The site of tenderness on palpation distinguishes these various overuse syndromes: In patellar tendinitis it is the patellar ligament that is tender and swollen, whereas in Sinding-Larsen-Johansson disease the site of tenderness is the inferior pole of the patella; in quadriceps tendinitis the local tenderness is at the proximal pole of the patella.[77–82]

Etiology. Repetitive loading of the knee in flexion and overtensioning of the knee extensor mechanism by a force that exceeds its tensile strength result in microtears, focal mucoid degeneration, and fibrinoid necrosis of the patellar ligament ("tendon") in patellar tendinitis.

Sinding-Larsen-Johansson disease presents as a stress fracture of the inferior pole of the patella with partial avul-

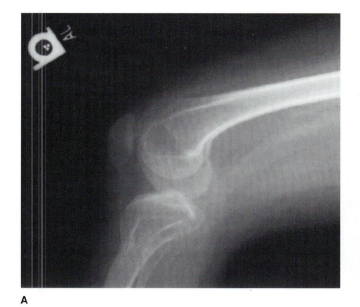

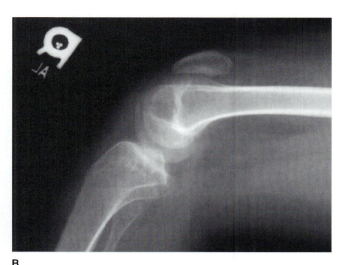

A   **B**

Figure 2–27. Lateral radiograms of the knee in an adolescent with spastic cerebral palsy. Note the knee flexion deformity and elongation of the patellar tendon with high-riding patella. **A.** Normal. **B.** High-riding patella.

sion of the patellar ligament from its patellar origin with subsequent soft tissue disruption. In the adolescent athlete a partial avulsion of the proximal pole of the patella or tear and degeneration of the quadriceps femoris at its attachment to the superior patella may occur. In children showing rapid growth spurts, similar changes develop at the tibial tuberosity (the Osgood-Schlatter lesion), which is discussed separately because it is so common.

Extensor tendinitis is also encountered in ambulating spastic children and adolescents with knee flexion deformity, quadriceps femoris contracture, and hamstring spasticity. In the spastic patient the patellar tendon is stretched and elongated with the patella riding high (patella alta). These children walk with a typical crouch gait and chronically complain of anterior knee pain.

Diagnosis. Ask the patient to point to the exact site of pain—is it diffuse or localized? The location of tenderness on palpation is the hallmark of this particular lesion. In patellar "tendinitis" the patellar tendon may be thickened and diffusely tender throughout its body. In Sinding-Larsen-Johansson disease the inferior pole of the patella is enlarged. Determine the location of the patella—is it riding high? Patella alta is commonly found in patellar "tendinitis." Is there hypermobility and laxity of the patella? Look for other findings of knee extensor malalignment. Ask the patient to extend the knee against resistance—it will be painful. Next, turn the patient to the prone position and hyperflex the knee—this elicits pain at the site of pathology.

Rule out contracture of the quadriceps femoris (Ely test), hamstrings (straight-leg raising and knee extension with the hip flexed to right angles), and triceps surae. Is there weakness of the ankle dorsiflexors?

Imaging. In Sinding-Larsen-Johansson syndrome, lateral radiograms of the knee disclose fragmentation with bony avulsion of the inferior pole of the patella with soft tissue calcification. The patellar tendon is elongated (Fig 2–27). In quadriceps tendinitis, similar findings are seen in the inferior pole of the patella. In patellar tendinitis the routine radiograms are normal; ultrasonography and MRI disclose the soft tissue pathology of the patellar tendon.

Treatment. Mild and chronic cases are managed by partial rest, curtailment of sports, and passive stretching and active strengthening exercises of the contracted quadriceps femoris and hamstrings. The triceps surae, if shortened, is stretched. Infrapatellar straps and taping of the inferior pole of the patella may be tried, but these are usually not tolerated by children and adolescents.

Acute painful knees are immobilized in an above-knee cylinder cast for 3 to 4 weeks, followed by an exercise and rehabilitation program. Very occasionally, intractable cases require surgical excision of the fragmented inferior pole of the patella. In spastic cerebral palsy, lengthening of the hamstrings may be indicated.

■ SYNOVIAL PLICA SYNDROME

In the embryo and fetus the knee joint is partitioned into suprapatellar, medial, and lateral compartments by synovial

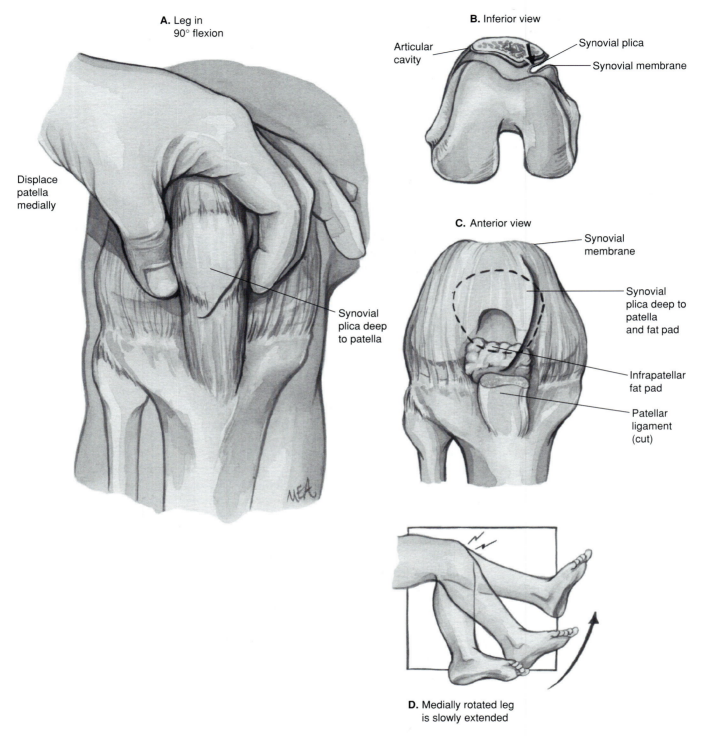

A. Leg in 90° flexion

Displace patella medially

Synovial plica deep to patella

B. Inferior view

Articular cavity

Synovial plica

Synovial membrane

C. Anterior view

Synovial membrane

Synovial plica deep to patella and fat pad

Infrapatellar fat pad

Patellar ligament (cut)

D. Medially rotated leg is slowly extended

Figure 2–28. Clinical test for medial plica. **A to D.** Flex the knee 90 degrees with the foot and leg held in medial rotation and the patella displaced medially with your fingers on its lateral border. Extend the knee slowly—at between 60 and 45 degrees of knee flexion a loud "pop" of the plica is heard as it slides over the femoral condyle. On palpation, a thickened synovial plica can be felt which is tender on palpation.

septa. In some individuals these septa fail to absorb and persist as medial patellar, suprapatellar, and infrapatellar synovial folds. Medial synovial shelves are more prevalent.[83]

Most plicae are asymptomatic and are incidental findings at arthroscopy performed for some other reason. These plicae glide freely and silently on flexion-extension of the knee. No treatment is indicated.

Occasionally following acute or chronic trauma, particularly in the adolescent athlete who runs and participates in jumping sports such as basketball or volleyball, the synovial plicae become inflamed and undergo progressive fibrosis and thickening. Most of these are medial patellar plicae. These patients complain of medial parapatellar pain. On flexion-extension of the knee, a snapping sensation can be felt. Flex the knee 90 degrees with the foot and leg medially rotated and push the patella medially; then extend the knee; between 60 and 45 degrees of knee flexion a loud "pop" is heard (Fig 2–28). One may be able to palpate the thick band of the plica over the medial femoral condyle. When the plica is inflamed, it is tender locally.[83–85,87]

Imaging.   Plain radiograms are normal. MRI detects the plica, but its routine use is not recommended. MRI is performed to rule out other lesions as the cause of knee pain.

Treatment.   Symptoms are usually relieved by restriction of vigorous physical activity and sports. Contracted muscles —the quadriceps, hamstrings, and triceps surae—are stretched by passive exercises.

When symptoms are severe and do not respond to conservative nonsurgical treatment, excision of the plica through the arthroscope relieves the symptoms.

■ STRESS FRACTURE OF THE PATELLA

With the increasing trend toward highly competitive sports in childhood and overuse of the extensor mechanism of the knee, stress fracture of the patella has become more common.

Clinically, it presents as pain after an overzealous repetitive sports activity in which the quadriceps muscle is overtensioned, such as playing hockey or basketball. The patient complains of pain in the region of the patella, which on examination has point tenderness. Active knee flexion against resistance aggravates the pain. Careful history-taking reveals chronic knee pain. Plain radiograms may disclose the stress fracture line or they may be normal. A bone scan with technetium-99m discloses linear increased uptake at the site of the fracture.

Treatment.   Treatment consists of immobilization of the knee in an above-knee cylinder cast with the knee in extension for a period of 6 weeks.

■ OSTEOCHONDRITIS DISSECANS OF THE PATELLA[91–93]

Segmental necrosis of the subchondral bone of the patella is caused by repetitive shear forces. Patients with recurrent subluxation of the patella are at risk. The osteochondral fragment may separate and cause pain; if it detaches, it floats as a loose body in the knee joint.

The presenting complaint is anterior knee pain, localized around the patella, and an antalgic limp. Compression of the patella against the femoral condyles is very painful, and there is painful crepitation of the patellofemoral joint on flexion-extension of the knee.

Axial radiograms of the patellofemoral joint disclose the osteochondral fragment. MRI shows the exact extent and location of the lesion. In children and young adolescents, conservative management is recommended in the form of immobilization of the knee in a cylinder cast. If nonoperative measures fail, the osteochondral fragment is drilled through the arthroscope, followed by immobilization of the knee for a period of 4 to 6 weeks in an above-knee cylinder cast.

■ OSTEOCHONDRITIS DISSECANS OF THE KNEE[94–101]

In osteochondritis dissecans a segment of subchondral bone with overlying articular cartilage separates from the surrounding osteocartilaginous tissues. The word *dissecans* is derived from "dis" (from) and "secare" (to cut out). The lateral aspect of the medial femoral condyle is the most common site of involvement. Repetitive trauma to subchondral bone weakened by a marginal blood supply is the most likely cause of osteochondritis dissecans. During medial rotation of the leg, the tibial spine impinges against the medial femoral condyle and produces fracture of the subchondral bone. Repetitive injury causes nonunion of the fracture. Initially the overlying articular cartilage is intact, but eventually the fragment with the articular cartilage separates and detaches. In children and adolescents a basic disturbance of osteogenesis of the femoral epiphysis may be present. Small accessory islets of osseous tissue separated from the main ossific nucleus are more vulnerable to trauma.

The presenting complaint is pain in the knee and "giving way" of the knee after strenuous physical activity such as running or other sports. There may be clicking or locking of the knee with effusion.

The salient physical finding is local tenderness over the site of the osteochondritis dissecans, which in the knee is commonly on the lateral surface of the medial condyle. Flex the knee acutely and with the tip of your index finger deeply palpate the medial and lateral surfaces of the sulcus of the femur. Next, with the patient supine and the knee flexed to a right angle, rotate the leg medially and then gradually extend the knee. At about 25 to 30 degrees of knee flexion the tibial spine impinges on the lateral surface of the medial condyle of the femur and the patient complains of pain. Rotate the leg laterally and the pain is relieved. This is referred to as Wilson's sign.[101]

Inspect and gently palpate the knee joint for effusion and synovial thickening and increased local temperature. Measure the distal thigh circumference; atrophy of the quadriceps is commonly present. Test range of motion of the knee: Is it full or restricted? Is there locking? When the osteochondritis dissecans fragment is partially or fully detached, a painful click may be elicited.

Imaging Findings. Radiograms of both knees are made in the AP, lateral, and intercondylar (or notch) projections. The radiographic appearance of osteochondritis dissecans is typical: A distinct subchondral fragment is separated from the surrounding bone by a radiolucent saucer-shaped line (Fig 2–29). Measure the size of the osteochondritis dissecans and determine its exact topography. Is it in the weight-bearing or non–weight-bearing area? The lateral condyle of the femur may be involved, although much less commonly than the medial condyle.

Do not misdiagnose irregular ossification of the femoral condyles as osteochondritis dissecans. Margins of the femoral condyles may be roughened, irregular, and indented, and foci of radiopaque ossification present beyond the boundaries of the main ossific nucleus of the femoral epiphysis. Occasionally an island of bone may be found inside the marginal irregularities of the femoral epiphysis. Be more suspicious when the posterior part of the lateral femoral condyle appears abnormal; most probably it is irregular ossification and normal.

Computed tomography clearly depicts the osteochondral fragment. It is performed when plain radiographs are suspicious but inconclusive or when one is uncertain whether the fragment is detached partially or completely. *Magnetic resonance imaging* clearly depicts the lesion and delineates the pathology of its overlying articular cartilage. It also demonstrates any other associated meniscal or soft tissue injuries. *Bone scan with technetium-99m* shows increased local uptake when the lesion is symptomatic; with healing of the lesion the increased uptake gradually decreases. Scintigraphy is indicated when symptoms persist in spite of conservative treatment.

Treatment. In a child under 12 years of age treatment should be conservative. The undetached osteochondritis dissecans will heal without surgical intervention. An above-knee cylinder cast is applied with the knee in a degree of flexion at which weight-bearing and loading to the lesional area are minimized. Ordinarily within 6 to 10 weeks the lesion heals and the symptoms subside. The cast is removed and gradual weight-bearing is allowed with crutch support.

When the diagnosis is made late and the osteochondritis dissecans is partially detached, arthroscopic examination and drilling of the lesion through the arthroscope

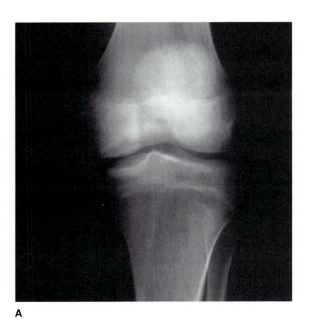

A

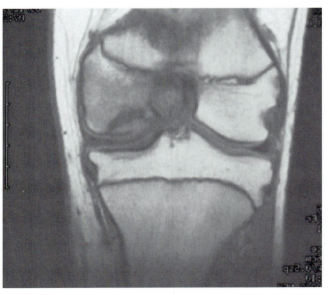

B

Figure 2–29. Osteochondritis of the medial condyle of the knee. Note the distinct fragment of subchondral bone separated from the surrounding bone by a radiolucent saucer-shaped line. **A.** AP radiogram. **B.** MRI.

under image intensifier radiographic control is carried out. In the occasional late case in which the fragment has come loose and is salvageable through the arthroscope, the crater is curetted down to bleeding bone and the fragment is reduced to its bed and pinned with two or more divergent pins (Kirschner wires or absorbable polyglycolide). The knee is immobilized in an above-knee cylinder cast for 6 to 8 weeks. When the loose body cannot be saved, it is removed through the arthroscope.

■ REFLEX SYMPATHETIC DYSTROPHY

Reflex sympathetic dystrophy (RSD) is a syndrome of autonomic nervous system overstimulation of unknown etiology. Psychological dysfunction has been implicated in its pathogenesis. In children and adolescents the knee is the most common site (more than 50 percent of the cases), with the foot and ankle next in frequency.

Symptoms often begin following a minor trauma, or there may be no history of antecedent injury. The cardinal symptoms are (1) *joint stiffness;* frequently in the knee there is loss of both flexion and extension; (2) *diffuse pain*—usually burning in nature and far out of proportion to the injury; (3) periarticular, nonspecific *swelling;* and (4) vasomotor changes consisting of *cyanosis* with mottled *discoloration* of the skin and decrease in skin *temperature* and *hypersensitivity.*

The course of untreated RSD runs in three stages: (1) *acute*—from onset of symptoms to 3 months, (2) *dystrophic*—from 3 to 6 months, and (3) *atrophic*—from 6 months on. Often the patient is seen late with moderate atrophy of the thigh.

Imaging Findings. Radiograms disclose diffuse osteoporosis of the distal femur and proximal tibia followed by patchy demineralization. Bone scan with technetium-99m shows increased local uptake and increased regional blood flow. In obscure cases an MRI of the knee is performed to rule out intra-articular and bony pathology.

Treatment. Early diagnosis and immediate treatment are vital. It behooves the surgeon to be acutely aware of the probability of RSD in its early acute stage, as immediate therapy shortens or averts its course and improves the eventual outcome.

Gentle physiotherapy in the form of active and passive range of motion exercises is performed to restore normal mobility of the knee and increase motor strength of muscles. Nonsteroidal anti-inflammatory medication (such as tolmetin or naproxen sodium) can be tried. They are particularly indicated for local or diffuse swelling of the knee joint. Analgesics in the form of beta-blocking agents can be given in resistant cases.

When the patient is seen later in the course of the RSD with persisting pain, rigidity of the knee joint, and moderate atrophy of the thigh and is not responding to the above measures, first perform a thorough neurologic examination to rule out intraspinal pathology. Beware! Spinal cord tumors may mimic RSD. Obtain appropriate neurologic consultation if indicated by the presence of positive neurologic findings. MRI of the knee is made to rule out pathology.

Then examine the knees under general anesthesia and document the range of knee motion by intraoperative radiograms. If there are positive clinical findings on examination of the knee under general anesthesia, should you perform arthroscopy? This should be individualized, depending upon the findings. Arthroscopy of a normal knee may aggravate RSD.

Immediately after manipulation of the knee, the patient is placed in a continuous passive motion machine to maintain range of motion. Aggressive physical therapy is carried out. It is best initially to admit the child to the hospital and then to follow with the continuous passive motion machine and therapy program on a home basis.

A psychology consultation and counseling are appropriate, with possible referral to a pain clinic. Bier block, sympathetic block, or epidural block is performed in resistant, persisting cases.[107]

■ DISCOID MENISCUS

A 6- or 8-year-old child presents with the chief complaint of "clunking" or "snapping" of the knee with a sensation of its "giving way" or "catching." In this abnormality of the knee, the shape of the meniscus is discoid instead of semilunar. The lateral meniscus is most commonly affected, and involvement is often bilateral. Only rarely is the medial meniscus discoid.[114–129]

Classification. There are two basic types of discoid meniscus—the hypermobile or ligament of Wrisberg type and the embryonal developmental type.

In the ligament of Wrisberg type, the posterior part of the lateral meniscus is not attached to the tibial plateau; its only posterior attachment is through the meniscofemoral ligament of Wrisberg, which is taut and inserts on the lateral surface of the medial femoral condyle. On extension of the knee, the lateral meniscus, having no attachment posteriorly to the tibial plateau, does not glide forward; instead it is pulled medially in the intercondylar area by the short meniscofemoral ligament (Fig 2–30A, B). On flexion of the knee the meniscofemoral ligament relaxes, and the displaced lateral meniscus returns to normal position by the contracting popliteus and coronary ligaments. With repetitive grinding and irritation between the tibial plateau and

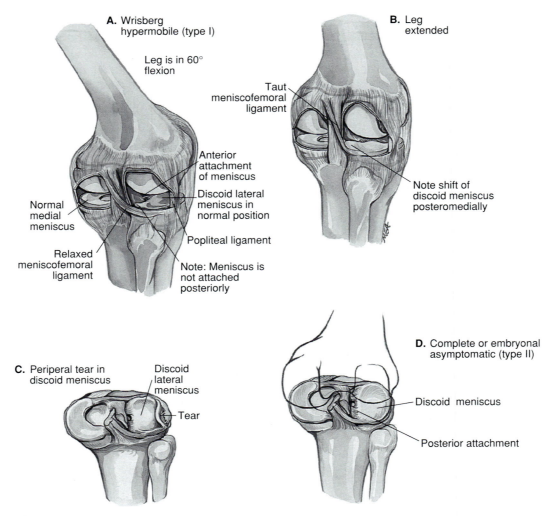

Figure 2–30. Classification and pathogenesis of discoid lateral meniscus. **A, B.** Wrisberg or hypermobility type. The lateral meniscus is not attached posteriorly. In 60 degrees of flexion the lateral meniscofemoral ligament is relaxed and the lateral meniscus is in its normal position over the tibial plateau. When the knee is extended, the contracted meniscofemoral ligament pulls the lateral meniscus posteromedially in the intercondylar region, producing the characteristic "clunk." On flexion the lateral meniscus returns to its normal position. **C, D.** The complete or embryonal type. The lateral meniscus is not hypermobile. Its posterior attachment is intact. Symptoms are produced by degeneration and peripheral tear of the lateral meniscus.

the femoral condyle, the lateral meniscus hypertrophies into a thick fibrocartilaginous mass. The clunk in the knee is produced by medial dislodging of the lateral meniscus when the knee is extended and relocation to its normal site when the knee is flexed.

The second type is the embryonal developmental type, which is subdivided by Watanabe into complete or incomplete types depending upon its source, the incomplete being smaller than the complete. In the embryonal type the meniscus is discoid and attached to the entire tibial plateau. Its attachments to the tibial plateau are intact; there is no hypermobility of the lateral meniscus (Fig 2–30C, D).

With increased wear and tear, mucoid and cystic degeneration of the discoid meniscus develops. Trauma may cause longitudinal or horizontal tears and/or peripheral detachment of the discoid meniscus.

History. Often the discoid meniscus is asymptomatic in the infant and young child. The parents' concern is the "snapping" or "clunking" sound on extension-flexion of the knee. Pain and locking of the knee usually are not clinical features until the child is an older juvenile or adolescent, when symptoms are precipitated by injury. Functional disability is minimal or none.

Examination. On inspection there is no atrophy of the thigh and no joint effusion. Palpation of the acutely flexed knee reveals some fullness at the lateral joint line. There is no synovial thickening and no increased local heat. On flexion-extension of the knee a loud "clunk" can be heard and felt. There may be slight restriction of full extension of the knee; forced hyperextension of the knee may elicit pain in the lateral compartment of the knee.

Differential Diagnosis. Consider and rule out the following: synovial plica, congenital subluxation of the tibiofemoral joint, abnormal mobility of the popliteal tendon, subluxation of the patellofemoral joint, and snapping tendons about the knee.

Imaging Findings. Plain radiograms are usually normal. In the markedly thickened discoid lateral meniscus the lateral tibiofemoral joint space is widened; occasionally the lateral femoral condyle is slightly flattened and the lateral aspect of the tibial plateau is cupped.

Diagnosis is made by MRI of the knee—the discoid shape and thickening of the lateral meniscus is clearly demonstrated. MRI is the imaging diagnostic tool of choice because it is noninvasive and does not use radiation. The only drawbacks of MRI are its cost and lack of availability. In the past arthrography of the knee was made to show the shape of the meniscus and to rule out tears.

Treatment. Most discoid menisci in children are asymptomatic and are periodically observed. When pain and functional disability are minimal, management is nonsurgical by physical therapy to strengthen the quadriceps femoris muscle, passive stretching of contracted muscles such as hamstrings, and restriction from strenuous physical sports.

Surgical treatment is instituted when the knee locks frequently and pain and functional disability are marked. When the discoid lateral meniscus is of the hypermobile Wrisberg type and/or when the meniscus is degenerated with cystic changes and torn, it is completely excised, often through an open surgical procedure, as it is quite difficult to do so through the arthroscope.

The discoid lateral meniscus is partially excised when its attachments are intact (i.e., the embryonal complete or incomplete type), when it is not hypermobile, and when tearing and degeneration are minimal. The central abnormal portion is removed and its peripheral rim is left intact to provide a cushioning effect (Fig 2–31). The procedure is best performed through an open lateral incision. Long-term results have shown that degenerative changes of the knee following total excision of the meniscus are marked, whereas with partial excision they are minimal.

■ PREPATELLAR BURSITIS

The pain is on the anterior aspect of the patella (Fig 2–32). Usually it is seen in patients who are retarded in motor development and who crawl on their knees.

■ PES ANSERINUS BURSITIS

The presenting complaint is pain in the upper medial tibia over the medial hamstring insertion following strenuous physical activity such as running—it is an overuse syndrome.

Examination reveals local tenderness and swelling of the pes anserinus bursa on the posteromedial aspect of the proximal metaphysis of the tibia. Flexion of the knee against resistance aggravates the symptoms. It occurs in the overzealous teenage athlete.

Plain radiograms are normal; they are made in the AP, lateral, and oblique projections to rule out other pathology as the cause of pain.

Treatment consists of curtailment of vigorous physical activity, partial rest, and nonsteroidal anti-inflammatory medication. Splinting of the knee in extension with a removable knee immobilizer is indicated for the acutely painful bursa. It is very rare that a persistent painful bursa is

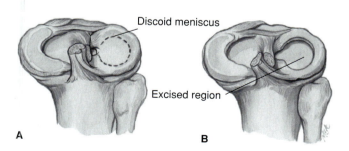

Figure 2–31. Partial excision of abnormal central portion of discoid lateral meniscus, leaving its peripheral rim intact. **A.** Note that its peripheral attachments are intact. The central portion is thickened, degenerated, and mucoid. **B.** Excision of the abnormal central part, leaving the peripheral rim intact, preserves the cushioning effect of the meniscus and minimizes degenerative changes of the knee joint.

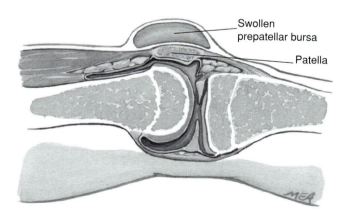

Figure 2–32. Prepatellar bursitis. Note the swollen adventitious bursa anterior to the patella. There is no intra-articular effusion.

injected with corticosteroids, followed by protection of the hamstring tendons and knee in an above-knee cylinder cast for 2 to 3 weeks.

Lateral Collateral Ligament Bursitis. In this overuse syndrome the pain and tenderness are at the posterolateral aspect of the knee, at or above the joint line. Manage as pes anserinus bursitis.

■ POPLITEAL CYST (BAKER'S CYST)

The presenting complaint is a soft tissue swelling behind the knee (Fig 2–33). It is usually asymptomatic and of insidious onset; occasionally the child complains of vague mild local discomfort. The common site is medial, originating in the gastrocnemius semimembranosus bursa immediately distal to the popliteal crease. Occasionally, the popliteal cyst is lateral in its location, and very rarely it may extend into the calf.

The cyst originates from the synovial sheaths of the tendons and contains clear viscous fluid. In contrast to adults, popliteal cysts in children ordinarily do not communicate with the knee joint and are not associated with intra-articular pathology.

Examination. On palpation the swelling is firm because it is distended with fluid and feels rubbery. Ask the patient to get up on his toes and hyperextend the knee—the swelling becomes more prominent. There is no local tenderness, increased heat, or pulsations. The cyst transilluminates. The knee has full range of motion and does not show any findings of internal derangement.

Imaging. AP, lateral, and oblique radiograms of the knee are made to rule out bony lesions such as osteochondroma. Ultrasonography shows that the swelling contains fluid and is not a solid mass.[131,133,134]

A lipoma, which should be considered in the differential diagnosis, shows as a radiolucent shadow in the radiogram. MRI is not indicated unless intra-articular pathology is suspected or the diagnosis is not clear.

Diagnosis. Fluid consistency on the ultrasonogram establishes the diagnosis. Aspiration or biopsy is rarely indicated.

Treatment. Simple observation at 3- to 6-month intervals is sufficient. Most cysts resolve in 1 to 2 years.[130,132] The recurrence rate is high following aspiration. Very occasionally surgical excision of the cyst is indicated in cases when, after several years of observation, the cyst does not regress but enlarges and causes symptoms.

■ SOFT TISSUE SWELLING AND EFFUSION IN THE KNEE

Synovitis and effusion of the knee joint are readily detected on inspection and palpation. When a child presents

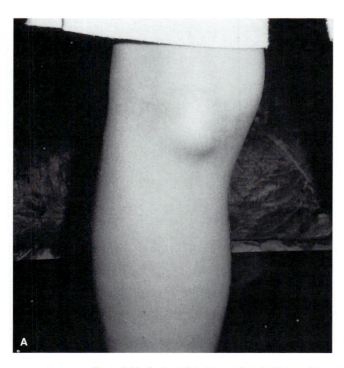
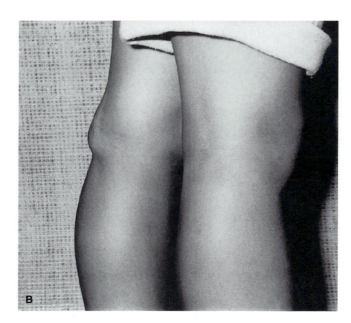

Figure 2–33. Popliteal (Baker's) cyst. Note that it is medial and just below the popliteal crease. **A.** Posterior view. **B.** Lateral view.

with a swollen and painful knee, one should inquire as to the following: the type of onset, whether insidious or acute; any history of trauma; any fever or increased local heat; whether the patient is able to bear weight on the lower limb; and the natural course of the swelling—whether acutely progressive or waxing and waning, decreasing with rest or increasing with activity and weight bearing. Specifically ask about any bleeding disorder. Not infrequently the initial manifestation of hemophilia is hemarthrosis of the knee. Has there been any exposure to a deer tick bite? Are any other joints swollen? Is there any family history of rheumatoid arthritis or immunologic disorder?

LYME ARTHRITIS

Lyme arthritis, named after the town of Old Lyme, Connecticut, where it was first described, is caused by the spirochete *Borrelia burgdorferi.* It is transmitted by the bite of the deer tick *(Ixodes dammini).*[135]

The presenting complaint is pain and swelling, usually in the knee. On specific query, about 50 percent of patients remember a characteristic circular erythematous migratory rash accompanied by joint pain, headaches, and malaise. Upon further questioning they have been in a wooded area with the presence of deer ticks. Examine all of the other joints, as there may be involvement of the elbows, hips, ankles, shoulders, or phalangeal joints.

On examination the patient has an antalgic limp with diffuse swelling of the knee joint anteriorly and some local synovial thickening and increased local heat. If not diagnosed and treated, the swelling becomes chronic. There may be associated neurologic and cardiac anomalies. With any knee joint swelling, one should include Lyme arthritis in the differential diagnosis. The diagnosis is made by demonstration of elevated titers of IgM and IgG antibodies against *Borrelia burgdorferi.* The sedimentation rate is elevated. Treatment consists of administration of antibiotics such as penicillin (phenormethyl) or tetracycline.

MONARTICULAR OR PAUCIARTICULAR ARTHRITIS

Monarticular or pauciarticular arthritis is a mild form of juvenile rheumatoid disease. It is characterized by the insidious onset of pain and swelling of the knee. Palpation reveals effusion and synovial thickening. Varying degrees of flexion contracture of the knee are present. Increased circulation causes growth stimulation of the distal femoral and proximal tibial physis and epiphysis. Examine all of the other joints, especially the fingers, to rule out tumefaction. Also examine the eyes to rule out iridocyclitis. Treatment consists of rest and protection of the knee with

splinting at night to prevent progressive flexion deformity and administration of nonsteroidal anti-inflammatory drugs. The prognosis is excellent with good local care of the joint. The disease is self-limited, usually subsiding over a period of 2 years.

Other rare causes of swelling and effusion in the knee joint are synovial chondromatosis and pigmented villonodular synovitis (on aspiration the joint fluid will be xanthochromatic.[136]

SEPTIC ARTHRITIS

Characteristic findings are acute pain, swelling and marked increased local heat, inability to bear weight on the lower limbs, and marked restriction of knee motion. When the joint effusion is marked, ballottement of the patella can be elicited (Fig 2–34). Aspiration of the knee yields serosanguinous fluid in the beginning and pus later.

Treatment consists of aspiration, lavage, and drainage through the arthroscope. Protection of the knee and physical therapy to re-establish full range of knee motion are important. With early diagnosis, effective treatment results are excellent.

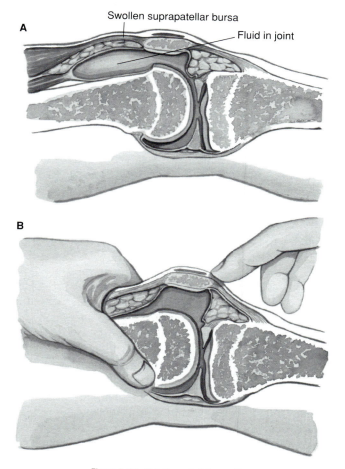

Figure 2–34. Ballottement of the patella.

Pain in the knee may also be caused by meniscal cruciate or collateral ligament injuries. The history of the patient sustaining a sports injury and physical findings of positive MacMurray, Apley, and Lachman tests and instability of the medial and lateral collateral ligaments make the diagnosis.

Rare conditions causing pain and swelling of the knee are reactive synovitis due to a lesion in the femoral condyles; tuberculous arthritis, which should always be kept on the list for the differential diagnosis in spite of its rarity in North America. Synovial chondromatosis, which is characterized on the radiogram by multiple areas of stippled calcification in the synovium, and hemangiomatosis of the synovium should be considered. Hemarthrosis due to bleeding disorders should always be kept in mind in the differential diagnosis.

■ ANGULAR DEFORMITIES OF THE LOWER LIMB

In the newborn and infant bowlegs and medial tibial torsion are normal; they represent the fetal position of the lower limbs. When the infant begins to stand and walk, the lower limbs straighten with a zero tibiofemoral angle by 18 months of age. Then, between 2 and 3 years of age, genu valgum gradually develops with an average lateral tibiofemoral angle of 12 degrees of valgus. Finally the knock-knees spontaneously correct by the age of 7 years to that of the adult valgus alignment of the lower limbs of 8 degrees in the female and 7 degrees in the male (Fig 2–35). The greater degree of valgus in females is due to their wider pelvis. This natural history of normal evolution of the alignment of the lower limbs is documented by the longitudinal clinical and radiographic study of Vankka and Salenius and previous reports of Böhm, Sherman, and Morley.[137,140–142] Extraneous and intrinsic factors may interfere with the swing of the "pendulum" from bowlegs to straight legs to knock-knees to normal alignment of the lower limbs.

PERSISTENT GENU VARUM IN THE OLDER CHILD

A 3-year-old child presents with bowlegs—with the ankles touching there is a wide space between the knees. The child has a rolling gait with lateral thrust at the knees and toes in due to the associated medial tibiofibular torsion. Gait abnormality and toeing-in increase when the child is tired, at the end of the day or after walking long distances. Parents are concerned. The pediatrician has assured them that bowlegs improve with growth. "It is not correcting—it is getting worse!" is a typical parental complaint. Bowlegs in a 3-year-old child are not normal. Does this represent persistence of severe physiologic bowlegs, a pathologic condition, or a growth disorder?

Assessment. *History.* Is there a family history of bowlegs or other limb deformities? If positive, were the legs bowed in early childhood and later straightened, or did they not straighten at all? How were they managed—simple observation, braces, special shoes, surgery? Inspect the legs of the parents and the siblings. Are the parents of short stature, indicating the possibility of bone dysplasia or generalized growth disorder?

When did they first notice the deformity in the child? Were the legs bowed at birth and in infancy, or did the bowlegs develop later on when the child started walking? Is the bowing improving, staying the same, or increasing in severity? Physiologic genu varum improves with growth, whereas pathologic bowing of the legs increases with skeletal growth. When did the child begin to stand and walk? Children with tibia vara (Blount's disease) are early walkers. Inquire as to the *previous treatment* and response to it.

Etiologic Factors. What has been the dietary and vitamin intake of the patient? Is there milk allergy? Any diet fads? Is there any history of trauma or infection? Inquire as to the possibility of exogenous metal intoxication, specifically lead and fluoride.

Examination. First measure the height of the child. Short stature suggests the possibility of vitamin D refractory (hypophosphatemic) rickets or bone dysplasia, such as achondroplasia or metaphyseal dysplasia.

Inspect the standing child from the front, back, and side. The appearance of bowlegs is exaggerated by lateral rotation of the hips and/or medial torsion of the tibiae and flexion posture of the knees (Fig 2–36A, B). Be sure the knees are straight and the patellae are facing straight forward. In apparent genu varum the bowlegged appearance of the lower limbs is corrected when the knees and hips are extended fully and the hips are rotated medially to neutral position with the patellae facing straight forward (Fig 2–36C). Check the alignment of the limbs for improvement of the bowlegged appearance with the patient standing and then supine.

Next clinically determine the degree of genu varum and deviation of the mechanical axis of the lower limbs. In stance and supine, measure the distance between the femoral condyles at the joint level with the ankles just touching each other. Be sure the knees are straight. Also measure the lateral thigh-leg angle, preferably with a long goniometer (Fig 2–37A). Project the center of gravity downward from the anterior superior iliac spine. Where does it fall? In the normally aligned lower limb it passes between the first and second metatarsals, whereas in genu varum it falls laterally toward the third, fourth, and fifth metatarsals (Fig 2–37B). Rule out deformity of the feet. Is there pes or metatarsus varus or valgus or are the feet normal?

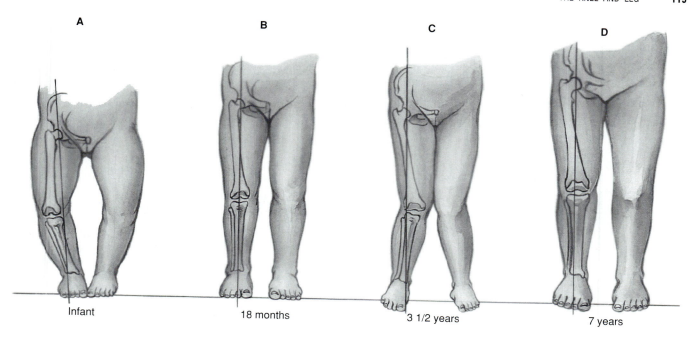

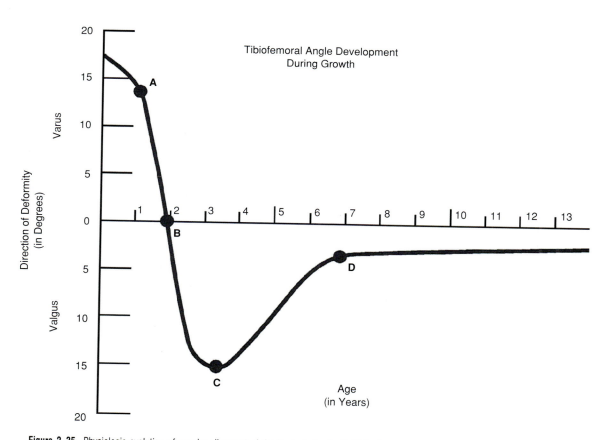

Figure 2–35. Physiologic evolution of angular alignment of the lower limbs. **A.** At birth. Note the bowlegs and medial tibiofemoral torsion. **B.** Eighteen months of age. The lower limbs are straight. **C.** Three and one-half years of age. Note the knock-knees. **D.** Seven years of age. Note that the genu valgum has corrected and the lateral femorotibial angle is normal, with valgus of 7 to 8 degrees.

A   B   C

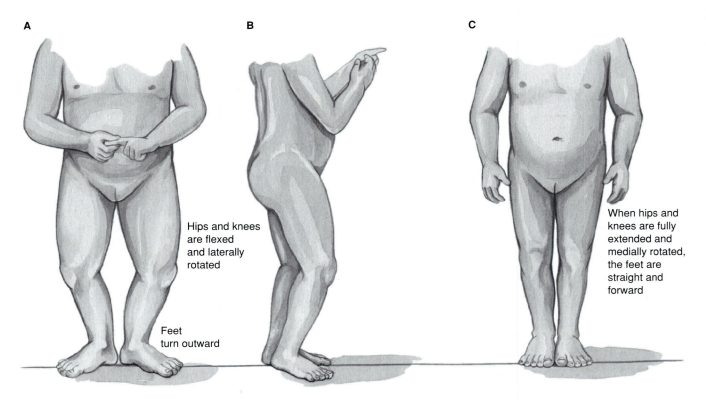

Hips and knees
are flexed
and laterally
rotated

Feet
turn outward

When hips and
knees are fully
extended and
medially rotated,
the feet are
straight and
forward

Figure 2–36. Apparent bowlegs. **A, B.** The lower limbs appear medially bowed because of the lateral rotation of the hips and legs and flexion deformity of the knees. **C.** When the knees are fully extended and the hips and legs are rotated medially so that the feet face straight forward, the apparent bowleggedness disappears.

Next determine the *site of varus angulation* (Fig. 2–38). Is it a gentle curve involving both the thigh and the leg with more pronounced bowing in the lower third of the femur and at the juncture of the middle and upper thirds of the tibia (seen in physiologic genu varum); is it at the knee joint, indicating ligamentous hyperlaxity; is it at the proximal tibial metaphysis with an acute medial angulation immediately below the knee (seen in Blount's disease); is it at the lower tibia at the junction of the middle and lower thirds (seen in the congenital familial form of tibia vara); is it in the proximal femur (seen in developmental or infantile coxa vara); or is it in the distal femoral metaphysis (seen in the very rare distal femoral vara)? When the lower tibiae are the sites of varus angulation, cross the ankles and lower legs; the upper tibial segment is straight and the lower segment angulated (Fig 2–38).

Next, inspect the gait and determine the foot progression angle; in genu varum the FPA may be medial or normal. Is there lateral thrust in the weight-bearing phase of gait? When laxity and incompetence of the lateral collateral ligament of the knee are present, the fibular head and upper tibia shift laterally (Fig 2–39). In tibia vara (Blount's disease) lateral thrust at the knee develops with progression

of the growth disorder, whereas in physiologic bowlegs there is no lateral thrust.

Next determine the stability of the medial and lateral collateral and cruciate ligaments of the knee. Then assess the torsion profile—range of rotation of the hips in prone posture, thigh–foot angle, tibial torsion, and transmalleolar axis (see Figs 2–64, 2–66, 2–68).

It is important to assess symmetry of involvement. In physiologic genu varum and congenital tibia vara it is usually bilateral and symmetric, whereas in Blount's disease it may be unilateral or bilateral, and when both tibiae are involved the degree of affection is often asymmetric.

Is there any disparity of the lower limb lengths? Are the iliac crests level in stance? Measure both the actual and apparent limb lengths and perform the Galeazzi and Ellis tests. In Blount's disease and in congenital longitudinal deficiency of the tibia, the involved or more severely affected limb is shorter than the contralateral one; in physiologic genu varum the lower limb lengths are even.

In the medially bowed leg, determine the level of the proximal fibula in relation to that of the tibia. Normally the upper border of the proximal fibular epiphysis is in line with the upper tibial growth plate—well inferior to the knee joint horizontal orientation line; whereas in Blount's

A. Genu varum measurement

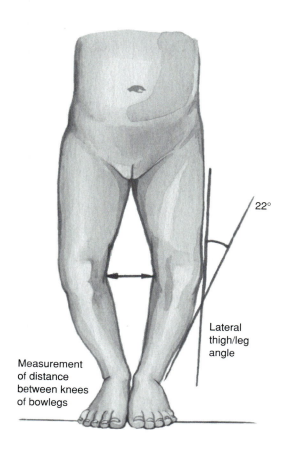

22°

Lateral
thigh/leg
angle

Measurement
of distance
between knees
of bowlegs

B. Center of gravity

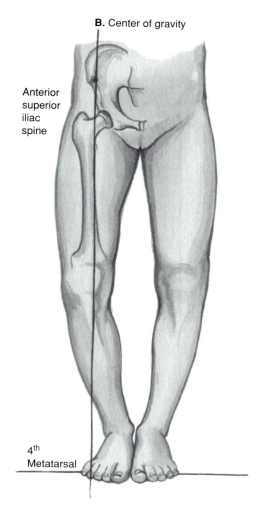

Anterior
superior
iliac
spine

4th
Metatarsal

Figure 2–37. Clinical determination of the degrees of genu varum. **A.** Medial malleoli just touching together. Measure the distance between the medial condyles of the femurs or the medial tibial or femoral condyles. Also measure the lateral thigh–leg angle. **B.** Project the center of gravity from the anterosuperior iliac spine to the femur. With the medial malleoli touching, note that in genu varum it falls lateral to the center of the foot.

disease, congenital longitudinal deficiency of the tibia, and achondroplasia demonstrate relative overgrowth of the fibula, and the fibular epiphysis is more proximal, near the joint line.

Palpate the epiphyses of the long bones at the ankles, knees, and wrists. In rickets (vitamin D refractory or vitamin deficiency) they are enlarged. Inspect the thoracic cage. Is there a "rachitic rosary" of the ribs because of enlargement of the osteochondral juncture, pectus carinatum deformity, or Harrison's groove—a horizontal depression of the lower ribs because of the pull of the diaphragm?

Imaging. Take radiograms when (1) a child is 3 years and older and the varus deformity is not improving or is getting worse, (2) the medial bowing is unilateral or asymmetric, (3) the site of varus angulation is acute in the proximal

tibial metaphysis immediately below the knee, and (4) the possibility of a pathologic condition is suggested by other clinical findings. The clinical stigmata suggesting pathologic genu varum are short stature (bone dysplasia), enlarged epiphysis and physis (rickets), history of trauma or infection (meningococcemia), short tibia and relatively long fibula, and history of possible metal intoxication (lead or fluoride).

Standing long films (AP and lateral) should be made to include the hips, knees, and ankles. Proper positioning is important—knees straight and patellae facing forward.

First in the plain radiograms, carefully look at the growth plates of the distal femur and proximal and distal tibia. In physiologic genu varum they are normal (Fig 2–40). In rickets the physes are markedly thickened, the

A. Distal third

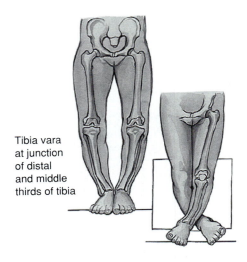

Tibia vara
at junction
of distal
and middle
thirds of tibia

B. Blount's disease

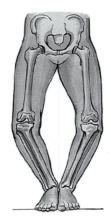

Angulation
presents
in medial
metaphysis
of proximal
tibia

C. Ligamentous insufficiency

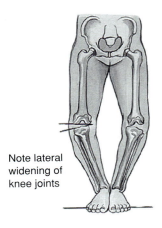

Note lateral
widening of
knee joints

D. Distal femoral vara

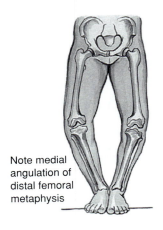

Note medial
angulation of
distal femoral
metaphysis

E. Physiologic genu varum

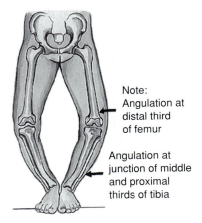

Note:
Angulation at
distal third
of femur

Angulation at
junction of middle
and proximal
thirds of tibia

F. Coxa vara

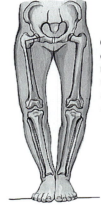

Coxa vara
exhibited at
reduced
neck-shaft
angle from 125° to
approximately 90°

Figure 2–38. Sites of varus angulation. **A.** At the juncture of the distal and middle thirds of the tibia (distal tibia vara). Note that upon crossing the ankles over one another, the lower limbs appear to be straight. **B.** In Blount's disease or tibia vara, the varus angulation is at the proximal tibial medial metaphysis. **C.** In ligamentous hyperlaxity of the knee, it is at the knee joint. **D.** In distal femoral vara, the varus angulation is at the distal medial femoral metaphysis. **E.** In physiologic genu varum there is a gentle bowing of the lower limb involving both the femur and the tibia. **F.** In coxa vara, varus angulation is at the femoral neck and shaft level.

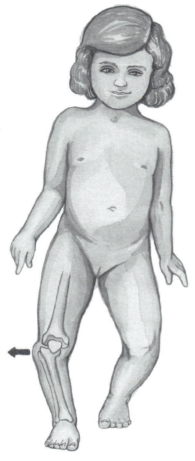

Proximal tibia and fibula move laterally during weight-bearing phase of gait

Figure 2–39. Lateral thrust. Note the lateral shift of the fibular head and upper tibia during the weight-bearing phase of gait because of laxity of the lateral collateral ligament of the knee.

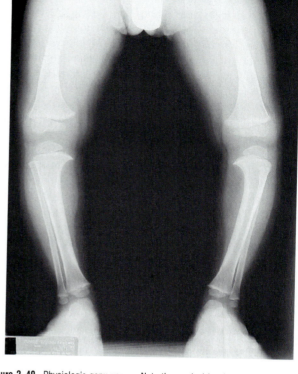

Figure 2–40. Physiologic genu varum. Note the marked bowing of the femurs and tibia. The growth plates are normal.

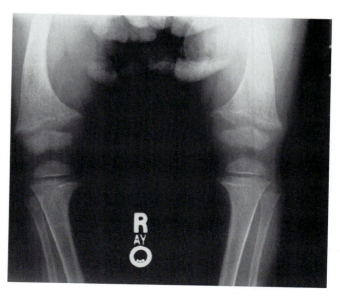

Figure 2–41. Genu varum in severe rickets. Note the wide growth plate and frayed physeal borders of the epiphyses.

physeal borders of the epiphyses are frayed with a brush-like pattern of the bone trabeculae, the epiphyses are enlarged, the bone trabeculae are coarse, and the cortices of the diaphyses of the femurs and tibiae have decreased bone density (Fig 2–41).

Second, inspect the epiphyses, metaphyses, and diaphyses. In physiologic genu varum there is no intrinsic bone disease and no sign of bone dysplasia. The medial cortices of the shafts of the femurs and tibiae are thick and sclerotic. The medial bowing of the lower limb is a gentle curve, taking place at the junction of the middle and proximal thirds of the tibiae and the distal thirds of the femurs. The horizontal joint lines of both the knee and ankle are tilted medially (Fig 2–42).

Measure the metaphyseal–diaphyseal angle. In physiologic genu varum it is less than 11 degrees, whereas in tibia vara it is greater than 11 degrees (Fig 2–43). A list of conditions that cause pathologic tibia vara is given in Table 2–3.

Treatment. Special shoes are of no value. Educate and assure the parents and follow the natural course of physiologic genu varum by reassessing the child in 6 months.

When severe genu varum is associated with severe medial tibial torsion and the metaphyseal–diaphyseal angle is 11 degrees or greater, a Fillauer bar or Denis Browne splint is prescribed with the feet (shoes) rotated laterally and with an 8- to 10-inch bar between the shoes. This is ordinarily worn only at night for a period of 3 to 6 months—not longer. The purpose is to expedite correction of excessive medial tibial torsion.

In the adolescent with severe genu varum with marked malalignment of the mechanical axis of the lower limbs, occasionally osteotomy of the tibia is indicated to correct the deformity or an asymmetric growth retardation of the lateral physis of the distal femur and/or proximal tibial physis. It is difficult to calculate the exact age for hemiepiphyseodesis. Stapling is preferred by this author.

TIBIA VARA (BLOUNT'S DISEASE)

The child with tibia vara presents with the chief complaint of bowlegs that are gradually progressing in severity and not improving spontaneously. The deformity is characterized by acute medial angulation of the tibia with excessive medial torsion immediately below the knee at the proximal metaphyseal region of the tibia.

Tibia vara develops in three age groups: (1) in the *infantile* or early onset—between 1 and 3 years of age, (2) in the *juvenile*—child between 4 and 10 years of age, and (3) in the *adolescent* (late onset)—11 years and older.

In the infantile and juvenile forms both legs are affected in 50 to 75 percent of the cases, whereas in the adolescent form involvement is unilateral in 80 percent of the cases.

Etiology. Tibia vara is caused by growth retardation of the medial and posterior part of the proximal tibial physis and epiphysis due to abnormal weight-bearing stress and compression forces on varus knees. Blount's disease does not develop in infants before walking age and is not observed in nonwalkers. Weight-bearing and walking are requisites for the development of tibia vara.

Children with tibia vara have severe genu varum and excessive medial tibial torsion and they are early walkers. A definite racial predilection to tibia vara occurs in Blacks and in children of the West Indies and West Africa who are early walkers and commonly have severe bowlegs.[152,153] Obesity is another pathogenic, aggravating factor.

Biomechanical finite element analyses have demonstrated that varus knees show marked increase in compres-

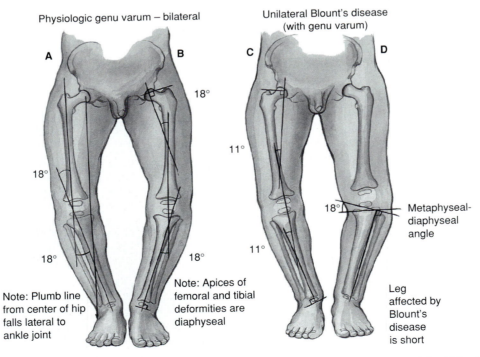

Figure 2–42. Physiologic genu varum and Blount's disease. Radiographic assessment of mechanical axis deviation and site of deformity. **Side A.** Tibiofemoral angle—measuring deformity at the knee. Note the gentle curve of the tibia and femur. **Side B.** Mechanical axis deviation test demonstrating involvement of both femur and tibia in malalignment. **Side C.** Mechanical axis deviation test for deformities of femoral and tibial diaphyses. **Side D.** Metaphyseal-diaphyseal angle—measurement for assessing Blount's disease.

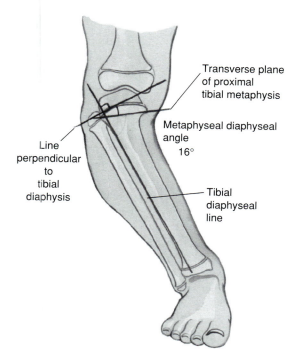

Figure 2–43. Metaphyseal-diaphyseal angle. (1) Draw a line parallel to the lateral border of the tibial diaphysis. (2) Draw a horizontal line in the plane of the proximal tibial metaphysis. (3) Draw a horizontal line perpendicular to the tibial diaphysis. The angle formed between lines 2 and 3 is the metaphyseal-diaphyseal angle.

sion forces across the medial part of the proximal tibial physis. Increase in body weight increases these forces.[147] It is a well-established fact that increases in compression forces on the physis and epiphysis inhibit growth, whereas increases in distraction and in tension forces stimulate growth.

When genu varum is associated with ligamentous hyperlaxity, the weight-bearing forces on the upper tibial epiphysis shift from perpendicular to oblique, which tends to displace the proximal tibial epiphysis laterally.

TABLE 2–3. SKELETAL AFFECTIONS THAT PRESENT AS BOWLEGS

1. *Apparent genu varum*
2. Physiologic genu varum
3. Congenital familial tibia vara
4. Tibia vara (Blount's disease)
5. Asymmetric growth arrest of medial part of distal femur and proximal tibia due to infection, fracture, or tumor
6. Rickets—vitamin D deficiency or refractory (hypophosphatemia)
7. Bone dysplasia, such as achondroplasia and metaphyseal dysplasia
8. Fibrocartilaginous dysplasia
9. Congenital longitudinal deficiency of the tibia with relative overgrowth of the fibula
10. Lead or fluoride intoxication

Pathogenesis of late-onset tibia vara is similar to that of the infantile type. Walking on varus knees and repetitive microtrauma of the growth plate may cause an osseous bridge to develop on the medial posterior part of the upper tibial physis.[158,174]

Pathology. The histopathologic studies of the infantile and late-onset (juvenile and adolescent) types have shown disruption of normal enchondral ossification, disorganization, and misalignment of the growth cartilage cell columns of the physis. The medial tibial plateau is depressed and deficient posteromedially.

The degree of varus of the tibia is greater in the infantile than in the adolescent type because the ossification center of the partially ossified epiphysis in the young child is more pliable than that of the ossified proximal tibial epiphysis of the adolescent. In the adolescent, eventually a bony bridge forms across the medial tibial physis.

Imaging Findings. The salient radiographic feature of tibia vara is the acute medial angulation of the tibia at its proximal metaphyseal region, with changes in the posteromedial portion of the proximal tibial metaphysis, physis, and epiphysis.

To measure the alignment of the lower limbs, standing radiograms are made in the AP and lateral projections, including the hips, knees, and ankles. Proper positioning of the child is crucial. Instruct the x-ray technician and supervise personally. Rotation of the limb and flexion posture of the knee alter the degree of varus. The AP view is made with the patient standing in front of a long cassette that shows the hips, knees, and ankles on the same film, with the knees in full extension and the knee (patella) facing straight forward. Children with tibia vara have excessive medial tibial torsion; when radiograms are made with the feet in straight forward position, significant errors in measurement are made. The degree and site of varus deformity are determined as follows: First, determine the mechanical axis (MA) of the lower limb by drawing a line from the center of the hip to the center of the ankle. Second, draw the MA of the tibia from the center of the ankle to the center of the knee; the anatomic axis and mechanical axis of the tibia are similar. Third, determine the mechanical axis of the femur by drawing a line from the center of the hip to the center of the knee and the anatomic axis of the femur by drawing a line from the periformis fossa to the center of the knee. Fourth, draw the orientation axis lines of the ankle, knee, and hip; a line drawn across the tibial plafond is the orientation line of the ankle joint; a line drawn across the subchondral bony plates of the medial and lateral femoral condyles is the orientation line of the knee joint; and a line drawn from the tip of the greater trochanter to the center of the femoral head is the orientation line of the hip joint.

In Blount's disease there is juxta-articular varus deformity of the tibia with a normal mechanical axis of the femur. Determine the degree and apex of the varus deformity as follows: Extend the mechanical axis of the femur distally and mechanical axis of the tibia proximally. The point of intersection of these two mechanical axes is the apex of the deformity, and the angle formed between the two lines is the degree of varus deformity (Fig 2–44A, B).

Blount's disease is usually associated with laxity of the knee joint ligaments, particularly the lateral collateral ligament. Determine the degree of varus deformity due to joint laxity first, by drawing a transverse line across the subchondral bony plate of the medial and lateral femoral condyle and second, by drawing a transverse line across the superior surface of the subchondral bony plate of the tibial plateau. This may be somewhat difficult when there is depression of the medial part of the proximal bony epiphysis of the tibia; use the lateral tibial plateau. Normally the femoral condyle and tibial plateau are parallel;

in tibia vara with lateral ligamentous joint laxity, the femoral condyle and tibial plateau lines are open laterally more than 7 degrees (Fig 2–45A, B).

Next measure the metaphyseal-diaphyseal angle of the proximal tibia according to the technique of Levine and Drennan (see Fig 2–43).[163] Draw a line parallel to the lateral cortex of the midshaft of the tibia; second, draw a line across the transverse plane of the proximal tibial metaphysis; third, draw a line perpendicular to the long axis of the tibial shaft. The angle formed between the metaphyseal transverse line and the perpendicular line to the tibial shaft is the metaphyseal–diaphyseal angle of the proximal tibia. It behooves the surgeon to remember that malrotation of the leg significantly alters the value of the metaphyseal–diaphyseal angle. It is imperative that the leg be in neutral rotation and a uniform measurement technique be employed.[150] In the early stage of tibia vara the lateral cortex of the tibia is straight, and during its natural course of progression the fibular shaft remains straight. When the metaphyseal–diaphyseal angle is

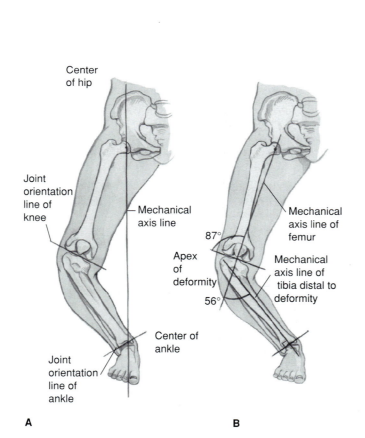

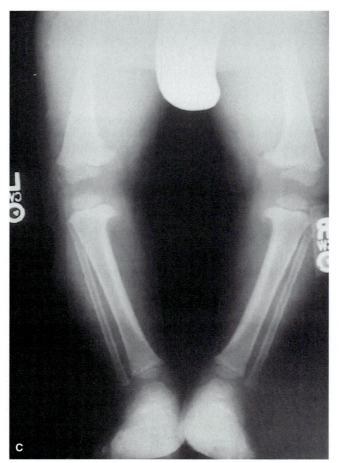

Figure 2–44. Mechanical axis deviation in tibia vara. **A, B.** See text. **C.** Radiogram of bilateral tibia vara.

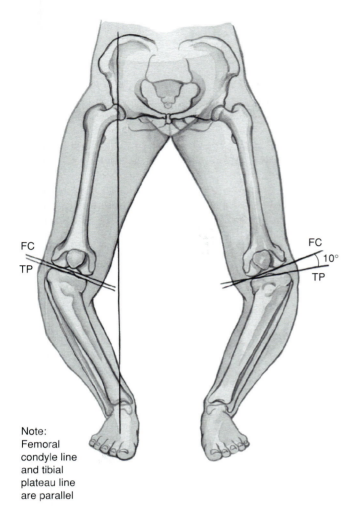

FC

TP

FC

TP

10°

Note:
Femoral
condyle line
and tibial
plateau line
are parallel

Figure 2–45. Determination of joint laxity in tibia vara. The right leg is normal. The left shows laxity of the lateral collateral ligament. Note the 10-degree lateral tibio-femoral angle.

the width of the physis of the proximal tibia; in tibia vara its lateral part is wider than its medial part. These changes, however, are subtle. The first radiographic sign of tibia vara is the development of radiolucencies and fragmentation in the medial part of the proximal metaphysis of the tibia. Gradually the medial part of the bony epiphysis becomes wedge-shaped. These findings are seen in the early stages of tibia vara (Langenskiöld I and II) (Fig 2–46). Tibia vara is a progressive disease leading to mild to moderate and severe medial angulation of the proximal tibia. The periods of progression are between 1 and 4 years and between 9 and 14 years—the preadolescent years. Occasionally between 2 and 4 years of age, spontaneous resolution occurs and the radiographic changes completely disappear. In the 5- to 8-year age group, the varus deformity either does not change or increases very slowly. This variability, of course, makes the effectiveness of orthotic treatment difficult to assess.

The appearance of a "shelf" in the metaphysis develops. This depression is filled with cartilage in the beak of the metaphysis. The bony epiphysis becomes more wedged medially, and the medial part of the physis becomes narrower. These changes correspond to stage III of Langenskiöld (Fig 2–46). When varus deformity is corrected by osteotomy, restoration and regeneration of normal bone structure are still possible, although not in all cases. Recurrence of the deformity may take place.

At this stage growth retardation of the medial column of the tibia becomes evident. The medial half of the tibial diaphysis is shorter than its lateral half. Relative overgrowth of the fibula occurs in relation to the medial half of the tibia; that is, the level of fibular physis-epiphysis appears to be higher than normal and more posterolateral in position.

With further maturation, the "metaphyseal shelf" increases in depth and the depression in the medial part of the metaphysis is filled in with the bony epiphysis. The upper tibial physis and epiphysis show medial inclination. The medial physeal slope is measured as follows: (1) Draw a line through the lateral aspect of the upper tibial physis, and (2) draw a line through the medial aspect of the tibial physis. The angle formed between these two lines is the degree of medial physeal slope; an angle greater than 60 degrees indicates a great probability of recurrent tibia vara after an osteotomy (Fig 2–47). The medial part of the physis is definitely narrowed. With fragmentation, the upper tibial epiphysis becomes progressively deformed and slopes medially. This corresponds to stage IV of Langenskiöld, which is seen between 5 and 10 years of age (Fig 2–46).

Between 9 and 11 years of age the metaphyseal "shelf" fills in further with bone, and a radiolucent band runs medially and inferiorly, giving the appearance of a

greater than 11 degrees, the probability of developing tibia vara is great.

Next it is important to assess the changes in the proximal tibia in the AP, lateral, and oblique projections—the epiphysis, physis, and metaphysis—and in the tibial and fibular diaphysis. Early radiographic changes are an indication of potential tibia vara. The trabecular lines of the medial part of the upper metaphysis of the tibia curve medially in response to alteration of weight-bearing forces in genu varum. Later the medial cortex of the upper tibial metaphysis angulates medially, whereas its lateral cortex is almost straight. Moderate to severe beaking of the medial part of the proximal tibial metaphysis is present. The medial cortex of the epiphysis of the tibia is more dense than its lateral part, with the proximal segment more sclerotic than the distal segment. Inspect

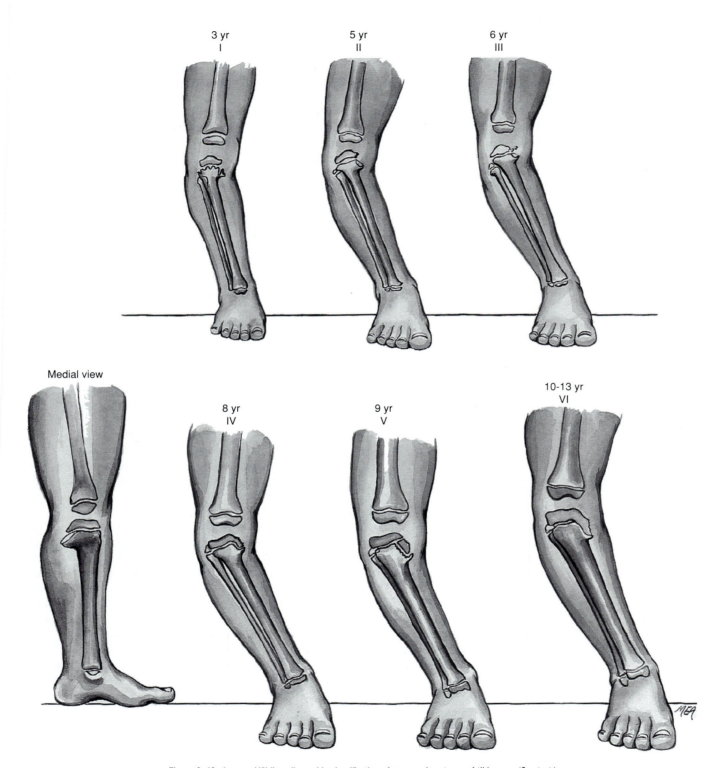

Figure 2–46. Langenskiöld's radiographic classification of progressive stages of tibia vara. (See text.)

Medial physeal slope

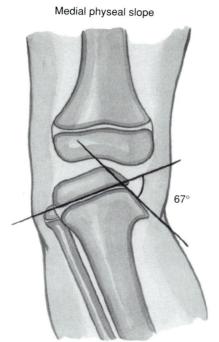

Figure 2–47. Medial physeal slope. Draw the following lines: First, draw a horizontal line across the lateral tibial diaphysis; second, draw a line parallel to the medial half of the tibial physis. Measure the angle between the two lines to determine the medial physeal slope.

Medial epiphyseal slope

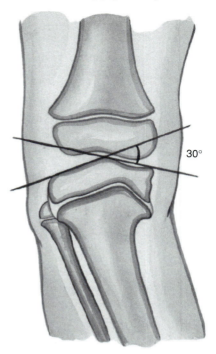

Figure 2–48. Medial epiphyseal slope.

double growth plate. There is definite joint incongruity (see Fig 2–46). The medial epiphyseal depression is measured by drawing a line parallel to the subchondral bony plate of the lateral epiphysis and another parallel to the subchondral bony plate of the medial epiphysis. The angle formed between the two lines medially is the degree of medial epiphyseal slope (Fig 2–48). Between 11 and 13 years of age the two arms of this apparent growth plate ossify (see Fig 2–46).

When a bony bridge forms across the medial tibial physis in the late-onset (juvenile-adolescent) tibia vara, the deformity becomes severe due to asymmetric growth. In the adult, untreated tibia vara results in joint instability, joint incongruity, and degenerative arthritis.[159,176,177] The importance of early correction of varus deformity prior to development of fixed joint incongruity and knee instability cannot be overemphasized.

Differential Diagnosis. In the differential diagnosis of tibia vara, one should consider physiologic bowing of the lower limbs (see pp. 118–120), congenital medial bowing of the tibia, and acquired pathologic conditions such as rickets, malunited fracture, osteomyelitis, focal fibrocartilaginous dysplasia, and Ollier's multiple enchondromatoses. Radiographic features of tibia vara distinguish it from the above.

Treatment. Management depends upon (1) the stage of the disease, (2) the age of the patient and the growth remaining, (3) the degree of varus deformity, (4) the health of the physis (absence or presence of an osseous bridge across the growth plate), (5) structural intra-articular deformation of the epiphysis, (6) the degree of the epiphyseal–physeal slope, (7) joint laxity, (8) weight of the patient, and (9) social conditions affecting compliance with treatment such as wearing orthotic devices.

It is crucial to diagnose early and treat when restoration of normal growth by correction of varus deformity is possible. Primary health care personnel should be instructed that persistent and progressive bowlegs in a child 2 to 3 years or older require orthopedic assessment and observation to rule out tibia vara.

Observation and Orthotic Management. The child between 2 and 3 years of age with persistent bowlegs—no improvement according to the parents or pediatrician—should have radiograms of the lower limbs made, especially if the child is (1) obese with body weight above the 90th percentile, (2) is an early walker, (3) is black and female, and (4) has excessive medial tibial torsion. These patients are observed and reassessed clinically and radiographically when (1) the varus deformity is juxta-articular at the proximal tibial metaphyseal region and less than 15 degrees, (2) they have marked to severe medial metaphyseal beak but no irregular radiolucencies, a metaphyseal–diaphyseal angle of the proximal tibia less than 11 degrees, (3) they have an exaggerated medial tibial torsion of less than 30 degrees on clinical assessment, and (4) in gait they have no lateral thrust at the knee on weight-bearing. Re-examine at 3- to 6-month intervals; if the varus is improving or is remaining unchanged, continue simple observation.

Orthotic management is recommended when the varus deformity is greater than 15 degrees and irregular radiolucency and fragmentation develop in the medial metaphyseal beak. When the medial tibial torsion is excessive—45 degrees or more—and there is no medial slope of the physis, a Fillauer bar 8 to 10 inches wide with the feet rotated laterally 30 to 45 degrees is prescribed to be worn at night only. Such an orthotic device assists in correction of severe medial tibial torsion. Reassess in 2 to 3 months clinically and radiographically.

When (1) irregular radiolucencies and a radiolucent "step" (depression filled with fibrocartilage) develop in the medial metaphyseal beak, (2) the varus increases with the metaphyseal–diaphyseal angle of greater than 11 degrees, (3) a medial slope of the physis develops, and (4) clinically there is a lateral thrust at the knee on weight-bearing in gait, a knee–ankle–foot orthosis (KAFO) is prescribed. Explain to the family that the objective of orthotic management is to attempt to decrease exaggerated abnormal compressive forces across the medial proximal tibial physis and epiphysis to prevent and possibly correct genu varum. It is questionable and controversial whether orthotic support can accomplish these goals. However, no bridges are burned in a child with stage I or II Langenskiöld tibia vara; the results of surgery (tibial osteotomy) are not compromised. The orthosis is a KAFO with a single medial upright (double upright in the very obese child), no hinge joint at the knee, and a strap-cuff at the knee pulling the proximal leg out of varus into valgus. At monthly intervals the medial upright is bent to pull the proximal leg into further valgus. The brace is worn when the child is up and around. The proximal medial growth plate of the tibia is protected from compressive growth retardation forces during standing and walking. At night a Fillauer bar with the feet rotated laterally is worn to correct tibial torsion. An attempt to prevent progression and correct varus deformity is made for 6 to 12 months. If there is no improvement or the deformity increases, the orthotic support should not be continued for more than 1 year.

Surgical Management. Valgization osteotomy of the proximal tibia and fibula is indicated in stage III Langenskiöld in a child 4 years or older who is not a candidate for orthotic support and in a child in whom orthotic treatment fails to improve or prevent progression of the tibia vara. When the child is 5 years or older with a Langenskiöld III or greater radiographic stage with a medial physeal slope of 60 degrees or greater, he or she is at risk for recurrence of varus deformity following valgization osteotomy. These children, particularly if they are obese, should have an MRI of the proximal tibia and knee made to rule out an osseous bridge across the physis and to determine the degree of medial-epiphyseal cartilaginous depression and incongruity. Computed tomography is an alternate way to ensure the health of the proximal tibial physis. If a physeal bony bridge is present, it is excised and fat interposed to prevent recurrence of deformity. The results of bony bridge resection are not consistently good; technically it is difficult to perform.

Epiphyseodesis or stapling of the lateral part of the proximal tibial physis is indicated in the older patient at the appropriate skeletal age; this can be combined with proximal tibial osteotomy. Elevation of the deformed medial plateau of the tibia and restoration of joint congruity are indicated in the older patient.

When lower limb length inequality is significant, limb length equalization by epiphyseodesis of the contralateral proximal tibia is indicated at the appropriate age. Near skeletal maturity, asymmetric physeal distraction with an external fixator (Ilizarov or modified Orthofix technique) may be performed for simultaneous correction of angular deformity and elongation of the limb.

TIBIA VARA DUE TO FOCAL FIBROCARTILAGINOUS DYSPLASIA

Unilateral acute medial angulation of the proximal tibia can be caused by focal fibrocartilaginous dysplasia on the medial aspect of the proximal tibia. The varus deformity occurs at the site of the lesion, which appears as a concave radiolucent defect on the medial metaphyseal–diaphyseal juncture. The deformity is progressive: The varus angulation increases with abnormal stresses of body weight. On gross examination the lesion appears as white, dense soft tissue; histologic examination shows dense acellular fibrous tissue with small areas of cartilaginous differentiation.[178–182]

Treatment consists of local *en bloc* excision of the lesion. When the varus deformity is not marked (less than 20 degrees) simple excision of the lesion and protection of the limb are adequate. With growth and remodeling the varus deformity spontaneously corrects. When the varus deformity is marked (more than 20 to 30 degrees) and is progressive, valgus osteotomy of the proximal tibia is performed simultaneously with excisional biopsy. The results of surgery are excellent.

PERSISTENT EXAGGERATED GENU VALGUM IN THE OLDER CHILD AND ADOLESCENT

Exaggerated genu valgum up to 7 years of age is physiologic and not pathologic. The problem is the adolescent or the child over 8 years of age who presents with moderate to severe knock-knees. The patient complains of pain in the thigh and/or calf and easy fatigability. Parents are concerned with his awkward gait: "He walks with his knees rubbing together, feet apart and one leg swinging around the other." With the quadriceps extensor mechanism malaligned, the patellae subluxate laterally due to an increased Q angle. The patellofemoral joints are unstable. Weightbearing forces on the ankle and foot are abnormal, evidenced by medial collapse of the upper of the shoes. The parents are told that the abnormal wear and tear at the knee will result in degenerative, crippling arthritis of the knee. They demand active treatment. How should you assess and manage such a problem?

First, determine the cause of abnormal genu valgum by careful history taking, diligent physical examination, and appropriate imaging studies. The various causes of genu valgum are listed in Table 2–4.

History. Is there a positive family history of abnormal knock-knees? Inspect the alignment of the lower limbs of the parents and siblings. Are there short-statured members in the family who suggest the presence of bone dysplasia, such as multiple epiphyseal, multiple enchondromatosis (Ollier's disease), or multiple hereditary exostosis, Ellis-Van Creveld syndrome, or Morquio's disease.

How was the alignment of the lower limbs at birth and in infancy? Were the legs bowed and then they gradually straightened and then became knock-knees, or was the genu valgum deformity noted at birth or in infancy? Is the deformity increasing, static, or improving? In developmental genu valgum when the child toes in in gait, he gradually improves the valgus deviation of the knees. Is there any dietary fad to suggest the possibility of vitamin D deficiency rickets? Is there any history of infection, trauma, or fracture that caused asymmetric growth retardation or stimulation? Were the knees ever swollen and hot, indicating rheumatoid arthritis? With increased circulation in the knee

TABLE 2–4. VARIOUS CAUSES OF GENU VALGUM

1. Developmental—physiologic, no intrinsic bone disease or congenital anomaly
2. Congenital—due to longitudinal deficiency of the fibula
3. Iliotibial band contracture
4. Trauma
   A. Malunion of fracture
   B. Growth stimulation by greenstick fracture of the proximal tibial metaphysis
   C. Asymmetric growth arrest due to fracture-separation involving the lateral segment of the upper tibial physis or distal femoral physis
5. Infection—causing asymmetric growth disturbance
6. Arthritis of knee—rheumatoid, hemophilia
7. Bone dysplasia—Morquio's syndrome, Ellis–Van Creveld syndrome, Ollier's disease (multiple enchondromatosis), multiple hereditary exostosis, metaphyseal dysplasia, multiple epiphyseal dysplasia
8. Osteogenesis imperfecta
9. Metabolic bone disease, particularly renal osteodystrophy

the tibia overgrows relative to the fibula. Is there any shortening of the limb with genu valgum? In congenital longitudinal deficiency of the fibula, genu valgum is common.

Examination. Measure the standing and sitting height of the patient to rule out short stature and bony dysplasia. Inspect the alignment of the lower limb in stance. Measure the degree of genu valgum with a goniometer on the lateral side of the thigh-leg, the distance between the medial malleoli with the knees just touching, and the line of the center of gravity projecting downward from the anterior superior of the iliac spine. In genu valgum it passes medial to the first metatarsal. Genu recurvatum causes an apparent increase in the degree of deformity.

Is the valgus deformity of the knee unilateral or bilateral? If both lower limbs are in valgus deviation, is it asymmetric or symmetric? Asymmetry or unilateral involvement is suggestive of pathologic genu valgum.

Ask the patient to walk. Is there protective toeing-in to shift the foot medially so that the center of gravity falls in the center of the foot?

Next, determine the stability of the collateral and cruciate ligament of the knee to rule out ligamentous laxity as the cause of knock-knees.

Determine the site of valgus angulation. Is it at the proximal tibia, such as seen in tibia valga or in greenstick fracture of the medial part of the proximal tibial metaphysis; is it at the knee, as seen in ligamentous hyperlaxity, congenital longitudinal deficiency of the fibula, or rheumatoid arthritis of the knee; or is it in the distal femur or in both the femur and the tibia, as seen in metabolic bone disease and bone dysplasia? Determine the degree of tibial torsion; tibia valga is usually associated with excessive lateral tibiofibular torsion.

Next, determine the range of motion of the hips, knees, and ankles. Do an Ober test to rule out iliotibial band contracture, which causes tibia valga. Is there increased heat or effusion in the knee joint to indicate rheumatoid arthritis? Carefully palpate the epiphysis and metaphysis and rule out exostosis. Rule out lower limb length inequality.

Imaging Findings. In developmental genu valgum the epiphysis, physis, and metaphysis are normal. The horizontal axis of the knees and ankles is tilted laterally. No intrinsic bone disease is present.

In pathologic genu valgum the radiographic features are usually characteristic, and diagnosis is readily made. When an osseous bridge across the lateral physis of the distal femur and proximal tibia is suspected, MRI should be performed. Bone age and CT of the lower limb studies are made if hemiepiphysiodesis is being planned.

Treatment. Special shoes are ineffective. If the feet are in valgus and foot strain is a complaint, foot orthotics, such as University of California Biomechancis Laboratory (UCBL) orthotics, are appropriate to support the foot. They do not correct the genu valgum but do relieve foot strain, easy fatigability, and foot–calf pain.

When the iliotibial band is contracted, it is stretched by passive stretching exercises.

Orthotics to control or correct genu valgum are of questionable value and controversial. I do not recommend it. The only indication for a KAFO is to support the knee ligaments and prevent them from overstretching. It is used in pathologic genu valgum.

In the adolescent with severe genu valgum with marked mechanical axis deviation, surgical correction is indicated. Two methods of management are available: (1) *Hemiepiphyseodesis* is done by stapling or fusing the medial part of the the distal femoral and/or proximal tibial growth plates. Appropriate timing is crucial. Despite all precautions, one may end up with overcorrection or undercorrection. I prefer stapling over epiphyseodesis because it allows a certain amount of flexibility of timing. (2) *Osteotomy* of the distal femur and proximal tibia is performed in the skeletally mature patient. Neurovascular structures, particularly the common peroneal nerve and tibial vessels, are at definite risk for injury. Gradual correction with an external fixator lessens the degree of neurovascular change.

CONGENITAL POSTEROMEDIAL ANGULATION OF THE TIBIA AND FIBULA

This deformity is obvious at birth. The contours of the anterior and lateral surfaces of the lower two thirds of the leg are concave, whereas the posterior and medial surfaces are convex.[185-189] The tibia and fibula are bowed posteriorly and medially at the juncture of their medial and distal thirds. A dimple in the skin at the apex of the bony deformity is often present; it may be associated with an extra transverse crease of the soft tissues, which may be mistaken for an annular band of the congenital constriction band syndrome. The calf is atrophied and the triceps surae muscle is weak.

The affected tibia and fibula are shorter than the contralateral normal leg, with an average percentile shortening of 13 percent and a range of 5 to 27 percent.

The foot is in calcaneovalgus deformity due to the posterior bowing of the tibia, weakness of the triceps surae, and contracture of the anterior tibial, extensor digitorum longus, and peroneus brevis and tertius. The ankle has no osseous or cartilaginous deformity. The subtalar and midtarsal joints have normal range of motion.

Etiology. The exact cause of this condition is not known. It appears to be a developmental defect taking place in the embryonic period. The angulation is not caused by intrauterine malposture. It is not hereditary and shows no gender predilection. Involvement is almost always unilateral.

Imaging Findings. The posteromedial bowing of the tibia and fibula is evident; the degrees of posterior and medial angulation are almost equal. The cortices on the anterior and lateral sides of the tibia are thickened. The osseous trabecular structure of the intramedullary cavity is normal; there is no narrowing of the intramedullary canal and no

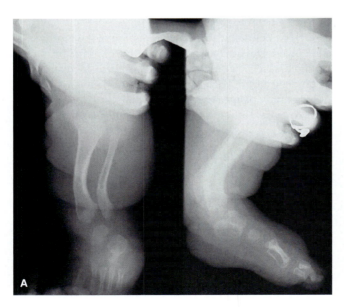
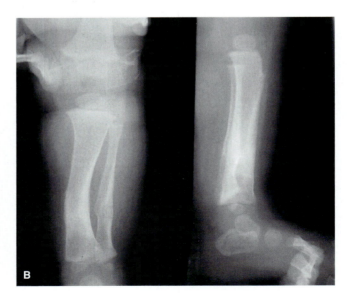

Figure 2–49. Posteromedial angulation of the tibia and fibula. **A.** Preoperative radiograms. **B.** Postoperative radiogram showing correction of deformity.

intramedullary sclerosis (Fig 2–49). Ossification of the distal tibial and fibular epiphyses is delayed. The proximal tibial and fibular epiphyses and physes are normal in growth.

Natural History. Risk for stress fractures is not increased: The patients with congenital posteromedial angulation of the tibia do not develop pathologic fracture and pseudarthrosis. This is in contrast to prepseudarthrosis of the tibia with anterior angulation, in which intramedullary sclerosis and narrowing of its canal occur.

The shortening of the tibia is progressive, with a constant proportional difference in length between the angulated tibia and the contralateral normal one. The average shortening increases throughout skeletal growth from 1.2 cm in the infant to 4.1 cm in the adult. The range of lower limb disparity at skeletal maturity is 3.3 to 6.9 cm.

Under the stresses of body weight the posteromedial angulation of the tibia and fibula decreases with bone growth. Spontaneous correction of the bowing is rapid in infancy—about 50 percent by 2 years of age. The rate of correction slows down after 3 years of age. Posterior angulation corrects more readily than medial bowing, and the angular deformity of the fibula corrects less than that of the tibia.

The calcaneovalgus deformity of the foot gradually improves by the time the infant begins to stand; however, pes planovalgus is commonly present in the adolescent.

Treatment. In the newborn calcaneovalgus deformity of the foot requires immediate attention. In *severe cases*—that is, when the foot cannot be plantar flexed to 20 degrees minus neutral—serial casts are applied to elongate the constricted capsule and ligaments on the anterior aspect of the ankle and the shortened muscles on the anterolateral aspect of the leg. The casts are changed once a week, and ordinarily within 3 weeks the deformity can be corrected. Then a KAFO is worn at night, and passive stretching exercises are performed to maintain the correction. In the *moderate* calcaneovalgus deformity—that is, the foot can be passively plantar flexed to neutral but is postured in dorsiflexion—passive stretching exercises bringing the foot into plantar flexion and inversion performed several times a day and night splinting in a KAFO are adequate to achieve and maintain the correction. In *mild* cases, only passive stretching exercises are performed.

Orthotic devices do not correct the posteromedial angulation of the tibia and fibula and should not be used. As stated, rapid correction takes place during the first 2 years of life. Anterior and lateral angulation osteotomy is performed if the posterior bowing exceeds 30 degrees after 3 or 4 years of age. Simultaneous lengthening of the tibia is not recommended because it is not well tolerated by the

young child. Bone healing is not a problem in congenital posteromedial angulation of the tibia and fibula.

Limb length disparity is corrected at the appropriate skeletal age by proximal tibial and fibular arrest of the contralateral leg when the projected disparity is 4 cm or less. If the projected limb length inequality is greater than 5 cm, elongation of the tibia is performed at age 8 to 10 years.

Persisting pes planovalgus is a problem in the older child. It is managed by supporting the foot in a UCBL foot orthosis. Rarely is surgical correction of severe flatfoot indicated.

CONGENITAL PSEUDARTHROSIS OF THE TIBIA

The presenting complaint is anterolateral bowing of the tibia at its distal one fourth or one third. Incipient or prepseudarthrosis shows no fracture and no pseudarthrosis. The affected tibia is slightly shorter than the contralateral normal one. A fracture may occur at the apex of the deformity; it fails to heal and pseudarthrosis develops. In severe cases the fracture is present at birth; often the fracture occurs when the infant begins to stand and walk.

The cause of congenital pseudarthrosis of the tibia is unknown. It is a bone dysplasia with defective formation of normal bone in the lower one half of the tibia; the bone weakens and angulates anterolaterally, and the intramedullary canal narrows, with hamartomatous tissue proliferation around the segment of the affected bone. Consequently, a pathologic fracture occurs at the apex of the deformity, and pseudarthrosis results because of failure of normal callus formation. Often the fibula is involved with the tibia.

The pathogenesis is complex. There seems to be a definite causal relationship to neurofibromatosis. Fortunately the complex affection of pseudarthrosis of the tibia is very rare; it occurs in 1 in 100,000 live births. Involvement is usually unilateral.

Classification. Congenital pseudarthrosis of the tibia manifests in varying degrees of severity. The most benign form—the late type—evidences mild to moderate anterolateral bowing of the tibia, with some atrophy and shortening of the leg. There is no association with or clinical stigmata of neurofibromatosis. Radiograms disclose intramedullary narrowing with sclerosis and anterolateral bowing of the tibia of varying degrees. This is the *incipient or prepseudarthrosis stage.* Following a minor trauma in early childhood stress fracture develops at the apex of the deformity; the fracture fails to unite and results in pseudarthrosis.

The name *congenital pseudarthrosis* is not correct in these cases; the term *developmental pseudarthrosis* of the tibia is more appropriate.

In the *cystic type* the anterolateral angulation of the tibia is not present at birth; it gradually develops in the first 6 months of life. The bowing is slight but definite. The pathologic fracture occurs between 4 and 12 months of age (average 8 months). Radiograms disclose cyst-like rarefaction in the lower third of the tibia and sometimes in the fibula. Narrowing of the diameter of the fibula is minimal and not significant. Most cases of the cystic type of pseudarthrosis of the tibia are not associated with neurofibromatosis.

The *dysplastic type,* on the other hand, is often associated with neurofibromatosis (in the Anderson series 100 percent and in the Morrissy series 11 of the 19 cases (about 60 percent).[191,200] At birth the tibia is bowed anterolaterally to a significant degree. Fracture may be present at birth or occur when the infant begins to crawl and stand. Ordinarily a definite pseudarthrosis develops by 1.5 years of age. Radiograms show an hourglass constriction of the lower third of the tibia at the apex of the deformity. The medullary cavity is partially or completely obliterated by sclerosis,

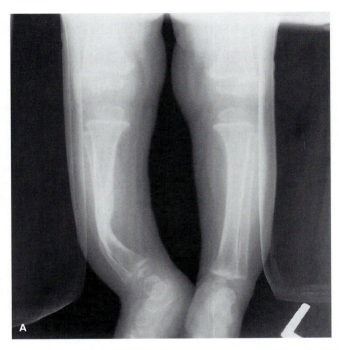

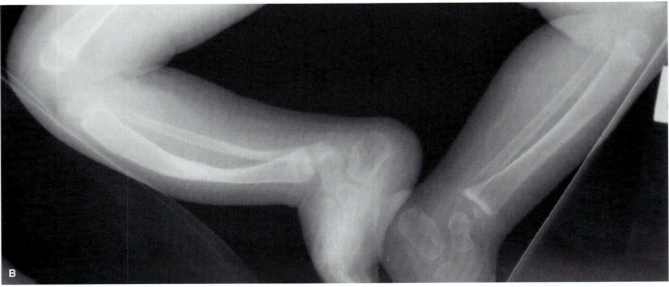

Figure 2–50. Radiographic appearance of congenital prepseudarthrosis of the tibia. **A, B.** Note the anterolateral bowing of the tibia with narrowing of its medullary canal and tapering of the shaft with decrease in its diameter.

and the diameter of the tibia is narrowed (Fig 2–50). The bone ends at the fracture site taper and are encased by hamartomatous fibrous tissue. Often the fibula is involved as well. Refracture and non-union are perpetual problems in the dysplastic type.

Treatment. The modality of management depends upon the type of congenital pseudarthrosis of the tibia and whether the pseudarthrosis is already present or is in its incipient phase. The problem is complex, often requiring multiple operations. The results are unpredictable, and at best the leg is short and dysplastic and prone to refracture and pseudarthrosis.

In the beginning it is best to explain the problems of obtaining and maintaining union, the complications, and the likelihood of eventual amputation to the parents.

In the incipient or prepseudarthrosis phase the objective of treatment is to prevent stress fracture of the anterolaterally bowed tibia whose medullary cavity is narrowed with partial to complete sclerosis. In the infant before standing, support the limb in an above-knee orthosis. Prior to walking age, perform a McFarland posterior autogenous bone graft bypass operation.[196,199] This reduces the risk of fracture but does not eliminate it. Continue to support the limb in an above-knee orthosis with an anterior shell support.

When fracture has taken place and definite pseudarthrosis has developed, one has to choose between (1) double-onlay bone grafting and intramedullary pin fixation, (2) Ilizarov technique of compression by bone transport, or (3) free vascularized fibular transplant. In every surgery, the hamartomatous and fibrous tissue at the pseudarthrosis site should be excised, the sclerotic bone should be removed, and the mechanical axis deviation of the anterolateral angulation should be corrected. At present I recommend the following: (1) Reserve free vascularized fibular transplant for failed cases. The procedure is a major one with the potential for serious complications and refracture. Use it only as a last resort. (2) In the dysplastic type, use the Ilizarov technique of compression and bone transport. After union is achieved, the limb is protected in an above-knee orthosis with an anterior shell. Despite protection in a brace, the incidence of refracture is high. Therefore, intramedullary pin fixation is performed after complete union is achieved.

In the cystic type, dual onlay graft with intramedullary fixation is an effective way to obtain union.

CONGENITAL PSEUDARTHROSIS OF THE FIBULA

The presenting complaint may be (1) local swelling and pain at the pseudarthrosis site (usually distal metaphyseal–diaphyseal region), and/or (2) eversion of the hindfoot due to ankle valgus, and (3) slight shortening of the leg due to concomitant involvement of the tibia with prepseudarthrosis. In infancy or early childhood, pseudarthrosis of the fibula may remain clinically silent. Close inspection reveals some lateral bowing of the fibula at the pseudarthrosis site, and the lateral malleolus rides high compared with the contralateral normal side and in relation to the medial malleolus.

Imaging. Radiographic findings depend upon the severity of involvement. The medullary canal is narrowed with sclerosis, the fibula is bowed laterally, the fibula is short with high-riding lateral malleolus and ankle valgus. Pseudarthrosis may be present at the fracture site. Pure pseudarthrosis of the fibula is very rare. Always carefully assess the tibia for intramedullary sclerosis and incipient pseudarthrosis (Fig 2–51).

Treatment. When the ankle joint is normally oriented or ankle valgus is minimal, pseudarthrosis of the fibula is treated by excision of the pseudarthrosis, bone grafting, and intramedullary fixation. When concomitant incipient pseudarthrosis of the tibia is present, posterior by-pass bone grafting is performed, with excision of the local hamartomatous soft tissue choking the tibia.

When there is progressive ankle valgus, distal fibular-tibial synostosis (Langenskiöld procedure) is performed. Severe ankle valgus is corrected by supramalleolar osteotomy.

CONGENITAL LONGITUDINAL DEFICIENCY OF THE FIBULA

The presenting complaint is a short leg with the foot twisted outward. The deformity is present at birth with varying degrees of severity. Congenital longitudinal deficiency of the fibula may vary in its manifestation from minimal hypoplasia to complete aplasia of the entire fibula. It is caused by failure of formation or arrest of development of the fibula. Because the anlage of the limb develops between the sixth and seventh week of embryonic life, the aberration of formation of the fibula must take place prior to 8 weeks of gestation. Its exact teratogenic cause is unknown. Heredity is not a factor.

Involvement often is unilateral; bilateral cases are rare. It is more prevalent in the female. Although it is a relatively uncommon anomaly, longitudinal deficiency of the fibula is the most common, followed in frequency by that of the radius.

Classification. Based upon the severity of the deficiency, Achterman and Kalamchi[212] classified congenital longitudinal deficiency of the fibula as follows: type IA—the entire

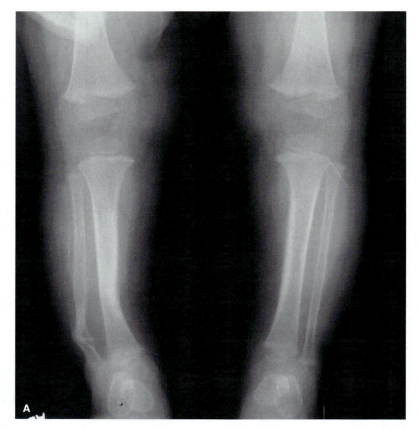

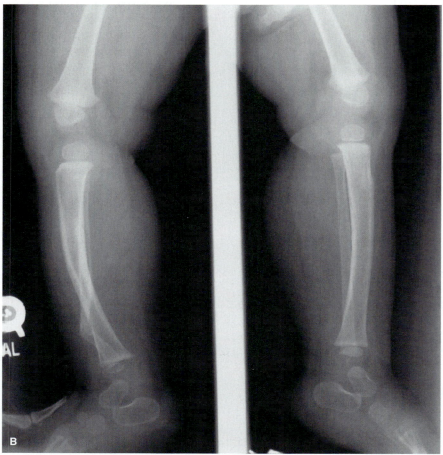

Figure 2–51. Congenital pseudarthrosis of the fibula with prepseudarthrosis of the tibia. **A, B.** AP and lateral views of the hip. Note the pseudarthrosis of the right fibula and the bowing of the tibia with intramedullary sclerosis. This was treated by excision of the pseudarthrosis of the fibula, grafting, and intramedullary fixation with an intramedullary nail. The hamartomatous tissue around the tibial prepseudarthrosis site was excised and a posterior bypass graft was applied. *(Continues)*

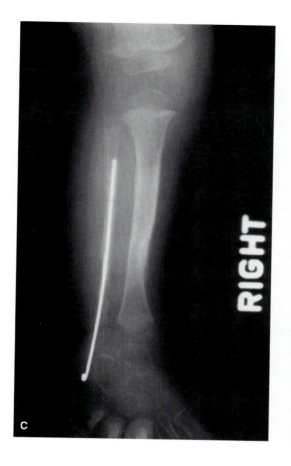

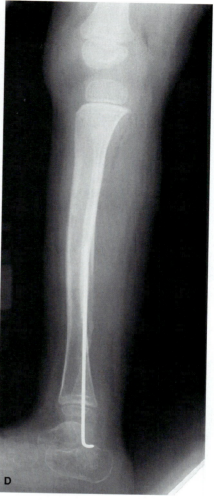

Figure 2–51 *(Continued)*. C, D. AP and lateral postoperative radiograms showing the healing of the pseudarthrosis and the posterior bypass graft.

fibula is present but hypoplastic and shortened with its upper epiphysis distal to the proximal physis of the tibia and the distal fibular physis proximal to the ankle joint (Fig 2–52A); type IB—the longitudinal deficiency is more severe, with one third to one half of the proximal fibula absent (Fig 2–52B); type II—only a distal vestigial fibrocartilaginous anlage of the fibula is present or the entire fibula is absent (Figs 2–52C-D, 2–53, and 2–54).[212]

Associated Anomalies. Congenital longitudinal deficiency of the fibula is not an isolated deformity but rather part of a wide spectrum of dysplasia of the entire lower limb. It represents a developmental field defect.

The tibia is almost always short and in type II deformities is bowed anteromedially. Other associated anomalies include absence of the lateral rays of the foot, coalition of the tarsal bones (especially talocalcaneal), equinovalgus deformity of the foot and ankle, ball-and-socket ankle joint, congenital shortening of the femur, genu valgum, absence of the anterior or posterior cruciate ligaments with anteroposterior instability of the knee, and hypoplastic and high-riding patella with instability of the patellofemoral joint. Other major but rare congenital malformations can occur in association with congenital longitudinal deficiency of the fibula, such as proximal focal femoral deficiency, absence of part or all of an upper limb, absence of ulnar rays in the hand, and syndactyly. Visceral abnormalities of the heart and kidney are very rare (Table 2–5). (See page 141.)

Clinical Features. Physical findings depend upon the type and severity of the deficiency of the fibula. Affected limbs in all cases are abnormally short with varying

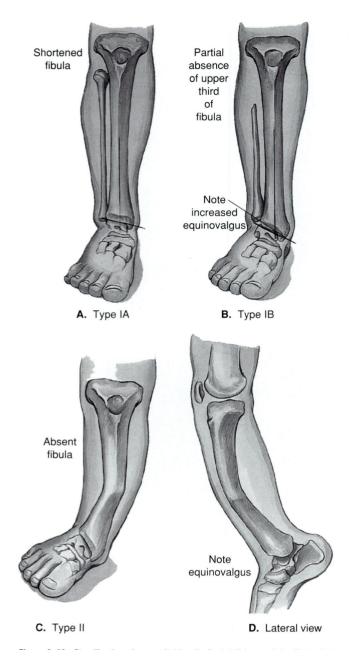

Shortened fibula

Partial absence of upper third of fibula

Note increased equinovalgus

A. Type IA

B. Type IB

Absent fibula

Note equinovalgus

C. Type II

D. Lateral view

Figure 2–52. Classification of congenital longitudinal deficiency of the fibula (Achterman and Kalamchi). **A.** Type IA. The entire fibula is present but hypoplastic. **B.** Partial absence of the upper third of the fibula. **C, D.** Type II. Entire fibula is absent, or only a distal fibrocartilaginous anlage of the fibula is present.

degrees of atrophy, and diminution in the girth of the calf.

When the entire fibula is present but hypoplastic, the shortening of the limb is minimal (less than 2 cm). The lateral malleolus is present but rides high. The ankle is in slight valgus and equinus but stable. Ordinarily the foot is normal. The knee joint is stable.

When the upper one third or one half of the fibula is absent, the predicted shortening of the tibia at skeletal ma-

turity is moderate (5 cm or less). The greater the deficiency of the fibula, the more severe the shortening of the tibia. The femur of the affected lower limb is short, ranging from 1 to 3 percent of the length of the contralateral normal femur. The tibia is slightly bowed anteromedially. Valgus deformity of the knee is present but minimal. The ankle and foot are in moderate equinovalgus deformity. Occasionally the midfoot and forefoot are in some degree of inversion and adduction to compensate for equinovalgus deformity of the ankle. The lateral malleolus is palpable, but it is high riding and small. Talocalcaneal coalition with a stiff hindfoot and ball-and-socket ankle joint may be present. One or occasionally two of the lateral rays of the foot may be absent.

When the fibular absence is total or only a vestigial distal fibular anlage is present, the shortening of the limb is marked to very severe. Both the tibia and femur are short.

Choi et al[217] classified the inequality between the lower limbs into three groups: *Group I*—The foot of the shorter limb is at the distal third of the contralateral normal limb with a shortening of 15 percent or less, with a predicted limb length inequality at skeletal maturity of 0.5 to 12 cm. *Group II*—The foot of the shorter limb is at the level of the middle third of the normal limb with a shortening between 16 and 25 percent with a predicted limb length disparity at maturity of 12.5 to 23 cm. *Group III*—The foot of the shorter limb is at the level of the proximal third of the contralateral normal limb with a shortening of greater than 26 percent with a predicted limb length inequality of greater than 23 cm.[217]

The short tibia is angulated anteromedially to a varying degree, with dimpling of the skin at the apex of the curve. The lateral malleolus is hypoplastic or high-riding or is absent and cannot be palpated. There is moderate to severe equinovalgus deformity of the foot and ankle. The fibrous or fibrocartilaginous anlage of the fibula acts as a lateral and posterior tether and deforming force, angulating the tibia anteromedially. Distally the fibrous anlage of the fibula inserts to the calcaneus and pulls the foot and ankle into equinovalgus. The fibrosed peroneals and contracted triceps surae are additional contributors to equinovalgus deformity of the foot and ankle. Ankle joint instability and lateral subluxation are often present due to absence of the lateral malleolus. Coalition of the talus and calcaneus with rigidity of the hindfoot and hypoplasia of the tarsal bones and atrophy of the foot are common.

In total absence of the fibula the lateral rays of the foot, ordinarily the fifth and fourth, are often absent. In very severe deficiency of the fibula the foot may be functionless, with absence of the third, fourth, and fifth rays and poor motor control of the foot and ankle.

The mechanical axis of the lower limb is displaced laterally due to medial angulation of the tibia at the juncture of its middle and distal thirds and to genu valgum deformity due to hypoplasia of the lateral condyle of the femur with

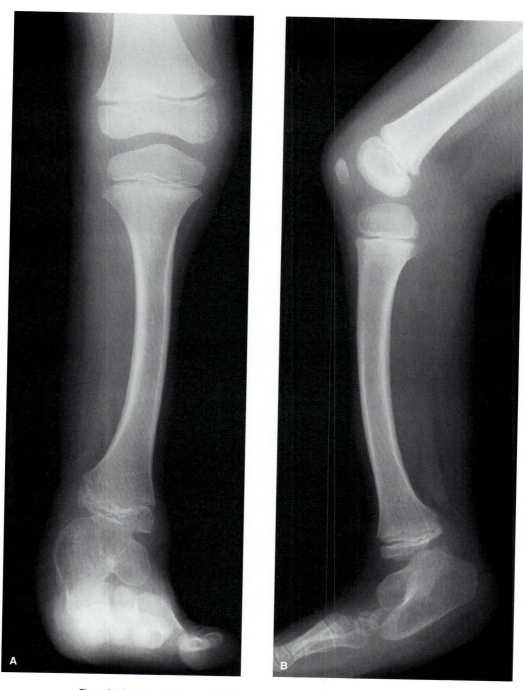

Figure 2–53. Congenital absence of fibula—type II. **A.** Anteroposterior view. **B.** Lateral view.

increase in medial-lateral condylar height ratio. The axis of the knee joint is not parallel to the floor; it is tilted laterally. Boakes et al have proposed that lateral femoral condylar hypoplasia and progressive genu valgum deformity are due to inhibition of growth caused by abnormal compression and stress in the lateral compartment of the knee.[214] The patella is hypoplastic, high-riding, and often subluxated laterally.

Anteroposterior knee instability is common and is caused by absence of either the anterior or posterior cruciates or both.

Treatment. The goals of treatment are provision of a plantigrade functional foot and equality of lower limb lengths.

In simple hypoplasia of the fibula and mild forms of partial absence of the proximal fibula with short tibia, the

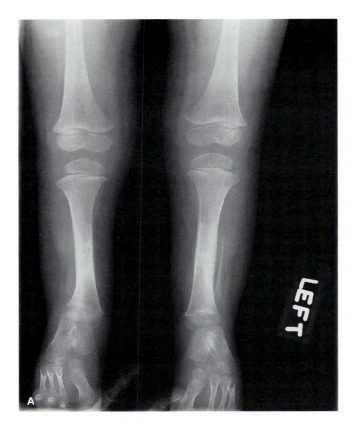

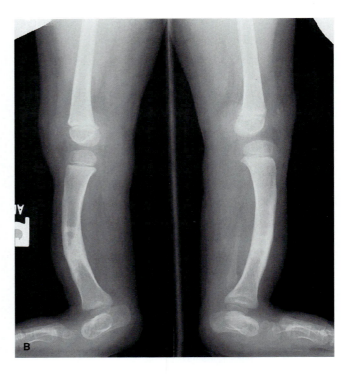

Figure 2–54. Bilateral absence of the fibula—type II on the right and type IB on the left. **A.** Anteroposterior view. **B.** Lateral view. Note that the distal fibula on the left is partially present but hypoplastic.

predicted lower limb disparity at skeletal maturity ordinarily is less than 4 to 5 cm, and the foot and ankle are quite functional. In these less severe forms of longitudinal deficiency of the fibula, treatment is relatively simple. In the infant and child, alignment of the foot and ankle is provided and maintained by passive exercises stretching the peroneals and triceps surae and splinting the foot and ankle in neutral position at night in an ankle–foot orthosis (AFO). When the child begins independent ambulation, a lift in the shoe is worn to compensate the spine and correct the short leg limp. Disparity of growth of the lower limbs is followed and at the appropriate skeletal age epiphyseodeses of the contralateral proximal tibia and fibula are performed to equalize limb lengths. Ankle valgus usually is not a problem; however, if it is progressive and exceeds 15 to 20 degrees, it is treated by supramalleolar varus angulation and medial displacement osteotomy of the tibia.

In severe deficiency with complete absence of the fibula or with only a vestigial anlage of the fibula present distally, management is difficult and complex. The problems are the marked lower limb inequality, the severity of deformity of the foot, the instability of the ankle, the degree of mechanical axis deviation of the lower limb due to medial and anterior bowing of the tibia at its distal third

and valgus deformity at the knee, the instability of the knee due to absence of the cruciate ligaments, the associated deformities of the femur and hip, and the psychosocial response of the patient and parents to amputation versus multiple surgical procedures and multiple hospitalizations.

Syme's amputation is performed when the foot is so severely deformed that a functional and plantigrade foot cannot be provided by surgery. Feet with only two rays, severe hypoplasia and absence of tarsal bones, or rigidity due to coalition of tarsal bones should be ablated.[219,220,223]

A foot with absence of the two lateral rays presents a difficult problem in decision-making. Syme's amputation is performed when the foot is hypoplastic and rigid, with coalition and absence of tarsal bones and poor motor control of the foot and ankle due to muscle atrophy and contracture. Ablation of the foot should be performed early before the infant begins to stand and walk independently. Syme's amputation provides proprioception in gait and an end-bearing stump that can be walked on. In children, revision of Syme's amputation is rarely necessary. In the prosthesis, cosmetic appearance and gait are very satisfactory.

The three- or four-ray foot is preserved when it is of adequate size, is flexible, and motor control is good. The

TABLE 2–5. ASSOCIATED ANOMALIES IN CONGENITAL LONGITUDINAL DEFICIENCY OF THE FIBULA

Common

Leg-Tibia	Short, bowed anteromedially
	Dimples of the skin at the apex of the anteromedial angulation of the tibia
Foot-Ankle	Valgus and equinus deformity
	Lateral subluxation of the ankle joint with interposition of deltoid ligament between medial malleolus and talus
	Ball and socket ankle joint
	Tarsal coalition, particularly of talus and calcaneus with rigidity of the hindfoot
	Absence of the lateral rays of the foot
	Delay in ossification of tarsal bones and distal tibial epiphysis
Knee-Leg	Genu valgum with deficiency of the lateral condyle of the femur and/or the lateral tibial epiphysis
	Absence of cruciate ligaments with anteroposterior instability of the knee
	Hypoplastic and high-riding patella with lateral subluxation
	Triceps surae—hypoplastic
Femur	Often congenitally short

Rare

Proximal femoral focal deficiency
Congenital longitudinal deficiency of the fibula of the contralateral limb (bilateral involvement)
Absence of part or all of the upper limb
Absence of ulnar rays of the hand
Syndactyly
Nail-patella syndrome—hereditary onycho-osteodystrophy
Peroneal muscles—fibrosed and weak

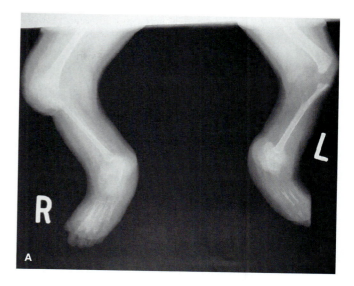

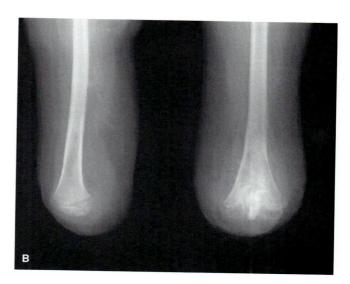

Figure 2–55. Congenital absence of the tibia treated by amputation. **A.** Preoperative radiograms. **B.** Postoperative radiograms.

equinovalgus deformity of the foot is corrected by sectioning of the contracted and fibrous peroneal tendons, calcaneofibular ligament, and fibrous anlage of the fibula. The lateral subluxation of the ankle joint is reduced, and the foot is anteriorly aligned under the distal end of the tibia. A plantigrade and functional foot is provided by passive stretching and active exercises and splinting of the foot–ankle in an AFO or KAFO at night.

Tibial lengthening is performed when the child is older, usually 8 to 10 years of age. The Ilizarov technique is preferred because with pins in the calcaneus one can control ankle valgus.[216] Dynamic splints are worn at night to prevent posterior subluxation of the knee.

CONGENITAL LONGITUDINAL DEFICIENCY OF THE TIBIA

The clinical manifestation varies with the severity of the deficiency. When the entire tibia is absent, the foot is in severe inversion and adduction (resembling clubfoot), the limb is short, and the knee is held in fixed flexion with the fibular head displaced proximally over a hypoplastic distal femur (Fig 2–55). The quadriceps muscle is deficient. This is type I of Kalamchi and Dawe's classification.[238]

When only the distal half of the tibia is absent, the limb is short to a lesser degree, the foot is inverted-adducted, and the medial malleolus is absent. The knee joint (femoral-tibial) is present but deformed, with 25 to 35 degrees of flexion deformity and a high-riding proximal fibular epiphysis. (This is type II—Kalamchi-Dawe.)

When the tibia is present but hypoplastic, the medial malleolus rides proximal to the fibular malleolus to a varying degree, the foot is held in varus with diastasis of the distal tibiofibular syndesmosis. The leg is short, and the knee is relatively normal. (This is type III.)

Absence of the tibia is a very rare anomaly, occurring in one per million live births. Often it is associated with other congenital anomalies, such as absence of the medial rays of the foot, proximal focal femoral deficiency, lobster claw hand, and congenital heart disease.

Treatment. When the tibia is totally absent, a knee disarticulation is performed and the limb is fitted with a conventional above-knee prosthesis. Esthetically and functionally it is best for the patient. Results of fibulofemoral arthroplasty are not satisfactory. In bilateral type I cases an attempt to preserve the foot and leg may be made by modified Browne fibulofemoral arthroplasty if quadriceps and hamstring muscle function is good. Parents should understand the drawbacks of persistent and progressive knee flexion contracture, difficulties with cumbersome orthotic or prosthetic external support, a cosmetically objectionable, very short lower leg, and a deformed, unstable ankle and foot.

In type II (absence of distal tibia), a side-to-side proximal tibiofibular arthrodesis is performed to provide stability to the knee joint. A modified Syme or Boyd amputation is performed, preserving the distal fibular physis.

In type III (present but hypoplastic tibia), the modality of treatment depends upon the degree of shortening and stability of the ankle joint. A synostosis of the distal tibia and fibula and Boyd ablation of the foot provide the best function.

■ ROTATIONAL MALALIGNMENT OF THE LOWER LIMBS

Toeing-in and toeing-out are the most common complaints in pediatric orthopedics. Often it is physiologic and not pathologic and of no clinical significance. It is vital to determine the cause and understand the natural history of the rotational malalignment and the effectiveness of various modalities of treatment. The various causes of toeing-in and toeing-out are listed in Tables 2–6 and 2–7.

The cause of toeing-in and toeing-out varies in different age groups. Often one can make a diagnosis of the rotational problem by the torsion profile and by the age of the child when first seen.

IN-TOEING

In the infant the most common cause of toeing-in is *metatarsus varus or adductus,* which often is combined with medial tibial torsion. Occasionally inward rotation-adduction of the foot is due to *talipes varus* (the hindfoot is inverted in addition to the forefoot varus) or *postural clubfoot* (the hindfoot and forefoot varus are accompanied by ankle equinus).

In the second year of life (toddler) toeing-in is due to *excessive medial tibiofibular torsion.* The toddler toes-in more on the left than on the right side. When the child is 3 years and older, in-toeing is usually bilateral and

TABLE 2–6. CAUSES OF TOEING-IN

Level	Deformity	Age Group
Foot-Ankle	Metatarsus varus or adductus—common	Infancy (untreated severe may persist into childhood)
	Talipes varus or postural clubfoot—infrequent	Infancy (untreated will persist into childhood)
Leg-Knee	Medial tibial torsion—common	Early childhood—1-2 years
	Protective toeing-in due to developmental genu valgum and flexible flatfoot (turns the foot inward so that the center of body weight from anterosuperior iliac spine falls on center of foot—common	Childhood 3 years and older
	Tibia vara associated with medial tibial torsion—infrequent	Less than 2 years
	Hypoplasia (congenital longitudinal deficiency) of tibia with relative overgrowth of fibula, often unilateral—rare	Toddler and older child
	Relatively long fibula in relation to tibia in bone dysplasia such as achondroplasia (bilateral and symmetric)—rare	Toddler and older child
Femur-Hip	Femoral antetorsion—common Splasticity of medial rotators, adductors of hip (cerebral palsy)—common	3-4 years and older When child begins to walk

TABLE 2–7. CAUSES OF TOEING-OUT

Level	Deformity	Age Group
Hip	Contracture of lateral rotators of the hip—very common, almost every baby	Infancy
	Developmental dislocation of the hip, congenital coxa vara (very rare)	When child begins to stand and walk
	Lateral femoral torsion, especially in the obese patient. Slipped capital femoral epiphysis?	Preadolescent and adolescent
	Neuromuscular disorders such as myelomeningocele and polio with paralysis of medial hip rotators	All age groups
Knee-Leg	Lateral tibial torsion—common. May be associated with genu valgum. Tibia valga—rule out contracture of iliotibial band.	Older child and adolescent
	Torsional malalignment—post-traumatic	All age groups
	Congenital longitudinal deficiency of the fibula with relatively long tibia—rare	All age groups
Foot-Ankle	Talipes calcaneovalgus and congenital convex pes valgus	Infancy
	Contracture of triceps surae causing pes valgus	Childhood
	Tarsal coalition with peroneal spastic flat foot	Childhood
	Neuromuscular disorders such as cerebral palsy with poor or absent cerebral control over anterior tibial muscle and/or contracture of the triceps surae	All age groups

symmetric; it is due to *femoral antetorsion*. The diagnosis of femoral antetorsion is readily made by observing the excessive medial rotation of the hips and restricted lateral rotation of the hips with the child lying prone with the hips extended; the child also prefers to sit in **W** or reverse tailor's position. Another common cause of toeing-in in childhood is *developmental genu valgum and flexible pes planovalgus*. In this condition toeing-in is protective: The child toes-in to shift the center of gravity to the center of the foot. When a child toes-in very severely, it often is due to a combination of torsional problems such as metatarsus varus with tibial medial torsion, or medial tibial torsion with femoral antetorsion, tibia vara (Blount's disease), or developmental genu varum combined with severe medial tibiofibular torsion. Occasionally three levels are affected—metatarsus varus plus medial tibial torsion plus femoral antetorsion.

In all age groups toeing-in may be *neuromuscular* in origin—due to spasticity of the posterior and/or anterior tibial muscles or spasticity of hip medial rotators and hip adductors. Always examine the child thoroughly to rule out spastic or athetoid cerebral palsy or upper motor lesions. A rare cause of toeing-in in all age groups is *relative overgrowth of the fibula in relation to the tibia*, seen in congenital longitudinal deficiency of the tibia (the involved leg is short—palpate the level of the proximal and distal fibular epiphyses). Relative overgrowth of the fibula is also seen in achondroplasia (it is symmetric, and other generalized features are diagnostic). Very occasionally in *tarsal coalition* (talocalcaneal or calcaneonavicular), the foot assumes a "spastic" varus posture and the child toes-in or the foot is inverted when the subtalar joint is affected by an inflammatory process such as rheumatoid arthritis. Examine the foot thoroughly and test subtalar motion—is it stiff? Ordinarily acetabular antetorsion is not a cause of in-toeing. The various causes of toeing-in are illustrated in Figure 2–56.

OUT-TOEING

When an infant lies supine and begins to stand and walk he or she toes out; this is due to contracture of the lateral rotators of the hips because of intrauterine fetal posture. It masks the effect of femoral anteversion. With time the lateral rotation contracture of the hips resolves and the degree of medial rotation of the hips increases (Fig 2–57). This is extremely common and is considered to be a normal finding.

Rare causes of toeing-out at the level of the hip in the young child who begins to walk are missed developmental dislocation of the hip (usually asymmetric and unilateral; when bilateral, the left side is worse than the right), and developmental (or congenital) coxa vara, in which the decreased femoral neck-shaft angle is associated with femoral retrotorsion. In the preadolescent and adolescent age group, particularly in the obese patient, lateral femoral torsion is

usually the cause of toeing-out. Caution! Examine the hips to rule out slipped capital femoral epiphysis. Flaccid paralysis of the medial rotators of the hip (in myelomeningocele and myotonia congenita) causes the child to toe out.

In the older child toeing-out is usually due to lateral tibiofibular torsion, which often is associated with some genu valgum or tibia valga. Perform the Ober test and rule out contracture of the iliotibial band. A rare cause of toeing-out at the level of the leg is congenital longitudinal deficiency of the fibula with relatively long tibia.

In the infant talipes calcaneovalgus and congenital convex pes valgus (vertical talus) cause valgus posture of the foot and ankle and toeing-out in gait. In the growing child pes valgus due to contracture of the triceps surae makes the child toe out. In the preadolescent and adolescent age group, tarsal coalition and peroneal spastic flat foot cause toeing-out in gait. Neuromuscular disorders (such as cerebral palsy) with equinus deformity of the foot and ankle and insufficiency of the anterior tibial muscle cause toeing-out. The various causes of toeing-out are shown in Figure 2–58.

HISTORY

Ask the parents the reason for the consultation. What is their concern? Do not be nonchalant—be thorough. The parents' concern is real. Are they afraid that the toeing-in or toeing-out will persist into adult life and cause problems such as arthritis of the knees and hips, or will it make it difficult for their child to participate in sports or function normally as an adolescent or adult?

Inquire about the pregnancy and birth history. Was there anything abnormal during pregnancy? What was the presentation at birth—vertex or breech? Was there any suggestion of intrauterine malposture?

Was the baby born full-term or premature? What was the birth weight? Medial tibial torsion does not occur in premature infants; because of their size, intrauterine molding and malposture are not problems. Premature infants toe out until late in childhood.[260]

What was the position of the feet at birth? Were they pointing inward, outward, or straight forward? Were the legs bowed? Was there any problem with the hips—subluxation or dislocation? Was there any patch of hair or hemangioma on the spine to suggest spinal dysrhaphism?

Take a developmental history. When did the infant begin to stand and walk? A delay in walking may suggest a neuromuscular disorder such as cerebral palsy (a spastic paraparesis or hemiparesis) or hypotonia (such as congenital amyotonia or Werdnig-Hoffman disease).

What is the upper limb function? Did the infant show any dominance of hand—left or right? The presence of hand dominance as an infant suggests hemiparesis of the contralateral side.

What has been the course of the rotational deformity? Is it improving, unchanged, or increasing in severity? Was any previous treatment given? What was the response to it?

A. Metatarsus varus

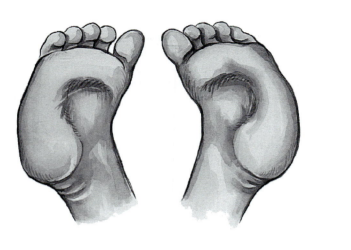

B. Protective toeing-in

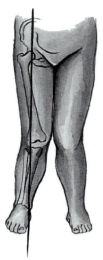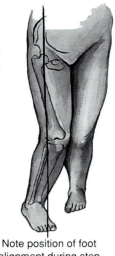

Note position of foot alignment during step

C. Medial tibial fibular torsion

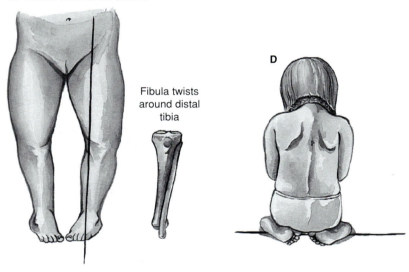

Fibula twists around distal tibia

D

E. Femoral antetorsion

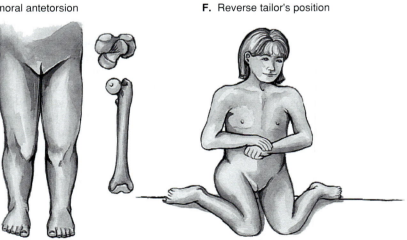

F. Reverse tailor's position

Figure 2–56. Common causes of toeing-in. **A.** Metatarsus varus. **B.** Protective toeing-in. **C, D.** Excessive medial tibial torsion. **E, F.** Femoral antetorsion and sitting posture.

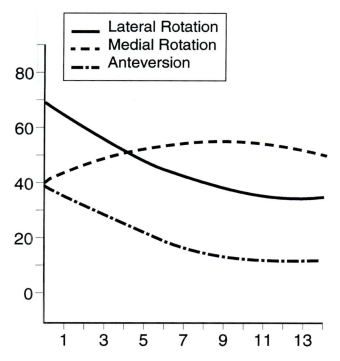

Figure 2–57. The natural history of the ranges of hip rotation and the degree of femoral anteversion (vertical axis) with increasing age (horizontal axis). (Courtesy of LT Staheli, personal communication.)

Ask the child and then the parents about the nature of the disability. A mild degree of in-toeing enables the child to run well, whereas severe toeing-in in the young child due to excessive medial tibial torsion may make the child trip and fall down. The running of a child with excessive femoral torsion is awkward. Toeing-out due to lateral torsion of the tibia is disabling; it causes medial foot strain, patellofemoral joint disability, and anterior knee pain.

ASSESSMENT

First, examine the entire child—the trunk, the upper limbs, and the lower limbs. Observe the child in stance, in gait, and while running. It is not uncommon that a mild hemiparetic cerebral palsied child presents with the chief complaint of toeing-in. Thorough examination reveals spasticity of the triceps surae and posterior tibial muscles. During running the upper limbs go into flexion at the elbow, and the slap test is uncoordinated on the affected side; there may be spasticity of the hamstrings and the hip adductors. Every so often a child who has just begun to walk and toe-out has dislocation of the hips. It behooves you to examine the hips thoroughly. This is especially a problem in bilateral dislocations because it often escapes notice in early life. Another cause of toeing-out is muscular dystrophy. Perform the Gower's test and if there is any suspicion of hypotonia, perform serum creatinine phosphokinase and serum aldolase studies.

In describing rotational alignment of the lower limbs, use the proper terminology.[282–286]

Version is defined as the normal twisting of a long bone on its anatomic longitudinal axis. Measurements that fall beyond (plus or minus) 2 standard deviations (SD) of the mean are referred to as *torsion*. Torsion is an abnormality—a deformity.

The line that joins designated bony landmarks at each end of a long bone is termed the *reference axis*. Version is neutral when these bony landmarks (reference axes) are located in the same plane. When the proximal reference axis is laterally twisted in relation to the distal axis, the rotational alignment is referred to as *anteversion;* when this rotation is greater than 2 SD from the mean, rotational malalignment is designated *antetorsion*. When the proximal reference (landmark) axis is medially rotated in relation to the distal reference landmark (or axis), the rotation is referred to as *retroversion*. When the rotation is beyond 2 SD of the mean, the rotational malalignment is referred to as *retrotorsion*. In the femur the terms *femoral anteversion* and *antetorsion* are used, whereas in the tibia the terms in common use are *medial version* or *torsion* and *lateral version* or *torsion*. In the tibia, instead of using the proximal reference point, the relationship of the distal to the proximal reference points is used to describe rotational alignment or malalignment.

Femoral version or torsion is the angle measured between the line joining the center of the femoral head with the center of the femoral shaft at the level of the lesser trochanter (proximal reference axis) and the line joining the most posterior points of the femoral condyles (distal reference axis) (Fig 2–59).

Tibial version or torsion is the angle measured between the transmalleolar axis and the bicondylar axis of the proximal tibia at the knee (Fig 2–60).

Torsion may involve one level such as the femur or the tibia, or it may affect both the femur and the tibia. Torsional deformity may be *additive*, such as the combination of femoral antetorsion and tibial medial torsion, or *compensatory*, such as when femoral antetorsion is combined with lateral tibiofibular torsion.

FETAL DEVELOPMENT AND NATURAL HISTORY OF LOWER LIMB ROTATION

The lower limb first manifests as a paddle bud on the ventrolateral body wall during the fourth to fifth week of gestation (Fig 2–61A). By the end of the sixth week the limb bud swelling flattens to form the foot plate, and the mesenchymal tissue condenses, outlining the pattern of the digits. Soon the tissue between the rays dissolves and notches are formed, deforming the digits. The great toes face preaxially (Fig 2–61B). The toes are fully formed in the 8-week embryo. The plantar surfaces of the feet appose in the so-called "praying feet" position

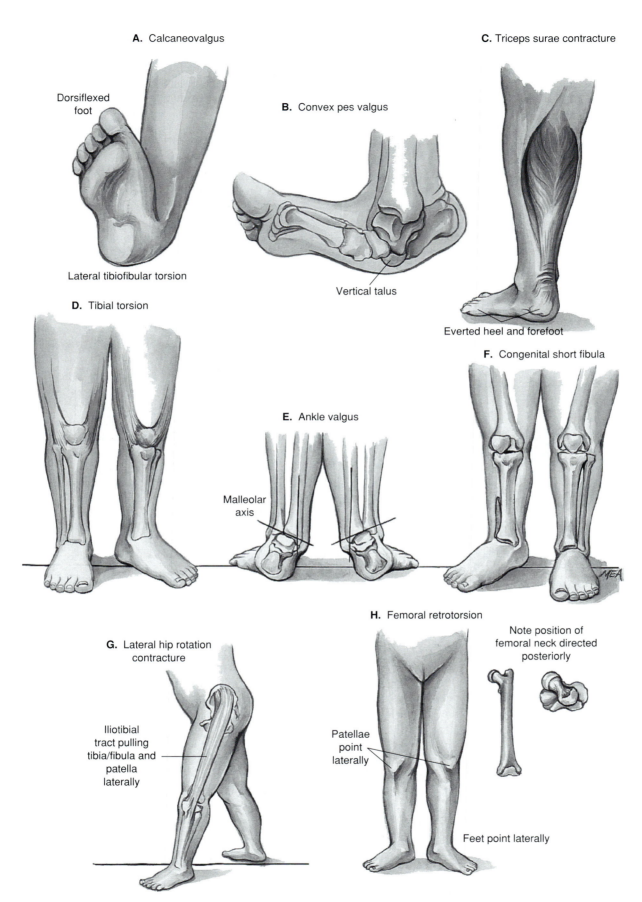

A. Calcaneovalgus

Dorsiflexed foot

Lateral tibiofibular torsion

B. Convex pes valgus

Vertical talus

C. Triceps surae contracture

Everted heel and forefoot

D. Tibial torsion

E. Ankle valgus

Malleolar axis

F. Congenital short fibula

G. Lateral hip rotation contracture

Iliotibial tract pulling tibia/fibula and patella laterally

H. Femoral retrotorsion

Note position of femoral neck directed posteriorly

Patellae point laterally

Feet point laterally

Figure 2–58. Causes of toeing-out. **A.** Calcaneovalgus deformity. **B.** Convex pes valgus (vertical talus). **C.** Contracture of triceps surae causing pes valgus. **D.** Lateral tibiofibular torsion. **E.** Ankle valgus. **F.** Congenital short fibula. **G.** Lateral hip rotation contracture. **H.** Femoral retrotorsion.

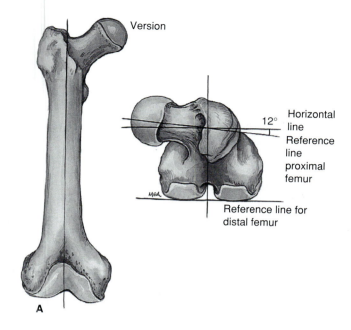

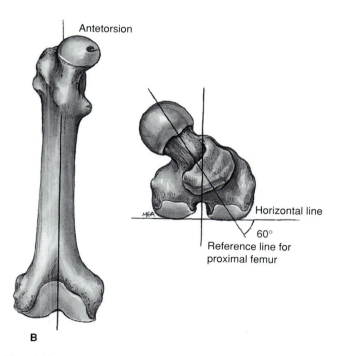

Figure 2–59. Femoral version and antetorsion. **A.** Femoral version is the angle measured by the line joining the center of the femoral head and the center of the femoral shaft and the line joining the posterior points of the femoral condyles. **B.** Femoral antetorsion.

of the fetus takes place: The femurs rotate laterally and the tibiae medially. After birth the degree of femoral anteversion continues to decrease; at 1 year of age the average femoral antetorsion measures 32 degrees and with growth it declines at 16 years of age to 16 degrees (Figs 2–62 and 2–63).

In a CT study of tibiofibular torsion in the growing fetus, Badelon et al found an increased lateral tibiofibular torsion in the early stages of fetal life; later on lateral torsion of the tibia gradually decreased and in the newborn the tibiofibular torsion was medial.[242] After birth the tibia rotates laterally; the average mean version of the tibia at skeletal maturity is 15 degrees lateral.

MEASUREMENT OF VERSION

Three methods are available for measuring limb rotation: (1) clinical; (2) imaging (radiographic, CT, ultrasonogram); and (3) cadaveric.

Cadaveric mensuration of rotation of a long bone is direct and exact because the anatomic landmarks for the proximal and distal reference axes are accessible. Anatomic measurement is used primarily as a research tool for determination of normal ranges of individual long bones. The values obtained by cadaveric measurements provide an exact base against which clinical assessments can be approximately compared. In an anatomic study of a cadaveric long bone, however, one is not assessing the rotational and axial alignment of the entire limb.

Clinical measurements are used in practice. They allow assessment of the rotational and angular alignment of the entire limb. Clinical determination of version provides approximate values because the bony landmarks are not readily accessible. Interobserver variation is wide. It is best to measure in 5-degree increments.

Tibial rotation is measured in several ways: First, with the child seated at the edge of the examining table with the knee flexed 90 degrees and the foot and ankle in neutral position. Bicondylar transverse axis of the tibia is parallel with the edge of the table; the transmalleolar axis of the ankle is measured by grasping the medial malleolus with the tip of the thumb and lateral malleolus with the index finger. Draw a visual line between the two malleoli and inspect the transverse crease of the ankle. The angular difference between the transcondylar axis of the tibia at the knee and the bimalleolar axis at the ankle is the degree of tibial torsion (Fig 2–64A, B).

The second method is determination of the thigh-foot angle. With the patient prone and the knee flexed at right angles, the foot and ankle in neutral position (i.e., foot at 90-degree angle to the tibia), measure the angle between the longitudinal axis of the thigh and the longitudinal axis of the foot (Fig 2–65).[282–287]

In the third method the child again lies flat on his abdomen with his knee flexed at 90 degrees and the foot

(Fig 2–61C). Soon afterwards, the lower limb rotates medially, bringing the great toe to the midline so that the feet are postured plantigrade (Fig 2–61D). Rotation of the lower limb takes place because of differential growth between its ectodermal and mesodermal layers. Soon mechanical intrauterine molding of the lower limbs

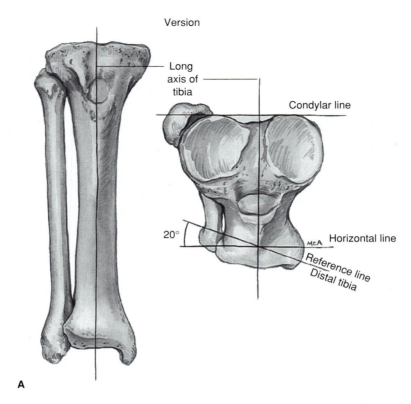

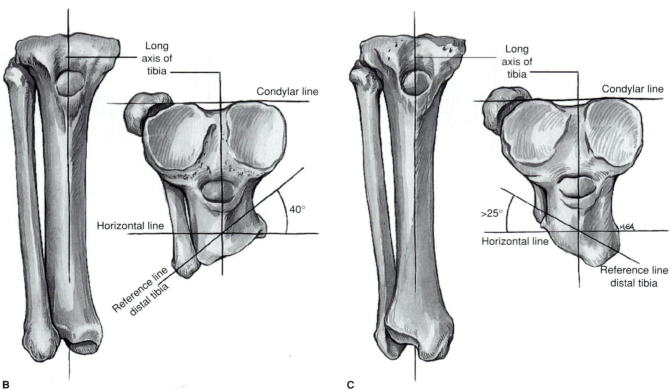

Figure 2–60. Rotational alignment of the tibia. **A.** Normal tibial version, the angle between the transmalleolar axis (distal reference axis) and the bicondylar axis of the proximal tibia at the knee (proximal reference axis). **B.** Medial tibiofibular torsion. **C.** Lateral tibiofibular torsion.

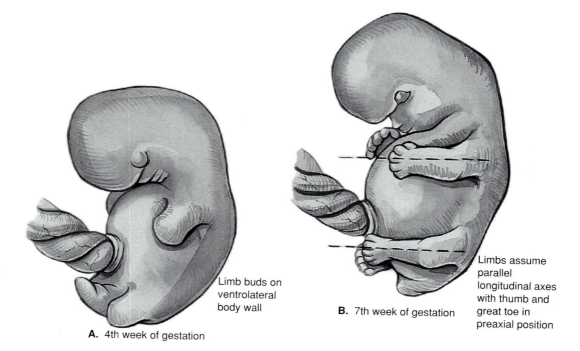

Limb buds on
ventrolateral
body wall

A. 4th week of gestation

B. 7th week of gestation

Limbs assume
parallel
longitudinal axes
with thumb and
great toe in
preaxial position

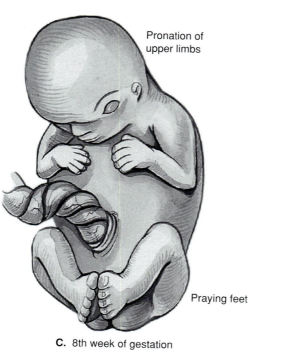

Pronation of
upper limbs

Praying feet

C. 8th week of gestation

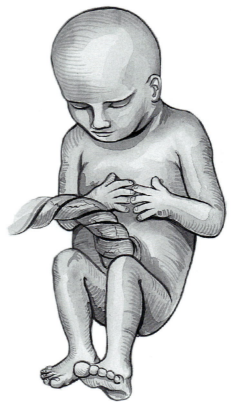

D. Feet become plantigrade with
medial rotation of lower limbs

Figure 2–61. Developmental and natural course of rotation of the lower limb in the fetus. **A.** At 4 weeks' gestation it appears as a paddle bud on the anterolateral body wall. **B.** At 7 weeks' gestation foot plate and digits form. The big toe faces preaxially. **C.** The "praying feet" position. The hips are rotated laterally. **D.** With further intrauterine development the lower limbs rotate medially and the feet assume plantigrade position.

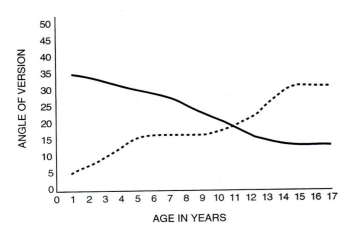

Figure 2-62. Femoral version *(solid line)* and tibial version *(dashed line)*. (Adapted from Staheli LT: Torsional deformities. *Pediatr Clin North Am* 24:800, 1977; with permission.)

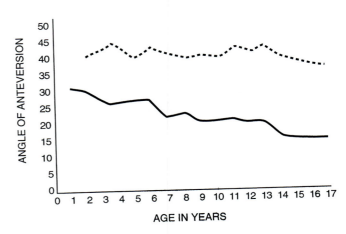

Figure 2-63. Values of normal femoral anteversion *(solid line)* and femoral antetorsion *(dashed line)* with increasing age. (Adapted from Fabry G, MacEwen GD, Shands AR: Torsion of the femur. *J Bone Joint Surg* 55A:1734, 1973; with permission.)

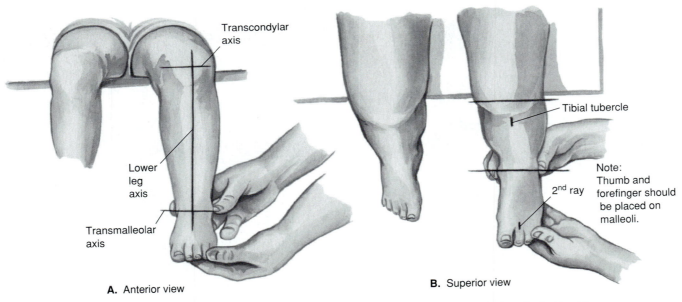

A. Anterior view

B. Superior view

Figure 2-64. Clinical measurement of tibial torsion. **A, B.** With the patient sitting at the edge of the table, determine the bicondylar axis of the knee and the bimalleolar axis of the ankle; the angular difference between the two axes is the degree of tibial torsion. **A.** Anterior view. **B.** Superior view.

and ankle in neutral position. The transcondylar axis of the tibia is parallel with the top of the table; the transmalleolar axis is determined as described above. The angle formed between the transcondylar and bimalleolar axis is the degree of tibial version. To be exact, when the bimalleolar axis is the distal reference axis, one is measuring tibiofibular torsion and not tibial torsion. When there is deformity of the ankle, such as ankle valgus with high-riding lateral malleolus in paralytic pes calcaneovalgus or post-traumatic malunion, an alternate method of determining tibial torsion is to use the tibial tubercle and the second metatarsal ray as anatomic landmarks; the foot should be normal (not in varus or valgus), the ankle at neutral, and the knee flexed at right angles with the patient sitting at the edge of the table (see Fig 2–64B).

The clinical method of determining *femoral torsion* is as follows: (1) Position of the patient is prone, lying flat on the examining table with his or her knee flexed 90 degrees. (2) Palpate the midpoint of the greater trochanter; in femoral antetorsion it lies posteriorly and in femoral retrotorsion anteriorly. In femoral antetorsion rotate the hip medially (i.e., the leg away from the axis of the body) away from the opposite leg until the greater trochanter reaches the most lateral position; the degree of medial hip rotation is the degree of femoral antetorsion. (3) In femoral retrotorsion rotate the hip laterally (i.e., the leg toward the center of the body, toward the opposite leg) (Fig 2–66).

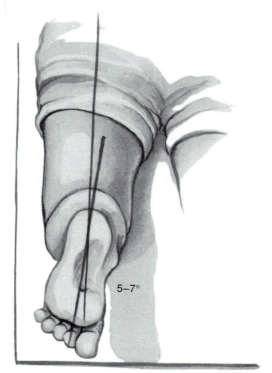

Thigh–foot angle

Figure 2–65. Thigh–foot angle to measure tibial torsion. With the patient prone and the knee flexed at right angles and the foot and ankle in neutral position, measure the angle between the longitudinal axis of the thigh and the longitudinal axis of the foot.

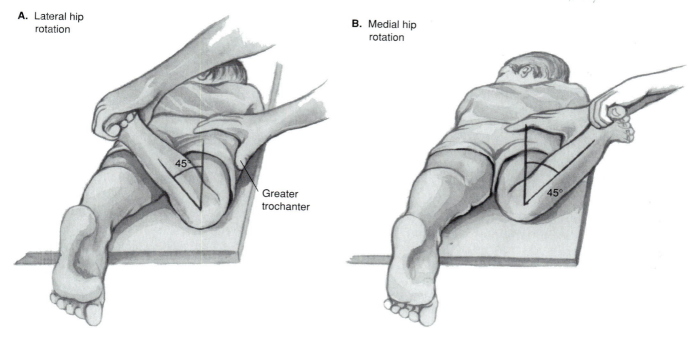

A. Lateral hip rotation

B. Medial hip rotation

Greater trochanter

Figure 2–66. Clinical method of determining femoral torsion. **A.** With the patient in prone position lying flat on the examining table, knees flexed 90 degrees, determine the midpoint of the lateral trochanter. In femoral retrotorsion, rotate the hip laterally. The degree of lateral rotation of the hip at which the midpoint of the greater trochanter becomes lateral is the degree of femoral retrotorsion. **B.** In femoral antetorsion, the midpoint of the greater trochanter lies posterior. Rotate the hip medially, i.e., the leg away from the center axis of the body. The degree of medial rotation at which the midpoint of the greater trochanter becomes straight lateral is the degree of femoral antetorsion.

Imaging techniques are used to determine femoral and tibial version. Computed tomography (CT) is the method of choice. It is accurate as long as the patient does not move (Fig 2–67). Its routine use is not recommended because of radiation, cost, and inconvenience. Computed tomography studies of torsion are performed when surgery is planned to correct the deformity.[257]

In the infant and young child ultrasonography measures torsion, particularly of the tibia. Accurate determination of the location of bony landmarks is difficult. Proper positioning of the patient is crucial; the child should not move. The accuracy of the method is technician dependent. Clinical determination is often adequate. Ordinarily ultrasonography is not indicated.[246,263,293]

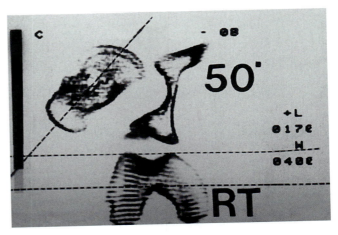

Figure 2–67. Computed tomography method of measuring femoral torsion.

NORMAL VALUES

The range of normal values varies, depending upon the technique used and variability of position of proximal and distal reference axes.

Femoral rotation averages 35 degrees (30 to 40 degrees) of anteversion at birth. With skeletal growth it progressively decreases, measuring an average of 8 degrees in the adult male and 14 degrees in the adult female. After the age of 8 years regression of femoral anteversion slows down markedly, but it does occur.

Tibial version alters with age; with skeletal growth the transmalleolar axis progressively rotates laterally. The average value of tibial version is 2 to 4 degrees lateral at birth and 10 to 20 degrees lateral in the adult.

Acetabular version measures about 13 degrees and remains relatively constant throughout childhood (as shown by CT studies) and during the first half of intrauterine life (as shown by histomorphic studies).[262]

ROTATIONAL PROFILE (STAHELI)

This is an efficient and accurate method to determine the level and severity of the rotational deformity. First, inspect the patient from the front with the feet facing straight forward. In excessive femoral antetorsion the patellae face medially (Fig 2–68A). Then rotate the feet laterally so that the patellae face straight forward. The degree of lateral rotation of the feet is an approximate assessment of femoral antetorsion (Fig 2–68B).

Next, ask the child to walk toward you and estimate the FPA, the angular difference between the long axis of the foot and the line of progression (Fig 2–68C). Ask the child to run and then walk. Observe the gait several times and then choose the average. Denote in-toeing by preceding it with a minus sign and out-toeing by a plus sign. Express the FPA in degrees. In the normal child the FPA is +10 degrees, with a wide range from −3 degrees to +20 de-

grees. The infant who has just begun walking toes out more than older children despite the fact that they have excessive femoral antetorsion. In these young children the lateral rotation of the hip is increased due to intrauterine flexion–adduction–lateral rotation posture of the hips, and medial rotation of the hips is restricted. As they get older the lateral rotation contracture of the hip resolves and their gait improves. Grade the severity of in-toeing: It is mild when −5 degrees to −10 degrees, moderate when −10 degrees to −15 degrees, and severe when greater than −15 degrees.

Second, determine the degree of medial and lateral rotation of the hip when the patient is prone with the pelvis level and the knees flexed 90 degrees. Do not push down on the pelvis. The legs (hips) are allowed to fall into normal medial and lateral rotation by forces of gravity alone. Do not use force! The angle between the vertical line and longitudinal axis of the leg is the degree of hip rotation (Fig 2–68D, E). When the leg moves away from the body toward the table it is medial rotation; when it moves toward the opposite leg it is lateral rotation. The degree of medial rotation of the hip decreases with increasing age; it is greater in girls than boys. According to Staheli, the degree of medial rotation of the hip is normally less than 70 degrees in girls and about 60 degrees in boys. The lower limit of lateral rotation of the hip is 25 degrees in both genders. A value of medial rotation of the hip greater than the above suggests excessive femoral antetorsion. The severity of femoral torsion is graded *mild* if the degree of medial rotation is 70 to 80 degrees and lateral rotation is 10 to 20 degrees. It is graded *moderate* if the medial rotation is 80 to 90 degrees and the lateral rotation is 0 to 10 degrees; it is *severe* if the degree of medial rotation of the hip is greater than 90 degrees and lateral rotation is less than 0 degrees.

Third, determine the *thigh-foot angle*, the angle formed between the longitudinal axis of the foot and the longitudinal axis of the thigh with the patient in prone position with the knees flexed 90 degrees and the foot and ankle in neutral position (Fig 2–68F). It measures the degree of tibial rotation. A negative value is given when the tibia is rotated medially (medial tibial torsion), and a positive value is given when the tibia is rotated laterally (lateral tibiofibular torsion).

In the infant the *thigh-foot angle* is medial (negative), but it becomes progressively lateral (positive) with increasing age. According to Staheli et al, in the middle of childhood the mean thigh–foot angle is about +10 degrees, with a range of normal values of −5 degrees to +30 degrees.[285]

Fourth, the angle of the *transmalleolar axis* is determined as follows: Place the patient prone, and flex the knees 90 degrees with the ankles in neutral position. Draw the transmalleolar axis by connecting the center points of the medial and lateral malleoli across the sole of the foot. Next, draw a line toward the heel perpendicular to the transmalleolar axis. The angle of the transmalleolar axis is the one formed between the longitudinal axis of the thigh and the line drawn across the heel perpendicular to the transmalleolar axis (Fig 2–68G). This determines the degree of hindfoot deformity. An abnormal transmalleolar axis denotes a rotation deformity of the foot rather than the tibia.

Last, assess alignment of the foot, whether there is metatarsus varus or calcaneovalgus deformity.

MEDIAL TIBIAL TORSION

Ordinarily medial tibial torsion is first noted by the parents when the child pulls up to standing or begins to walk. The presenting complaint is that he is pigeon-toed and toes-in in gait. Involvement is often bilateral; in unilateral cases the left side is more commonly involved. Examine the feet and the entire lower limb; medial tibial torsion is often associated with metatarsus varus, genu varum, or tibia vara. With the patellae facing straight forward, the feet point inward, with the medial malleolus lying posterior to the lateral malleolus. In the prone position, the thigh–foot angle is medial. In stance the center of gravity falls lateral to the second ray. The FPA is medial. The natural history of medial tibial torsion is spontaneous correction with growth. The young child with excessive medial tibial torsion may trip and fall, but spontaneous resolution is rapid in early childhood and there should be no residual disability. The medial tibial torsion that persists in the older child or adolescent does not cause any disability; in fact, mild toeing-in facilitates running because it places the toes in functional position to assist in ankle push-off.

FEMORAL ANTETORSION

This deformity usually presents as a cause of in-toeing at 3 to 4 years of age. It is present at birth but is camouflaged by the contracture of the lateral rotation of the hip. In-toeing due to femoral antetorsion increases up to 5 to 6 years of age and then gradually decreases. It is more common in the female and is familial. Femoral antetorsion is often symmetric. On inspection in stance the patellae and knees are turned inward because of medial rotation posture of the hips; the heels are rotated laterally. With the feet facing straight forward and the knees in full extension, the lower limbs have a bow-legged appearance; when the feet are rotated laterally so that the patellae point straight forward, the bow-legged appearance disappears.

The child prefers to sit in W or reverse tailor's position. In gait the FPA is medial to varying degrees. When the child is tired, the in-toeing becomes more pronounced. Running is clumsy and awkward; during the swing phase the thighs are rotated medially and the legs and feet are rotated outward. When toeing-in is excessive, the child may trip and fall because of crossing-over of the feet.

Next, place the child in prone position with the hips in full extension and the knees flexed 90 degrees. The characteristic physical finding of femoral antetorsion is excessive medial rotation of the hips (as much as 90 degrees) and restriction of lateral rotation of the hips (usually to neutral position). When the child is supine with the hips flexed, the lateral rotation of the hips is increased because the anterior capsule of the hip and the Bigelow ligament are relaxed.

As the child gets older, compensatory lateral rotation of the tibia develops. This combination of excessive medial femoral antetorsion and lateral tibiofibular torsion is referred to as torsional malalignment syndrome (Fig 2–69). It causes increase in the Q angle, patellofemoral joint instability, and anterior knee pain.

In the past it was speculated that excessive femoral antetorsion causes degenerative arthritis of the hip; however, recently it has been demonstrated that this is not true because the degree of femoral antetorsion in patients with degenerative arthritis of the hip is equal to that in a control group of patients without arthritis. Also, it has been claimed that increased femoral antetorsion impairs running ability; however, Staheli et al showed that physical performance of adolescents and adults with increased femoral antetorsion is equivalent to that of a control group of persons with normal femoral torsion.[287]

LATERAL TIBIAL TORSION

Lateral tibial torsion is usually first noted in the juvenile or preadolescent patient who is presented with the chief complaint of pain in the instep of the foot or anterior knee pain. Often lateral tibial torsion is secondary to compensation for excessive femoral antetorsion or is due to contracture of the

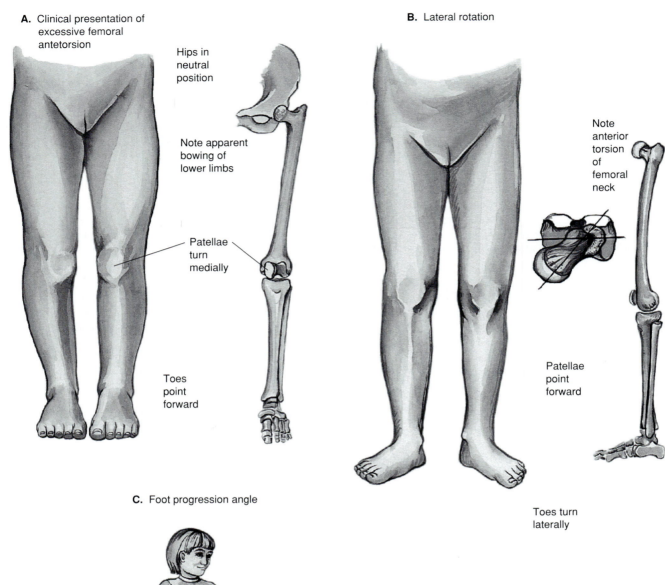

A. Clinical presentation of excessive femoral antetorsion

Hips in neutral position

Note apparent bowing of lower limbs

Patellae turn medially

Toes point forward

B. Lateral rotation

Note anterior torsion of femoral neck

Patellae point forward

Toes turn laterally

C. Foot progression angle

Feet point medially

Figure 2–68. Rotation profile. **A, B.** Inspect the patient standing with the feet facing forward and note the position of the patellae. In femoral antetorsion they are facing inward. When the feet are rotated laterally, the patellae face straight forward. **C.** Foot progression angle. *(Continues)*

D. Lateral hip rotation

E. Medial hip rotation

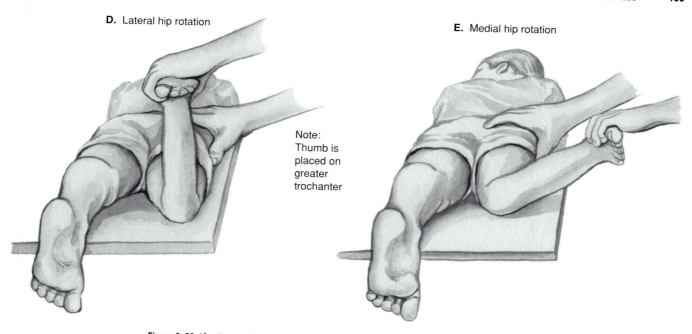

Note:
Thumb is
placed on
greater
trochanter

Figure 2–68 *(Continued).* Clinical methods of measuring tibial torsion **D, E.** Hip rotation *(Continues).*

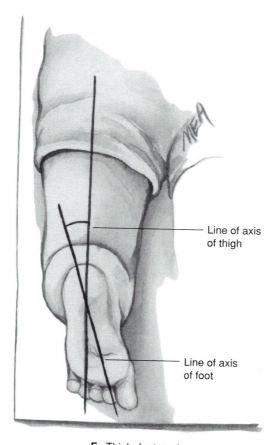

Line of axis
of thigh

Line of axis
of foot

F. Thigh–foot angle

Figure 2–68 *(Continued).* **F.** Thigh–foot angle. *(Continues)*

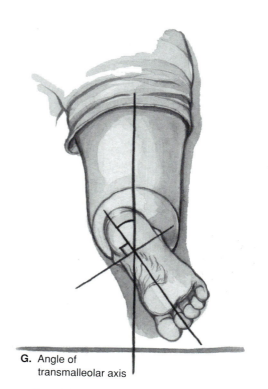

G. Angle of
transmalleolar axis

Figure 2–68 *(Continued).* **G.** Transmalleolar angle.

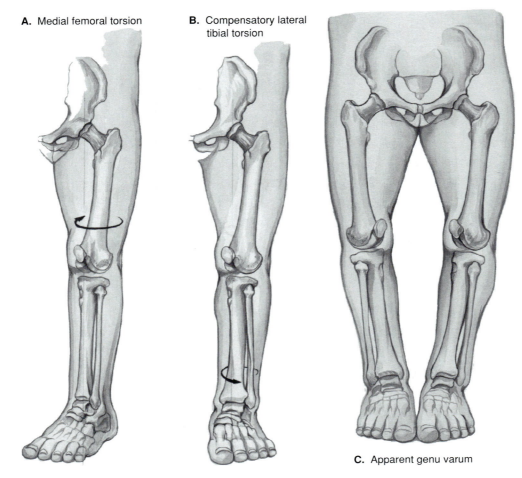

A. Medial femoral torsion

B. Compensatory lateral tibial torsion

C. Apparent genu varum

Figure 2–69. Apparent genu varum caused by excessive femoral antetorsion and compensatory lateral tibial torsion. **A.** Femoral antetorsion with the medial rotation of the knee and patella. **B.** Lateral tibial torsion to compensate for the femoral antetorsion. **C.** Anterior view of the patient with apparent genu varum.

iliotibial band. Occasionally it is a primary developmental deformity. One or both sides may be involved.

On inspection with the patient standing with his or her patellae facing straight forward, the feet point laterally and the center of gravity falls medial to the first metatarsal. It may be associated with genu valgum, tibia valga, and/or pes planovalgum. In the prone position with the hips extended and the knees flexed 90 degrees, the feet point laterally with a lateral thigh–foot angle. Determine the position of the lateral malleolus. In lateral tibial torsion it lies posterior to that of the medial malleolus. Perform Ober's test to rule out contracture of the iliotibial band. Determine the degree of femoral antetorsion in the prone position. Determine range of dorsiflexion of the ankle to rule out contracture of the triceps surae as a cause of out-toeing.

Lateral tibial torsion does not resolve spontaneously with growth, but rather tends to increase in severity. In the adolescent and adult it does cause medial foot strain and patellofemoral joint instability and pain.

FEMORAL RETROTORSION OR DECREASED ANTETORSION

This rotational malalignment of the femur is rare but does occur and is overlooked as a cause of hip pain. It may be a primary developmental deformity or secondary to slipped capital femoral epiphysis.[294]

On examination in stance the patellae and the feet point outward. The FPA is lateral. In the prone position with the hips in extended position, medial rotation of the hips is restricted whereas lateral rotation is excessive. CT and true lateral radiographic projection of the hips show the femoral retrotorsion. In the primary developmental form there is coxa valga, whereas in slipped capital femoral epiphysis the femoral neck-shaft angle is decreased.

Femoral retrotorsion does not correct with growth; it may increase and cause osteoarthritis of the hip.

TREATMENT

Treatment of *medial tibial torsion* and *femoral antetorsion* is unnecessary because these deformities resolve spontaneously in more than 80 percent of cases. The first step of management, therefore, is education and reassurance of the parents. Do not be nonchalant! Take the concerns of the parents seriously. Examine the child thoroughly to determine the correct cause. Explain the natural history of medial tibial torsion with femoral antetorsion to the parents and the fact that only very occasionally (probably 1 in 1000) does it cause disability in adult life. Also explain that you will follow the child every 6 to 12 months to ensure that with skeletal growth the deformity is improving and that if it does not it can be corrected surgically when the child is 10 to 14 years of age. Reassure the parents by such a "wait and see" approach that you are not "burning bridges"; instead, this approach prevents unnecessary surgery with its potential problems and complications.

The parents will question you about *nonsurgical measures.* Shoe wedges or wearing the right shoe on the left foot and the left shoe on the right foot does not improve torsional malalignment. They camouflage the deformity in the eyes of the parents and neighbors; but they cause and aggravate flatfoot. With femoral antetorsion tell the parents not to harass their child if he or she sits with the lower limbs in W position; there is no scientific evidence that changing the W sitting posture to sitting with legs dangling on a chair alters the natural course of femoral antetorsion. What about twister cables? Explain to the family that they will do harm by forcing the femoral heads anteriorly; the hip joint will subluxate anteriorly and cause hip pain. Night hip splints do not reduce femoral antetorsion. Exercises and gait training to alter in-toeing are ineffective and a waste of time.

A controversial issue is the use of rotational splints for excessive medial tibial torsion. On the basis of positive clinical impressions, many orthopedic surgeons, including this author, prescribe a Denis Browne or Fillauer bar (or any of the other commercially available designs). They are solid bars attached to open-toed, laced shoes either by clips or preferably by bolting the bar to the shoe. The feet point out to the desired degree. In some of the new designs the bars are hinged, allowing the child to kick. Because they are less restraining they are supposed to be more comfortable, but they are more expensive.

Barlow and Staheli experimentally simulated night splinting in a growing rabbit model using skeletal markers. The splinting did not produce rotational change in the tibia or femur.[243] However, in rabbits, Wilkinson could produce torsional changes in the femur by forced rotation of the hips.[299] In the human, however, there are no published reports of prospective studies objectively demonstrating by CT the effect of rotating splints on tibial torsion. Clinically rotating splints improve in-toeing gait when applied at a young age—between 6 months and 2.5 years of age. It is questionable whether the so-called derotation splints exert any torsional force on the tibia; instead the forces may be transmitted to the knee. Derotating splints may cause rotational instability at the knee. Clinically they are ordinarily not tolerated after the age of 3 years. This author prescribes derotation splints when medial tibial torsion is greater than 60 degrees in a young child of 1.5 to 2 years of age; they are to be worn only at night. Initially the feet should be rotated out 20 to 30 degrees; the degree of lateral rotation is then gradually increased but should not exceed 45 degrees. The bar between the shoes should not be too wide—no longer than 6 to 8 inches—as it will cause medial instability of the knee and genu valgum. The use of Denis Browne splints for more than 3 to 4 months is not recommended. Problems with Denis Browne or Fillauer bar splints are (1) loose laces on the shoe and the child kicks off the braces; (2) pain in the knee because of ligamentous stretch; (3) inability of the child to sleep at night; (4) pressure sores from the shoes. In the older child who gets out of the crib, walking on Denis Browne splints should not be allowed because the child may fall down and sustain a fracture—warn the parents.

Tibial osteotomy is rarely indicated to correct medial tibial torsion. This is performed only in cerebral palsy and myelomeningocele and occasionally in clubfoot patients who have excessive medial tibiofibular torsion. Proximal tibial rotational osteotomy has the potential for serious complications of peroneal nerve palsy and compartment syndrome. Therefore, most surgeons prefer to perform the surgery distally in the supramalleolar region. Recently the trend is to correct torsional deformities with an Ilizarov apparatus, which allows correction of valgus and varus deformities and also enables a short limb to be lengthened simultaneously.

Femoral osteotomy should not be performed until the child is 9 years of age and older. When the degree of femoral antetorsion is greater than 45 degrees, clinically the hip cannot be rotated laterally to neutral position and there is a definite functional disability. The procedure should not be performed for cosmetic reasons. One should always take into consideration the degree of lateral tibial torsion and the

FPA. The objective is to provide a normal FPA and not to make the child toe out. A subtrochanteric osteotomy is the level of choice.

REFERENCES

Congenital Dislocation of the Knee

1. Austick DH, Dandy DJ: Early operation for congenital subluxation of the knee. *J Pediatr Orthop* 3:85, 1983
2. Bell MJ, Atkins RM, Sharrard WJW: Irreducible congenital dislocation of the knee. *J Bone Joint Surg* 69B:403, 1987
3. Bensahel H, DalMonte A, Hjelmstedt A, Bjerkreim I, Wientroub S, Matasovic T, Porat S, Bialik V: Congenital dislocation of the knee. *J Pediatr Orthop* 9:174, 1989
4. Curtis BH, Fisher RL: Heritable congenital tibio-femoral subluxation. *J Bone Joint Surg* 52A:104, 1970
5. Ferris B, Aichroth P: The treatment of congenital knee dislocation. *Clin Orthop* 216:135, 1987
6. Finder JA: Congenital hyperextension of the knee. *J Bone Joint Surg* 46B:783, 1964
7. Iwaya T, Sakaguchi R, Tsuyama N: The treatment of congenital dislocation of the knee with the Pavlik harness. *Int Orthop (SICOT)* 7:25, 1983
8. Jacobsen K, Vopalecky F: Congenital dislocation of the knee. *Acta Orthop Scand* 56:1, 1985
9. Johnson E, Audell R, Oppenheim WL: Congenital dislocation of the knee. *J Pediatr Orthop* 7:194, 1987
10. Katz MP, Grogono BJS, Soper KC: The etiology and treatment of congenital dislocation of the knee. *J Bone Joint Surg* 49B:112, 1967
11. Larsen LJ, Schottstaedt ER, Bost FC: Multiple congenital dislocation associated with characteristic facial abnormality. *J Pediatr* 37:574, 1950
12. Leveuf J, Pais C: Les dislocations congenitales du genou (genu recurvatum, subluxation, luxation). *Rev Orthop* 32:313, 1946
13. McFarland BL: Congenital dislocation of the knee. *J Bone Joint Surg* 11:281, 1929
14. Munk S: Early operation of the dislocated knee in Larsen's syndrome. A report of 2 cases. *Acta Orthop Scand* 59:582, 1988
15. Niebauer JJ, King DE: Congenital dislocation of the knee. *J Bone Joint Surg* 47A:207, 1960
16. Nogi J, MacEwen GD: Congenital dislocation of the knee. *J Pediatr Orthop* 2:509, 1983
17. Parsch K, Schulz R: Ultrasonography in congenital dislocation of the knee. *J Pediatr Orthop* (B) 3:76, 1994
18. Roach JW, Richards BS: Congenital dislocation of the knee (clinical conference). *J Pediatr Orthop* 8:226, 1988
19. Roy DR, Crawford AH: Percutaneous quadriceps recession: A technique for management of congenital hyperextension deformities of the knee in the neonate. *J Pediatr Orthop* 9:717, 1989
20. Seringe R, Reneaud I: Congenital dislocation of the knee in the newborn. *J Pediatr Orthop* (B) 1:182, 1992
21. Silverman FN: Larsen's syndrome: Congenital dislocation of knees and other joints, distinctive facies and frequently, cleft palate. *Ann Radiol* 15:297, 1972

Knee Hyperextension (Genu Recurvatum) and Flexion Deformity

22. Broughton NS, Wright J, Menelaus MB: Range of knee motion in normal neonates. *J Pediatr Orthop* 13:263, 1993
23. Coon V, Donato G, Houser C, Bleck E: Normal ranges of hip motion in infants six weeks, three months, and six months of age. *Clin Orthop* 110:256, 1975
24. Hoffer MM: Joint motion limitation in newborns. *Clin Orthop* 148:94, 1980
25. Reade E, Hom L, Hallum A, Lopopolo R: Changes in popliteal angle measurement in infants up to one year of age. *Dev Med Child Neurol* 26:774, 1984

Congenital Absence of the Patella

26. Bernhang AM, Levine SA: Familial absence of the patella. *J Bone Joint Surg* 55A:1088, 1973
27. Kutz ER: Congenital absence of the patellae. *J Pediatr* 34:760, 1949

Congenital Dislocation of the Patella

28. Gao G-X, Lee EH, Bose K: Surgical management of congenital and habitual dislocation of the patella. *J Pediatr Orthop* 10:255, 1990
29. Jones RDS, Fischer RL, Curtis BH: Congenital dislocation of the patella. *Clin Orthop* 119:177, 1976
30. Langenskiöld A, Ritsila V: Congenital dislocation of the patella and its operative treatment. *J Pediatr Orthop* 12:315, 1992
31. Stanisavljevic S, Zemenick G, Miller D: Congenital, irreducible, permanent lateral dislocation of the patella. *Clin Orthop* 116:190, 1976
32. Walker J, Rang M, Daneman A: Ultrasonography of the unossified patella in young children. *J Pediatr Orthop* 11:100, 1991

Bipartite Patella

33. Echeverria TS, Bersani FA: Acute fracture simulating a symptomatic bipartite patella. *Am J Sports Med* 8:48, 1980
34. Green WT: Painful bipartite patellae. A report of three cases. *Clin Orthop* 110:197, 1975
35. Ogden JA, McCarthy SM, Jokl P: The painful bipartite patella. *J Pediatr Orthop* 2:263, 1982
36. Schmidt DR, Henry JH: Stress injuries of the adolescent extensor mechanism. *Clin Sports Med* 8:343, 1989
37. Weaver JK: Bipartite patellae as a cause of disability in the athlete. *Am J Sports Med* 5:137, 1977

Patellofemoral Joint

38. Brattstrom H: Shape of the intercondylar groove normally and in recurrent dislocation of patella. *Acta Orthop Scand* (Suppl) 68:1, 1964

39. Butler-Manuel PA, Guy RL, Heatley FW, Nunan TO: Scintigraphy in the assessment of anterior knee pain. *Acta Orthop Scand* 61:438, 1990

40. Carson WG, James SL, Larson RL, Singer KM, Winternitz WW: Patellofemoral disorders: Physical and radiographic evaluation. Part II. Radiographic examination. *Clin Orthop* 185:165, 1984

41. Dowd GSE, Bentley G: Radiographic assessment in patellar instability and chondromalacia patellae. *J Bone Joint Surg* 68B:297, 1986

42. Ficat RP, Hungerford DS: *Disorders of the Patellofemoral Joint.* Baltimore, Williams & Wilkins, 1977

43. Fulkerson JP, Schutzer SF, Ramsby GR, Bernstein RA: Computerized tomography of the patellofemoral joint before and after lateral release or realignment. *J Arthroscopy* 3:19, 1987

44. Inoue M, Shino K, Hirose H, Horibe S, Ono K: Subluxation of the patella. Computed tomography analysis of patellofemoral congruence. *J Bone Joint Surg* 70A:1331, 1988

45. Insall J: "Chondromalacia patellae": Patellar malalignment syndrome. *Orthop Clin North Am* 10:117, 1979

46. Insall J, Salvati E: Patella position in the normal knee joint. *Radiology* 101:101, 1971

47. Kennedy JC (ed): *The Injured Adolescent Knee.* Baltimore, Williams & Wilkins, 1979

48. Kolowich PA, Paulos LE, Rosenberg TD, Farnsworth S: Lateral release of the patella: Indications and contraindications. *Am J Sports Med* 18:359, 1990

49. Kujala UM, Osterman K, Kormano M, Komu M, Schlenzka D: Patellar motion analyzed by magnetic resonance imaging. *Acta Orthop Scand* 60:13, 1989

50. Lancourt JE, Cristini JA: Patella alta and patella infera. *J Bone Joint Surg* 57A:1112, 1975

51. Laurin CA, Dussault R, Levesque HP: The tangential x-ray investigation of the patellofemoral joint. *Clin Orthop* 144:16, 1979

52. Laurin CA, Levesque HP, Dussault R, Labelle H, Peides JP: The abnormal lateral patellofemoral angle. *J Bone Joint Surg* 60A:55, 1978

53. Malghem J, Maldague B: Depth insufficiency of the proximal trochlear groove on lateral radiographs of the knee: Relation to patellar dislocation. *Radiology* 170:507, 1989

54. McConnell J: The management of chondromalacia patellae: A long-term solution. *Aust J Physiother* 2:215, 1986

55. Merchant AC, Mercer RL, Jacobsen RH, Cool CR: Roentgenographic analysis of patellofemoral congruence. *J Bone Joint Surg* 56A:1391, 1974

56. Minkoff J, Fein L: The role of radiography in the evaluation and treatment of common anarthrotic disorders of the patellofemoral joint. *Clin Sports Med* 8:203, 1989

57. Schutzer SF, Ramsby GR, Fulkerson JP: Computed tomographic classification of patellofemoral pain patients. *Orthop Clin North Am* 17:235, 1986

58. Shellock FG, Mink JH, Fox JM: Patellofemoral joint: Kinematic MR imaging to assess tracing abnormalities. *Radiology* 168:551, 1988

59. Smillie IS: *Injuries of the Knee Joint,* 5th ed. New York, Churchill Livingstone, 1978

60. Thabit G III, Micheli LJ: Patellofemoral pain in the pediatric patient. *Orthop Clin North Am* 23:567, 1992

61. Walsh WM: Patellofemoral joint. In DeLee JC, Drez DD: *Orthopaedic Sports Medicine. Principles and Practice.* Philadelphia, WB Saunders Co, 1994, pp 1163–1248

62. Williams PF: Orthopedic Pediatric Management in Childhood. London, Blackwell Scientific, 1982

Osgood-Schlatter Lesion

63. Ehrenborg G: The Osgood-Schlatter lesion. Clinical and experimental study. *Acta Chir Scand* (Suppl) 288:1, 1962

64. Ehrenborg G, Engfeldt B: Histologic changes in the Osgood-Schlatter lesion. *Acta Chir Scand* 121:328, 1961

65. Ehrenborg G, Engfeldt B: The insertion of the ligamentum patellae on the tibial tuberosity. Some news in connection with the Osgood-Schlatter lesion. *Acta Chir Scand* 121:491, 1961

66. Fericot CF: Surgical management of anterior tibial epiphysis. *Clin Orthop* 5:204, 1955

67. Kujala UM, Kvist M, Heinonen O: Osgood-Schlatter's disease in adolescent athletes: Retrospective study of incidence and duration. *Am J Sports Med* 13:236, 1985

68. Lynch MC, Walsh HPJ: Tibia recurvatum as a complication of Osgood-Schlatter's disease: A report of two cases. *J Pediatr Orthop* 11:543, 1991

69. Mital MA, Matza RA, Cohen J: The so-called unsolved Osgood-Schlatter lesion. A concept based on fifteen surgically treated lesions. *J Bone Joint Surg* 62A:732, 1980

70. Ogden JA: Radiology of postnatal skeletal development. X. Patella and tibial tuberosity. *Skeletal Radiol* 11:246, 1984

71. Ogden JA, Southwick WO: Osgood-Schlatter's disease and tibial tuberosity development. *Clin Orthop* 116:180, 1976

72. Osgood RB: Lesions of the tibial tubercle occurring during adolescence. *Boston Med Surg J* 148:114, 1903

73. Rostron PKM, Calver RF: Subcutaneous atrophy following methylprednisone injection in Osgood-Schlatter epiphysitis. *J Bone Joint Surg* 61A:627, 1979

74. Schlatter C: Verletzungen des schnabelformigen Forsatzes der oberen Tibiaepiphyse. *Beitr Klin Chir* 38:874, 1903

75. Stirling RI: Complications of Osgood-Schlatter's disease. *J Bone Joint Surg* 34B:149, 1952

76. Woolfrey BF, Chandler EF: Manifestations of Osgood-Schlatter's disease in late teen age and early adulthood. *J Bone Joint Surg* 42A:327, 1960

Knee Extensor Tendinitis

77. Batten J, Menelaus MB: Fragmentation of the proximal pole of the patella. *J Bone Joint Surg* 67B:249, 1985

78. Blazina ME, Kerlan RK, Jobe FW, Carter VS, Carlson GJ: Jumper's knee. *Orthop Clin North Am* 4:665, 1973

79. Ferretti A, Ippolito E, Mariani P, Puddu G: Jumper's knee. *Am J Sports Med* 11:58, 1983

80. Kelly DW, Carter VS, Jobe FW, Kerlan RK: Patellar and quadriceps tendon ruptures—Jumper's knee. *Am J Sports Med* 12:375, 1984

81. Medlar RC, Lyne ED: Sinding-Larsen-Johansson disease: Its etiology and natural history. *J Bone Joint Surg* 60A:1113, 1978

82. Roels J, Martens M, Mulier JC, Burssens A: Patellar tendinitis (jumper's knee). *Am J Sports Med* 6:362, 1978

Synovial Plica Syndrome

83. Broom MJ, Fulkerson JP: The plica syndrome: A new perspective. *Orthop Clin North Am* 17:179, 1986

84. Mital MA, Hayden J: Pain in the knee in children: The medial plica shelf syndrome. *Orthop Clin North Am* 10:713, 1979

85. Patel D: Arthroscopy of the plicasynovial folds and their significance. *Am J Sports Med* 6:217, 1978

86. Pipkin G: Lesions of the suprapatellar plica. *J Bone Joint Surg* 32A:363, 1950

87. Vaughan-Lane T, Dandy DJ: The synovial shelf syndrome. *J Bone Joint Surg* 64B:475, 1982

Stress Fracture of the Patella

88. Devas MB: Stress fractures of the patella. *J Bone Joint Surg* 42B:71, 1960

89. Dickason JM, Fox JM: Fracture of the patella due to overuse syndrome in a child: A case report. *Am J Sports Med* 10:248, 1982

90. Iwaya T, Tukatori Y: Lateral longitudinal stress fracture of the patella: Report of three cases. *J Pediatr Orthop* 5:73, 1985

Osteochondritis Dissecans of the Patella

91. Edwards DH, Bentley G: Osteochondritis dissecans patellae. *J Bone Joint Surg* 59B:58, 1977

92. Smillie IS: *Osteochondritis Dissecans.* Edinburgh, E & S Livingston, 1960

93. Stougaard J: Osteochondritis dissecans of the patella. *Acta Orthop Scand* 45:111, 1974

Osteochondritis Dissecans of the Knee

94. Caffey J, Madell SH, Royer C, Morales P: Ossification of the distal femoral epiphysis. *J Bone Joint Surg* 40A:647, 1958

95. Cahill BR, and Berg BC: 99m-Technetium phosphate compound joint scintigraphy in the management of juvenile osteochondritis dissecans of the femoral condyles. *Am J Sports Med* 11:329, 1983

96. Fairbanks HAT: Osteo-chondritis dissecans. *Br J Surg* 21:67, 1933

97. Green WT, Banks HH: Osteochondritis dissecans in children. *J Bone Joint Surg* 35A:26, 1953

98. Guhl J: Osteochondritis dissecans. In Shahriaree H (ed): *O'Connor's Textbook of Arthroscopic Surgery.* Philadelphia, JB Lippincott, 1984, pp 211–226

99. Smillie IS: *Osteochondritis Dissecans.* Baltimore, Williams & Wilkins, 1960

100. Smillie IS: *Injuries of the Knee Joint.* Edinburgh, Livingstone, 1970

101. Wilson JN: A diagnostic sign in osteochondritis dissecans of the knee. *J Bone Joint Surg* 49A:477, 1967

Reflex Sympathetic Dystrophy

102. Alioto JT: Behavioral treatment of reflex sympathetic dystrophy. *Psychosomatics* 22:539, 1981

103. Cooper DE, DeLee JC, Ramamurthy S: Reflex sympathetic dystrophy of the knee. *J Bone Joint Surg* 71A:365, 1989

104. Dietz FR, Matthews KD, Montgomery WJ: Reflex sympathetic dystrophy in children. *Clin Orthop* 258:225, 1990

105. Katz MM, Hungerford DS: Reflex sympathetic dystrophy affecting the knee. *J Bone Joint Surg* 69B:797, 1987

106. Kozin F, McCarty DJ, Sims J, Genanth K: The reflex sympathetic dystrophy syndrome. *Am J Med* 60:321, 1976

107. Ladd AL, DeHaven KE, Thanik J, Patt RB, Feuerstein M: Reflex sympathetic imbalance. Response to epidural blockade. *Am J Sports Med* 17:660, 1989

108. Lankford LL, Thompson JE: Reflex sympathetic dystrophy, upper and lower extremity: Diagnosis and management. *AAOS Instr Course Lect* 26:163, 1977

109. Ogilvie-Harris DJ, Roscoe M: Reflex sympathetic dystrophy of the knee. *J Bone Joint Surg* 69B:804, 1987

110. Schutzer SF, Gossling HR: The treatment of reflex sympathetic dystrophy syndrome. *J Bone Joint Surg* 66A:642, 1984

111. Sherry DD, Weissman R: Psychologic aspects of childhood reflex neurovascular dystrophy. *Pediatrics* 81:582, 1988

112. Silber TJ, Majd M: Reflex sympathetic dystrophy syndrome in children and adolescents. *Am J Dis Child* 142:1325, 1988

113. Simon H, Carlson D: The use of bone scanning in the diagnosis of reflex sympathetic dystrophy. *Clin Nucl Med* 5:116, 1980

Discoid Meniscus

114. Aichroth PM, Patel DV, Marx CL: Congenital discoid lateral meniscus in children. A follow-up study and evolution of management. *J Bone Joint Surg* 73B:932, 1991

115. Beals RK: The "snapping knee" of infancy. *J Bone Joint Surg* 60A:679, 1978

116. Bellier G, Dupont JY, Larrain M, Caudron C, Carlioz H: Lateral discoid menisci in children. *Arthroscopy* 5:52, 1989

117. Clark CR, Ogden JA: Development of the menisci of the human knee joint. Morphological changes and their potential role in childhood meniscal injury. *J Bone Joint Surg* 65A:538, 1983

118. Dimakopoulos P, Patel D: Partial excision of discoid meniscus. Arthroscopic operation of 10 patients. *Acta Orthop Scand* 61:40, 1990

119. Engber WD, Mickelson MR: Cupping of the lateral tibial plateau associated with a discoid meniscus. *Orthopaedics* 4:904, 1981

120. Fritschy D, Gonseth D: Discoid lateral meniscus. *Int Orthop* 15:145, 1991

121. Fujikawa K, Iseki F, Mikura Y: Partial resection of the discoid meniscus in the child's knee. *J Bone Joint Surg* 63B:391, 1981

122. Hall FM: Arthrography of the discoid lateral meniscus. *AJR* 128:993, 1977
123. Kaplan EB: Discoid lateral meniscus of the knee joint: Nature, mechanism, and operative treatment. *J Bone Joint Surg* 39A:77, 1957
124. Lloyd EI: Clicking knee in childhood. *Lancet* 1:525, 1933
125. McGinty JB, Geuss LF, Marvin RA: Partial or total meniscectomy. *J Bone Joint Surg* 59A:763, 1977
126. Silverman JM, Mink JH, Deutsch AL: Discoid menisci of the knee: MR imaging appearance. *Radiology* 173:351, 1989
127. Smilie IS: The congenital discoid meniscus. *J Bone Joint Surg* 30B:671, 1948
128. Smilie IS: *Injuries of the Knee Joint,* ed 4. Baltimore, Williams & Wilkins, 1970, pp 39–97
129. Watanabe M, Takeda S, Ikeuchi H: *Atlas of Arthroscopy,* ed 2. Tokyo, Igaku Shoin, 1969

Popliteal Cyst (Baker's Cyst)

130. Dinham JM: Popliteal cysts in children. *J Bone Joint Surg* 57B:69, 1975
131. Gompels BM, Darkington LG: Evaluation of popliteal cysts and painful calves with ultrasonography; comparison with arthrography. *Ann Rheum Dis* 4:355, 1982
132. MacMahon EB: Baker's cysts in children—is surgery necessary? *J Bone Joint Surg* 55A:1311, 1973
133. Rudikoff JC, Lynch JJ, Phillips E, Clapp PR: Ultrasound diagnosis of Baker's cyst. *JAMA* 235:1054, 1976
134. Szer IS, Klein-Gitelman M, DeNardo BA, McCauley RG: Ultrasonography in the study of prevalence and clinical evolution of popliteal cysts in children with knee effusions. *J Rheumatol* 19:458, 1992

Soft Tissue Swelling and Effusion in the Knee

135. Culp RW, Eichenfield AW, Davidson RS, Drummond DS, Christoferson MR, Goldsmith DP: Lyme arthritis in children. *J Bone Joint Surg* 69A:96, 1987
136. Ogilvie-Harris DJ, McLean J, Zarnett ME: Pigmented villonodular synovitis of the knee. The results of total arthroscopic synovectomy, partial, arthroscopic synovectomy, and arthroscopic local excision. *J Bone Joint Surg* 74A:119, 1992

Angular Deformities of the Lower Limb

137. Böhm M: Infantile deformities of the knee and hip. *J Bone Joint Surg* 15:574, 1933
138. Kling TF Jr: Angular deformities of the lower limbs in children. *Orthop Clin North Am* 18:513, 1987
139. Kling TF Jr, Hensinger RN: Angular and torsional deformities of the lower limbs in children. *Clin Orthop* 176:136, 1983
140. Morley AJM: Knock knees in children. *Br Med J* 2:976, 1957
141. Sherman M: Physiologic bowing of the legs. *South Med J* 53:830, 1960
142. Vankka E, Salenius P: Spontaneous correction of severe tibiofemoral deformity in growing children. *Acta Orthop Scand* 53:567, 1982

Tibia Vara (Blount's Disease)

143. Blount WP: Tibia vara. Osteochondrosis deformans tibiae. *J Bone Joint Surg* 19:1, 1937
144. Blount WP: Tibia vara, osteochondrosis deformans tibiae. *Curr Pract Orthop Surg* 3:141, 1966
145. Bradway JK, Klassen RA, Peterson HA: Blount disease: A review of the English literature. *J Pediatr Orthop* 7:472, 1987
146. Carter JR, Leeson MC, Thompson GH, Kalamchi A, Kelly CM, Makley JT: Late-onset tibia vara: A histopathologic analysis. A comparative evaluation with infantile tibia vara and slipped capital femoral epiphysis. *J Pediatr Orthop* 8:187, 1988
147. Cook SE, Lavernia CJ, Burke SW, Skinner HB, Haddad RJ Jr: A biomechanical analysis of the etiology of tibia vara. *J Pediatr Orthop* 3:449, 1983
148. de Pablos J, Franzreo M: Treatment of adolescent tibia vara by asymmetrical physeal distraction. *J Bone Joint Surg* 75B:592, 1993
149. Erlacher P: Deformerierende Prozesse der epiphysengegend bei Kindern. *Arch Orthop Unfallchir* 20:81, 1922
150. Feldman MD, Schoenecker PL: Use of the metaphyseal-diaphyseal angle in the evaluation of bowleg. *J Bone Joint Surg* 75A:1602, 1993
151. Ferriter P, Shapiro F: Infantile tibia vara: Factors affecting outcome following proximal tibial osteotomy. *J Pediatr Orthop* 7:1, 1987
152. Golding JSR: Tibia vara. *J Bone Joint Surg* 44B:216, 1962
153. Golding JSR, McNeil-Smith JD: Observations on the etiology of tibia vara. *J Bone Joint Surg* 45B:320, 1963
154. Greene WB: Infantile tibia vara. Review. *J Bone Joint Surg* 75A:130, 1993
155. Henderson RC, Greene WB: Etiology of late-onset tibia vara: Is varus alignment a prerequisite? *J Pediatr Orthop* 14:143, 1994
156. Henderson RC, Kemp GJ: Assessment of the mechanical axis in adolescent tibia vara. *Orthopedics* 14:313, 1991
157. Henderson RC, Kemp GJ, Greene WB: Adolescent tibia vara: Alternatives for operative treatment. *J Bone Joint Surg* 74A:342, 1992
158. Henderson RC, Kemp GJ, Hayes PR: Prevalence of late-onset tibia vara. *J Pediatr Orthop* 13:255, 1993
159. Hoffman A, Jones RE, Herring JA: Blount's disease after skeletal maturity. *J Bone Joint Surg* 64A:1004, 1982
160. Langenskiöld A: Tibia vara. Osteochondrosis deformans tibiae. A survey of 23 cases. *Acta Chir Scand* 103:1, 1952
161. Langenskiöld A: Aspects of the pathology of tibia vara. *Ann Chir Gynaecol Fenn* 44:58, 1955
162. Langenskiöld A: Tibia vara: Osteochondrosis deformans tibiae. Blount's disease. *Clin Orthop* 158:77, 1981
163. Levine AM, Drennan JC: Physiologic bowlegs and tibia vara. *J Bone Joint Surg* 64A:1158, 1982
164. Loder RT, Johnston CE. II. Infantile tibia vara. *J Pediatr Orthop* 7:639, 1987
165. Loder RT, Schaffer JJ, Bardenstein MB: Late-onset tibia vara. *J Pediatr Orthop* 11:162, 1991
166. Sasaki T, Yagi T, Monji J, Yasuda K, Kanno Y: Transepiphyseal plate osteotomy for severe tibia vara in child-

ren: Follow-up study of four cases. *J Pediatr Orthop* 6:61, 1986

167. Schoenecker PL, Meade WC, Pierron RL, Sheridan JJ, Capelli AM: Blount's disease: A retrospective review and recommendations for treatment. *J Pediatr Orthop* 5:181, 1985

168. Sevastikoglou JA, Erickson I: Familial infantile osteochondrosis deformans tibiae: Idiopathic tibia vara. *Acta Orthop Scand* 38:81, 1967

169. Siffert RS: Intraepiphyseal osteotomy for progressive tibia vara: Case report and rationale of management. *J Pediatr Orthop* 2:81, 1982

170. Siffert RS, Katz JF: The intra-articular deformity in osteochondrosis deformans tibiae. *J Bone Joint Surg* 52A:800, 1970

171. Smith CF: Tibia vara (Blount's disease). *J Bone Joint Surg* 64A:630, 1982

172. Stren H: Operative elevation of the medial tibial joint surface in Blount's disease. One case observed for 18 years after operation. *Acta Orthop Scand* 40:788, 1970

173. Takatori Y, Iwaya T: Orthotic management of severe genu varum and tibia vara. *J Pediatr Orthop* 4:633, 1984

174. Thompson GH, Carter JR: Late-onset tibia vara (Blount's disease). Current concepts. *Clin Orthop* 255:24, 1990

175. Wenger DR, Mickelson M, Maynard JA: The evolution and histopathology of adolescent tibia vara. *J Pediatr Orthop* 4: 78, 1984

176. Zayer M: *Natural History of Osteochondritis Tibiae.* Mb. Blount. Lund, Gleerups, 1976

177. Zayer M: Osteoarthritis following Blount's disease. *Int Orthop* 4:63, 1980

Tibia Vara Due to Focal Fibrocartilaginous Dysplasia

178. Bell SN, Campbell PE, Cole WG, Menelaus MB: Tibia vara caused by focal fibrocartilaginous dysplasia. *J Bone Joint Surg* 67B:780, 1985

179. Bradish CF, Davies SJ, Malone M: Tibia vara due to focal fibrocartilaginous dysplasia. The natural history. *J Bone Joint Surg* 70B:106, 1988

180. Husien AM, Kale VR: Tibia vara caused by focal fibrocartilaginous dysplasia. *Clin Radiol* 40:104, 1989

181. Kariya Y, Taniguchi K, Yagisawa H, Ooi Y: Focal fibrocartilaginous dysplasia: Consideration of healing process. *J Pediatr Orthop* 11:545, 1991

182. Olney BW, Cole WG, Menelaus MB: Three additional cases of focal fibrocartilaginous dysplasia causing tibia vara. *J Pediatr Orthop* 10:405, 1990

Genu Valgum

183. Bowen JR, Leahey JL, Zhang ZH, MacEwen GD: Partial epiphysiodesis at the knee to correct angular deformity. *Clin Orthop* 198:184, 1985

184. Howorth MB: Knock knees: With special reference to the stapling operation. *Clin Orthop* 77:233, 1971

Congenital Posteromedial Angulation of the Tibia and Fibula

185. Badgley CE, O'Connor SJ, Kudner DF: Congenital kyphoscoliotic tibia. *J Bone Joint Surg* 34A:349, 1952

186. Heyman CH, Herndon CH, Heiple KG: Congenital posterior angulation of the tibia with talipes calcaneus. A long-term report of eleven patients. *J Bone Joint Surg* 41A:476, 1959

187. Hofmann A, Wenger DR: Posteromedial bowing of the tibia. Progression of discrepancy in leg lengths. *J Bone Joint Surg* 63A:384, 1981

188. Pappas AM: Congenital posteromedial bowing of the tibia and fibula. *J Pediatr Orthop* 4:525, 1984

189. Yadav SS, Thomas S: Congenital posteromedial bowing of the tibia. *Acta Orthop* 51:311, 1980

Congenital Pseudarthrosis of the Tibia

190. Anderson DJ, Schoenecker PL, Sheridan JJ, Rich MM: Use of an intramedullary rod for the treatment of congenital pseudarthrosis of the tibia. *J Bone Joint Surg* 74A:161, 1992

191. Andersen KS: *Congenital Pseudarthrosis of the Tibia.* Thesis, Copenhagen, 1978

192. Baker JK, Cain TE, Tullos HS: Intramedullary fixation for congenital pseudarthrosis of the tibia. *J Bone Joint Surg* 74A:169, 1992

193. Boyd HB, Sage FP: Congenital pseudarthrosis of the tibia. *J Bone Joint Surg* 40A:1245, 1958

194. Crossett LS, Beaty JH, Betz RR, Warner W, Clancy M, Steel HH: Congenital pseudarthrosis of the tibia. Long-term follow-up study. *Clin Orthop* 245:18, 1989

195. Dormans JP, Krajbich JI, Zuker R, Demuynk M: Congenital pseudarthrosis of the tibia: Treatment with free vascularized fibular grafts. *J Pediatr Orthop* 10:623, 1990

196. Eyre-Brook AL, Baily RAJ, Price CHG: Infantile pseudarthrosis of the tibia; three cases treated successfully by delayed autogenous by-pass graft, with some comments on the causative lesion. *J Bone Joint Surg* 51B:604, 1969

197. Fern ED, Stockley I, Bell MJ: Extending intramedullary rods in congenital pseudarthrosis of the tibia. *J Bone Joint Surg* 72B:1073, 1990

198. Lloyd Roberts GC, Shaw NE: The prevention of pseudarthrosis in congenital kyphosis of the tibia. *J Bone Joint Surg* 51B:100, 1969

199. McFarland B: Pseudarthrosis of the tibia in childhood. *J Bone Joint Surg* 33B:36, 1951

200. Morrissy RT, Riseborough EJ, Hall JE: Congenital pseudarthrosis of the tibia. *J Bone Joint Surg* 63B:367, 1981

201. Paley D, Catagni M, Argnani F, Prevot J, Bell D, Armstrong P: Treatment of congenital pseudarthrosis of the tibia using the Ilizarov technique. Clin Orthop 280:81, 1992

202. Plawecki S, Carpentier E, Lascombes P, Prevot J, Robb JE: Treatment of congenital pseudarthrosis of the tibia by the Ilizarov method. *J Pediatr Orthop* 10:786, 1990

203. Purvis GD, Holder JE: Dual bone graft for congenital pseudarthrosis of the tibia: Variations of technic. *South Med J* 53:926, 1960

204. Simonis RB, Shirali HR, Mayou B: Free vascularized fibular grafts for congenital pseudarthrosis of the tibia. *J Bone Joint Surg* 73B:211, 1991

205. Sofield HA, Millar EA: Fragmentation, realignment, and intramedullary rod fixation of deformities of the long bones in children. A ten-year appraisal. *J Bone Joint Surg* 41A: 1371, 1959

206. Uchida Y, Kojima T, Sugioka Y: Vascularized fibular graft for congenital pseudarthrosis of the tibia. Long-term results. *J Bone Joint Surg* 73B:846, 1991

207. Weiland AJ, Weiss AP, Moore JR, Tolo VT: Vascularized fibular grafts in the treatment of congenital pseudarthrosis of the tibia. *J Bone Joint Surg* 72:654, 1990

Congenital Pseudarthrosis of the Fibula

208. Dooley BJ, Menelaus MB, Paterson DC: Congenital pseudarthrosis and bowing of the fibula. *J Bone Joint Surg* 56B:739, 1974

209. Hsu LCS, O'Brien JP, Yau ACMC, Hodgson AR: Valgus deformity of the ankle in children with fibular pseudarthrosis: Results of treatment by bone-grafting of the fibula. *J Bone Joint Surg* 56A:503, 1974

210. Langenskiöld A: Pseudarthrosis of the fibula and progressive valgus deformity of the ankle in children: Treatment by fusion of the distal tibial and fibular metaphyses; a review of three cases. *J Bone Joint Surg* 49A:463, 1967

211. Merkel KD, Peterson HA: Isolated congenital pseudarthrosis of the fibula: Report of a case and review of the literature. *J Pediatr Orthop* 4:100, 1984

Congenital Longitudinal Deficiency of the Fibula

212. Achterman C, Kalamchi A: Congenital absence of the fibula. *J Bone Joint Surg* 61B:132, 1979

213. Bensahel H, Baum C: Aplasie congénitale du perone. *Ann Chir Infant* 15:103, 1974

214. Boakes JL, Stevens PM, Moseley RF: Treatment of genu valgus deformity in congenital absence of the fibula. *J Pediatr Orthop* 11:721, 1991

215. Boyd HB: Amputation of the foot with calcaneotibial arthrodesis. *J Bone Joint Surg* 21:997, 1939

216. Catagni MA: Management of fibular hemimelia using the Ilizarov method. *AAOS Instr Course Lect* 41:431, 1992

217. Choi IH, Kumra SJ, Bowen JR: Amputation or limb-lengthening for partial or total absence of the fibula. *J Bone Joint Surg* 72A:1391, 1990

218. Coventry MB, Johnson EW Jr: Congenital absence of the fibula. *J Bone Joint Surg* 34A:941, 1952

219. Davidson W, Bohne WHO: The Syme amputation in children. *J Bone Joint Surg* 57A:905, 1975

220. Epps CH Jr, Schneider PL: Treatment of hemimelias of the lower extremity. Long-term results. *J Bone Joint Surg* 71A:273, 1989

221. Exner GH, Ruttimann B: Fibular aplasia. *Int Orthop* 229:1991

222. Harris RI: Syme's amputation. The technical details essential for success. *J Bone Joint Surg* 38B:614, 1956

223. Herring JA: Syme's amputation for fibular hemimelia: A second look in the Ilizarov era. *AAOS Instr Course Lect* 41:435, 1992

224. Hootnick D, Boyd NA, Fixsen JA, Lloyd-Roberts GC: The natural history and management of congenital short tibia with dysplasia or absence of the fibula. *J Bone Joint Surg* 59B:267, 1977

225. Jansen K, Andersen KS: Congenital absence of the fibula. *Acta Orthop Scand* 45:446, 1974

226. Letts M, Vincent N: Congenital longitudinal deficiency of the fibula (fibular hemimelia). Parental refusal of amputation. *Clin Orthop* 287:160, 1993

227. Maffulli N, Fixen JA: Fibular hypoplasia with absent lateral rays of the foot. *J Bone Joint Surg* 73B:1002, 1991

228. Pappas AM, Hanawalt BJ, Anderson M: Congenital defects of the fibula. *Orthop Clin North Am* 3:187, 1972

229. Thomas IH, Williams PH: The Gruca operation for congenital absence of the fibula. *J Bone Joint Surg* 69B:587, 1987

230. Tuli SM, Barma BP: Congenital diastasis of tibio-fibular mortise. *J Bone Joint Surg* 54B:346, 1972

231. Westin GW, Sakai DN, Wood WL: Congenital longitudinal deficiency of the fibula. *J Bone Joint Surg* 58A:492, 1976

Congenital Longitudinal Deficiency of the Tibia

232. Bose K: Congenital diastasis of the inferior tibiofibular joint. *J Bone Joint Surg* 58A:886, 1976

233. Brown FW: Construction of a knee joint in congenital total absence of the tibia. A preliminary report. *J Bone Joint Surg* 47A:695, 1965

234. Epps CH Jr, Tooms RE, Edholm CD, Kruger LM, Bryant DD III: Failure of centralization of the fibula for congenital longitudinal deficiency of the tibia. *J Bone Joint Surg* 73A:858, 1991

235. Grissom LE, Harcke HT, Kumar SJ: Sonography in the management of tibial hemimelia. *Clin Orthop* 251:266, 1990

236. Hootnick D, Boyd NA, Fixsen JA, Lloyd Roberts GC: The natural history and management of congenital short tibia with dysplasia or absence of the fibula. *J Bone Joint Surg* 59B:267, 1977

237. Jones D, Barnes J, Lloyd Roberts GC: Congenital aplasia and dysplasia of the tibia with intact fibula. *J Bone Joint Surg* 60B:31, 1978

238. Kalamchi A, Dawe RV: Congenital deficiency of the tibia. *J Bone Joint Surg* 67B:581, 1985

239. Loder RT, Herring JA: Fibular transfer for congenital absence of the tibia: A reassessment. *J Pediatr Orthop* 7:8, 1987

240. Schoenecker PL, Capelli AM, Millar EA, Sheen MR, Haher T, Aiona MD, Meyer LC: Congenital longitudinal deficiency of the tibia. *J Bone Joint Surg* 71A:278, 1989

241. Tuli SM, Varma BP: Congenital diastasis of the tibio-fibular mortise. *J Bone Joint Surg* 54B:346, 1972

Rotational Malalignment of the Lower Limbs

242. Badelon O, Bensahel H, Folinais D, Lassale B: Tibiofibular torsion from the fetal period until birth. *J Pediatr Orthop* 9:169, 1989

243. Barlow DW, Staheli LT: Effects of lateral rotation splinting on lower extremity bone growth: An in-vivo study in rabbits. *J Pediatr Orthop* 11:583, 1991

244. Bennett JT, Bunnell WP, MacEwen GD: Rotational osteotomy of the distal tibia and fibula. *J Pediatr Orthop* 5:294, 1985

245. Blumel J, Eggers GWN, Evans EB: Eight cases of hereditary bilateral medial tibial torsion in four generations. *J Bone Joint Surg* 39A:1198, 1957

246. Butler A, Guy RL, Heatley FW: Measurement of tibial torsion—a new technique applicable to ultrasound and computed tomography. *Br J Radiol* 65:119, 1992

247. Cahuzac JP, Hobatho MC, Baunin C, Boulot J, Darmana R, Autefage A: Classification of 125 children with rotational abnormalities. Part B. *J Pediatr Orthop* 1:59, 1992

248. Cooke TDV, Price N, Fisher B, Hedden D: The inwardly pointing knee. An unrecognized problem of external rotational malalignment. *Clin Orthop* 260:56, 1990

249. Crane L: Femoral torsion and its relation to toeing-in and toeing-out. *J Bone Joint Surg* 41A:421, 1959

250. Eckhoff DG: Effect of limb malrotation on malalignment and osteoarthritis. *Orthop Clin North Am* 25:405, 1994

251. Eckhoff DG, Montgomery WK, Kilcoyne RF, Stamm ER: Femoral morphometry and anterior knee pain. *Clin Orthop* 302:64, 1994

252. Engel GM, Staheli LT: The natural history of torsion and other factors influencing gait in childhood. A study of the angle of gait, tibial torsion, knee angle, hip rotation and development of the arch in normal children. *Clin Orthop* 99:12, 1974

253. Fabry G, MacEwen GD, Shands AR Jr: Torsion of the femur. A follow-up study in normal and abnormal conditions. *J Bone Joint Surg* 55A:1726, 1973

254. Fabry G, Cheng LX, Molenaers G: Normal and abnormal torsional development in children. *Clin Orthop* 302:22, 1994

255. Galbraith RT, Gelberman RH, Hajek PC, Baker LA, Satoris DJ, Rab GT, Cohen MS, Griffin PP: Obesity and decreased femoral anteversion in adolescence. *J Orthop Res* 5:523, 1987

256. Guidera KJ, Ganey TM, Keneally CR, Ogden JA: The embryology of lower-extremity torsion. *Clin Orthop* 302:17, 1994

257. Hernandez RJ, Tachdjian MO, Poznanski AK, Dias LS: CT determination of femoral torsion. *AJR* 137:97, 1981

258. Herzenberg JE, Smith JD, Paley D: Correcting torsional deformities with Ilizarov's apparatus. *Clin Orthop* 302:36, 1994

259. Hubbard DD, Staheli LT, Chew DE, Mosca VS: Medial femoral torsion and osteoarthritis. *J Pediatr Orthop* 8:540, 1988

260. Hunziker UA, Largo RR, Duc G: Neonatal metatarsus adductus, joint mobility, axis and rotation of the lower extremity in preterm and term children 0-5 years of age. *Eur J Pediatr* 148:19, 1988

261. Hutter CG Jr, Scott W: Tibial torsion. *J Bone Joint Surg* 31A:511, 1949

262. Jacquemier M, Jouve JL, Bollini G, Panuel M, Migliani R: Acetabular anteversion in children. *J Pediatr Orthop* 12:373, 1992

263. Joseph B, Carver RA, Bell MJ, Sharrard WJ, Levick RK, Aithal V, Chacko V, Murthy SV: Measurement of tibial torsion by ultrasound. *J Pediatr Orthop* 7:317, 1987

264. Kate BR: Anteversion versus torsion of the femoral neck. *Acta Anat* 94:457, 1976

265. Katz K, Krikler R, Wielunsky E, Merlob P: Effect of neonatal posture on later lower limb rotation and gait in premature infants. *J Pediatr Orthop* 11:520, 1991

266. Katz K, Naor N, Merlob P, Wielunsky E: Rotational deformities of the tibia and foot in preterm infants. *J Pediatr Orthop* 10:483, 1990

267. Khermosh O, Lior G, Weissman SL: Tibial torsion in children. *Clin Orthop* 79:25, 1971

268. Knittel G, Staheli LT: The effectiveness of shoe modifications for intoeing. *Orthop Clin North Am* 7:1019, 1976

269. Krengel WF III, Staheli LT: Tibial rotational osteotomy for idiopathic torsion. A comparison of the proximal and distal osteotomy levels. *Clin Orthop* 283:285, 1992

270. LeDamany P: La torsion du tibia. Normale, pathologique, expérimentale. *J Anat Physiol* 45:598, 1909

271. Lee J, Jarvis J, Unthoff HK, Avruch L: The fetal acetabulum. A histomorphometric study of acetabular anteversion and femoral head coverage. *Clin Orthop* 281:48, 1992

272. McNicol D, Leong JCY, Hsu LCS: Supramalleolar derotation osteotomy for lateral tibial torsion and associated equino-varus deformity of the foot. *J Bone Joint Surg* 65B:166, 1983

273. McSweeny A: A study of femoral torsion in children. *J Bone Joint Surg* 53B:90, 1971

274. Mosca VS, Staheli LT: Surgical management of torsional and angular deformities of the lower extremities, in Chapman MW (ed): *Operative Orthopedics.* Philadelphia, JB Lippincott, 1988, p 2227

275. Pitkow EB: External rotation contracture of the extended hip. A common phenomenon of infancy obscuring femoral neck anteversion and the most frequent cause of out-toeing gait in children. *Clin Orthop* 110:139, 1975

276. Pizzutillo PD, Eidelson SG: Persistent femoral anteversion and knee pain in the second decade of life. *Orthop Trans* 13:555, 1989

277. Reikeras O: Is there a relationship between femoral anteversion and leg torsion? *Skeletal Radiol* 20:409, 1991

278. Reikeras O: Patellofemoral characteristics in patients with increased femoral anteversion. *Skeletal Radiol* 21:311, 1992

279. Reikeras O, Hoiseth A: Torsion of the leg determined by computed tomography. *Acta Orthop Scand* 60:330, 1989

280. Ruwe PA, Gage JR, Ozonoff MB, DeLuca PA: Clinical determination of femoral anteversion. A comparison with established techniques. *J Bone Joint Surg* 74A:820, 1992

281. Schrock RD Jr: Peroneal nerve palsy following derotation osteotomies for tibial torsion. *Clin Orthop* 62:172, 1969

282. Staheli LT: Rotational problems of the lower extremities. *Orthop Clin North Am* 18:503, 1987

283. Staheli LT: Low positional deformity in infants and children. A review. *J Pediatr Orthop* 10:559, 1990

284. Staheli LT, Clawson DK, Hubbard DD: Medial femoral torsion: Experience with operative treatment. *Clin Orthop* 146:222, 1980

285. Staheli LT, Corbett M, Wyss C, King H: Lower-extremity rotational problems in children. Normal values to guide management. *J Bone Joint Surg* 67A:39, 1985

286. Staheli L, Engel GM: Tibial torsion: A method of assessment and a survey of normal children. *Clin Orthop* 86:183, 1972

287. Staheli LT, Lippert F, Denotter P: Femoral anteversion and physical performance in adolescent and adult life. *Clin Orthop* 129:213, 1977

288. Stroud KL, Smith AD, Kruse RW: The relationship between increased femoral anteversion in childhood and patellofemoral pain in adulthood. *Orthop Trans* 13:555, 1989

289. Stuberg W, Temme J, Kaplan P, Clarke A, Fuchs R: Measurement of tibial torsion and thigh–foot angle using goniometry and computed tomography. *Clin Orthop* 272:208, 1991

290. Svenningsen S, Apalset K, Terjesen T, Anda S: Osteotomy for femoral anteversion. Complications in 95 children. *Acta Orthop Scand* 60:401, 1989

291. Svenningsen S, Apalset K, Terjesen T, Anda S: Regression of femoral anteversion. A prospective study of intoeing children. *Acta Orthop Scand* 60:170, 1989

292. Svenningsen S, Terjesen T, Auflem M, Berg V: Hip rotation and in-toeing gait. A study of normal subjects from 4 years until adult age. *Clin Orthop* 251:177, 1990

293. Terjesen T, Anda S, Ronningen H: Ultrasound examination for measurement of femoral anteversion in children. *Skel Radiol* 22:33, 1993

294. Tönnis D, Heinecke A: Diminished femoral antetorsion syndrome. A cause of pain and osteoarthritis. *J Pediatr Orthop* 11:419, 1991

295. Turner MS: The association between tibial torsion and knee joint pathology. *Clin Orthop* 302:47, 1994

296. Turner MS, Smillie LS: The effect of tibial torsion on the pathology of the knee. *J Bone Joint Surg* 63B:396, 1981

297. Wedge JH, Munkacsi I, Loback D: Anteversion of the femur and idiopathic osteoarthrosis of the hip. *J Bone Joint Surg* 71A:1040, 1989

298. Weseley MS, Barenfeld PA, Eisenstein AL: Thoughts on intoeing and out-toeing: Twenty-years' experience with over 5000 cases and a review of the literature. *Foot Ankle* 2:49, 1981

299. Wilkinson JA: Femoral anteversion in rabbits. *J Bone Joint Surg* 44B:386, 1962

300. Winter WG Jr, Lafferty JF: The skiing sequelae of tibial torsion. *Orthop Clin North Am* 7:231, 1976

301. Wynne-Davies R: Talipes equinovarus. A review of 84 cases after completion of treatment. *J Bone Joint Surg* 46B:464, 1969

302. Yagi T: Tibial torsion in patients with medial-type osteoarthrotic knees. *Clin Orthop* 302:52, 1994

THE HIP

Deformities and diseases of the hip vary in different age groups. In the newborn, developmental dysplasia of the hip and postural deformities are the most common problems.

In infancy, septic hip and osteomyelitis of the proximal femur are the most serious problems that require immediate diagnosis and treatment. With delay of diagnosis, the hip joint is destroyed with devastating deformities. Rare deformities in infancy and in the young child are developmental coxa vara, proximal femoral focal deficiency, and congenital shortening of the femur.

Between 2 and 4 years of age, transient synovitis of the hip or irritable hip is the most common. In the child between 4 and 8 years of age, Perthes' disease is the most frequent hip disorder. In the preadolescent, slipped capital femoral epiphysis is the most common presenting condition.

■ DEVELOPMENTAL DYSPLASIA OF THE HIP

The presenting complaint of developmental dysplasia of the hip varies depending upon the degree of displacement, upon whether the hip is subluxatable, dislocatable, or dislocated, and upon the age of the patient. Dysplasia implies a developmental, progressive deformation of the hip in which the proximal femur, the acetabulum, and the capsule are defective. The displacement of the femoral head occurs in utero (fetal or prenatal), at birth (perinatal), or after birth (postnatal). The clinical and imaging findings and pathologic changes depend upon the time of dislocation.

Developmental dislocation of the hip falls into two major categories: *teratologic,* which is associated with other severe malformations such as myelomeningocele, arthrogryposis multiplex congenita, lumbosacral agenesis, and chromosomal abnormalities, and *typical,* which occurs in an otherwise normal infant. In this section, only typical dislocation of the hip is discussed.

Typical dislocation of the hip is subdivided into three types: (1) the dislocated hip, in which the femoral head is completely out of the acetabulum; the dislocation may be reducible by simple flexion-abduction of the hip, or it may be irreducible; (2) the dislocatable hip, in which the femoral head is still located in the acetabulum but can be easily displaced out of it by adduction and extension of the hip; and (3) the subluxatable hip, in which the femoral head can be partially displaced out of the acetabulum, but not completely. The subluxatable hip manifests a ''giving'' sensation but no clunk, whereas the dislocatable hip demonstrates a definite clunk when the hip is displaced in and out of the acetabulum. The unstable hip may be dislocatable or subluxatable. The subluxated hip may be loose and easily reducible or rigid and irreducible.

Incidence. Developmental dysplasia of the hip has definite predilection for the female, occurring six to eight times more often in girls than in boys. Definite racial and geographic variations are also found occurring in 0.1 per 1,000 in Chinese, 1.7 per 1000 in the Swedish, and 75 per 1000 in Yugoslavians. The incidence is very high in American Indians. The left hip is involved in about 60 percent of the cases and the right hip in 20 percent; 20 percent are bilateral. When both hips are involved, the left hip is more severely affected than the right. The greater involvement on the left side is the result of the intrauterine posture of the lower limbs of the fetus, with the tendency to lie with his or her back toward the mother's left side.

Etiology. The cause of developmental dysplasia of the hip is multifactorial: (1) ligamentous hyperlaxity, (2) excessive femoral antetorsion, (3) acetabular antetorsion and/or deficiency, and (4) intrauterine malposture, supported by its high incidence in breech presentation and in twin or multiple pregnancies, and its high association with other postural deformities of the limbs and trunk.

Newborns at risk. The index of suspicion should be high for the presence of hip dislocation when (1) there is a positive family history; (2) the patient is the first-born female; (3) a cesarean section has been performed because of breech presentation; (4) oligohydramnios due to premature rupture of the membranes or other causes is present; (5) intrauterine crowding has occurred because of twin or multiple pregnancy; (6) the presentation at birth is frank breech; (7) the knee has been in extended posture in utero (Fig 3–1).

Clinical Findings. These vary with the age of the infant, the degree of displacement of the femoral head (subluxatable, dislocatable, or dislocated), and whether the dislocation is prenatal, perinatal, or postnatal.

Birth to Two Months of Age. Examine the whole baby. In the newborn the diagnosis of dislocated hip is made by the Ortolani test and the dislocatable hip by the Barlow test.

Prior to performing these tests, look for the following findings, which are often associated with developmental dysplasia of the hip: (1) metatarsus varus, (2) pes calcaneovalgus, (3) torticollis, (4) plagiocephaly, and (5) extension contracture of the knee (Fig 3–2). Their presence should alert the pediatrician to the possible presence of hip dislocation.

Next, carefully examine the hip and lower limbs for the following physical findings:

1. *Asymmetrical thigh folds and popliteal creases* do occur in the newborn; they are due to pelvic obliquity with abduction contracture of one hip and sometimes adduction contracture of a varying degree of the opposite hip (Fig 3–3A, B). Caution! The adducted hip may be dysplastic. Do not overdiagnose these cases as developmental dislocation

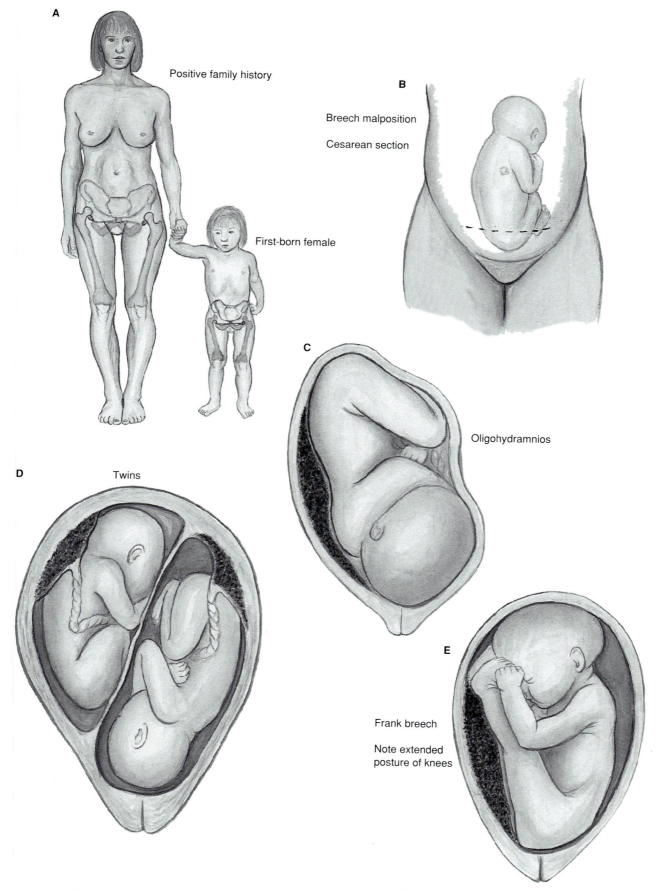

Figure 3–1. Newborn infants at high risk for developmental dysplasia of the hip. **A.** Positive family history—female and first born. **B.** Breech malposture and cesarean section. **C.** Oligohydramnios. **D.** Intrauterine crowding such as with twins or multiple pregnancy. **E.** Frank breech presentation with extended posture of the knees.

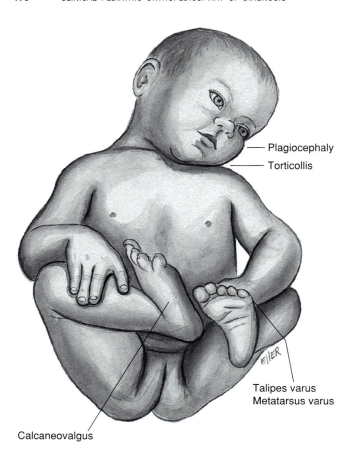

Plagiocephaly

Torticollis

Talipes varus
Metatarsus varus

Calcaneovalgus

Figure 3–2. Musculoskeletal deformities associated with developmental dysplasia of the hip are torticollis, plagiocephaly, calcaneovalgus, metatarsus or pes varus, and extension contracture of the knee. (Not illustrated.)

of the hip, and do not overtreat. Ultrasound examination often shows a low alpha angle.

2. *Apparent shortening of the femur (positive Galeazzi sign)* is usually not found in the newborn unless the dislocation has developed in utero. Be cautious! Be sure the hips are in symmetric position. When one hip is tilted into abduction, the leg of the adducted hip appears shorter. A congenital short femur should not be misdiagnosed as a dislocated hip because of a positive Galeazzi sign (Fig 3–3C).

3. *Asymmetry of inguinal folds.* Normally the inguinal folds are symmetric and they stop short of the anal aperture posteriorly (Fig 3–3D). When the femoral head is dislocated posteriorly and displaced superiorly, the inguinal folds are asymmetric. On the involved side the inguinal fold extends posteriorly and laterally beyond the anal aperture (Fig 3–3E, F). When both hips are dislocated, the inguinal folds may be symmetric, but they extend posteriorly beyond the anal aperture (Fig 3–3G).[3]

4. *Extension "looseness" of the hip and knee.* A newborn baby has 15 to 20 degrees of hip and knee flexion contracture—this is a normal finding (Fig 3–4A). Ordinarily by 2 to 3 months of age, the flexion deformity of the hips and knees disappears. Perform the Thomas test to demonstrate the normal flexion deformity of the hip, and extend the knees maximally to show flexion deformity of the knee (Fig 3–4B). When the hip is dislocated, the hip and knee extend fully or hyperextend (Fig 3–4C, D). Hip-knee extension "looseness" is a very probable sign of hip dislocation. It is simple to elicit. Caution! The baby should not cry and fight the examiner.

When the hip is frankly dislocated, the following lines are projected on the patient to determine the superior displacement of the proximal femur.

5. The *Klisić line* is drawn between the tip of the greater trochanter and the anterior superior iliac spine and extended superomedially toward the umbilicus. In the normal hip the line bisects the umbilicus (Fig 3–5A), whereas in the dislocated hip it passes inferior to the umbilicus (Fig 3–5B).

6. *Nélaton's line* is drawn between the ischial tuberosity and anterior superior iliac spine. Determine the position of the greater trochanter. In the normal hip the tip of the greater trochanter lies at or below Nélaton's line (Fig 3–6A), whereas in the dislocated hip it lies superior to Nélaton's line (Fig 3–6B).

ORTOLANI TEST. This was originally described by Le-Damany.[88] Place the infant on a firm mattress or examining table. The baby should be relaxed and not crying and resisting the examiner. Examine one hip at a time. With one hand, stabilize the pelvis and thigh with the hip abducted and the pelvis flat on the table; with the other hand, place the long and index fingers on the greater trochanter and the thumb across the knee. Do not place the thumb on the femoral triangle because it is painful and causes the baby to cry. Be gentle! Do not dig in with your fingertips! (Fig 3–7A, B).

Abduct the 90-degree flexed hip and with your index finger lift the femoral head to the acetabulum. You hear a *clunk* as the hip is reduced—this is the *"clunk of entry"* (Fig 3–7C).

Next adduct the hip. The femoral head displaces out of the acetabulum with a clunk, referred to as the *"clunk of exit"* (Fig 3–7D). Caution: The Ortolani test may be negative in antenatal in utero dislocations; this is particularly a problem in bilateral dislocations.[123,124]

A click should not be confused with a clunk. The click is a short, high-pitched sound or a dry crunch. It is caused by a ligamentous or myofascial "pop" from the iliotibial band or gluteal tendons or by a vacuum phenomenon in the hip. A subluxating patella may cause a click at the knee. A click is not a sign of developmental dysplasia of the hip.

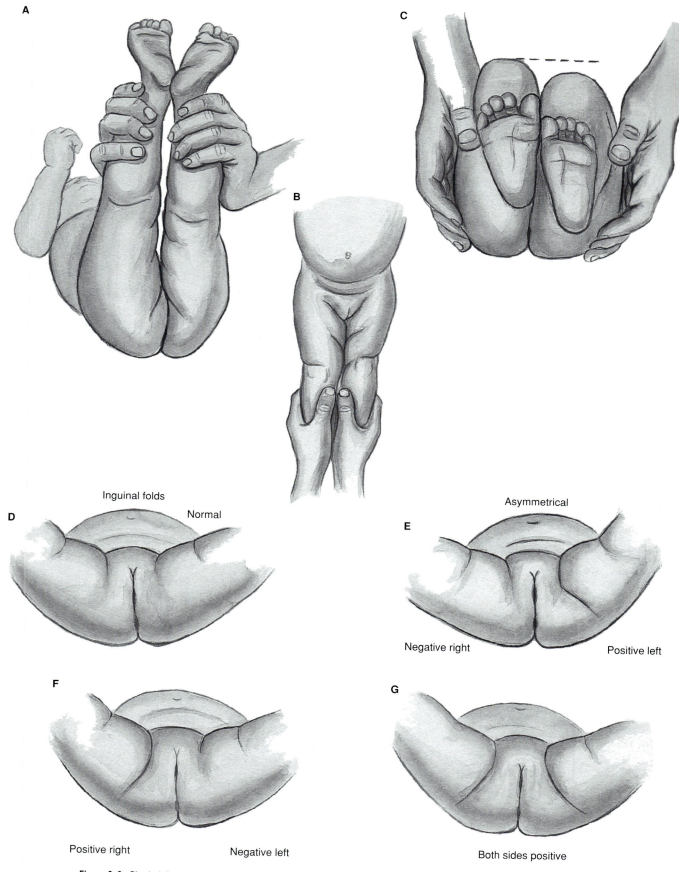

Figure 3–3. Physical findings suggesting developmental dysplasia of the hip. **A, B.** Asymmetric thigh folds and popliteal creases. **C.** Apparent shortening of the femur (positive Galeazzi sign). **D.** Normal inguinal folds. **E.** Asymmetric inguinal folds. Note that the left side is positive. The inguinal fold extends beyond the anal aperture. The right hip is normal. **F.** The inguinal fold is extending beyond the anal aperture on the right but not on the left. **G.** On both sides the inguinal folds extend beyond the anal aperture, suggesting bilateral posterior dislocation of the hips.

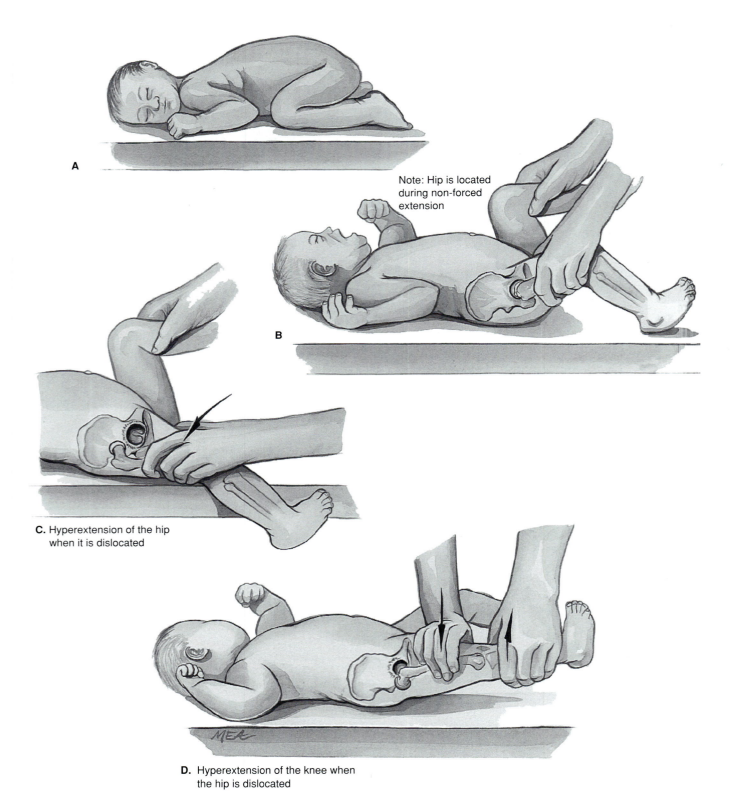

Note: Hip is located
during non-forced
extension

C. Hyperextension of the hip
when it is dislocated

D. Hyperextension of the knee when
the hip is dislocated

Figure 3–4. Extension "looseness" of the hip and knee. **A.** The normal posture of a newborn. Note that the hips and knees are in flexion. **B.** On the Thomas test, note the hip flexion contracture of 20 degrees and the knee flexion posture. **C, D.** When the hip is dislocated posteriorly, the hip and knee extend fully or hyperextend.

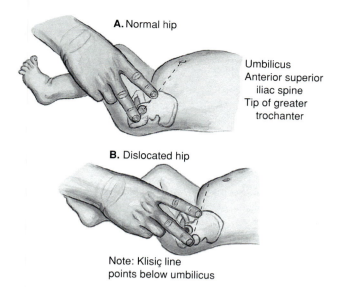

A. Normal hip

B. Dislocated hip

Umbilicus
Anterior superior
iliac spine
Tip of greater
trochanter

Note: Klisiç line
points below umbilicus

Figure 3–5. The Klisiç line. Project a line between the tip of the greater trochanter and the anterosuperior iliac spine and extend it superomedially toward the umbilicus. **A.** Normal hip. Note that the line bisects the umbilicus. **B.** Dislocated hip. The line passes inferior to the umbilicus.

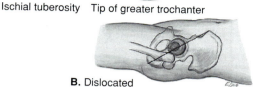

A. Normal

Anterior superior iliac spine

Note: Tip of greater trochanter lies at or below Nélaton's line

Ischial tuberosity   Tip of greater trochanter

Note: Tip of greater trochanter is superior to Nélaton's line

B. Dislocated

Figure 3–6. Nélaton's line. It is drawn between the ischial tuberosity and the antero-superior iliac spine. **A.** Normal hip. The tip of the greater trochanter is below Nélaton's line. **B.** In the dislocated hip the tip of the greater trochanter is above Nélaton's line.

BARLOW'S TEST. This test is performed to determine whether a hip is dislocatable. The posture of the infant is similar to that for the Ortolani test—supine on a firm mattress. Extension of the hip increases its instability, whereas hyperflexion of the hip makes the hip more stable. Hold the untested hip in 90 degrees of flexion and 45 degrees of abduction. The hip to be tested is held in 45 degrees of flexion and 5 to 10 degrees of adduction, an unstable position. With the long and index fingers over the greater trochanter on the proximal upper thigh and the thumb over the medial aspect of the lower thigh above the knee (not over the lesser trochanter), push the femoral head posteriorly and laterally in an attempt to dislocate the hip. When the hip is dislocatable the femoral head slips out of the acetabulum with a *clunk*—the "clunk of exit" (Fig 3–8A, B). Next release the posterolateral force and gently flex and abduct the hip. The femoral head is reduced into the acetabulum with a clunk—the "clunk of entry" (Fig 3–8C).[12,13] In questionable cases test the hip in greater extension and adduction—a position of greater hip instability.

In the unstable subluxatable hip, the femoral head cannot be pushed out of the acetabulum; there is no clunk of exit. Only a sliding, telescoping movement is felt. These hips stabilize spontaneously. Be gentle! Do not cause iatrogenic dislocation.

Three to Twelve Months of Age. With progressive posterolateral and superior displacement of the femoral head, the following physical findings develop:

1. Adduction contracture of the hip. The range of passive abduction of the dislocated hip in 90 degrees of hip flexion is progressively limited.

2. Apparent shortening of the thigh—positive Galeazzi sign. With the hips and knees flexed at right angles with the infant lying flat on a firm table, the knee on the dislocated side is at a lower level.

3. Laterally rotated posture of the lower limb with the hip and knee in extension.

4. Asymmetry of the thigh and inguinal folds and popliteal creases is more marked in unilateral dislocations. The inguinal folds extend posteriorly beyond the anal aperture.

5. Positive telescoping sign or piston mobility. To test, grasp the lower thigh and knee with one hand and hold the greater trochanter with the other hand. With the hip in some adduction, move the femur up and down in a piston fashion and note the excessive abnormal motion of the greater trochanter. Test the hip in flexion and extension (Fig 3–9).

After Walking Age. In addition to the previous findings, the child walks with a gluteus medius lurch, toes out, and has a short leg and toe-heel gait (Fig 3–10). In stance the lumbar lordosis is excessive, with prominent greater trochanters and widened perineum. The Trendelenburg test is positive. With increasing adduction contracture of the hips, there is compensatory genu valgum. The physical findings in different age groups are summarized in Table 3–1.

Imaging. *Ultrasonography.* The hip of the neonate and young infant (up to 6 months of age) is best assessed by ultrasonography, which depicts the cartilaginous parts of the acetabulum and femoral head and neck. Two methods are used to evaluate the hip: (1) nonstress static technique of Graf, and (2) the dynamic stress technique.[49]

In the Graf nonstress technique, a direct single coronal image of each hip is made with the baby lying in lateral

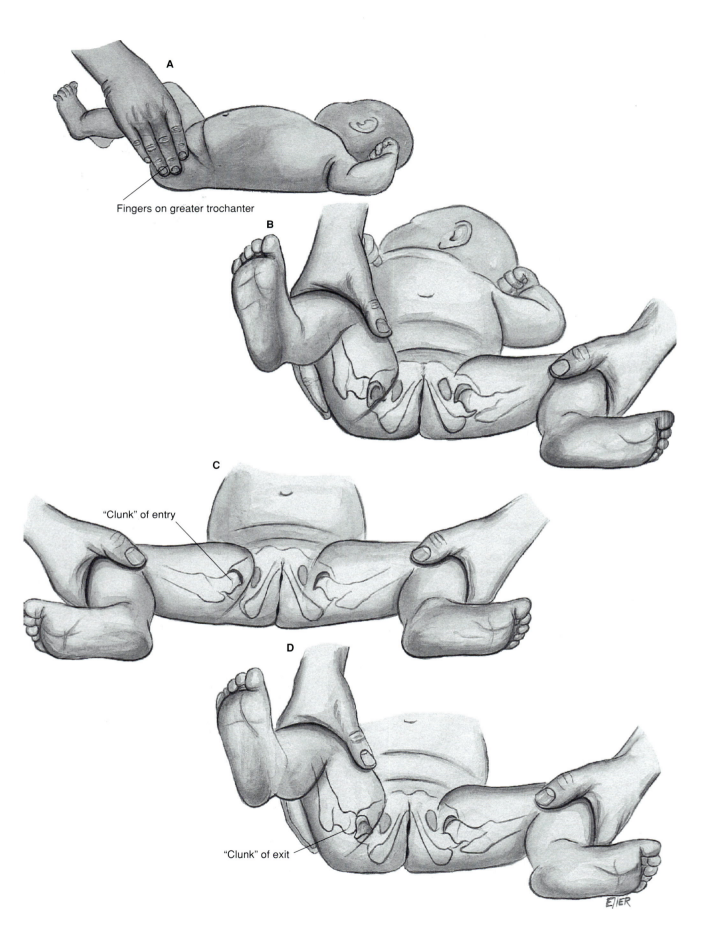

A

Fingers on greater trochanter

B

C

"Clunk" of entry

D

"Clunk" of exit

Figure 3–7. Ortolani test. **A, B.** Position of the patient. The right hip is being tested. Note that the left hand stabilizes the contralateral hip and thigh. The examiner's right hand tests the hip. Note that the tips of the index and long fingers are over the tip of the greater trochanter and the thumb is over the medial aspect of the lower thigh, not in the groin. **C.** Note that on abduction of the hip the femoral head locates into the acetabulum and there is a "clunk of entry." **D.** On adduction of the hip and some extension, the femoral head displaces out of the acetabulum, producing a clunk—the "clunk of exit."

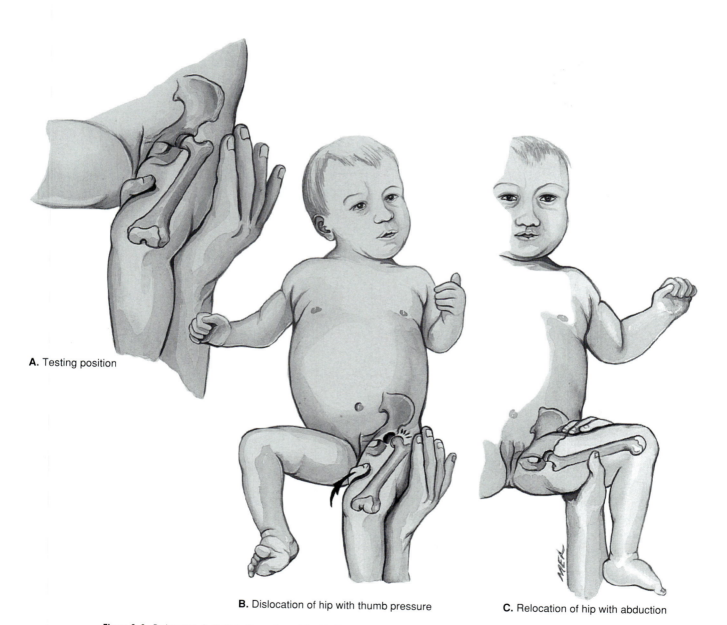

A. Testing position

B. Dislocation of hip with thumb pressure

C. Relocation of hip with abduction

Figure 3–8. Barlow test. **A, B.** Note the posture of the hip. The hip to be tested is in 45 degrees of flexion and 5 to 10 degrees of adduction. This is an unstable position. In the dislocatable hip, when the femoral head is pushed posteriorly, it slips out of the acetabulum with a clunk. **C.** On releasing the pressure, and flexing and abducting the hip, the femoral head spontaneously reduces into the acetabulum. Increasing the degree of hip extension makes the hip more unstable.

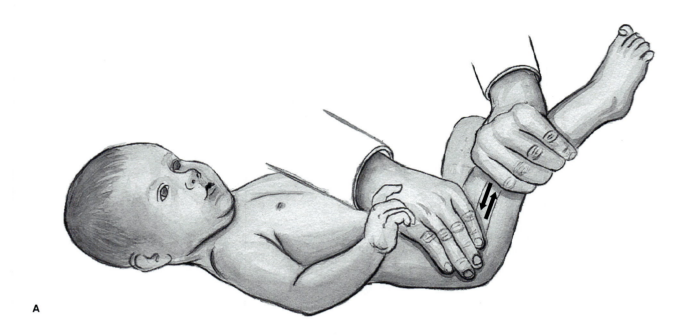

A

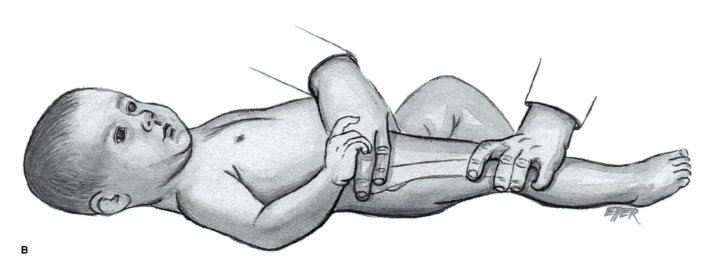

B

Figure 3–9. Telescoping or piston mobility sign. **A, B.** On push and pull of the femur with the hip in flexion and extension, the greater trochanter moves up and down.

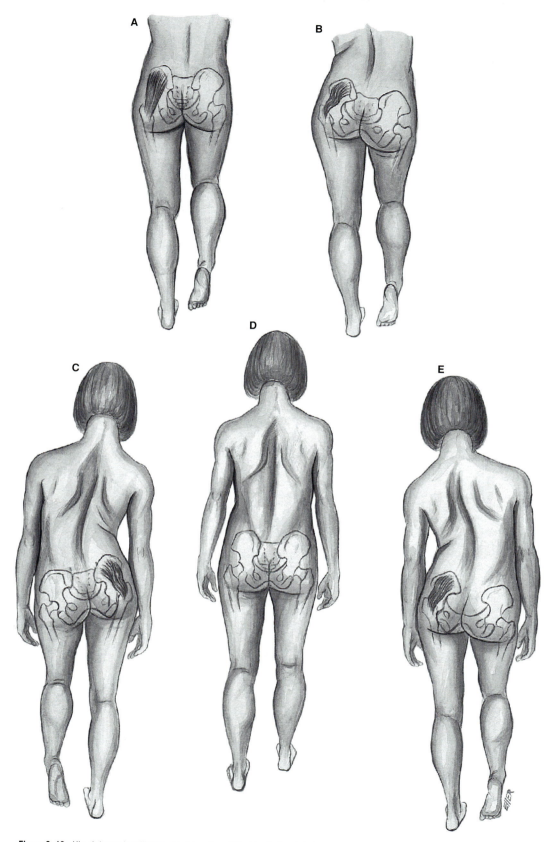

Figure 3–10. Hip abductor insufficiency in dislocation of the hip. **A.** Trendelenburg test. When standing on the normal hip, the opposite pelvis does not drop down. **B.** When standing on the dislocated hip, the opposite pelvis drops. **C to E.** Gluteus medius lurch.

TABLE 3–1. CLINICAL FINDINGS IN DEVELOPMENTAL DISLOCATION OF THE HIP

Birth to Two Months

A. Associated findings
  1. Metatarsus varus
  2. Pes calcaneovalgus
  3. Torticollis
  4. Plagiocephaly
  5. Extension contracture of the knee

B. Suggestive signs
  1. Asymmetric thigh folds and popliteal creases
  2. Apparent shortening of the femur (positive Galeazzi sign)
  3. Asymmetry of inguinal folds
  4. Extension "looseness" of hip and knee (i.e., loss of normal flexion deformity of hip and knee)
  5. Klisiç's line projection passing inferior to umbilicus
  6. Tip of the greater trochanter above Nélaton's line

C. Diagnostic tests
  1. Positive Ortolani (or LeDamany) test for dislocation of hip
  2. Positive Barlow test for dislocatable hip

  Caution! Ortolani and Barlow tests may be negative in rigid antenatal dislocations and after the age of 3 months.

Three to Twelve Months of Age

  1. Limitation of hip abduction in 90 degrees of hip flexion (progressive adduction contracture of hip)
  2. Positive Galeazzi sign
  3. Laterally rotated posture of the lower limbs with apparent shortening with the hip–knee in extended posture
  4. Marked asymmetry of the thigh and inguinal folds and popliteal creases
  5. Piston mobility or telescoping sign
  6. Lateral prominence of the greater trochanter
  7. Ortolani test—may be either negative or positive

After Walking Age

  1. Posture—excessive lumbar lordosis, protuberant abdomen, prominent greater trochanter
  2. Gluteus medius lurch
  3. Positive Trendelenburg sign
  4. Short leg limp. Toe–heel gait and out-toeing
  5. Increasing adduction contracture of the hips with compensatory genu valgum

position with the hips flexed 35 to 45 degrees and medially rotated 10 to 15 degrees. The following structures are determined: (1) the distal part of the ossified ilium in the roof of the acetabulum, (2) the ossified medial wall of the acetabulum, (3) the triradiate cartilage, (4) the cartilaginous femoral head and its ossific nucleus if developed, (5) the cartilaginous roof of the acetabulum and the labrum, (6) the capital femoral physis, and (7) the ossified metaphysis of the femoral neck (Fig 3–11A, B).

Subjectively, by inspection, assess the position of the femoral head, the appearance of the bony acetabulum, the configuration of the acetabulum, the position of the cartilaginous labrum, and the shape of the cartilaginous roof.

Next draw the following lines: (1) a vertical line parallel to the ossified lateral wall of the ilium (this is the reference line), (2) a tangent line to the bony roof of the acetabulum from the osseous margin of the acetabulum at the roof of the triradiate cartilage to the lowest point of the ilium at the center of the hip joint (this is the bony roof line), and (3) a line from the lateral bony edge of the acetabulum to the labrum (the cartilaginous roof line).

The *alpha* angle is the angle formed between line one—the reference line—and line two—the bony roof line. In the normal hip the alpha angle should be 60 degrees; the smaller the alpha angle, the greater the dysplasia of the hip (Fig 3–11C). The *beta* angle is the angle formed between the reference line (line 1) and the cartilaginous roof line (line 3). It objectively determines the decentering or lateral-superior subluxation of the hip. When the beta angle is greater than 77 degrees, the hip is subluxated and the labrum is everted (see Fig 3–11C).

TABLE 3–2. GRAF HIP TYPES

Type	Description	Alpha Angle	Beta Angle	Comments	Treatment
I	Normal hip	>60°	<77°	Stable; never dislocates (unless biomechanics are altered [e.g., meningomyelocele, cerebral palsy])	None
II	Concentric position				
a	Physiologic immaturity (age <3 mo.)	50–60°	<77°		Should be observed until change to type I
b	Delayed ossification (age >3 mo.)	50–60°	<77°		Evaluation by orthopedic surgeon
c	Concentric position with very deficient acetabulum	43–49°	<77°		Evaluation by orthopedic surgeon
d	Subluxation	43–49°	>77°	Labrum everted	Required
III	Low dislocation	<43°	>77°	Bony roof deficient; labrum everted	Required
IV	High dislocation	Not measurable	>77°	Flat bony acetabulum; labrum interposed between head and ilium	Required

Courtesy of Dr. James Donaldson.

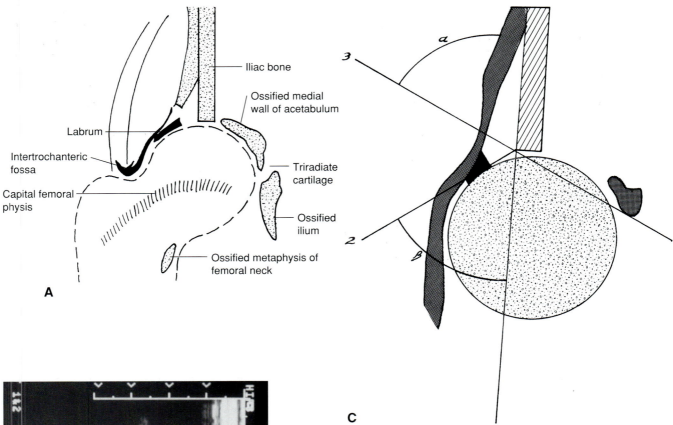

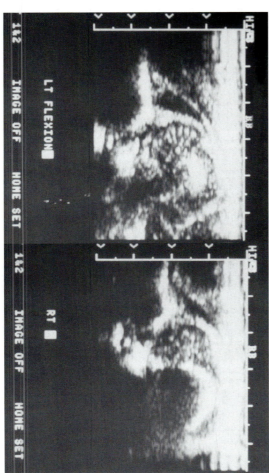

Figure 3–11. Ultrasonographic findings of the normal hip of an infant. **A.** Diagram of an ultrasonogram of a normal left hip. **B.** Ultrasonogram. **C.** Diagram showing the alpha and beta angles. Determine the following in this single coronal image. Note the reference line parallel to the lateral wall of the ilium and the bony roof, which is a tangent line drawn from the osseous margin of the acetabulum at the roof of the triradiate cartilage to the lowest point of the ilium at the center of the hip joint, and the cartilaginous roof line, which is a line from the lateral bony edge of the acetabulum to the labrum. The alpha angle is the angle formed between the reference line and the tangent line. It should be 60 degrees. The beta angle is the angle formed between the reference line and the cartilaginous roof line. It should be less than 77 degrees.

Depending upon these objective measurements and visual, subjective assessment, Graf has given the following classification with treatment recommendations: type I—the hip is normal; type II—it is concentrically reduced but immature and delayed in ossification (its severity varies with the age of the child and the degree of hip dysplasia); type III—the hip is subluxated or has a low dislocation; type IV—the dislocation is high (Table 3–2).

Because of the small size of the bony acetabular roof in the premature infant, the alpha angle may be measured to be normal; in 2 to 4 weeks, with further ossification of the acetabulum, the Graf technique becomes reliable. A 2- to 5-degree variation between examiners is inconsequential. A dysplastic hip cannot be made to look normal by the Graf technique.

The Dynamic Stress Method. With the infant supine, each hip is imaged in the transverse plane, with the examiner performing the Barlow maneuver with his or her free hand if the hip is dislocatable and the Ortolani test if the hip is dislocated to test reducibility. Note the articular relationship of the femoral head to the acetabulum.[56,118]

In the left hip up to 6 mm of motion is normal, and in the right hip 4 mm of motion is normal.

Dynamic stress assessment of the hip with ultrasonography is performed in the transverse plane with the hip in neutral and in the coronal plane.

Simultaneous Anterior Imaging of Both Hips with Ultrasonography (Suzuki technique).[170,171] Examination is performed with both hips extended and then flexed and abducted. It can be performed with a Pavlik harness on or in a plaster cast to demonstrate maintenance of reduction. It depicts the relationship between the femoral head and acetabulum and the degree and direction of displacement of the femoral head—lateral, anterior, posterior, and proximal.

The position of the patient is supine. First ultrasonography is performed with the hip extended. Place the transducer on the pubis and obtain a cross-sectional view perpendicular to the axis of the body. Move the transducer proximally until both pubic bones and femoral heads are displayed. The image of the ossified metaphysis of the femoral neck assists in locating the position of the cartilaginous femoral head. This is the *standard plane.* First, draw the *P (or pubic) line* along the anterior surface of the pubic bones.

Second, draw the *E line* from the lateral margin of the pubic bone perpendicular to the P line. Third, draw the *center line* midway between the pubic bones (Fig 3–12). The examination is then repeated with the hips in flexion and abduction.

In the normal hip with the hips extended and in neutral position—that is, in the standard plane—the whole femoral head, showing its maximum diameter, is located posterior to the P line, with a narrow space between its anterior surface and the P line. Medially no space exists between the femoral head and the E line touching it or extending beyond it. When the hips are flexed-abducted, the position of the femoral heads does not change.

When the hip is subluxated or dislocated in the extended position (standard plane) the femoral head moves anterior to the P line and displaces laterally, with a space developing between the medial margin of the femoral head and the E line. In the extended position the femoral heads are not dislocated posteriorly.

In flexion and abduction, when the hip is dislocated or subluxated, the femoral head displaces posteriorly. Suzuki has classified the degree of posterior displacement of the femoral head into three grades.[170] Type A—the femoral head is displaced posteriorly and laterally, but it is still in contact with the inner wall of the acetabulum. Type B—the femoral head is displaced posteriorly and laterally, with loss of contact with the inner wall of the acetabulum but still in contact with the posterior margin of the acetabulum and center of the femoral head lying at or anterior to the

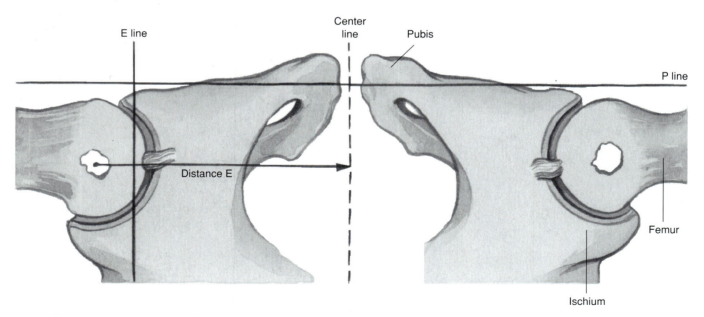

Figure 3–12. Diagram of a normal hip. Simultaneous anterior imaging (Suzuki technique). Note the following lines: (1) the P or pubic line on the anterior surface of the pubic bones, (2) the E line, which is drawn from the lateral margin of the pubic bone and perpendicular to the P line, and (3) the center line drawn midway between the pubic bones. Note that the cartilaginous femoral heads are located posterior to the P line, with a very narrow space between the head and the P line. Also, medially there is no space between the cartilaginous femoral head and the E line.

posterior edge of the acetabulum. Type C—the femoral head is displaced out of the acetabulum with its center posterior to the posterior rim of the acetabulum (Fig 3–13).

Radiographic Findings. In the newborn and young infant, the femoral head is not ossified and a greater part

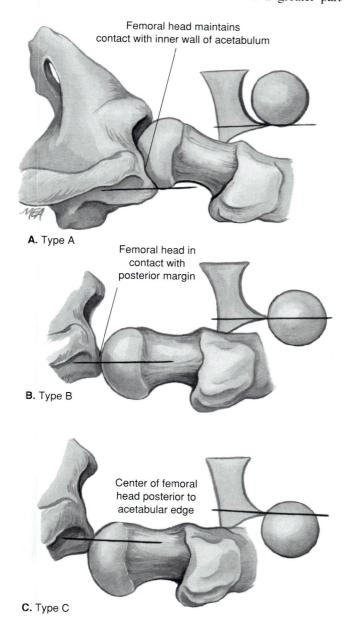

A. Type A

Femoral head maintains contact with inner wall of acetabulum

Femoral head in contact with posterior margin

B. Type B

Center of femoral head posterior to acetabular edge

C. Type C

Figure 3–13. Suzuki classification of types of posterior displacement of the femoral head in developmental dysplasia of the hip. Diagram of ultrasonogram of the hips made in the frontal transverse plane with the hips flexed and abducted.
 A. In type A note that the posteriorly displaced femoral head is still in contact with the inner wall of the acetabulum. **B.** In type B, note that the posteriorly displaced femoral head is in contact with the posterior rim of the acetabulum with its center at or anterior to the edge of the posterior acetabulum. **C.** In type C note that the femoral head is dislocated outside of the acetabulum with its center posterior to the acetabular rim. Ultrasound and the Pavlik harness in congenital dysplasia of the hip. (*J Bone Joint Surg* 75B:483, 1993.)

of the acetabulum is cartilaginous. In order to assess the development of the acetabulum and superolateral displacement of the femoral head, draw the following lines: *Hilgenreiner's line or the Y line*—a horizontal line through the upper margin of the radiolucent triradiate or Y cartilage, and *Ombredanne's vertical or Perkins' line*—a vertical line from the most lateral ossific margin of the roof of the acetabulum to transect perpendicularly and through the Y line, thereby forming quadrants around each hip.[63,122,132] In the normal hip the medial end of the ossified upper femoral metaphysis lies medial to Perkins' line and inferior to Hilgenreiner's line. In the subluxated hip it lies lateral to Perkins' line. In the dislocated hip the medial end of the ossific metaphysis of the femoral neck lies lateral to Perkins' line and superior to Hilgenreiner's line (Fig 3–14).

Next draw *Shenton's line* between the superior border of the obturator foramen and the medial border of the femoral neck; this forms an even, continuous arc in the normal hip. It is broken and interrupted when the femoral head is displaced superolaterally (Fig 3–15). Caution! When the hip is laterally rotated or adducted, Shenton's line may be slightly broken.

The *U figure or teardrop of Koehler* is delayed in ossification in developmental subluxation or dislocation of the hip because of lack of or inadequate stimulation from the capital epiphysis. The teardrop ossifies normally when the infant is a few months old. In persisting hip dysplasia the width of the teardrop shadow is greater than normal, and its lateral border, which corresponds to the inner wall of the acetabulum, does not ossify (Fig 3–16). With concentric reduction, the width of the teardrop decreases.

The *acetabular index* is the angle formed between Hilgenreiner's Y line and a tangential line to the lateral ossific margin of the roof of the acetabulum (Fig 3–17).

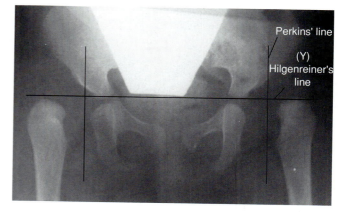

Perkins' line

(Y) Hilgenreiner's line

Figure 3–14. AP radiogram of bilateral dislocation of the hips and the quadrants formed by the Hilgenreiner (Y) and Perkins' lines. Note that the medial end of the ossific metaphysis of the femoral necks lies lateral to the Perkins' line and superior to the Hilgenreiner line.

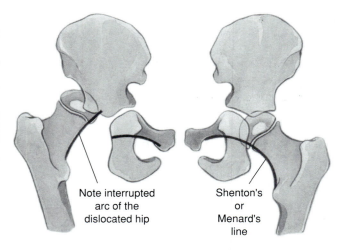

Figure 3–15. Shenton's line as seen in an AP diagram of the hips. It is drawn between the superior border of the obturator foramen and the medial border of the femoral neck. Note that in the normal hip it forms an even, continuous arc, whereas in the dislocated hip it is interrupted with superior displacement of the femoral head.

The acetabular index alters with axial and sagittal plane rotation of the pelvis. An acetabular index of 25 to 35 degrees in newborns and infants is within normal limits; an index of greater than 40 degrees implies acetabular dysplasia.

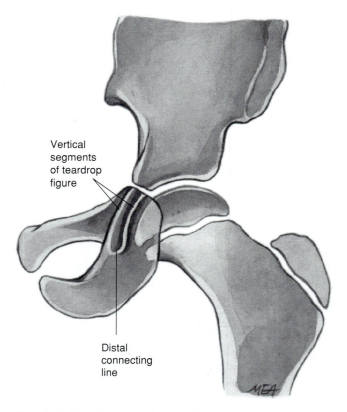

Figure 3–16. The ∪ figure or teardrop of Koehler. In hip subluxation or dislocation it is delayed in ossification and wide.

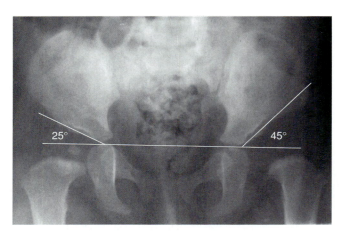

Figure 3–17. Acetabular index is the angle formed between the Hilgenreiner (Y) line and a tangential line to the lateral ossification roof of the acetabulum.

The *acetabular notch* appears as a cup-shaped defect in the lateral iliac wall immediately above the acetabulum; the notch is demarcated medially by a line of sclerotic bone (Fig 3–18). When present with a steeply inclined acetabular roof, it indicates an unstable or subluxated hip.[138]

Arthrography, a commonly performed procedure in the past, is being replaced by the newer imaging technology—ultrasonography, computed tomography (CT) scan, and magnetic resonance imaging (MRI). Some surgeons still prefer to use it because arthrography defines the limits of the capsule, showing whether it is stretched out or adherent to the lateral wall of the ilium or floor of the acetabulum. Arthrography shows the hourglass constriction of the capsule by the iliopsoas tendon. It also

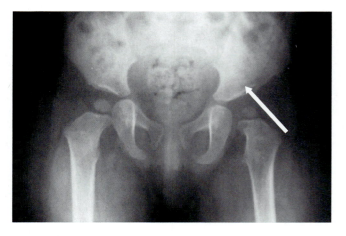

Figure 3–18. Acetabular notch. Note the cup-shaped defect on the lateral wall of the ilium immediately above the acetabular margin and its medial demarcation by a line of sclerotic bone. The acetabular roof is dysplastic and the hip is unstable.

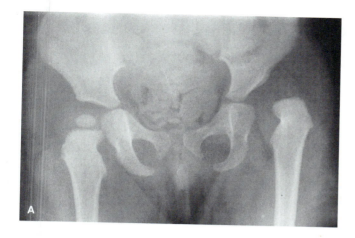

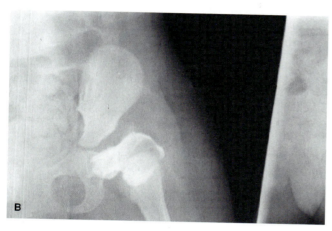

Figure 3–19. Arthrogram of the hip. **A.** Radiogram shows dislocation of left hip in a 1.5-year-old female. **B.** Arthrogram showing the medial pooling of the dye and hourglass constriction of the capsule by the psoas tendon.

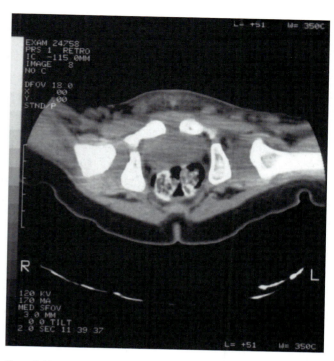

Figure 3–20. CT scan of both hips in developmental dysplasia of the left hip. Note the neck of the femur sitting laterally and the marked femoral antetorsion and acetabular torsion with posterior deficiency of the acetabulum.

of the acetabulum. Prior to performing innominate osteotomy such as a Salter procedure, it is vital to perform a CT three-dimensional reconstruction study to depict the acetabular pathology. Also, a CT study is performed to determine femoral torsion.

depicts whether reduction is concentric or inadequate due to intra-articular obstacles of reduction such as inverted limbus or hypertrophic and redundant ligamentum teres or pulvinar (Fig 3–19). The drawback of arthrography is that it is an invasive procedure that requires general anesthesia.[4,50,67] I occasionally perform it on a patient who is under general anesthesia for closed reduction of the hip when the safety zone is very poor and I cannot decide whether simple adductor myotomy or a medial approach to the hip should be carried out to achieve concentric reduction.

CT scan shows the concentricity of reduction and whether the hip is displaced posteriorly in the cast.[24,60] Whenever a closed reduction is performed under general anesthesia and a hip spica cast is applied, a CT scan is performed with the cast on to determine the adequacy of concentric reduction (Fig 3–20). A CT scan also shows the degree of acetabular antetorsion, and posterior deficiency

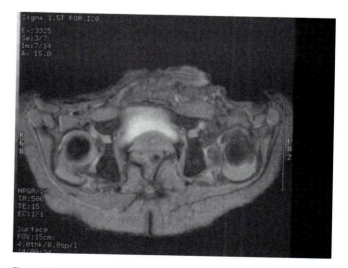

Figure 3–21. Postreduction MRI of both hips in developmental dislocation of the left hip. The right femoral head sits concentrically in the acetabulum, whereas the left sits laterally, with soft tissue interposition between the femoral head and the socket.

MRI is performed to delineate the cartilaginous and soft tissue pathology of the hip, the adequacy of reduction, and any ischemic process of the femoral head or neck (Fig 3–21).[52]

Treatment. Management of typical dislocation of the hip varies according to the degree of displacement of the femoral head—subluxatable, dislocatable, or dislocated—and the age of the child. Treatment depends on the age of presentation and degree of displacement.

Birth to Two Months of Age. When the dislocation is perinatal and easily reduced by the Ortolani maneuver, the reduction is maintained dynamically in a Pavlik harness (Fig 3–22). It is a dynamic splint that allows active hip flexion and abduction, provides stability to the hip, and promotes normal development of the acetabulum.[116,129]

Make AP radiograms of the hip with the Pavlik harness properly adjusted to determine the position of the femoral heads in relation to the acetabulum. A common pitfall is inadequate hip flexion. Ultrasonography of the hips is performed from the front to check concentricity of reduction.

In Suzuki type A hip subluxation with minimal posterolateral displacement, there is no bony or significant soft tissue obstruction to concentric reduction; the weight of the lower limb abducts the hip and relocates the femoral head deep into the acetabulum. Type C (Suzuki) dislocation cannot be reduced by the Pavlik harness; reduction is obstructed by a taut iliopsoas, capsular isthmus, and intra-articular obstacles. In type B (Suzuki), reduction by the Pavlik harness can be attempted. If reduction cannot be achieved within 1 or 2 weeks, the use of the harness should be discontinued. In type B cases, when the Pavlik harness is used in flexion-abduction, the femoral head may further displace posteriorly, converting type B into type C. In such an instance, the use of the Pavlik harness should be discontinued[170] (see Fig 3–13).

The use of a Pavlik harness is contraindicated when (1) the child is 6 months or older, (2) the hips and knees are stiff, (3) the dislocation is antenatal, (4) ultrasonogram of the hip joint shows complete dislocation (type C Suzuki), (5) there has been failure to concentrically reduce type B Suzuki in 1 or 2 weeks, and (6) severe, generalized ligamentous hyperlaxity is present, increasing the risk of obturator or anterior dislocation and causing neurovascular compromise.

Close monitoring—initially twice a week and then once a week—is crucial. Follow the patient and rule out possible development of complications such as femoral, brachial, or facial nerve palsy; medial instability of the knee; and anterior or inferior (obturator) dislocation of the hip.[116] Forced abduction of the hips in prone position should be avoided; alternate the position between supine and semilateral (not lying on the dislocated side). The infant

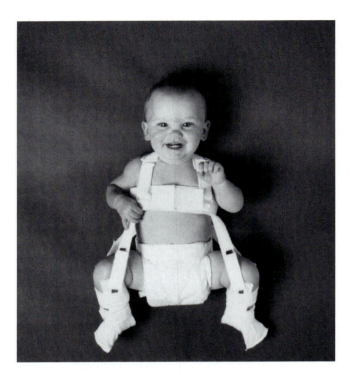

Figure 3–22. Pavlik harness as manufactured by Wheaton Brace Company, Carol Stream, Illinois.

should be able to kick his or her legs actively. Inability to extend the knee indicates femoral nerve palsy. At each visit, determine the degree of flexion of the hip. Avoid hyperflexion because it causes inferior dislocation. An abducted, stiff, and painful hip signals the possibility of anterior dislocation of the hip. Examine the knees for mediolateral instability and subluxation. Be sure the anterior stirrups (straps) are in the axillary line and the posterior straps are loose, not forcing the hips in extreme abduction.

The *dislocated hip* is maintained in a Pavlik harness 24 hours of the day for 1 month, at which time ultrasonography of the hip is repeated. Often, in 1 month the hip stabilizes, both clinically and by ultrasonographic findings. When the hip is stable, allow the infant to be out of the Pavlik harness 1 to 2 hours per day for the following 2 weeks and then 3 to 4 hours per day for an additional 2 weeks. Assess maintenance of reduction and maturation of the hip clinically and by ultrasonography. If the hip is stable, the Pavlik harness is worn only at night for an additional 2 to 4 weeks. Ordinarily the total period of wear for a Pavlik harness is 2 to 3 months, depending upon the age at diagnosis and the clinical and ultrasonographic response to dynamic retention in the Pavlik harness.

Other types of hip abduction-flexion splints made of fiber glass or other plastic materials are commercially available, such as the Craig, Ilfed, and Von Rosen splints.

In the newborn and young infant with a *dislocatable hip,* the Pavlik harness is used to stabilize the hip, but the duration of splinting is shorter. When the hip is *subluxatable* and unstable, triple diapers are ordinarily adequate.

Three to Six Months of Age.   The modality of treatment in this age group depends upon the degree of lateral and superior displacement of the femoral head and the severity of contracture of the hip adductors and flexors.

THE DISLOCATED HIP.

When the femoral head can be concentrically reduced by simple flexion-abduction of the hip with a wide zone of stability (safe zone), the Pavlik harness is used to retain the reduction. When the zone of safety of reduction is narrow, with or without hip adduction contracture, the Pavlik harness may be tried for 1 or 2 weeks. It is vital to perform ultrasonography with the harness on to determine the position of the femoral head in relation to the acetabulum. When the reduction is concentric, the Pavlik harness stabilizes the hip. When the femoral head is more than 50 percent displaced posteriorly in the Pavlik harness, it is best to perform a closed reduction and retain the reduction in a hip spica cast. The zone of safety of reduction is determined by recording the degree of hip flexion-abduction and rotation at which the femoral head is reduced into the acetabulum and then reversing the maneuver and recording the degree of hip abduction, flexion, and rotation at which the femoral head redislocates.

Dislocated hips that fail to be reduced or stabilized by the Pavlik harness are treated by closed reduction and retention in a hip spica cast for a period of 2 to 3 months and then treated with a hip flexion-abduction splint, from which they are gradually weaned.

DISLOCATABLE HIPS.

These hips are treated in a hip abduction splint. In the noncompliant family, particularly when the acetabulum is dysplastic, it may be wise to apply an above-knee hip spica cast for a period of 4 to 6 weeks initially and then use a hip abduction splint.

Six to Twelve Months of Age.   Dislocated Hip.   Closed reduction is performed under general anesthesia. When the femoral heads are riding high, a preliminary period of skin traction is appropriate, but it should not exceed 2 weeks. Recently some controversy has arisen concerning the value of traction, but I strongly recommend it.[27,38,75,139,152,188,191] It lowers the femoral heads distally and stretches out associated hip adductor and flexor contractures.

The objective is to obtain concentric and stable reduction. When the "safe zone" is narrow, it can be increased by adductor tenotomy-myotomy. The adequacy of reduction is determined by intraoperative ultrasonography in the transverse plane. Also, an AP radiogram is made prior to application of the hip spica cast. Extreme positions of the hip, such as abduction and medial or lateral rotation, should be avoided because of the high risk of avascular necrosis. The hips should be in the human and not the frog-leg position. Ninety degrees of hip flexion with 45 to 60 degrees of hip abduction and neutral rotation is the ideal posture of the hips. After application of a hip spica cast, make another AP radiogram of the hips to make sure that the femoral head and neck are pointing toward the acetabuli. I strongly recommend that a CT scan be made to rule out posterior subluxation or dislocation. In the past, true lateral radiograms of the hip were made in the cast, but those were often inadequate to determine the position of the femoral heads in relation to the acetabuli in the AP plane. The total period of cast immobilization after closed reduction is ordinarily 3 and sometimes 4 months. The cast is changed every 4 to 6 weeks under general anesthesia, depending upon the growth of the infant and the snugness of the cast, with intraoperative clinical examination and ultrasonographic and radiographic assessment of the maintenance of reduction and acetabular development.

OPEN REDUCTION.

This is indicated when one is unable to achieve a concentric reduction by closed methods. Obstacles to closed reduction are (1) a taut iliopsoas tendon constricting the hip capsule (hourglass constriction), (2) a transverse acetabular ligament, (3) a large limbus, (4) a thickened pulvinar, (5) marked hypertrophy of the ligamentum teres, (6) capsular adhesions to the lateral wall of the ilium, and (7) taut hip adductors.

Open reduction by a medial approach is performed when obstacles to reduction are medial, that is, the iliopsoas tendon, transverse acetabular ligament, and contracted inferoanterior capsule of the hip joint. An adductor myotomy of the hip can be performed at the same time. The disadvantage of the medial approach is that one cannot plicate a stretched, lax capsule. When the capsule is very lax, the hip is exposed through an anteromedial approach and the stretched capsule is plicated and tautened. Following open reduction, the patient is immobilized in a hip spica cast for 6 to 8 weeks. The anterolateral approach for open reduction of the hip is rarely indicated in a child less than 1 year of age except when it is an antenatal dislocation or when the acetabulum is very deficient and acetabuloplasty is indicated to stabilize the hip.

After Walking Age.   In this age group, the intra-articular and extra-articular obstacles to reduction become greater. The capsular constriction by the iliopsoas tendon is stiffer and more severe. The femoral head is displaced more superiorly and the capsule is adherent to the lateral wall of the ilium. The transverse acetabular ligament with the inferior anterior capsule of the hip is pulled against the acetabulum, thereby preventing concentric reduction. The labrum is thicker and more deformed and infolded. In order to achieve concentric reduction, these obstacles must be overcome. It is important to individualize each case and not to make decisions based solely on the age of the patient. One may succeed in obtaining concentric reduction by closed methods in a child after walking age, but an open reduction is often necessary.

An important decision to make in this age group is whether prereduction traction should be used. This is an individual decision that the surgeon must make. In a high dislocation that is rigid and, on the telescoping maneuver, has no mobility, I believe that it is best to manage it by femoral shortening. This facilitates concentric reduction, reduces compressive forces on the femoral head, and diminishes the risk of avascular necrosis. The older the child and the more rigid the dislocation, the greater the need for femoral shortening at the time of open reduction of the hip. These cases should not have preoperative traction. The borderline cases are children between 1 and 2 years of age. I prefer traction because in my experience it facilitates reduction, and the probability of success by closed reduction increases. The period of traction should not exceed 2 weeks and skeletal traction should not be used.

Under general anesthesia, when the hip reduces easily and reduction is concentric as confirmed by ultrasonography and/or arthrography and there is a wide zone of safety, open reduction should not be performed. The period of cast immobilization after walking age when treated by closed methods is 6 months, with cast changes every other month.

Problems and Complications. *Persisting instability of the hip.* When the infant begins to stand and bear weight on the reduced hip and begins walking, the femoral head progressively displaces posterolaterally and superiorly, in the weight-bearing position. This may be due to severe ligamentous hyperlaxity, excessive femoral antetorsion, and/or acetabular antetorsion or deficiency of the acetabulum anterosuperiorly and/or posteriorly.

Clinically, severe ligamentous hyperlaxity is readily determined. Imaging studies are performed to determine the torsional deformity of the acetabulum and femur. A CT scan delineates the anatomic pathology of deficiency of the acetabulum and the degree of antetorsion of the acetabulum and femur.

Subluxation of the hip may be reducible or irreducible. Make an AP radiogram of the hips in neutral position and then abduction and medial rotation. When the hip is reducible, the child should be treated with a hip abduction-flexion orthosis, which should be worn at night and during the day. A device that is commonly available or can readily be manufactured is the Scottish Rite hip abduction orthosis. The clinical stability of the hip is assessed after 2 months, and radiograms are made in weight-bearing position at 2-month intervals to assess whether hip stability is improving. If no improvement is seen within 6 to 12 months, surgical correction of the anatomic factors causing hip instability should be considered. If the subluxated hip is not reducible, two options are available: (1) MRI of the hips, which, if not available, may make arthrography of the hips necessary.[67] The intra-articular obstacles to concentric reduction are determined, and the appropriate surgical measures are taken to correct them.

Persisting Acetabular Antetorsion. When severe in a child 18 months of age or older and not responding to orthotic management, this condition is corrected by Salter's innominate osteotomy. It provides coverage of the femoral head with an acetabular roof consisting of hyaline cartilage, which is biologically physiologic. A definite advantage of Salter's innominate osteotomy is that it does not disturb growth of the acetabulum at the triradiate cartilage or the growth zone of the acetabular rim.

Concentric reduction of the hip is a requisite, and the hip should have nearly normal range of motion with no myostatic contracture of the iliopsoas muscle or hip adductors.

The Salter innominate osteotomy (Fig 3–23) is a derotation osteotomy and does not change the capacity of the acetabulum.[146–149] When the acetabulum is shallow and deficient in a child 2 to 5 years of age, a pericapsular acetabuloplasty is performed to provide coverage of the head.[32,66] This is illustrated in Figure 3–24.

Periacetabular osteotomy is performed by drilling multiple holes and then connecting them with an osteotome. Next the acetabular roof is mobilized inferiorly, laterally, and anteriorly, thereby decreasing the acetabular capacity and providing full coverage of the femoral head. Wedges of bone graft are inserted at the gaping osteotomy site. Internal fixation is not required. The danger of this procedure is disturbance of the growth of the rim of the acetabulum. It is vital to stay superior to it.

Pemberton's periacetabular innominate osteotomy corrects the deficiency of the anterior and superolateral walls of the acetabulum.[130,131] The advantage of the procedure is that it tautens the marked laxity of the capsule and stiffens the hypermobile hip joint. The osteotomy extends to the posterior rim of the triradiate cartilage, but the fulcrum of the rotation and angulation is located at the triradiate cartilage. This is a drawback because of the risk of growth arrest of the triradiate cartilage. Because of this potential problem, some surgeons do not favor this method of correction of the shallow deficient acetabulum. The patient should be between 2 and 6 years of age. The principle and technique of Pemberton's osteotomy are illustrated in Figure 3–25.

When the acetabulum is deficient and the femoral head is large, an Albee shelf arthroplasty is performed which covers the head anteriorly and laterally.[1] Bone grafts inserted at the osteotomy site extend beyond the rim of the

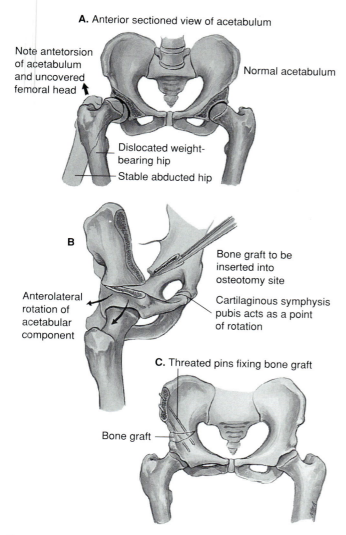

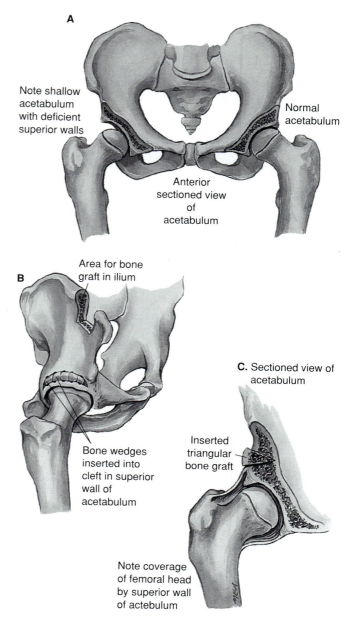

Figure 3–23. Salter's innominate osteotomy to correct acetabular antetorsion. **A.** Note that in weight-bearing position, the right femoral head is not covered. When the right hip is abducted 20 to 30 degrees and medially rotated 10 to 15 degrees, the femoral head is fully contained in the acetabulum. **B.** The technique of osteotomy. The iliac bone is sectioned from the greater sciatic notch toward a point immediately above the anteroinferior iliac spine. The distal segment of the ilium is rotated laterally and downward, and the wedge of autogenous iliac bone graft is inserted at the osteotomy site. **C.** The divided iliac bones and the graft are transfixed with two threaded Steinmann pins. Note the complete coverage of the right femoral head in the weight-bearing position.

Figure 3–24. Pericapsular acetabuloplasty. **A.** The acetabulum is shallow and deficient superiorly and anteriorly on the right. Note the space between the femoral head and the acetabular roof as compared with the normal acetabulum on the left. **B, C.** Anterior and lateral views showing the pericapsular acetabuloplasty performed and grafted with autogenous wedges of iliac bone. Note that the femoral head is fully covered by the acetabulum—no space between the femoral head and the acetabular roof.

acetabulum, thereby enlarging the acetabulum so that it can cover the large femoral head fully. A danger of this procedure is disturbance of growth of the rim of the acetabulum (Umba zone). Stay above it! The principle of the procedure is illustrated in Figure 3–26.

Excessive Femoral Antetorsion and Coxa Valga. Ordinarily, with splinting of the hips in abduction and flexion, femoral antetorsion corrects up to the age of 4 to 5 years. Femoral

derotation osteotomy is being performed less and less. At present, when femoral shortening is carried out in a young child with a delayed diagnosis of developmental dysplasia of the hip, derotation of the proximal femur is simultaneously performed to correct antetorsion. In neuromuscular paralytic dislocation of the hip, intertrochanteric derotation varization osteotomy is often performed.

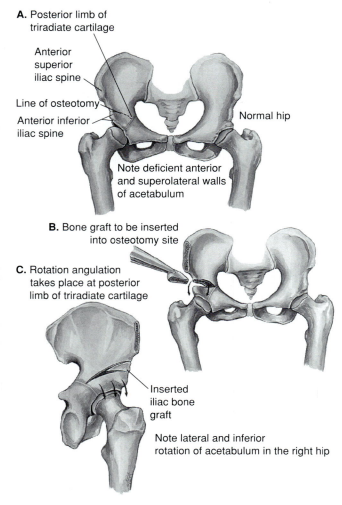

A. Posterior limb of triradiate cartilage

Anterior superior iliac spine

Line of osteotomy

Anterior inferior iliac spine

Normal hip

Note deficient anterior and superolateral walls of acetabulum

B. Bone graft to be inserted into osteotomy site

C. Rotation angulation takes place at posterior limb of triradiate cartilage

Inserted iliac bone graft

Note lateral and inferior rotation of acetabulum in the right hip

Figure 3–25. Pemberton periacetabular innominate osteotomy. **A.** Note the deficient acetabulum and the space between the femoral head and the roof of the socket. The line of innominate osteotomy extends to the posterior limb of the triradiate cartilage to a point immediately above the anteroinferior iliac spine. **B, C.** The distal segment of the ilium is tilted downward, anteriorly, and laterally and transfixed with an autogenous wedge of iliac bone graft. Note the decrease in the acetabular capacity and the adequate coverage of the femoral head.

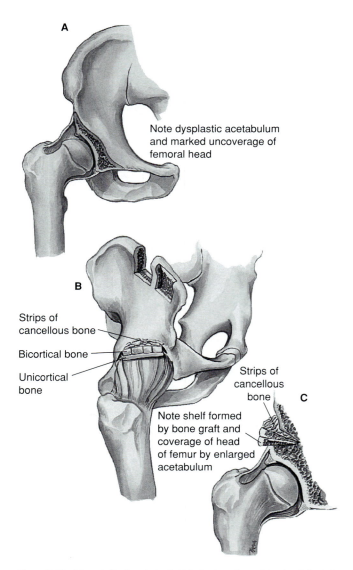

A

Note dysplastic acetabulum and marked uncoverage of femoral head

B

Strips of cancellous bone

Bicortical bone

Unicortical bone

Strips of cancellous bone

C

Note shelf formed by bone graft and coverage of head of femur by enlarged acetabulum

Figure 3–26. Albee shelf arthroplasty. **A.** Note the large femoral head and the deficient dysplastic acetabulum. **B, C.** A pericapsular osteotomy is performed and the wedges of bone graft extend beyond the rim of the acetabulum, which is tilted inferolaterally and anteriorly. Note the full coverage of the femoral head.

When the capsule is very lax, a capsulorrhaphy is indicated. Failure to do so results in resubluxation.

Ischemic Necrosis of the Femoral Head. This is an iatrogenic complication caused by excessive hip abduction and rotation of the hip in spica cast or splint, forceful manipulation, and inadvertent division of the retinacular or circumflex vessels during surgery. Marked abduction of the hip compresses the medial circumflex artery between the taut iliopsoas tendon and either the hip adductors or the pubic ramus. Extreme abduction of the hip compresses the posterosuperior branches of the medial circumflex artery as the greater trochanteric fossa impinges on the rim of the acetabulum. Extreme medial rotation of the hip stretches and occludes the medial circumflex vessels. These extreme

positions of the hip do not affect the lateral circumflex vessels, and the blood supply of the greater trochanter is unaffected.[119,120]

The deformities produced by ischemia depend upon the age of the patient, the anatomic site of vascular occlusion, and whether the capital epiphysis or physis or both are affected.

Ischemic necrosis of the femur in developmental dysplasia of the hip is classified as follows according to Kalamchi and MacEwen.[77]

GROUP I.   Only the femoral head is involved. There is delay of ossification or temporary fragmentation of the cap-

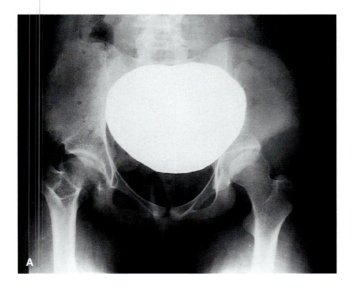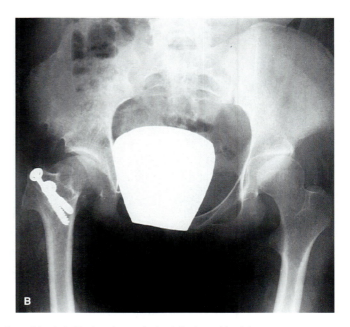

Figure 3–27. Type II Kalamchi-MacEwen ischemic necrosis of the femoral head. **A.** The lateral part physis of the femoral head is closed, whereas the medial part is open. The femoral head is tilted out of the acetabulum. Note the shortening of the femoral neck, uncoverage of the femoral head, and relative overgrowth of the greater trochanter. **B.** A distal transfer of the greater trochanter was performed to place the tip of the greater trochanter in the center of the femoral head, thereby establishing normal biomechanics of the hip and gluteus medius muscle function. Note that the femoral head is still uncovered. This requires a shelf arthroplasty.

tital femoral ossific nucleus. It is caused by temporary interruption of the blood supply by the medial circumflex artery due to extracapsular occlusion. The capital epiphysis reossifies rapidly with minimal deformity. There may be slight coxa magna and/or decreased height of the epiphysis.

GROUP II. The lateral segment of the capital physis is affected by occlusion of the posterosuperior branches of the medial circumflex artery. The lateral part of the growth plate arrests prematurely, whereas its medial part is open. This asymmetric growth arrest of the capital physis causes valgus tilting of the femoral head out of the acetabulum, marked uncovering of the femoral head, and a short femoral neck (Fig 3–27).

GROUP III. This is characterized by central closure of the capital physis and symmetric growth retardation and a short femoral neck—coxa breva (Fig 3–28). The femoral head remains round and contained in the acetabulum, and the femoral neck-shaft angle remains normal; there is no coxa vara. With cessation of growth from the capital femoral physis, progressive shortening (1/8 inch per year) and moderate limb length disparity of the lower limbs occur. Relative overgrowth of the greater trochanter is present, along with gluteus medius insufficiency and Trendelenburg lurch.

GROUP IV. The entire blood supply of both the proximal femoral epiphysis and physis is obstructed (Fig 3–29). The resultant deformation of the upper femur is severe, with

marked delay in ossification of the femoral head with coxa magna, flattening of the femoral head, and hip joint incongruity. The sequela is severe osteoarthritis of the hip in young adult life.

Hip Dysplasia in the Adolescent. This may manifest in the following four forms: (1) stable and congruous but dysplastic, (2) unstable and subluxating, (3) subluxated and congruous but reducible, or (4) subluxated and irreducible, with marked incongruity. In the adolescent patient, usually a female, who presents with pain and gluteus medius lurch, treatment depends upon the type and severity of dysplasia. If the hip is stable and congruous, it is observed at 3- to 6-month periodic assessments. When the hip is subluxating and dysplastic but congruous and reducible, innominate osteotomy is performed to cover the femoral head. If the hip can be contained by 20 to 25 degrees of hip abduction, a triple innominate osteotomy is the procedure of choice.[165,179] This is illustrated in Figure 3–30. Triple innominate osteotomy does not enlarge the acetabular capacity.

When the hip joint is congruous or slightly incongruous and the femoral head is large and uncovered by a dysplastic shallow acetabulum, shelf arthroplasty is performed which enlarges the acetabulum and covers the large femoral head. This is illustrated in Figure 3–31.

When the hip joint is subluxated and markedly incongruous and the femoral head is large, a Chiari medial displacement osteotomy is performed.[64,107] The innominate bone is divided between the anteroinferior iliac spine and

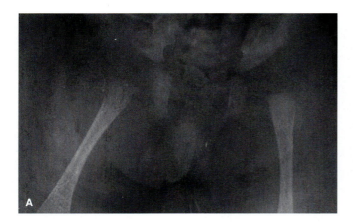

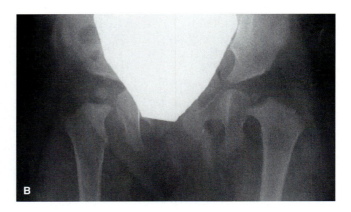

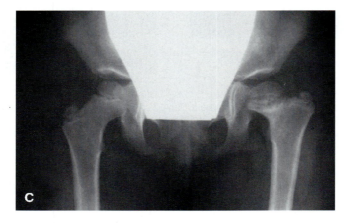

Figure 3–28. Group III Kalamchi-MacEwen ischemic necrosis of the proximal femur. **A.** AP radiogram showing dislocation of the left hip at 1 month of age treated by closed reduction and immobilization in a hip spica cast. **B.** AP radiogram of the hips at one year of age. The physeal injury of the left femoral head is beginning to show. **C.** At 4 years of age, note the short left femoral neck. The growth plate is irregular, showing evidence of avascular injury. The capital epiphysis is round and contained in the acetabulum. Also note the relative overgrowth of the greater trochanter.

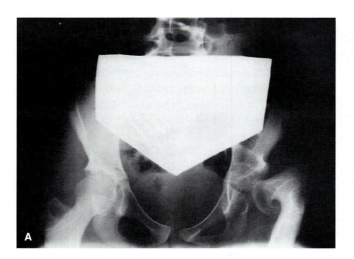

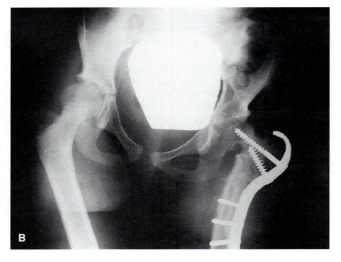

Figure 3–29. Group IV Kalamchi-MacEwen ischemic necrosis. **A.** AP radiogram showing severe deformity of the left hip due to total necrosis of the epiphysis and the physis. Note the flattening and deformity of the femoral head, severe coxa vara, and relative overgrowth of the greater trochanter. **B.** Postoperative AP radiogram of the hips. A valgization intertrochanteric osteotomy was performed with distal and lateral transfer of the greater trochanter. This procedure increases the longevity of the left hip and delays the onset of arthritis.

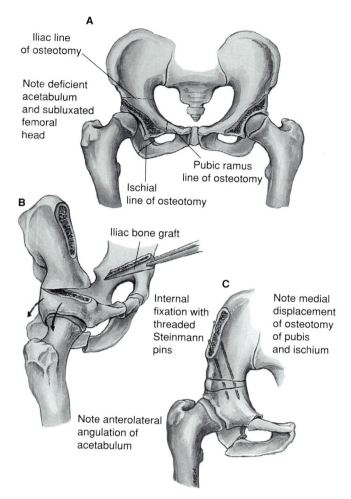

Iliac line
of osteotomy

Note deficient
acetabulum
and subluxated
femoral
head

A

Pubic ramus
line of osteotomy

Ischial
line of osteotomy

B

Iliac bone graft

Internal
fixation with
threaded
Steinmann
pins

C

Note medial
displacement
of osteotomy
of pubis
and ischium

Note anterolateral
angulation of
acetabulum

Figure 3–30. Steel's triple innominate osteotomy. **A.** The innominate bone is sectioned at three sites—the ilium, the pubis, and the ischium. **B, C.** The distal segment of the innominate bone is tilted anterolaterally to cover the femoral head fully. The iliac osteotomy is grafted with an autogenous iliac bone graft and transfixed with two threaded Steinmann pins or AO cannulated screws.

the greater sciatic notch immediately above the attachment of the capsule of the hip joint. The inferior segment of the innominate bone is displaced medially, and the upper segment of the innominate bone becomes the shelf covering the femoral head. A curvilinear cut of the ilium covers the head anteriorly, superiorly, and laterally. When there is gluteus medius lurch, Chiari medial displacement osteotomy may be combined with distal lateral transfer of the greater trochanter (Fig 3–32). This requires a transtrochanteric surgical approach.

■ CONGENITAL ABDUCTION CONTRACTURE OF THE HIP AND PELVIC OBLIQUITY

This common deformity, particularly in the first-born infant, is due to intrauterine malposture of the fetus. This

packaging deformity is also referred to as windblown syndrome of the hips.

The presenting complaint is asymmetry of the thigh and popliteal creases when the lower limbs are held parallel and vertical in supine or prone position. The lower limb on the side of the hip abduction contracture appears long because the ipsilateral pelvis is tilted inferiorly and the anterior superior iliac spine and the iliac crest are tilted downward. The opposite hip may have an adduction contracture of varying degrees. Postural flexible varus or valgus deformities of the feet are common. Severe cases may present with postural scoliosis due to the infrapelvic obliquity. Occasionally associated postural torticollis and plagiocephaly may be present.

Is the contralateral adducted hip stable? Rule out hip subluxation or dislocation. Perform the Barlow and Ortolani tests—they are negative in congenital pelvic obliquity. The Galeazzi test is negative; that is, the knee levels are even when the infant is supine with the pelvis level and the hips and knees flexed 90 degrees. Caution! Be sure the hips are in neutral position, not abducted or adducted, as the thigh of the adducted hip appears shorter on the Galeazzi test.

Perform the Thomas test. In congenital pelvic obliquity the hips have the normal flexion deformity, whereas in congenital dislocation of the knee the hip on the dislocated side hyperextends. Extend the knees; in congenital pelvic obliquity the knees have a normal flexion deformity, whereas in congenital dislocation of the hip the knee on the dislocated side hyperextends or extends fully.

In the neonate and young infant it is difficult to perform the Ober test because they wiggle, cry, and resist. Instead, with the infant in prone position, stabilize the pelvis with one hand and hold the opposite limb out of the way and with your other hand hold the knee and lower thigh of the hip to be tested. Be gentle—do not squeeze with your fingers (no finger prints!). Lift the knee of the tested side toward the ceiling (extend the hip), and bring the thigh toward the opposite side. Record the degree of abduction contracture of the hip. Next, with the hip extended manually, adduct and rotate the hip medially (i.e., away from the center of the body) and record the degree of lateral rotation contracture of the hip (Fig 3–33). Then perform the same prone abduction–lateral rotation test on the opposite side and demonstrate it to the parents. Let them do it; they will be performing this procedure as a passive stretching exercise to correct the abduction contracture.

Next, flex and abduct the hips in frog position and inspect the inguinal folds. In abduction contracture they will stop short of the anus, whereas in congenital dislocation of the hip they will extend posterior to the anus.

Inspect the spine carefully for external stigmata of spinal dysrhaphism—any midline patch of hair, hemangioma, or sinus? Is there scoliosis? When scoliosis is present, is it postural; it disappear when the pelvis is level by abducting the hip on the side of the abduction contracture? Test flexibility of the spine.

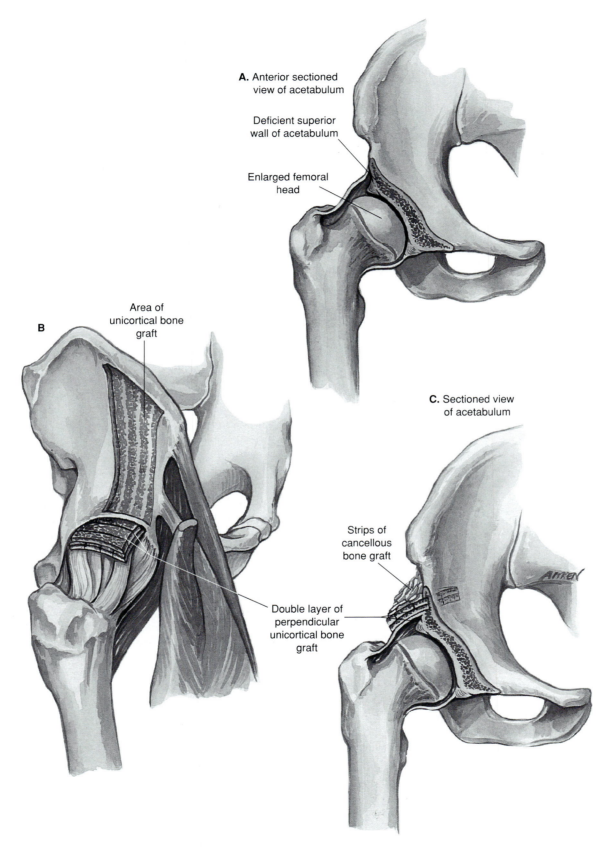

A. Anterior sectioned
view of acetabulum

Deficient superior
wall of acetabulum

Enlarged femoral
head

Area of
unicortical bone
graft

B

C. Sectioned view
of acetabulum

Strips of
cancellous
bone graft

Double layer of
perpendicular
unicortical bone
graft

Figure 3–31. Staheli's shelf arthroplasty. **A.** Note the deficient superior wall of the acetabulum and uncoverage of the enlarged femoral head. **B, C.** Note the layers of unicortical bone graft covering the head of the femur and enlarging the acetabulum.

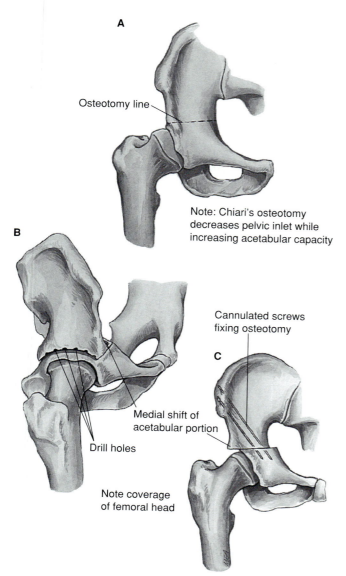

A.

Osteotomy line

Note: Chiari's osteotomy decreases pelvic inlet while increasing acetabular capacity

B

Cannulated screws fixing osteotomy

C

Medial shift of acetabular portion

Drill holes

Note coverage of femoral head

Figure 3–32. Chiari medial displacement osteotomy. **A.** Note the incongruous hip with uncoverage of the large deformed femoral head and the dysplastic acetabulum. **B, C.** Following division of the iliac bone between the anteroinferior iliac spine and the greater sciatic notch, the distal segment of the innominate bone is displaced medially. The superior segment of the ilium covers the femoral head as a biologically alive shelf. Internal fixation is with threaded Steinmann pins or cannulated screws.

In the occasional infant with associated torticollis, palpate the sternocleidomastoid muscle. In congenital muscular torticollis the sternocleidomastoid muscle is fibrotic and contracted, whereas in postural torticollis, it is soft and flexible; there is no "tumor" and no fibrotic contracture.

When there is associated plagiocephaly, palpate the fontanelles and rule out cranial synostosis. Perform a quick neuromuscular examination to rule out spasticity of the upper and lower limbs.

Imaging Findings. A plain radiogram—only an AP view of the pelvis—is made to rule out congenital deformity of the upper femur such as developmental coxa vara or proximal femoral focal deficiency.

An ultrasonogram shows normal hips or some immaturity of the hip opposite to the side of the abduction contracture. There is no subluxation or dislocation.

Treatment. Treatment consists of passive stretching exercises performed in four sessions per day, 20 to 30 times each session (see Fig 3–33). When performed faithfully, within 3 to 4 weeks the abduction contracture and pelvic obliquity are completely corrected. These exercises are performed once a day for an additional 4 to 8 weeks in order to prevent recurrence. As a rule it is best to re-examine the infant when he or she starts independently walking to rule out any out-toeing gait abnormality.

What is the natural history of the hips if they are left alone? It depends upon the severity of the abduction contracture. If mild, it spontaneously resolves. If moderate, when the child begins to walk he or she toes out and may develop genu valgum and malalignment of the quadriceps due to persisting contracture of the iliotibial band. If severe, in addition to the above problems, the opposite adducted hip may subluxate.[198]

■ DEVELOPMENTAL COXA VARA

The presenting complaint is a lurching limp that may be unilateral or bilateral in a child who is 2 to 3 years of age. The limp is not antalgic; that is, it is painless and the weight-bearing phase is not shortened. The involved femur is short, the amount of shortening depends upon the degree of coxa vara; ordinarily it does not exceed 2 to 3 cm. The thigh and popliteal creases are uneven. The Trendelenburg test is positive. Lumbar lordosis is exaggerated, especially in bilateral coxa vara. Measure the height of the child; these children are usually short in stature. When coxa vara is associated with bone dysplasia, the height of the child is excessive (5th to 10th percentile). On testing range of hip motion, abduction and medial rotation are limited. With varus angulation of the femoral head and neck, the tip of the greater trochanter is elevated in relation to the center of the femoral head. Determine the relation of the tip of the greater trochanter to Nélaton's line—it is slightly higher. The hip is stable and the Barlow maneuver and Ortolani test are negative.

In the normal hip the mean neck-shaft angle of the femur is 150 degrees at birth, 145 degrees in the 3-year-old, 140 degrees at 6 years of age, 135 degrees at 10 years of age, and 120 degrees in the adult.[213] In developmental coxa vara there is abnormal decrease in the femoral neck-shaft angle due to a primary defect in enchondral ossification in the medial part of the femoral neck. The defective part of the femoral neck consists of

A

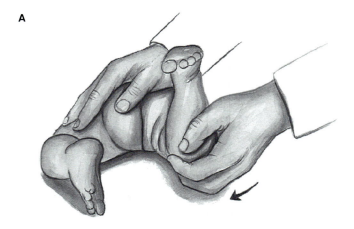

B

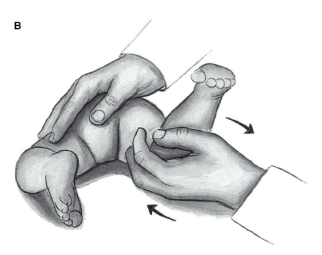

Figure 3–33. Passive stretching exercises for correction of abduction contracture of the hip. **A.** The infant is in prone position lying flat on his abdomen. The pelvis and opposite thigh are stabilized with one hand. With the other hand, the knee and thigh on the side of the abducted hip are held gently. The thigh is pushed medially. **B.** The hip is laterally rotated as it is held in adduction to the count of 5 and released. This is also the method to determine the degree of abduction and lateral rotation deformity of the affected hip.

fibrous or abnormal fibrocartilaginous tissue. Under the stresses of body weight and muscle forces, the anatomically weakened neck deflects into progressive varus. The plane of the upper femoral physis changes from horizontal to vertical.

Developmental coxa vara is rare, occurring in 1 in 25,000 live births. There is no racial or gender predilection. One or both hips may be involved, unilateral cases being more common.

Often developmental coxa vara is misdiagnosed as developmental dislocation of the hip. The clinical finding that distinguishes the two conditions is the restriction of medial rotation of the hip in coxa vara because of the associated femoral antetorsion. In developmental dislocation of the hip, medial rotation of the hip is normal or often excessive.

Developmental coxa vara should also be distinguished from congenital short femur with coxa vara, a mild form of proximal femoral focal deficiency; in the latter the shortening, adduction, and lateral rotation contractures of the hips are marked and the condition is evident at birth.

Coxa vara may also occur in various bone dysplasias such as spondyloepiphyseal dysplasia or Morquio's disease. A radiographic skeletal survey establishes the diagnosis.

Imaging Findings. In the plain AP radiogram of the hip, the abnormal decrease of the neck-shaft angle of the femur is noted (Fig 3–34). The defective area of enchondral ossification in the medial part of the femoral neck is radiolucent; it gives the appearance of an inverted V with the radiolucent capital femoral physis tilted into a vertical position by the varus angulation of the upper femur.

Caution! In the radiogram when the hips are laterally rotated the femoral neck-shaft angle increases. Be sure the AP radiogram is made with the hips in neutral or slight medial rotation. Look for the prominence of the lesser trochanter.

Coxa vara may also be acquired as a result of growth retardation or arrest of the capital femoral epiphysis due to avascular necrosis such as in Perthes' disease or as a complication of dislocation of the hip or septic hip. It may also be due to malunion of a femoral neck fracture or a residual deformity of slipped capital femoral epiphysis.

Determine the Hilgenreiner-epiphyseal (HE) angle in the AP radiogram of the pelvis. The Hilgenreiner line is the horizontal line drawn between the triradiate cartilage; the epiphyseal line is the vertical-oblique line drawn through the metaphyseal side of the defect in the femoral neck. The angle formed between these two lines is the HE angle (Fig 3–35). In a retrospective review of coxa vara, Weinstein et al found that (1) if the HE angle is greater than 60 degrees, the varus angulation increases, (2) if the HE angle is between 40 and 45 degrees, the coxa vara improves, (3) if the HE angle is less than 60 degrees and greater than 45 degrees, the "zone was gray"—the coxa vara could increase or remain stationary—and the hip should be observed.[214]

Treatment. Operative treatment in the form of intertrochanteric abduction–medial rotation osteotomy is indicated when the HE angle is greater than 60 degrees. The femoral neck (with the capital physis and the defect) is tilted from vertical to horizontal position, thereby relieving the shearing stresses on the weak medial defect of the femoral neck, stimulating ossification and healing of the defect of the femoral neck, and returning the muscle physiology of the hip abductors and mechanics of the hip to normal. There is

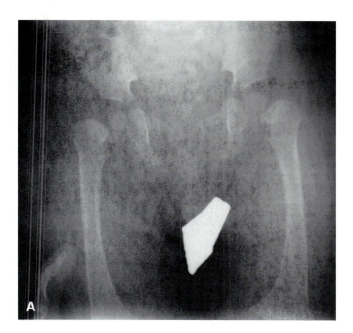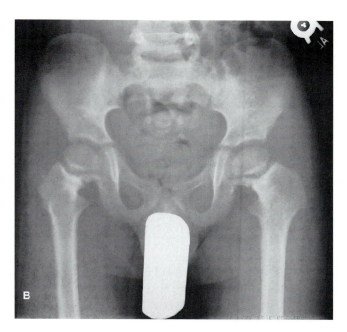

Figure 3–34. Bilateral developmental coxa vara of both hips in a 2-year-old child. Note the abnormal decrease in the neck-shaft angle, which is about 100 degrees, and the fibrocartilaginous defect in the metaphysis of the neck of the femur forming a V with the capital physis. **A.** Preoperative. **B.** Postoperative bilateral valgization-derotation osteotomies.

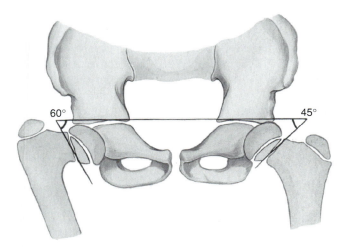

Figure 3–35. The Hilgenreiner-epiphyseal angle (HE) is the angle that is formed by the Hilgenreiner Y line and a line drawn through the metaphyseal site defect in the femoral neck. When greater than 60 degrees, the coxa vara deformity increases; when the angle is between 40 and 45 degrees, the coxa vara improves with growth; and when it is between 45 and 60 degrees, it may increase or remain stationary.

some variance of opinion as to timing of surgery. I believe that it is best to correct the deformity soon after the child begins to walk—between 18 and 24 months of age. Numerous techniques are described in the literature.[199,212]

Nonoperative measures such as orthotic devices do not prevent progression of varus deformity. Unilateral coxa vara tends to be progressive with growth; secondary dysplastic changes of the posterior acetabulum and degenerative arthritis of the hip develop in adult life.

■ CONGENITAL SHORTENING OR HYPOPLASIA OF THE FEMUR

This form of longitudinal deficiency of the femur is quite common; the femur is simply miniature—just short; the femoral neck-shaft angle and the hip joint are normal. No other associated skeletal defects, such as tarsal coalition or absence of the fibula, are present. Occurrence is sporadic. Only one side is involved, and the severity of involvement varies.

The presenting complaint varies according to the age of the patient. In the infant the affected lower limb lies in lateral rotation. On performing the Galeazzi test, the shortening of the femur is evident by the uneven level of the knees. Caution! Be sure the pelvis is not tilted to either side. The thigh and popliteal creases are uneven. Is it developmental dislocation of the hip? Perform the Ortolani and Barlow tests; they are negative in the congenitally short femur. Determine passive range of abduction-adduction and medial-lateral rotation of the hip. In simple hypoplasia of the femur, range of hip abduction is normal; there is no adduction contracture of the hip (a finding common in developmental dislocation of the hip). In the short femur there is restriction in range of medial rotation and abduction of the hip; in developmental dislocation of the hip, hip adduction and medial rotation are normal or hypermobile. Turn the patient on her side and determine the relationship of the tip of the greater trochanter to Nélaton's line (drawn between the anterosuperior iliac spine and the ischium). In the congenitally short femur, the tip of the greater trochanter is at or below Nélaton's line, whereas in the dislocated hip it is above Nélaton's line.

In the short femur the thigh often bows laterally at its middle third. Look for skin dimples; they are present in proximal femoral focal deficiency but absent in the congenitally short femur.

When the child starts to stand and walk, the short leg limp is evident. The shoulder dips inferiorly in the weight-bearing phase of gait; the knee of the long limb is flexed and the ankle and foot of the short limb are in equinus posture.

Imaging Findings. The femur is small but otherwise normal. There may be delay in ossification of the capital femoral epiphysis, but eventually it develops normally. In the occasional case with lateral bowing of the femur, the apex of the angular deformity is in its middle third. The medullary canal is normal; it is not narrowed by intramedullary sclerosis.

Treatment. The ratio of longitudinal growth of the short femur to the long femur remains the same throughout growth.[215] The total predicted shortening at skeletal maturity is calculated as follows:

1. Predict the length of the long femur at completion of skeletal growth by the Green Anderson chart or from the straight line graph of Moseley.
2. Determine the percentile ratio between the short and long femur at present; for example, the long femur is 20 cm and the short femur is 18 cm. The short femur is in the 90th percentile in length in relation to the long femur.
3. At skeletal maturity, the length of the long femur is 40 cm; the short femur is $40 \times .9 = 36$ cm. The total shortening is $40 - 36 = 4$ cm.

Mild deformities of lower limb length (less than 2 cm) are managed by a shoe lift; moderate deformities (i.e., 2 to 5 cm) are treated by equalization of limb lengths by epiph-yseodesis of the distal femur of the long limb at the appropriate skeletal age. Severe deformities of limb length (i.e., greater than 5 cm) are treated by elongation of the short femur.

■ PROXIMAL FEMORAL FOCAL DEFICIENCY

This major congenital malformation of the upper femur is readily diagnosed at birth by its typical clinical picture. The thigh is short and bulky, with flexion-abduction lateral rotation contracture of the hip. The degree of shortening of the femur varies; the lower limb length disparity may be of great magnitude.

Classification. Various radiographic classifications are given in the literature.[216,217,221,222,233,236] Aitken's classification is simple.[216] In type A the femur is short with coxa vara and is bowed laterally at the subtrochanteric region or at its upper third. The hip joint is always stable with a femoral head in a normal acetabulum. In the infant with type A proximal femoral focal deficiency, the femoral head and neck and upper fourth of the femoral shaft are cartilaginous and not visible in plain radiograms. The lower two thirds of the femoral shaft is ossified; its upper end is bulbous and not spiked (Fig 3–36A).

In type B the shortening of the femur is great. The femoral head and acetabulum are present but delayed in ossification. The upper end of the femoral shaft is bulbous, is displaced laterally, and lies above the femoral head. The connection between the femoral head and neck and the shaft is by defective cartilage. The degree of coxa vara deformity is severe (Fig 3–36B).

In type C the acetabulum is very shallow and the femoral head absent or markedly hypoplastic. The upper end of the femoral shaft is tapered into a spike and is sclerotic. The hip is very unstable, with an absent or defective articular relationship between the femur and acetabulum (Fig 3–36C).

In type D the femoral shaft is extremely short, with an absent acetabulum and femoral head (Fig 3–36D).

Proximal femoral focal deficiency cases may be subdivided into two general groups: (1) those with an absent or abnormal hip joint with severe coxa vara, and (2) those with a good hip joint.

Fixsen and Lloyd Roberts classified proximal femoral focal deficiency according to the appearance of the proximal end of the ossified femoral shaft.[221] In *type I* the upper end of the femoral shaft is truly *bulbous*. These femurs develop continuity of the femoral head and neck and greater trochanter with the femoral shaft and result in a stable hip. The acetabulum is normal. Occasionally a pseudarthrosis may develop at the subtrochanteric region which heals spontaneously or after bone grafting. The prognosis is good

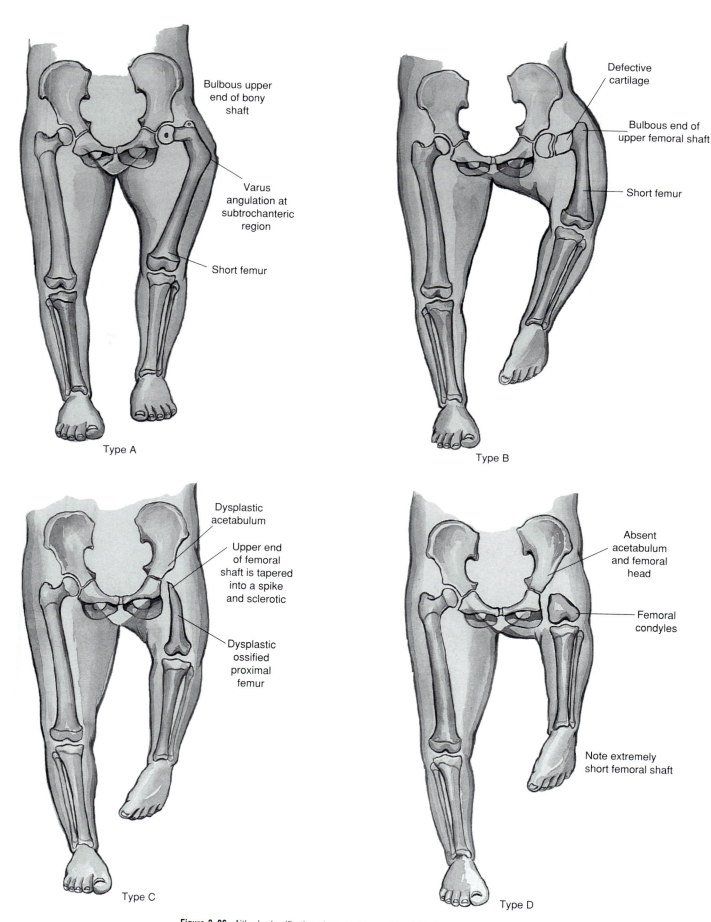

Figure 3-36. Aitken's classification of proximal femoral focal deficiency. See text.

for a functional lower limb (Fig 3–37). In type II the upper end of the femoral shaft is *blunt* and separated from an ossified cap by a cartilaginous zone. The acetabulum is good. These hips are unstable, and their prognosis and function are guarded. In type III the upper end of the femoral shaft is *pointed* into a spike with some sclerosis. The acetabulum is dysplastic and coxa vara is severe. The hip is very unstable and the prognosis is poor. Sanpera and Sparks assessed various classifications of proximal femoral focal deficiency and found the Fixsen-Lloyd Roberts classification sound in predicting the functional outcome of the femur and hip.[235]

In the newborn and young infant, sonography accurately depicts the morphology and deformity of the acetabulum, the femoral head and neck, the femoral neck-shaft angle, the shortening and angulation of the femur, and the stability of the hip joint. Every newborn and young infant with proximal femoral focal deficiency should have sonography of the hip performed.[225]

Associated Anomalies. Proximal femoral focal deficiency is caused by a multifocal teratogenic process. Examine the entire lower limb and the whole child. Associated malformations are found in about 80 percent of the cases. These include (1) congenital longitudinal deficiency of the fibula, (2) congenital shortening of the tibia, (3) flexion deformity of the knee, (4) absence of the cruciate ligaments of the knee, (5) absent or hypoplastic patellae that are riding high and are displaced laterally, (6) tarsal coalition, and (7) absence of rays of the foot or absence of a part of the upper limb.

Treatment. Factors to consider in management are (1) the magnitude of the lower limb length disparity as predicted at skeletal maturity, (2) whether the hip is stable or unstable, (3) malrotation of the entire lower limb, and (4) severity of the associated deformities.

The femur is lengthened at the appropriate age when the hip is stable; the foot–ankle function is adequate and the projected shortening at skeletal maturity is less than 20 cm (Fig 3–38). Several lengthenings are required to equalize limb lengths at 8 years of age, at 12 years of age, and possibly at 14 years of age. Psychosocial factors should be considered in decision-making.

A conversion surgery is performed to provide a stump that can be fitted into a conversion prosthesis when the limb length shortening is greater than 20 cm, and/or the foot is so deformed that it is not functional. The type of conversion recommended is a rotationplasty of the lower limb through the knee with simultaneous knee fusion (Torode and Gillespie procedure).[236] When a decision is made to perform a Syme's amputation, it should be done before 1 year of age because of emotional considerations. Bilateral cases should not have rotationplasty.

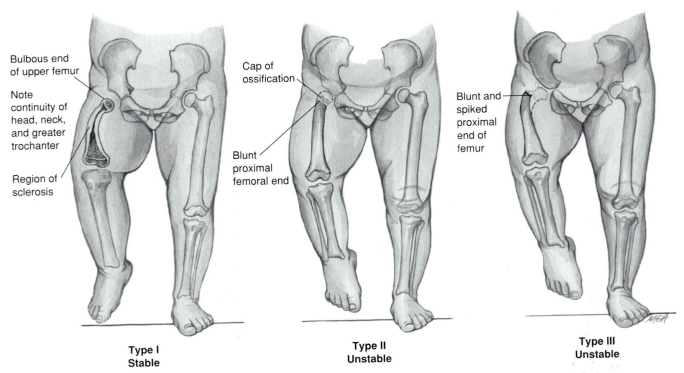

Bulbous end of upper femur

Note continuity of head, neck, and greater trochanter

Region of sclerosis

Cap of ossification

Blunt proximal femoral end

Blunt and spiked proximal end of femur

Type I
Stable

Type II
Unstable

Type III
Unstable

Figure 3–37. Fixsen and Lloyd Roberts' classification of proximal femoral focal deficiency. See text.

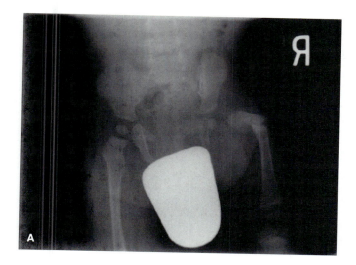

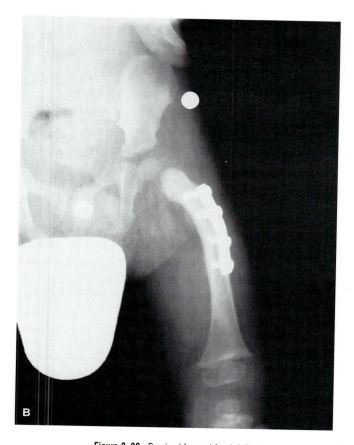

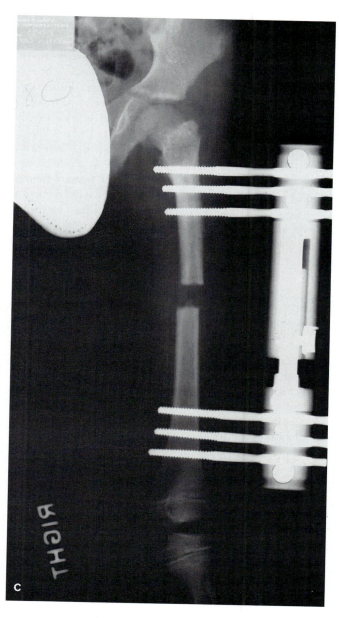

Figure 3–38. Proximal femoral focal deficiency of the femur with coxa vara. **A.** Preoperative. **B.** Following valgization osteotomy of the proximal femur. **C.** The femur is being lengthened with a unilateral Orthofix apparatus.

■ THE PAINFUL HIP

Pain originating from the hip is felt on the anterior aspect of the hip and radiates to the anteromedial aspect of the thigh and knee. Pain on the posterolateral aspect of the hip and thigh is due to lumbosacral or pelvic bone pathology. Upper lumbar lesions may refer pain to the anterior aspect of the hip and thigh.

A multitude of conditions cause hip pain; some diseases are more common in certain age groups, whereas others have no age predilection. By careful history-taking, physical examination, and localization of the maximum site of tenderness and appropriate laboratory and imaging studies, one may make an accurate diagnosis. According to etiologic categories of disease, the possible causes of pain are given in Table 3–3 and illustrated in Figure 3–39.

■ ACUTE SUPPURATIVE (OR SEPTIC) ARTHRITIS OF THE HIP

Inflammation of the hip caused by pus-forming bacteria is the most common site of septic arthritis. It is sometimes referred to as ''Tom Smith's arthritis'' because Smith emphasized the serious nature and crippling sequelae of the disease caused by destruction of the articular cartilage and interruption of the blood supply.[253]

It occurs primarily in neonates, infants, and young children between 2 and 3 years of age. The infection is blood borne. The metaphysis of the neck of the femur is intracapsular; pathogenic organisms may liberate into the hip joint when the osteomyelitis focus breaks through the cortex of the femoral neck or the organisms may lodge primarily in the synovial tissues (Fig 3–40).

Clinical Picture. In the neonate and young infant, systemic reaction to septicemia may be absent or minimal. The newborn infant with sepsis may not be feverish. The baby is irritable, refuses to feed, and fails to gain weight. Look for an open wound or focus of infection such as otitis media. The limbs of a newborn in the nursery, particularly if premature, should be examined almost daily for joint or bone infections.

In the older child the onset of pain and fever is acute, and the child refuses to bear weight on the lower limbs or walks with an antalgic limp. The anterior aspect of the hip is warm on palpation and appears swollen.

The hip, in response to marked effusion, distention of the capsule, and increased hydrostatic pressure, assumes the position of maximum hydrostatic pressure. It is held in 30 to 60 degrees of flexion, 10 to 15 degrees of lateral rotation, and 10 degrees of abduction (not adduction) (Fig 3–41A). With lateral and upward displacement of the femoral head, the thigh and popliteal and inguinal creases become asym-

TABLE 3–3. CAUSES OF PAINFUL HIP

I. Infection
  A. Septic arthritis of the hip
  B. Osteomyelitis of proximal femur, femoral neck, or upper femoral shaft
  C. Osteomyelitis of pelvic bones—often the ilium posteriorly over the sacroiliac joint
  D. Psoas abscess or infected iliopsoas bursitis
II. Inflammation
  A. Toxic synovitis or irritable hip
  B. Rheumatoid arthritis
  C. Osteitis pubis
  D. Bursitis—greater or lesser trochanter, iliopectineal
III. Vascular compromise—avascular necrosis
  A. Perthes' disease
  B. Post-traumatic
  C. Sickle cell disease
  D. Idiopathic
IV. Trauma—stress fracture
  A. Slipped capital femoral epiphysis
  B. Fracture—acute trauma or stress
    1. Femoral neck
    2. Intertrochanteric
    3. Anterior superior, or inferior iliac spine
    4. Greater trochanter, lesser trochanter
    5. Ischium, pubis, or ilium
V. Tumors or tumorous conditions
  A. Benign—osteoid osteoma, osteoblastoma, eosinophilic granuloma, aneurysmal bone cyst
  B. Malignant—Ewing's sarcoma, osteogenic sarcoma
  C. Leukemia—diffuse pain

metric (Fig 3–41B). Range of motion of the hip is markedly restricted and painful (Fig 3–41C to E). The hip is acutely tender anteriorly. In osteomyelitis of the femoral neck, the maximum tenderness is posterior. A crescendo in intensity and pitch of the cry is the telltale sign of severe pain. Observe the gluteal creases; if they extend posterior to the anal aperture, suspect septic hip subluxation or dislocation (Fig 3–41F).

Laboratory Findings. The white blood cell count is elevated, with a shift to the left on differential. The erythrocyte sedimentation rate (ESR) and C-reactive protein are also elevated. The newborn and infant, however, may show a lack of systemic response to infection, and white blood count and ESR may be normal. Lactic acid levels will be elevated up to 2000 to 3000 m. per cc. in the septic joint fluid when the pathogenic organisms are gram positive coxi and gram negative rods. The low pH of the joint fluid reduces the effectiveness of antibiotics, especially aminoglycosides.

Imaging Findings. Ultrasonography shows marked distention of the hip joint capsule with effusion (Fig 3–42). Both the radiograms and ultrasonograms demonstrate varying degrees of lateral displacement of the femoral head.

On scintigraphy with technetium-99m there is diffuse periarticular uptake. Pinhole and SPECT imaging detects associated osteomyelitis of the femoral neck, if present, by the intense focal accumulation of the radionuclide. In complex cases in which active suppurative inflammation should be distinguished from other processes, a scan with gallium-67 citrate is performed. This radionuclide labels the white blood cells as it binds to serum proteins and localizes primarily in inflammatory tissue. Its accuracy of detection of pyogenic arthritis is very high. Its routine use is not recommended because of the large ionizing radiation dose.

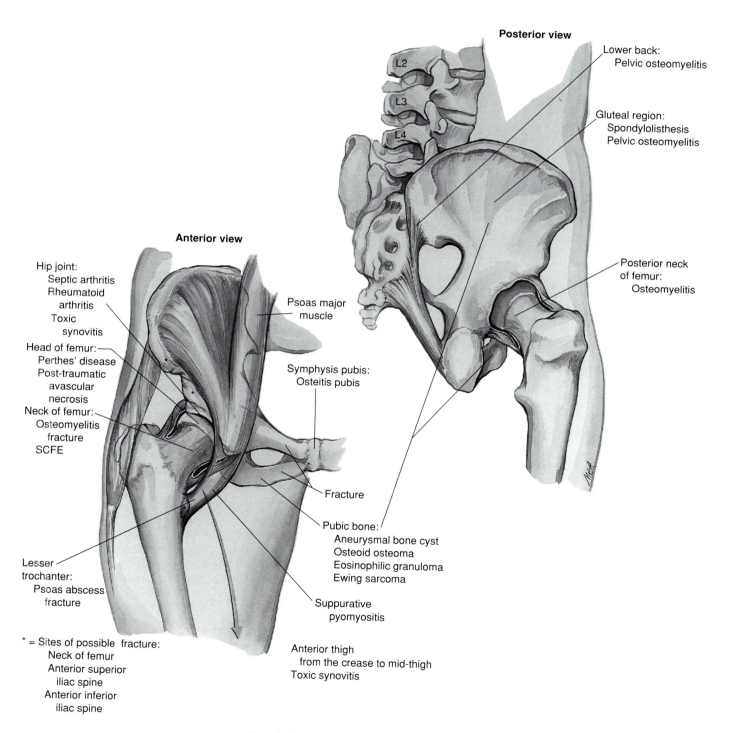

Posterior view

Lower back:
Pelvic osteomyelitis

Gluteal region:
Spondylolisthesis
Pelvic osteomyelitis

Posterior neck
of femur:
Osteomyelitis

Anterior view

Hip joint:
Septic arthritis
Rheumatoid
arthritis
Toxic
synovitis

Head of femur:
Perthes' disease
Post-traumatic
avascular
necrosis

Neck of femur:
Osteomyelitis
fracture
SCFE

Lesser
trochanter:
Psoas abscess
fracture

* = Sites of possible fracture:
Neck of femur
Anterior superior
iliac spine
Anterior inferior
iliac spine

Psoas major
muscle

Symphysis pubis:
Osteitis pubis

Fracture

Pubic bone:
Aneurysmal bone cyst
Osteoid osteoma
Eosinophilic granuloma
Ewing sarcoma

Suppurative
pyomyositis

Anterior thigh
from the crease to mid-thigh
Toxic synovitis

Figure 3–39. Possible sources of hip pain. See text.

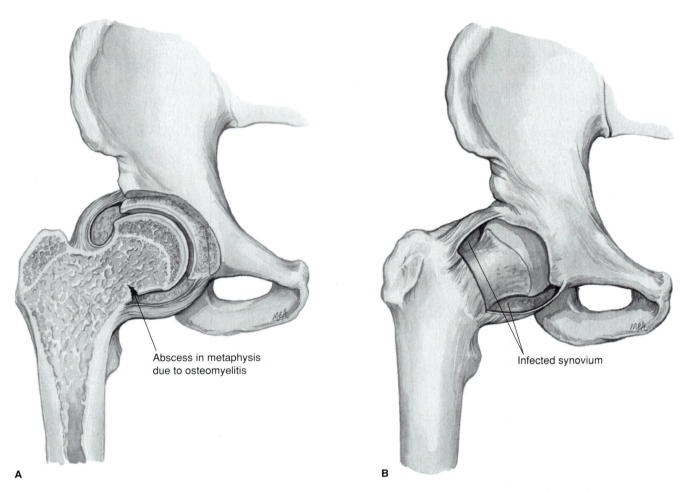

Figure 3–40. Routes of infection in suppurative arthritis of the hip. **A.** Note that the metaphysis of the femoral neck is intracapsular; an osteomyelitic force in the femoral neck may break through its cortex and infect the hip joint. **B.** Pathogenic organisms may lodge in the synovial tissues primarily from the blood.

Diagnosis. Clinically, *osteomyelitis of the femoral neck* with sympathetic effusion in the hip joint is difficult to differentiate from septic arthritis. Carefully palpate for the point of maximal tenderness. In osteomyelitis it is posterior over the metaphysis of the femoral neck, whereas in septic arthritis it is anterior over the joint. In septic arthritis the hip joint motion is very painful or markedly restricted, whereas in osteomyelitis of the femoral neck, limitation of hip motion and pain are much less. In septic arthritis the normal swelling and increased local heat are over the hip anteriorly, whereas in osteomyelitis the entire proximal thigh is swollen and warm.

Acute rheumatic fever (rare, but it does occur) may manifest initially as acute painful swollen hip joint. Suspect it when there is migrating arthralgia, erythema marginatum, and pericarditis. *Acute transient synovitis* and *juvenile rheumatoid arthritis* are other inflammatory conditions of the hip to consider in the differential diagnosis. Extracapsular infections, which may mimic in-

fection of the hip, are osteomyelitis of the acetabulum or ilium, infectious sacroiliitis, infection of the iliopectineal bursa, and pyomyositis of the hip adductor muscles. In infectious iliopsoas bursitis the hip is held in flexion and medial rotation and the maximal site of tenderness is over the lesser trochanteric region. CT, MRI, and technetium-99m and gallium-67 citrate scintigraphy establish the diagnosis in these conditions.

Aspiration of the hip joint should be performed as soon as septic arthritis is suspected by the acute painful joint and the marked restriction of motion. Sedation and proper restraint of the child are important. Use image intensifier radiographic control to guide your needle and to document that it is in the joint. An 18- or 20-gauge lumbar puncture needle with a stylet inside prevents inadvertent breaking of the tip of the needle and plugging of the needle with fibrin or inflamed synovial tissue. Use air and not radiopaque dye for verification that the tip of the needle is in the joint, as the dye is bactericidal and should not be in-

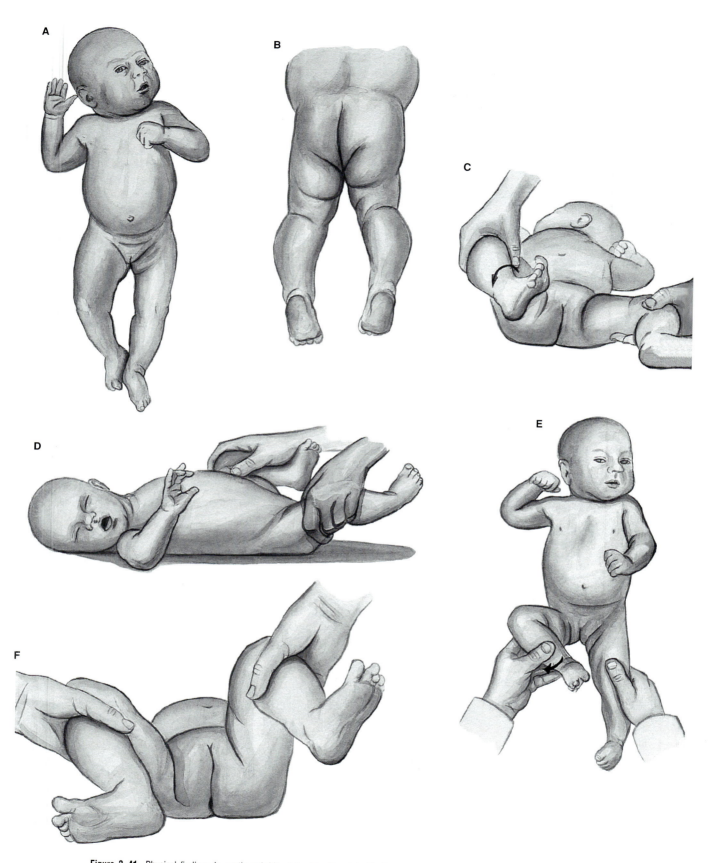

Figure 3–41. Physical findings in septic arthritis of the hip. The right hip is infected. **A.** The hip is abducted, flexed, and laterally rotated, assuming the position of maximum hydrostatic pressure of the joint. **B.** Note the asymmetry of the thigh and popliteal and gluteal folds—on the right they are displaced upward. **C to E.** Abduction, extension, and medial rotation of the hip are restricted. **F.** Note that the right thigh is swollen anteriorly. The inguinal crease extends posteriorly beyond the anal aperture, indicating hip subluxation.

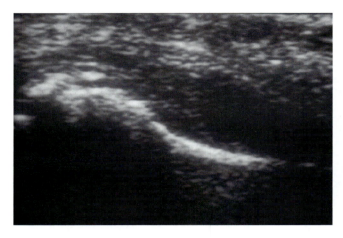

Figure 3–42. Ultrasonographic findings of septic hip. Note marked effusion-distention of the hip joint anteriorly.

stilled prior to obtaining fluid for culture. The route of aspiration varies with the preference of the surgeon. I prefer the adductor approach, but alternate routes are anterior (one finger lateral to the femoral vessels and one finger distal to Poupart's ligament), lateral, or superior. Initially the joint fluid is serosanguinous, but soon it becomes cloudy. Remember, turbid fluid in the joint is not always pus; acute effusion of rheumatoid arthritis may be cloudy. Make a smear with Gram's stain and culture for identification of pathogenic organism with sensitivity studies. Joint fluid cell count is markedly elevated, sugar is reduced, and mucin is poor.

Treatment. When the diagnosis of septic hip is made by aspiration of the joint, it should be drained immediately and appropriate antibiotics administered intravenously.

Complications of septic arthritis are very serious; they include avascular necrosis of the femoral head due to tamponade of blood supply by increased hydrostatic pressure in the hip joint, relative overgrowth of the greater trochanter and shortening of the femur, pathologic dislocation of the hip, destruction of the femoral head by the pyogenic processes, and severe arthritis.

■ PYOMYOSITIS OF ADDUCTOR MUSCLES OF THE HIP

This very rare infection may mimic septic arthritis of the hip. The child walks with an antalgic gait, holding the affected hip in adduction and flexion. The diagnostic physical finding is painful swelling and local tenderness of the involved muscles. When an abscess forms, the muscles may become fluctuant. MRI shows the muscle swelling and the extent of involvement and delineates the abscess. Treatment

consists of incision and drainage and administration of intravenous antibiotics.

■ PSOAS ABSCESS AND INFECTED ILIOPSOAS BURSITIS

These occur rarely in children. The hip is painful, medially rotated, and flexed. Extension and lateral rotation of the hip are painful. When the iliopsoas bursa is infected, the local tenderness is over the lesser trochanteric region.

CT or MRI demonstrates the pathology. Treatment consists of intravenous antibiotics and incision and drainage when an abscess is found.

■ OSTEOMYELITIS

The presenting complaints vary, depending upon the age of the patient—that is, neonate, infant, or child; the bone involved (long bone, flat bone, or vertebra); the anatomic site in the long bone (metaphysis, diaphysis, or epiphysis); onset (acute or subacute—in the latter the epiphysis may be involved); the pathogenic organism and its virulence; the immune resistance of the host; and the route of infection—hematogenous or direct inoculation.

Osteomyelitis should be suspected and ruled out in any patient who complains of pain in long or flat bones and walks with an antalgic limp. Often associated systemic signs are present such as fever, chills, and vomiting with dehydration. Systemic response to bone infection, however, may be absent or minimal in the neonate or young infant. There may be a history of injury or the presence of other infection such as otitis media or chickenpox. Inquire about antibiotic therapy for ear infection and temperature elevations. Inadequate antibiotic treatments mask the infection and make the diagnosis difficult.

The hallmark of osteomyelitis is *local pain* in the affected bone, ordinarily in the metaphyseal region of a long bone; the pain is constant and intense and rapidly increases in severity. The slightest motion of the limb aggravates the pain; therefore, the child keeps his limb motionless—"pseudoparalysis." Not infrequently the primary care physician makes an erroneous diagnosis of paralysis. When the femur or tibia is affected, the child refuses to bear weight on the affected lower limb. The pain is due to the tremendous pressure in bone produced by the inflammatory exudate. When the regional cortex perforates and the subperiosteal abscess ruptures, the intense pain subsides.

Gently palpate the affected bone. In osteomyelitis there is acute localized *tenderness* over the *metaphysis* of long bones. When the proximal femoral metaphysis is involved, the tenderness is best elicited posteriorly over the hip joint in the metaphysis; in septic arthritis of the hip the maximal tenderness is anterior over the hip. In osteomyelitis of the proximal femur the upper thigh is swollen. Other findings are increased local heat and redness. Protective muscle spasms posture the hip in varying degrees of flexion. Sympathetic sterile effusion may be present in the hip.

Laboratory Findings. The white blood cell count may be elevated with a shift to the left on the differential; it may be normal in the ill child with poor systemic response. Leukocytosis is nonspecific and unreliable.

Erythrocyte sedimentation rate and C-reactive protein are elevated. C-reactive protein levels rise and fall rapidly; they are an excellent indication of the activity of the infectious process and its response to treatment. Always obtain a culture of the blood and infected foci, if present, before starting antibiotic therapy.

Imaging. When signs and symptoms suggest acute osteomyelitis, plain radiograms in the AP, lateral, and oblique projections and bone scan with technetium-99m are performed.

Radiograms portray the bone and soft tissues in two dimensions. During the early stages inspect the radiograms for soft tissue changes. Osteomyelitis causes edema in the deep muscle layers adjacent to the affected long bone. Initially the radiolucent plane representing adipose tissue between muscles is displaced away from bone. Later, edema in the fatty planes shows similar density to muscles, and the displaced radiolucent lines disappear in the radiogram.

In order to detect changes in lucent muscle planes, identical views of the contralateral limb are made for comparison. Use a soft tissue technique (30 percent reduction of bone density) to more clearly depict soft tissue changes.

A frequent problem is distinguishing cellulitis from osteomyelitis. In the latter, the deep tissues are swollen, whereas in the former the superficial soft tissues are swollen.

In 1 to 2 weeks when osteomyelitis is untreated, spotty, irregular areas of rarefaction appear in the affected bone. This is due to destruction and absorption of the bone trabeculae and local hyperemia. When the infection spreads to the regional cortex, subperiosteal abscess forms. This is best seen on an ultrasonogram, which, in addition, shows the soft tissue edema.[264,292,294,297] Later changes in the course of osteomyelitis are the formation of involucrum (new bone) and sequestrum (dead bone).

CT scan localizes the infection, especially in the pelvic bone and vertebral column. A bone scan with technetium-99m shows increased local uptake at the site of the osteomyelitis during the first 2 days of the onset of infection. It portrays the pathophysiologic response of bone to infection but is not diagnostic for osteomyelitis.[302,305,309] Increased uptake may be caused by numerous other conditions. Bone scan may be negative in osteomyelitis in children.[267,268] Bone scan is of definite value in locating multifocal osteomyelitis.[277,292,293] Gallium citrate indium-labeled leuko-

cyte scanning is specific for an inflammatory process but not diagnostic of infection; increased radiation exposure, time consumption, and expense are its drawbacks. In difficult cases when a differential diagnosis between Ewing's sarcoma and osteomyelitis is being considered, MRI is performed.

Treatment. Every effort should be made to identify the organism, select the proper antibiotic, and deliver the antibiotic in sufficient concentration and duration to the affected bone to control progressive bone destruction.

Aspiration is crucial to confirm the diagnosis by demonstrating the pathogenic organism by Gram's stain or culture. It also has its therapeutic implications because pus in the bone or a subperiosteal abscess requires surgery to prevent progressive bone destruction. Perform bone aspiration prior to starting antibiotics. In about 90 percent of cases, the pathogenic organism can be demonstrated when osteomyelitis is present. Use a lumbar puncture needle with a stylet inside. Aspirate the most tender area. If subperiosteal aspiration is negative, proceed to intraosseous aspiration. The procedure is very painful, and the proper analgesics should be administered.

Antibiotic therapy is started after cultures are made and an educated guess is made as to the most likely organism and its sensitivity. Factors to consider are the age of the patient, the predisposing cause, and the Gram stain. Once the culture results and sensitivity are available, the initial antibiotic is changed to the most effective one as necessary. Table 3–4 lists the choices of antibiotics for initial therapy for osteomyelitis.

Should antibiotic delivery be oral or parenteral? The initial treatment must always be intravenous. One should remember that antibiotics penetrate into live bone but not into dead bone. The efficacy of antibiotic therapy markedly diminishes in the presence of pus or other products of inflammation and tissue destruction. In general, intravenous antibiotics are delivered for a minimum of 5 to 7 days (preferably for 2 to 3 weeks), and then, depending upon the response, are changed to oral therapy for an additional 5 to 6 weeks. It is best to use a PIC line. Factors to consider in changing from an intravenous to an oral route are the clin-

TABLE 3–4. INITIAL ANTIBIOTIC THERAPY FOR OSTEOMYELITIS IN INFANTS AND CHILDREN

Neonates	Probable Organism	Antibiotic
Neonates <2 months	Group B streptococcus, *Staphylococcus aureus,* or gram-negative rods *Haemophilus influenzae*	Nafcillin + aminoglycoside Cefadyl + aminoglycoside Ceftriaxone or Cefotaxime Cefuroxime
Infants >2 months <3 years	*S. aureus* (90% of cases)	Cefuroxime
Children	*S. aureus* (90% of cases)	Nafcillin

ical response, the verification of adequate serum levels when given orally, the reliability of the parents, and the ability to swallow and retain the medication.

Surgical drainage is indicated when pus is found on aspiration and bone destruction is seen in the radiogram and when there is no clinical response to antibiotic therapy after 36 to 48 hours. The purpose of surgery is to remove dead bone and inflammatory products by debridement and to ensure that the antibiotics reach the site of infection. Make small incisions in the periosteum and do not extensively strip the periosteum because it devascularizes the regional bone. Make a small window for debridement, lavage the infected site copiously, and drain it for 24 to 48 hours.

The overall prognosis for treatment of osteomyelitis is good. Prognostic factors are the age of the patient (poor in the neonate and young infant), the time between onset of symptoms and the beginning of treatment (the sooner the better), and the type of organism and its sensitivity.

NEONATAL OSTEOMYELITIS

In the neonate and the young infant up to 18 months of age, the blood vessels between the metaphysis and epiphysis communicate (Fig 3–43A, B). In the child over 1½ years of age the physis serves as a functional barrier to the spread of infection from the metaphysis into the epiphysis; the blood vessels of the metaphysis and epiphysis do not communicate (Fig 3–43C). In the neonate and young infant this communication of the blood supply between the metaphysis and epiphysis results in two devastating complications: (1) the infectious process usually extends to the epiphysis and involves the adjacent joint, and the pus destroys the epiphysis; (2) involvement and destruction of the physis cause major growth disturbance.

Osteomyelitis in the neonate differs from that of the child in several other ways.[289] Because the immune system and inflammatory response in the neonate are weak, infection tends to spread rapidly and involve multiple sites. Also, clinically, temperature, white blood cell count, and ESR may be normal or only slightly elevated. This lack of systemic response to infection should always be remembered when examining a fussy neonate with a swollen limb who cries acutely when you touch or move the limb.

The causative organism in the neonate and young infant is often group B streptococcus. Other probable organisms are gram-negative rods *(Haemophilus influenzae)* or *Staphylococcus aureus;* therefore, the selection of the initial

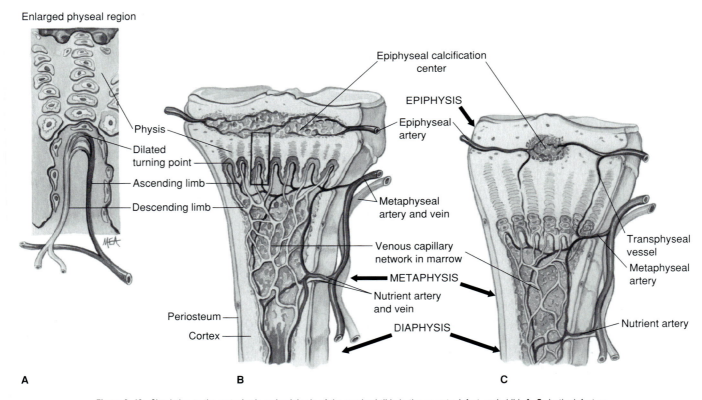

Enlarged physeal region

Epiphyseal calcification center

EPIPHYSIS

Epiphyseal artery

Physis

Dilated turning point

Ascending limb

Descending limb

Metaphyseal artery and vein

Venous capillary network in marrow

METAPHYSIS

Nutrient artery and vein

Transphyseal vessel

Metaphyseal artery

Periosteum

Cortex

DIAPHYSIS

Nutrient artery

A B C

Figure 3–43. Circulation to the metaphysis and epiphysis of the proximal tibia in the neonate, infant, and child. **A, B.** In the infant up to 18 months of age, the blood vessels of the epiphysis and metaphysis communicate between the transphyseal vessels. **C.** In the child over 1½ years of age, note that the growth plate acts as a barrier, and the epiphyseal and metaphyseal vessels do not communicate.

antibiotic to provide coverage prior to the results of culture are cefotaxime, oxacillin, or gentamicin.

The most common site of neonatal osteomyelitis is the proximal femur; next is the proximal humerus (Fig 3–44). When diagnosis and treatment are delayed, the result is destruction of the femoral or humeral head. Remember, in 40 percent of neonatal osteomyelitis cases, multiple sites are affected. It behooves the physician to

examine the entire skeletal system daily, if not twice a day. Technetium-99m bone scanning detects multiple sites of infection.

Early diagnosis and treatment are crucial. Delay in effective treatment results in destruction of the epiphysis, physis, and joint.

Suspicious sites (bone or joint) are aspirated. When pus is obtained, prompt surgical drainage is carried out. Appropriate antibiotics are administered intravenously, usually through a central PIC line. With early diagnosis and immediate treatment, the prognosis is good.

SUBACUTE OSTEOMYELITIS

The presenting complaint is mild pain of insidious onset with minimal functional impairment and little or no fever or systemic illness. When the proximal femur is involved, the patient complains of mild anterior hip or thigh pain of several weeks duration. Restriction of range of hip motion is minimal. On deep palpation there is local tenderness over the affected site.

In subacute osteomyelitis there is a modified relationship between the host (increased resistance) and pathogen (decreased virulence). In about 40 percent of the cases, the host-pathogen relationship is modified by prior antibiotics that the patient has received for infections other than osteomyelitis.[287,288,295,301]

The initial radiogram in subacute osteomyelitis is often abnormal. The epiphysis, metaphysis, and diaphysis of the long bones or the vertebral column may be involved. Bone scan with technetium-99m shows increased uptake. The classification of Roberts et al. is given in Figure 3–45.[300]

Diagnosis. Blood cultures are usually negative. Bone cultures obtained at biopsy are positive in 60 percent of the cases. Often *S. aureus* is the pathogenic organism. Many patients undergo biopsy because of the suspicion of a bone tumor. A conclusive diagnosis is made by histologic demonstration of chronic inflammation in bone from the biopsy specimen and positive culture.

Treatment. When the imaging findings are typical and aspiration of the lesions yields a positive culture, some bone lesions heal with antibiotics alone. When the lesion fails to respond to antibiotic therapy, surgery is indicated in the form of biopsy, culture, and curettage. Antibiotics are given in addition to surgical measures. The prognosis is good. Symptoms disappear rapidly, and the bone lesion heals without residual deformity.

CHRONIC MULTIFOCAL OSTEOMYELITIS

This is a rare inflammatory affection of childhood occurring between the ages of 4 and 14 years. The presenting com-

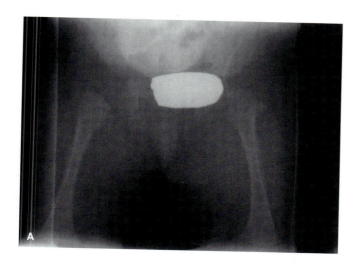

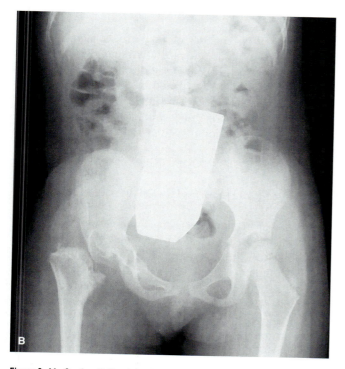

Figure 3–44. Septic arthritis of the right hip in a neonate. **A.** Note the lateral subluxation of the hip joint. This was diagnosed late and the hip joint was not drained, resulting in total destruction of the femoral head. **B.** AP radiograms of both hips showing the destroyed femoral head and superolateral subluxation of the proximal femur.

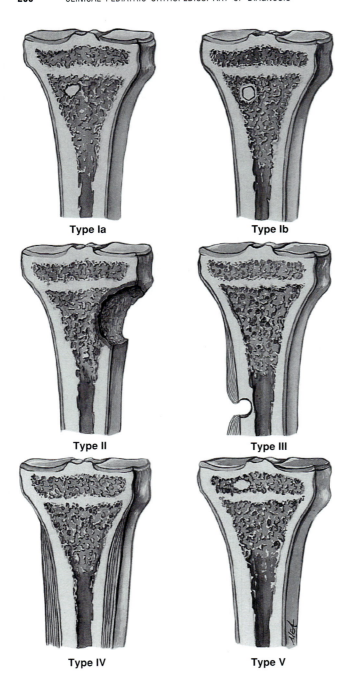

Type Ia

Type Ib

Type II

Type III

Type IV

Type V

Figure 3–45. Classification of subacute osteomyelitis (according to Roberts et al). Type I is an area of radiolucency located in the metaphysis of the long bones with intact adjacent cortical bone. Type I is subdivided into two subtypes. Type Ia is a punched-out radiolucency of varying size with no surrounding reactive bone. It resembles eosinophilic granuloma. In Type Ib the metaphyseal radiolucency is surrounded by a sclerotic margin. It represents the classic Brodie abscess.

In Type II, the area of radiolucency is in the metaphysis, with erosion and loss of the regional cortex. In the radiogram it appears as an aggressive lesion, suggesting osteolytic osteogenic sarcoma.

In Type III, the osteomyelitis is diaphyseal in location with marked cortical and subperiosteal reaction; its appearance suggests osteoid osteoma.

Type IV is diaphyseal in location and is characterized by onion-skin layering of subperiosteal bone; its appearance is similar to early Ewing's sarcoma.

Type V is located in the epiphysis of long bones and appears as a concentric area of radiolucency. Its appearance is similar to benign chondroblastoma, eosinophilic granuloma, or enchondroma.

Type VI (not illustrated—see the chapter on the Spine) involves the vertebral body, which appears collapsed with erosion. Its radiographic picture suggests tuberculosis.

pelvis. Bone scan with technetium-99m shows increased local uptake and detects bone lesions that initially are clinically silent.

Immunologic studies have not shown any deficit. Histologic examination of the tissues is essential for diagnosis. Bone cultures are usually negative. Biopsy is often performed.

Treatment. This consists of nonsteroidal anti-inflammatory drugs to provide symptomatic relief. Antibiotics are given empirically as a therapeutic trial, but if symptoms persist after 2 weeks they should be discontinued. Steroids may be given. Surgical treatment is rarely necessary. The long-term prognosis is good, with no evidence of disturbance of growth or joint destruction or angular deformity of the long bones.

OSTEOMYELITIS OF THE INNOMINATE BONE

In children and adolescents the *ilium* is most commonly involved; the area next to the sacroiliac joint is the usual site of onset of the infection. Clinical presentation depends upon the direction of spread of the infection.[266,273,280,281]

When the infectious process extends anteriorly to involve the inner wall of the ilium, the presenting symptoms and signs are *abdominal* pain and tenderness, mimicking acute appendicitis. Misdiagnosed patients have undergone exploration of the abdomen and removal of a normal appendix. The astute clinician applies firm lateral pelvic compression, a maneuver that elicits and aggravates the pain. On careful palpation the local tenderness is over the posterior part of the ilium, near the sacroiliac joint. On gentle rectal examination the tenderness is over

plaint is gradual onset of pain and local tenderness at the sites of infection, predominantly at the metaphysis of long bones, but occasionally in the vertebral bodies, sacroiliac joint, or medial end of the clavicle. The bone lesions are often symmetric and sometimes sequential in onset. Symmetry of involvement is not essential for diagnosis. Chronic multifocal osteomyelitis may be associated with polyarthritis, psoriasis, and palmoplantar pustulosis.[265,271,274,286]

Imaging. Plain radiograms show typical features of osteomyelitis, but these may be difficult to see in the spine and

the inner wall of the ilium posteriorly and not the region of the appendix.

When the outer cortex of the ilium is invaded and perforated by the inflammatory process, the presenting complaint is pain in the buttocks. Local tenderness is present over the affected ilium. When the diagnosis is delayed, a subgluteal soft mass may be palpated due to formation of an abscess. Neurologic examination is normal; straight-leg raising elicits hamstring muscle spasm and pain in the posterior thigh.

The upper trunk of the lumbar plexus may be irritated when the inner cortex of the ilium is perforated by the septic process and the abscess extends deep and inferiorly into the anterior wall of the sacrum and pelvis. In such cases the presenting complaint is low back pain, sciatica, and an antalgic limp. Straight-leg raising is positive. The patellar tendon reflex may be depressed or absent. The hip has full range of motion. Deep palpation reveals tenderness over the posterior wall of the ilium near the sacroiliac joint. When the pelvis is laterally compressed the patient complains of intense pain in the buttocks.

Imaging Findings. Initially, plain radiograms are normal. Perform bone scan with technetium-99m; it shows intense localized uptake. Early diagnosis is crucial. When bone scan is positive and radiograms are normal, CT is performed. It may be normal or may show soft tissue abscess or lytic areas in bone. The problem is differentiation of iliac osteomyelitis from Ewing's sarcoma, especially later on when lytic lesions in bone and soft tissue mass form. MRI is of definite value in distinguishing the two.

Management. Aspirate the lesion under image intensifier radiographic control and obtain blood culture (in spite of benign systemic findings of infection) to identify the pathogenic organism.

Next, with the clinical diagnosis of infection and not tumor, administer an intensive course of intravenous antibiotic therapy. In the case of osteomyelitis, dramatic response is seen within 24 to 48 hours. When no immediate response to antibiotic therapy is seen, a biopsy should be obtained to confirm the diagnosis of infection and rule out tumor.

When an abscess is formed, the affected osteomyelitic bone should be surgically drained.

■ ACUTE TRANSIENT SYNOVITIS OF THE HIP

A child, ordinarily between 3 and 6 years of age, presents with an antalgic limp and pain in the anteromedial aspect of the thigh and knee. There may be a history of recent upper respiratory infection or allergic rhinitis. The onset of hip irritation is often acute but may be gradual. The cause of this nonspecific inflammation of the hip is unknown.

Diagnosis is made by exclusion and by the natural course of the disease, which is short-lived and ephemeral. The condition is self-limited, and the symptoms disappear within a few weeks.[310–331]

On physical examination medial rotation of the hip in flexion is restricted; there is also some limitation of hip abduction (both in flexion and extension) and hip extension, with varying degrees of flexion deformity of the hip. There may be local tenderness on the anterior aspect of the hip joint. Toxic symptoms are absent or minimal, with temperature elevation less than 100°F.

Imaging Findings. Ultrasonography detects and measures the degree of joint effusion (Fig 3–46). The patient is placed in the supine position with both hips in neutral extension, rotation, and abduction-adduction. The normal hip is scanned first and then the irritable hip. The probe is placed longitudinal to the axis of the femoral neck. The distance between the anterior margin of the joint capsule and the femoral neck is the ultrasonographic joint space (UJS)—it is anechoic. In the normal hip the capsule lies immediately adjacent on the anterior aspect of the femoral neck. In synovitis of the hip with effusion, in the beginning the capsule is anterior and then medial. When the UJS is greater than 6 mm or when there is a difference of 3 mm or more between the normal and the involved hip, abnormal capsular distention is present. The capsule may be distended by fluid (effusion type) or hypertrophy of the synovium (synovitis type). In the effusion type the increased UJS is anechoic and homogeneous, whereas in the synovitis type UJS is anechoic but irregular. In acute transient synovitis the capsular distention is produced by synovial effusion (it is homogeneous), whereas in Perthes' disease it is produced by synovial thickening (it is irregular). Therefore the finding of capsular distention with the joint space showing irregular areas of high echogenicity is highly suggestive of Perthes' disease.[314]

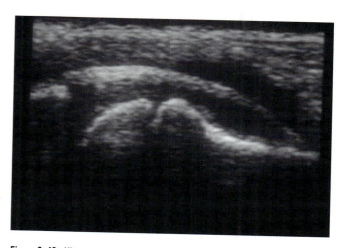

Figure 3–46. Ultrasonogram of acute transient synovitis. Note the marked distention of the joint capsule.

Next place the probe vertical to the surface of the femoral head and determine the thickness of its articular cartilage. Measure the width of the anechoic space between the subchondral bone of the femoral head and the deep contour of the labrum; it is the thickness of the cartilage of the femoral head. Thickening of the cartilage of the femoral head is common in Perthes' disease, whereas femoral epiphyseal cartilage thickening is rare or much less in acute transient synovitis.

Thickening of the articular cartilage in Perthes' disease has also been demonstrated by arthrography and MRI. The cartilage is thickened due to either swelling caused by pathologic changes in osmotic pressure, hypertrophy as a response to avascular necrosis of bone and subsequent subchondral fracture, or both.

Accurate differential diagnosis between transient synovitis and Perthes' disease cannot be made based solely on ultrasonographic examination. Ordinarily symptoms of transient synovitis subside and disappear within 2 weeks with bed rest and restriction of physical activity. However, if symptoms persist and a repeat ultrasound study shows persistent effusion and capsular distention, Perthes' disease should be strongly suspected and scintigraphy with technetium-99m should be performed.

In acute toxic synovitis of the hip, *bone scan with technetium-99m* shows slight diffuse uptake which disappears with subsidence of the synovitis, whereas in Perthes' disease the bone scan shows decreased uptake of the radionuclide in the avascular and fragmentation stages of the disease.

Plain radiograms of the hip are normal in transient synovitis. The superolateral bulging of the soft tissues around the hip is due to abnormal posture of the hip in adduction and lateral rotation and not to capsular distention.[312] Widening of the medial articular cartilage space due to lateral displacement of the femoral head is very rare in transient synovitis. When it is present, rule out septic arthritis of the hip by aspiration of the hip joint.

CT and MRI are not indicated in transient synovitis of the hip. These studies are performed only in the rare case in which a lesion of the acetabulum or femoral head and neck is suspected as the cause of persisting and increasing symptoms.

Laboratory Studies. These are performed to rule out other causes of synovitis of the hip, such as sepsis, rheumatoid arthritis, and tubercular arthritis. Complete blood count, ESR, and skin tests for tuberculosis are normal, and latex fixation and other immunologic tests for rheumatoid arthritis are negative.

Aspiration of the hip joint is performed only in the rare case when symptoms and capsular distention persist with lateral displacement of the femoral head and the presence of toxic signs of fever, elevated ESR, and leukocytosis.

Treatment. This consists of bed rest at home with restriction of physical activities and administration of nonsteroidal anti-inflammatory medications such as naproxen sodium. The noncompliant hyperactive child may have to be admitted to the hospital and placed in counterpoised split Russell traction.

Recurrence of acute transient synovitis of the hip may occur. Reassure the parents. Explain to them that synovium in the hip is similar to the upper respiratory tract and may have repeated "colds."

In the past the literature stated that 2.5 to 10 percent of children with acute transient synovitis develop Perthes' disease. Recent studies have shown this to be false.[319,323] It is recommended, however, that children with acute transient synovitis be followed and reassessed 2 and 6 months after the initial episode.

■ LEGG-CALVÉ-PERTHES DISEASE

Legg-Calvé-Perthes' disease is a self-limited affection of the hip characterized by aseptic necrosis of the whole or part of the femoral head produced by interruption of its blood supply, followed by subchondral fracture, revascularization, and repair of the dead bone. Legg and Calvé and Perthes described the condition independently in 1910, but it is often referred to in its abbreviated synonym, Perthes' disease, because of its brevity and the fact that Perthes, in 1913, gave a precise description of the disease and recognized its ischemic nature.[348,439–441,465,466] Historically, however, Waldenström in 1909 described this disorder of the hip but regarded it as tuberculous in nature and therefore forfeited eponymous immortality.[519]

The age incidence of Perthes' disease is quite narrow; most cases occur between 3 and 9 years of age, with an average of 6 years and a span of 2 to 13 years. It is more common in boys, with a male to female ratio of 4:1. It is very rare in blacks, Indians, and Polynesians. There is a definite geographic variation, with a reported incidence of 1:1200 in Massachusetts and 1:5590 in Scotland.[351,455] In one out of ten, involvement is bilateral. When both hips are involved, it behooves the surgeon to rule out epiphyseal dysplasia, hypothyroidism, Gaucher's disease, and other causes of aseptic necrosis of the femoral head.

History. The presenting complaint is an antalgic limp and mild pain on the anteromedial aspect of the thigh and knee. The limp and pain are insidious in onset, of several weeks' duration, and usually intermittent, being aggravated by physical activity and relieved by rest. In some cases a history of definite injury can be obtained with symptoms beginning after the trauma.

Occasionally Perthes' disease is asymptomatic; it is diagnosed during a radiographic examination made for some other reason such as a diagnostic study of the kidney or bladder. There is a high association of Perthes' disease with urinary tract abnormalities, undescended testicles, and hernia. Rule them out—do not hesitate to inspect and palpate the groin and the scrotum.

In the history, inquire as to whether the child has congenital heart disease or epilepsy or had pyloric stenosis; they are rare concomitant anomalies.

Genetic factors do not play a role in the pathogenesis of Perthes' disease. When there is a family history and involvement is bilateral, the child likely has epiphyseal dysplasia.

Etiology. Perthes' disease is produced by impairment of the blood supply to the femoral head. Biopsy specimens have shown different stages of repair in the different parts of the femoral head, indicating that there has been more than one ischemic episode. Experimentally, multiple episodes of infarction are required to produce the pathologic picture of Perthes' disease.[376,415,494] The exact cause of interruption of circulation to the femoral head remains obscure.

Numerous theories speculating on the pathogenesis of the disease have been proposed. Increased intra-articular pressure and tamponade compression of the retinacular vessels around the femoral neck and a causal relationship between acute transient synovitis of the hip and Perthes' disease have been speculated upon. Bone scan studies with technetium-99m in transient synovitis of the hip have not shown a cold femoral head; instead there is often a slight diffuse increased uptake of the radionuclide due to regional hypervascularity. Acute transient synovitis does not cause Perthes' disease; instead, the subchondral fracture in Perthes' disease causes synovitis of the hip.

Increased blood viscosity in patients with Perthes' disease has been reported by Kleinman and Bleck.[431] The venous drainage of the femoral neck is disturbed in Perthes' disease, as shown by the increased interosseous venous pressure and abnormal intraosseous venogram.[392,509]

Constitutional factors have been implicated because of short stature and delayed skeletal maturation of the patients with Perthes' disease.[345] It is the lower legs and forearms which are primarily short. After healing of the disease, the bone age returns to normal. Patients with Perthes' disease have decreased levels of Somatomedin C (IGF1).

Imaging Findings. Radiographic images depict the anatomic changes in the femoral head and neck. The pathogenesis of deformation of the femoral head is illustrated in Figure 3–47. In the *initial stage,* enchondral ossification of the ossific nucleus of the femoral head stops due to interruption of the blood supply and infarction of the bony epiphysis. The result is a smaller size of the ossific nucleus of the femoral head compared with that of the contracted normal hip. The articular cartilage of the femoral head continues to grow because it derives its nutrition from the synovial fluid; the femoral head cartilage enlarges on both its medial and lateral aspects. With overgrowth of articular cartilage of the femoral head, the medial articular cartilage space between the ossific nucleus and the teardrop of the acetabulum gradually widens (Fig 3–48A, B, p. 215).

The second radiographic sign in Perthes' disease is the *subchondral fracture,* which is seen as a crescentic subchondral radiolucent line in the femoral head (Fig. 3–47C, D). This is referred to as "Caffey's sign" because he was the first to describe its nature in Perthes' disease.[346,347] It is best seen in the Lowenstein lateral projection. Beginning in the anterior part of the femoral head, it extends posteriorly in the subchondral zone to a varying distance; depending upon the extent of necrosis and fracture of the trabecular bone (Fig 3–49A, B, p. 216).

Good quality radiograms are essential for visualization of the subchondral fracture. The clinical onset of Perthes' disease is triggered by the subchondral fracture. In the radiograms it is a temporary finding, seen early in the course of the disease. In 2 to 6 months, with resorption and enchondral ossification, the subchondral fracture line disappears in the radiogram. The subchondral fracture is best shown in the MRI.

The next radiographic finding in Perthes' disease is increased opacity of the femoral head (Fig 3–50, p. 218). This increased density of the ossific nucleus is due mostly to calcification of the necrotic marrow and partly to appositional new bone formation and fracture, collapse, and crowding of the crushed avascular bone.

Anatomically, in the initial stages of Perthes' disease the physis is abnormal, with disarray and irregularity of the cellular column of the growth plate and increased calcified cartilage in the primary spongiosa. The articular cartilage and physeal abnormalities are best visualized in the MRI and not in the plain radiograms.

Once the fracture of the infarcted bone occurs, the process of revascularization and repair begins. The loose necrotic trabeculae of bone are resorbed by invasion of fibrous vascular tissue and replaced by fibrocartilage, a process termed "creeping substitution." In the plain radiogram this repair process is depicted as fragmentation of the dense bone by radiolucent patchy areas (Fig 3–51, p. 218).

With enchondral ossification from the live subchondral bone plate, islands of new bone form and extend into the thickened articular cartilage of the femoral head. In the plain radiogram, these islands of new bone are depicted as "calcification" lateral to the epiphysis. With further bone growth these islands of new bone enlarge and fuse with the main ossific nucleus of the femoral head.

Streaks of unossified cartilage may extend from the growth plate into the subjacent metaphysis and give a cystic appearance (Figs 3–52 and 3–53 pp. 218–219). An assessment of metaphyseal changes by MRI scan have

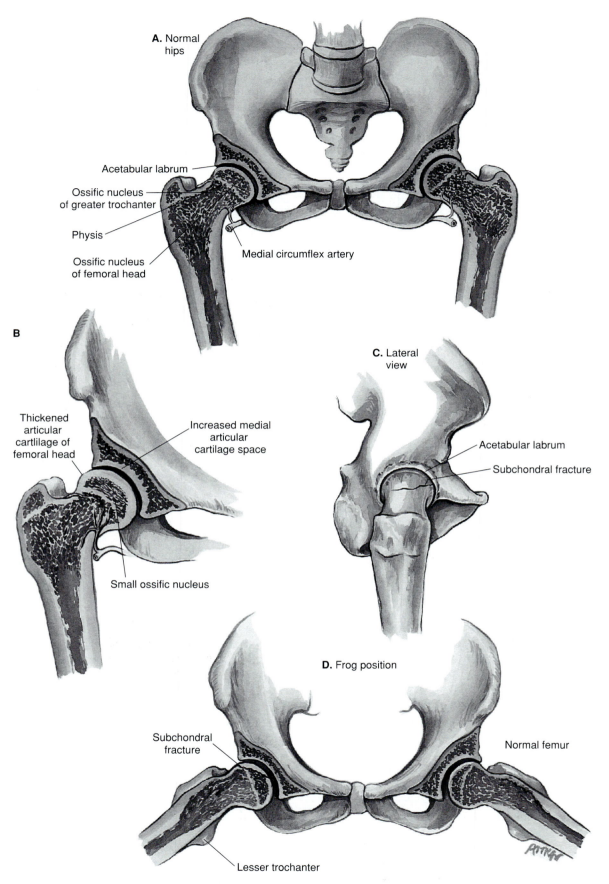

A. Normal hips

Acetabular labrum

Ossific nucleus of greater trochanter

Physis

Ossific nucleus of femoral head

Medial circumflex artery

B

Thickened articular cartilage of femoral head

Increased medial articular cartilage space

Small ossific nucleus

C. Lateral view

Acetabular labrum

Subchondral fracture

D. Frog position

Subchondral fracture

Normal femur

Lesser trochanter

Figure 3–47. Pathogenesis of femoral head deformity in Perthes' disease. **A.** Normal hips. **B.** Perthes' disease of the right hip. Note that the ossific nucleus of the femoral head is small, the articular cartilage of the femoral head is thickened, and the medial articular cartilage space is increased. **C, D.** Lateral and frog-leg views showing the subchondral fracture. **(Continues)**

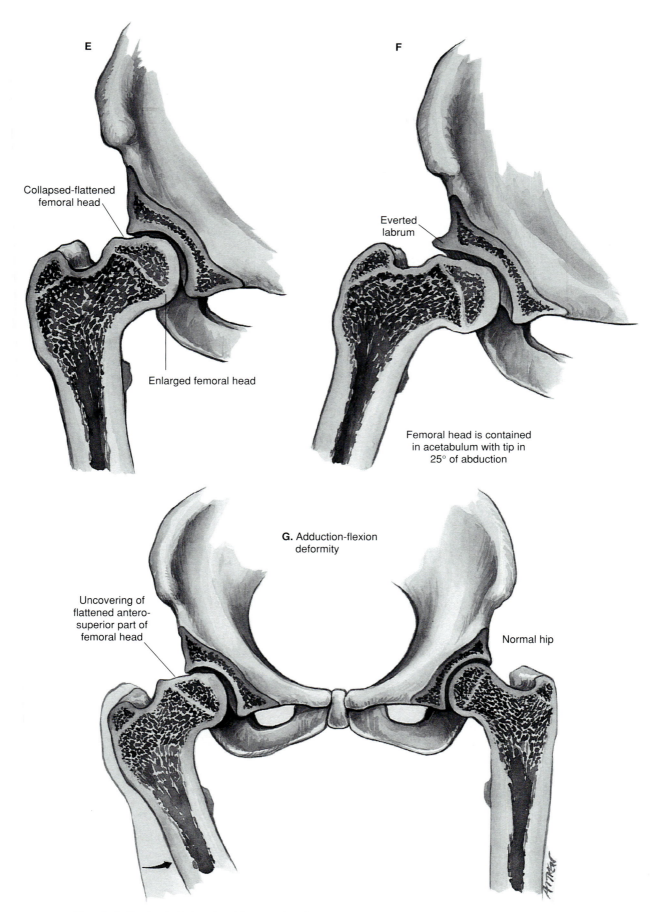

Figure 3–47 *(Continued)*. **E.** Anterolateral flattening of the femoral head in the weight-bearing position. **F.** Superior displacement of the femoral head with eversion of the labrum. Note: In 20 degrees of abduction, the femoral head is contained in the acetabulum. **G.** The hip is held in progressive flexion-adduction with further uncovering of the femoral head, which is flattened and extruded anterolaterally in weight-bearing. *(Continues)*

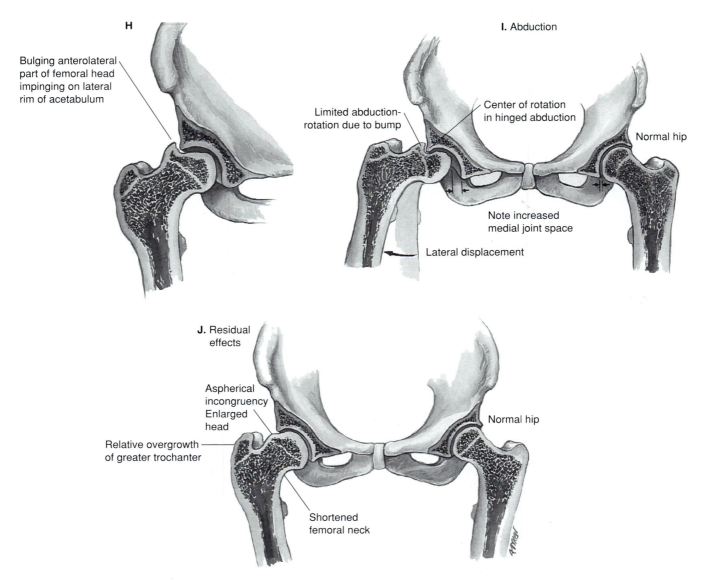

Figure 3–47 *(Continued)*. **H.** In weight-bearing position, the anterolateral part of the femoral head bulges upward and impinges on the rim of the acetabulum. **I.** Hip abduction is limited and blocked by the bump on the femoral head. Note the increased medial joint space. **J.** Residual deformities: (1) enlarged femoral head—coxa magna; (2) short femoral neck—coxa breva; (3) relative overgrowth of the greater trochanter.

demonstrated that most of these so-called metaphyseal cysts are physeal and epiphyseal irregularities and not true metaphyseal cysts.[413]

In the reparative phase, gradual reossification takes place. The anterolateral part of the femoral head is last to reform. When necrosis is extensive, the round femoral head converts to oval in shape.

Ultrasonography. Anterior and lateral views are obtained with the patient supine and the lower limbs in neutral rotation.[510,512] Ultrasonography shows: (1) effusion in the hip (which, when persistent, should make one suspicious of Perthes' disease), (2) thickening and enlargement of the articular cartilage of the epiphysis, (3) lateral and anterior uncoverage of the femoral head, flattening of the femoral head, and (4) irregularity and deformation of the bony epiphysis.

Scintigraphy with Technetium-99m. The concentration of technetium-99m in bone depends upon the regional blood flow and bone metabolism. Pin-hole imaging is made in both the AP and lateral projections. In Perthes' disease, at

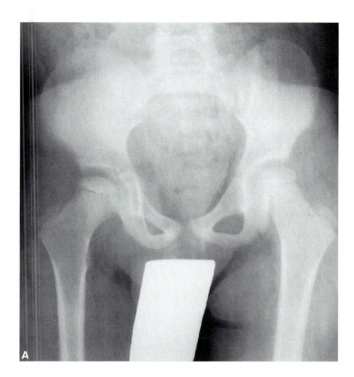

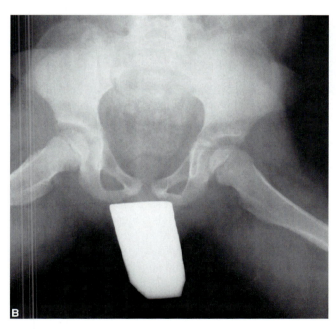

Figure 3–48. Initial finding in the plain radiogram of the hips in Perthes' disease. **A.** AP and **(B)** frog lateral projections of both hips. Note that the ossific nucleus of the left femoral head is smaller than the opposite normal right hip. Also note the widening of the articular cartilage space between the ossific nucleus of the femoral head and the teardrop of the acetabulum. This is due to effusion and cartilage hypertrophy.

the site of avascular necrosis of the femoral head absence or decrease of uptake of the nuclide is seen (Fig 3–54A). Revascularization of the dead bone is accompanied by progressive increase in uptake of the nuclide from the periphery. With full vascularization the uptake of the nuclide is normal (Fig 3–54B).[349]

During the course of Perthes' disease, the following stages are seen in the bone scan: *stage 1*—the whole ossific nucleus appears avascular; *stage 2*—when revascularization takes place by recanalization, a lateral column is seen on the bone scan; this is a good prognostic sign (Fig 3–55). Failure of revascularization of the lateral column is a poor prognostic sign. *Stage 3*—the anterolateral part of the epiphysis gradually fills; and *stage 4*—with complete healing, the bone scan returns to normal.

Magnetic Resonance Imaging. MRI directly assesses all that constitutes bone marrow—fat, hematopoietic cells, water, and mineral. In T1-weighted images, epiphyseal and apophyseal ossification centers have high signal intensity because hematopoietically they are inactive. Mineral diminishes the signal intensity because of lack of mobile proteins.

Both coronal and sagittal planes are examined in T1- and T2-weighted sequences. They depict the infarcted zone in the femoral head exactly before changes are evident in the plain radiogram. MRI shows total ischemia of the femoral head prior to the subchondral fracture. When the subchondral fracture occurs, it is shown in the MRI as a subchondral low-intensity line. In the plain radiograms the subchondral fracture line is a transient finding seen in the early stages of the disease and not in all hips, whereas in the MRI subchondral fracture is depicted in all hips and is present well beyond the early phase of the disease. MRI determines the extent of the infarcted bone (Fig 3–56).

When repair takes place in the T1-weighted images, the fibrous repair tissue is shown as a semilunar or cup-shaped low-intensity band. The outer zone of the repair tissue interface is of low intensity on both T1- and T2-weighted images, demarcating living bone from necrotic bone. In the MRI, healing is shown by an increase of the normal signal intensity. Bos et al. performed follow-up MRI scans at 6-month intervals which reflected the developmental stages of the repair process of each group classified according to Catterall.[341]

MRI demonstrates the contour of the cartilaginous femoral head, whether round or flattened, the exact degree of extrusion and uncoverage of the femoral head, the degree of superolateral displacement of the femoral head (subluxation), the eversion of the labrum of the acetabulum, and the extent of necrosis.

For serial follow-up for assessing the extent of healing of the femoral head, plain radiography is performed—it is

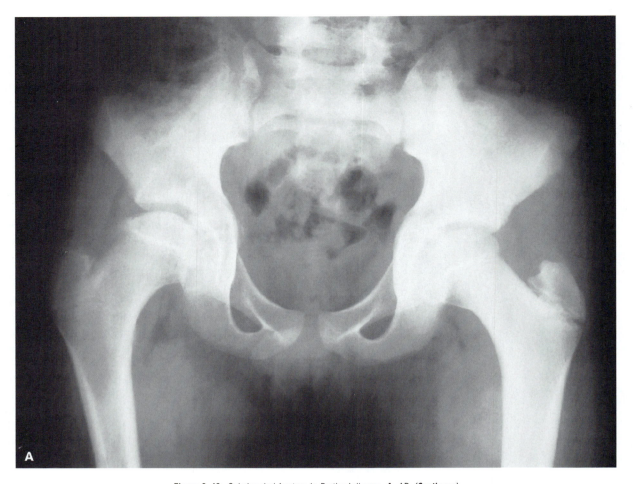

Figure 3-49. Subchondral fracture in Perthes' disease. **A.** AP. *(Continues)*

just as good as MRI. When progressive deformation of the femoral head is suspected, MRI is performed instead of arthrography, as the latter is an invasive procedure that often requires general anesthesia.

The drawbacks of MRI are cost, availability, and the need for sedation of the child because of the requirement of immobility during examination. Because of these disadvantages I recommend its use in class B (Salter-Thompson) and group B and C in the lateral pillar classification of Herring.

Arthrography is indicated when there is the suggestion of hinged abduction, osteochondritis dissecans, or a torn labrum. In the past, arthrography was used to assess deformation of the femoral head, however, at present, MRI is performed to delineate the cartilaginous epiphysis. Arthrography should be performed in the operating room under strict sterile conditions and technique. Infection and anaphylactic reaction to the radio-opaque dye are rare complications.

Classification. The degree of involvement in Perthes' disease varies. At present there are three plain radiographic classifications: (1) subchondral fissure of Salter-Thompson; (2) lateral pillar of Herring; and (3) Catterall's grouping. Conway has proposed a biologic classification based upon the bone scan findings with technetium-99m.[351,352,360,361,412,493]

Extent of Subchondral Fracture (Salter-Thompson). This is detected in the early stages of the disease before resorption of the femoral head begins. It is a transient radiographic finding, not seen in all cases. It is important to take good quality radiograms in both the standard AP and Lowenstein frog-lateral projections. In *Class A,* the extent of subchondral fracture is less than half of the femoral head; in *Class B,* the extent of subchondral fracture is more than half of the femoral head. Class A correlates with Catterall's groups I and II, and class B with Catterall's

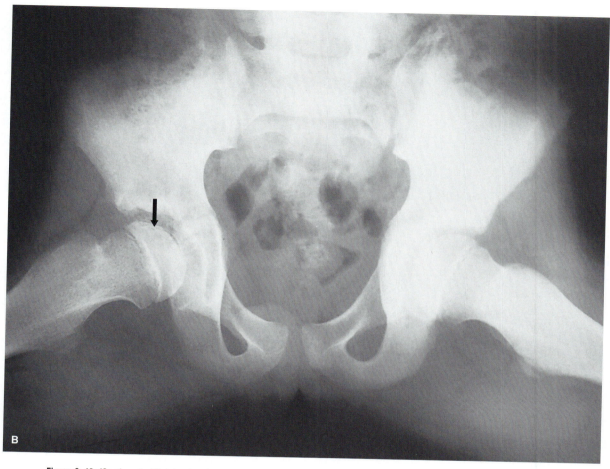

Figure 3–49 *(Continued).* **(B)** Lateral projections showing the subchondral radiolucent line in the anterior part of the right femoral head. It extends posteriorly.

groups III and IV. In class A there is an intact, viable lateral capital femoral epiphyseal margin which shields the epiphysis from stress and lessens the possibility of collapse and deformity, whereas in class B such a supporting column is absent.[493]

Lateral Pillar Classification. Herring et al. developed lateral pillar classification; the lateral pillar is defined as the lateral 15 to 30 percent of the capital epiphysis on the AP radiograph. In group A the lateral pillar is normal; in group B, greater than 50 percent of the original height of the lateral pillar is preserved and is intact with some radiolucency. In group C less than 50 percent of the original height of the lateral pillar is preserved and is intact with radiolucency (Fig 3–57, p. 220). This classification is accurate, reproducible, and easy to use.[412] Lateral pillar group A corresponds to Catterall group I and possibly group II; lateral pillar group B corresponds to Catterall group II and possibly III; and lateral pillar group C corresponds to Catterall groups III and IV.

Catterall Classification. Catterall proposed a classification (groups I, II, III, and IV) according to the extent of the involvement of the femoral head, based upon the radiographic appearance at the time of maximum epiphyseal resorption[351,352] (see Table 3–5). Its prognostic value is limited in the early stages.

Scintigraphic Classification (Conway). Conway gave a biologic classification based upon the bone scan findings with technetium-99m.[360,361] Two forms of the healing process are delineated: *A tract,* characterized by early lateral column formation, and *B tract,* in which a lateral column does not form. The prognosis is poor when a lateral column is absent 2 to 3 months after the onset of symptoms. *A tract* heals with recanalization, which may occur rapidly: *stage*

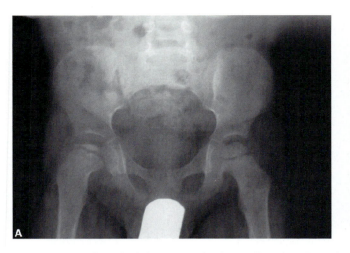
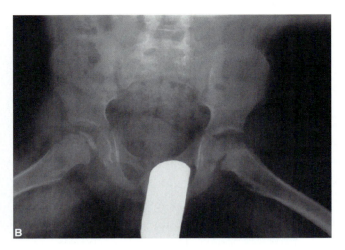

Figure 3–50. Increased opacity of the ossific nucleus of the right femoral head in Perthes' disease. **A.** AP and **(B)** lateral radiograms of the hips.

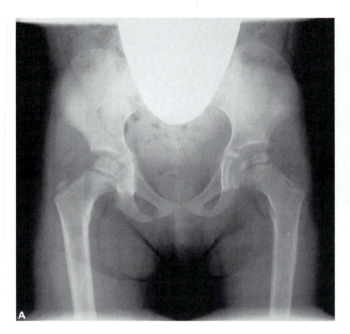
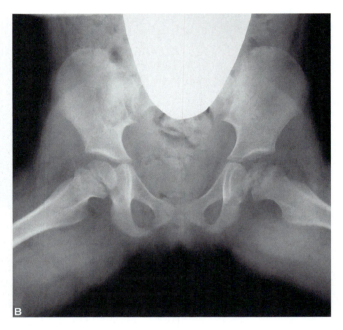

Figure 3–51. Fragmentation of the ossific nucleus of the femoral head in Perthes' disease. **A.** AP and **(B)** frog lateral radiogram of both hips. Note the patchy areas of rarefaction and fragmentation in the left femoral head.

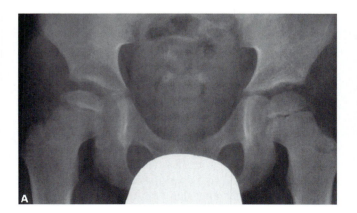
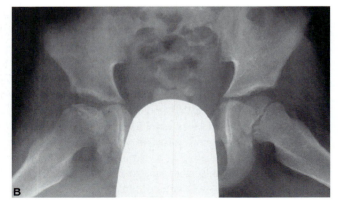

Figure 3–52. Metaphyseal rarefaction in Perthes' disease. **A.** AP and **(B)** frog lateral views.

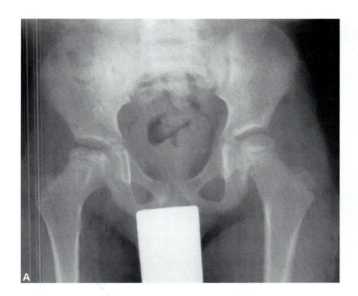

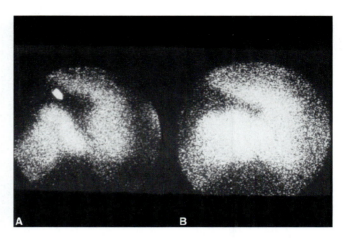

Figure 3–54. Bone imaging with technetium-99m in Perthes' disease. **A.** Initial stage showing absence of local uptake of the nuclide in the femoral head. **B.** One year later showing revascularization and full uptake of the nuclide.

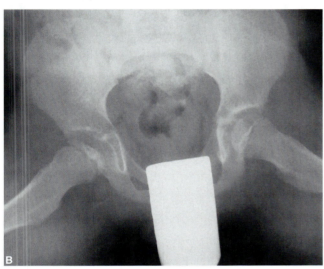

Figure 3–53. Large metaphyseal cyst, which is located anteriorly next to the physis with irregular rarefaction in the head of the femur. **A.** AP view. **B.** Frog lateral view.

Differential Diagnosis. Consider the following conditions of the hip: (1) transient synovitis, (2) pyogenic arthritis; (3) juvenile rheumatoid arthritis; (4) rheumatic fever; (5) tuberculous arthritis and (6) tumors such as eosinophilic granuloma, osteoid osteoma, benign osteoblastoma, and lymphomas. When both hips are affected, one should rule out multiple epiphyseal dysplasia, hypothyroidism, trichorhinophalangeal syndrome, and Gaucher's disease.

Treatment. The goal in management of Perthes' disease is to obtain a normal femoral head and neck and a congruous hip with normal range of hip motion and to prevent degenerative arthritis of the hip in adult life. About 60 percent of patients do well without definitive treatment and about 40 percent require surgical management. What

1A (whole head)—0 to 2 months; *stage 2A* (lateral column)—3 months; *stage 3A* (anterior extrusion)—6 months; and *stage 4A*—more than 1 year. *B tract* heals with neocanalization; these patients display head-at-risk radiographic signs at follow-up studies: *stage 1B* (whole head)—0 to 1 year; *stage 2B* (base filling)—more than 1 year; *stage 3B* (mushroom)—more than 1 to 2 years; and *stage 4B* (healed)—1 to 4 years. The bone scan classification precedes the radiographic "head-at-risk" sign by an average of 5 months.

I recommend using the Conway bone scan, Salter subchondral fracture, and Herring's lateral pillar classification in the *early stages* and Catterall's classification later in the course of the disease.

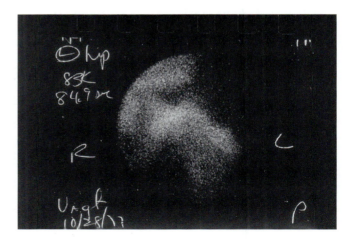

Figure 3–55. Technetium-99m scintigraphy findings in Perthes' disease. Note the lateral column. This is stage II (Conway). It is a good prognostic sign.

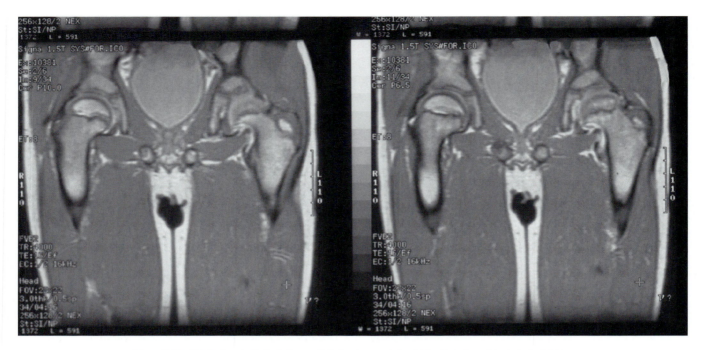

Figure 3–56. MRI findings in Perthes' disease. Note the decreased signal intensity in the epiphysis in the left hip.

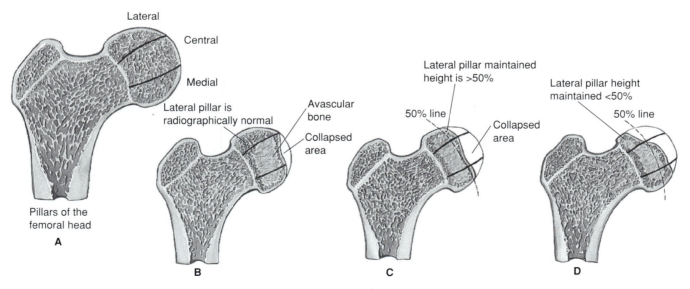

Figure 3–57. Lateral pillar classification of Herring. **A.** The three pillars as seen in the AP projection of the hip. The lateral 15 to 30 percent of the capital epiphysis is the lateral pillar. **B.** Group A—the lateral pillar is normal. **C.** Group B—greater than 50 percent of the original height of the lateral pillar is preserved. **D.** Group C—less than 50 percent of the lateral column is preserved.

TABLE 3–5. CATTERALL'S GROUPS

	I	II	III	IV
Epiphyseal signs				
Sclerosis	No	Yes	Yes	Yes
Subchondral fracture line	No	Anterior	Posterior	Complete
Junction		Clear	Clear	Sclerotic—no
Involved/uninvolved segments			Often "V"	
Viable bone on growth plate		Anterior margin	Anterior half	Posterior half—no
Triangular appearance to medial/lateral aspects		No	No	Occasional—yes
Metaphyseal signs				
Localized rarefaction	No	Anterior	Anterior	Anterior or central
Diffuse rarefaction	No	No	Yes	Yes
Posterior remodeling	No	No	No	Yes

Courtesy of Dr. A. Catterall.

are the features that determine the outcome of Perthes' disease?

1. *Gender and age of the child at clinical onset.* The older the patient, the worse the prognosis. Patients between 2 and 6 years of age have the least amount of residual deformity because they have more time to remodel the epiphysis and acetabulum with bone growth. Patients 10 years of age and older have the worst prognosis. The hips of boys do better than those of girls because girls have a more extensive form of the disease.

2. *Extent of necrosis of the femoral head.* The greater the involvement, the poorer the prognosis. The extent of subchondral fracture correlates with the extent of bone resorption. Group A hips (in which the subchondral fracture extends through less than one half of the femoral head) do well, whereas group B hips (subchondral fracture involves more than half of the femoral head) do poorly. In Catterall group I and II patients, the outlook is good, whereas in Catterall groups III and IV the prognosis is poor.

3. *The degree of anterolateral protrusion (or extrusion) of the femoral head out of the acetabulum.* When epiphyseal extrusion is more than 20 percent, the prognosis is poor. Epiphyseal extrusion is assessed in the plain radiogram. Loss of containment of the capital femoral epiphysis results in increased stress concentration on the femoral head in weight-bearing.

4. *Superolateral subluxation.* Crushing of the trabeculae and flattening of the epiphysis result in upward and anterolateral displacement of the femoral head. When the Shenton's line is broken and the femoral head is flattened and extruded superiorly, the outlook is poor. This can be readily detected in the MRI. Arthrography is an invasive procedure requiring general anesthesia or deep sedation; arthrography is performed only when hinged abduction is suspected.

5. *Stage in the natural course of the disease and phase of deformation of the femoral head.* The earlier in the natural course of the disease treatment is commenced, the better the prognosis. The spherical femoral head becomes ovoid in shape because of loss of epiphyseal height due to trabecular fracture and overgrowth of the articular cartilage. The ball-and-socket hip joint is converted from *spherical congruency* to *aspherical congruency.* Under mechanical forces when the femoral head collapses and flattens progressively, a "roller-bearing" shape of the hip joint develops; this is referred to by Stulberg as *aspherical incongruency.*[506,507] On clinical examination the development of a roller-bearing shape of the hip can be detected on flexion-extension of the hip—the hip adducts in extension and abducts and laterally rotates in flexion.[351] Untreated, with growth of the anterolateral extruded femoral head, "hinge abduction" develops (see Fig 3–47 H, I). Results of long-term studies have shown that hips with spherical congruency do not develop degenerative arthritis in adult life; those hips with aspherical congruency often develop mild to moderate arthritis beyond 50 years of age, whereas hips with aspherical incongruency usually develop degenerative arthritis before the age of 50 years.

6. *Persistent loss of hip motion.* A stiff hip in Perthes' disease is a poor prognostic sign. In the early stages it is due to muscle spasm and soft tissue contracture and later in the course of the disease is due to deformation of the femoral head and hinged abduction. Rigid contracture of the medial capsule of the hip is another pathogenic factor. Restoration and maintenance of full range of hip motion are essential to obtain a good result.

7. *Growth disturbance of the capital femoral physis.* Premature closure of the growth plate of the femoral head causes relative overgrowth of the greater trochanter and shortening of the femur.

8. *Body weight.* The hip of the obese child does not do well because of increased mechanical loading of the hip.

Of the various factors determining the outcome of Perthes' disease, the orthopedic surgeon can control only a few. The age, gender, and extent of involvement are uncontrollable; early diagnosis, provision of full mobility of the hip, and containment are controllable by adequate treatment. Growth disturbance of the capital femoral physis and of the cartilage of the femoral head cannot be controlled; they result in residual deformity. The longevity of the hip can be prolonged by correction of the residual deformities of the hip.

Phases of Management. *1. Restoration and Maintenance of Full Concentric Motion.* This can be accomplished by placing the patient in traction, preferably bilateral Russell's traction with a medial rotation strap on the thigh of the affected hip. The period of traction required may be 1 to 2 weeks. Active and gentle passive exercises are performed several times a day. Nonsteroidal anti-inflammatory medications, such as naproxen sodium (Naprosyn) and tolmetin sodium (Tolectin) may be given to control synovitis of the hip.

2. Containment. Keep the femoral head within the acetabulum and maintain mobility of the hip through a normal range. Plasticity of the femoral head allows molding by the acetabulum. During this period of containment, forces through the hip joint are reduced in order to minimize the risk of further trabecular fracture and deformation of the femoral head.

Concentric containment of the hip can be achieved by orthosis or by surgery—innominate osteotomy, intertrochanteric varus osteotomy, or a combination of pelvic and femoral osteotomies. Orthotic containment and surgical containment are parallel and not sequential; that is, avoid the pitfall of using orthosis first and, when it fails, proceeding to surgical containment. The results of Salter's innominate osteotomy or varus femoral osteotomy are poor when performed late after a serious deformity of the femoral head has already developed.

Containment is indicated when a child is 6 years or older with more than 50 percent of the femoral head involved—that is, Salter-Thompson group B, Herring groups B and C, or Catterall's groups III and IV. For containment to succeed, the hip should have good to full range of motion with no irritability and the femoral head should be spheroid or only slightly collapsed.

The Scottish Rite Hospital orthosis is the most common brace used at present. It abducts the hip and contains the femoral head in the acetabulum and allows flexion-extension motion of the hip. Its drawback is failure to control hip rotation and pelvic obliquity. Despite the challenge of effectiveness of the abduction orthosis in recent studies, I use orthotic containment; it slows the child down and contains the femoral head.

A Petrie or abduction cast is indicated as a prelude to surgery in patients who present late with an extruded and deformed femoral head. Soft tissue surgery (adductor myotomy and medial capsulotomy) reduces the femoral head into the acetabulum, and the Petrie cast maintains the reduction for 2 to 3 months. Following restoration of mobility of the hip and improved sphericity of the femoral head, innominate osteotomy and/or proximal femoral osteotomy is performed to contain the femoral head.

OPERATIVE CONTAINMENT. *Pelvic osteotomy (Salter)* is preferred by this author over intertrochanteric proximal femoral osteotomy because it provides adequate anterolateral coverage of the femoral head without shortening the femur. Instead it lengthens the lower limb by 1 to 2 cm and also improves gluteus medius lurch. Other advantages of Salter's innominate osteotomy are that metal removal is easier and there is no risk of fracture through a screw hole in the femur.[334,366,487–489,491,503,504] It is indicated in children over 6 years of age with class B Salter-Thompson or Herring B and C groups and also in the younger child who presents late with beginning collapse of the femoral head and a break in Shenton's line. A vital requisite of Salter's innominate osteotomy is adequate range of hip motion.[488–492]

Proximal femoral varus osteotomy is preferred by some surgeons because it is technically simpler to perform and postoperative stiffness is less of a problem than with a Salter innominate osteotomy.[332,333,350,351,359,423,449,451,462,475] The disadvantages of femoral osteotomy are that (1) it further shortens the affected lower limb; (2) it increases the "functional" coxa vara; following femoral osteotomy, the neck-shaft angle should not be less than 110 degrees; (3) it causes aggravation of the Trendelenburg lurch; and (4) metal removal is a major operative problem with risk of stress fracture through the screw holes.

Combined pelvic and femoral osteotomy is preferred by some surgeons in the older child with severe involvement; it provides adequate coverage of the femoral head without creating a deformity of the proximal femur and without uncovering the femoral head posteriorly.[362] These severe cases of coxa magna are best managed primarily by shelf augmentation acetabuloplasty.

Residual Deformities. *Lower limb length disparity* develops primarily as a result of ischemia and retardation of growth from the proximal femoral physis. Subchondral fracture and collapse and flattening of the femoral head augment the shortening. When treated by intertrochanteric femoral varus osteotomy, the shortening is further increased. The disparity of limb length becomes clinically significant if it exceeds 2.5 cm (1 inch).[496] Limb lengths are equalized by epiphyseodesis of the contralateral femur at the appropriate skeletal age.

Relative Overgrowth of the Greater Trochanter and Short Femoral Neck. These are caused by growth retardation or arrest of the capital femoral physis and continued normal growth of the greater trochanteric apophysis. The result is gluteus medius limp and Trendelenburg lurch. The deranged mechanics of the hip are treated by distal and lateral transfer of the greater trochanter. The results of growth arrest of the greater trochanter are unpredictable, especially after the age of 7 years, and the procedure does not elongate the femoral neck functionally.

Extrusion and Uncoverage of the Femoral Head. If the uncoverage of the femoral head is more than 25 percent and the hip joint is relatively congruous, it is treated by shelf augmentation.[435] When the hip joint is incongruous and painful, Chiari's medial displacement osteotomy of the innominate bone is performed; it is best to use the transtrochanteric surgical approach and simultaneously transfer the greater trochanter distally and laterally in order to correct or prevent Trendelenburg lurch.[335,355,432] The line of osteotomy should be curvilinear. Use three-dimensional CT scan to delineate the pathologic anatomy for appropriate preoperative planning.

Hinged Abduction of the Hip. The femoral head collapses and displaces superolaterally. The articular cartilage on the anterolateral part of the femoral head overgrows and bulges out and upward from under the lateral rim of the acetabulum. The hip assumes an adducted posture; on attempting hip abduction the extruded enlarged anterolateral part of the femoral head impinges on the anterolateral border of the acetabulum and does not slide into the socket of the acetabulum. The patient complains of pain and a clunking sensation. The hip develops progressive adduction deformity, with apparent shortening of the lower limb. Make plain radiograms with the hip in (1) neutral, (2) maximal abduction, and (3) varying degrees of adduction. Abduction of the hip is markedly restricted; on forcing the hip into abduction, the medial articular cartilage space widens. The pathologic anatomy of the hip is best demonstrated by arthrography of the hip.

An abduction-extension intertrochanteric osteotomy is performed. Requisites are a hip joint that is congruent in adduction (usually 15 to 30 degrees) and some flexion (10 to 30 degrees) and the presence of functional range of hip adduction beyond the congruent point.[477] The lower limb is aligned in the middle of the arc of movement, and congruity of the femoral head within the acetabulum is restored. The hinging is relieved and the femoral head is rounded by remodeling.

Osteochondritis Dissecans. Seven to 10 years after healing of Perthes' disease, the patient, commonly an adolescent male, presents with pain and progressive restriction of hip motion. Some patients complain of a clicking or catching sensation in the hip. Plain radiograms of the hips show a localized area of bone in the superolateral aspect of the femoral head, separated by a radiolucent zone from the remainder of the femoral head. CT scan and MRI depict the pathology and the exact site of the osteochondral fragment.

Osteochondritis dissecans in Perthes' disease often results from persistence of an unhealed necrotic fragment; occasionally it may represent a living ossific nucleus that failed to unite with the adjoining part of the femoral head.[375,394,395,399,422,505]

The type of management depends upon whether the osteochondral fragment is loose or not. This is determined by arthrography of the hip. When the contrast dye does not dissect deep in the radiolucent zone between the osteochondritis dissecans and the femoral head and the articular cartilage covering the femoral head is smooth, the osteochondral fragment is not detached and it may heal without surgical intervention. Protect the affected hip with a three-point toe-touch crutch gait. The prognosis is good for healing, which may take 6 to 12 months. If the osteochondral fragment is loose, as shown by the contrast dye dissecting deep to the dissecans fragment and by motion of the fragment on manipulation of the hip, surgical treatment is indicated. Pin the fragment if it is large and loose. If it is small, it is excised and its base is drilled. Intertrochanteric flexion-adduction osteotomy may be indicated in some cases to enhance healing by removing weight-bearing stresses on the lesion.

Torn acetabular labrum is a very rare problem. It manifests as hip pain and an area of rarefaction of the lateral roof of the acetabulum. The torn labrum is best demonstrated by arthrography. Treatment consists of excision of the torn labrum.

■ SLIPPED CAPITAL FEMORAL EPIPHYSIS

An adolescent who presents with an unexplained limp and pain in the anteromedial aspect of the thigh and knee without a history of significant trauma should be under suspicion for the development of *chronic slipped capital femoral epiphysis.* Do not pass off the complaints lightly and make the misdiagnosis of a torn muscle or sprained knee. A common pitfall is to make radiograms of the knee, with the finding that "They are normal—there is nothing seriously wrong with your boy." It is vital to make the diagnosis in the early stage of the slipping process and prevent progressive displacement of the capital epiphysis.

The *limp* is antalgic, that is, the painful type with a quick, short step on the involved side and a long step on the contralateral side. In moderate or severe slips there may be a short leg limp and a gluteus medius lurch (on the weight-bearing phase). The shoulder dips down and the patient leans to the affected side. The foot progression angle is lateral; that is, in gait the child toes-out.

The *pain* is dull and often of several weeks' or months' duration; it is exaggerated by strenuous physical activity such as running or other vigorous sports.

Inspect the physical habitus of the patient. Often it is of the adiposogenital type (obese with underdeveloped genitalia), or less frequently the patients are thin and tall, indicating a very rapid growth spurt.

Assess the posture of the lower limb in stance and supine on the examining table. It is held in lateral rotation (Fig 3–58A). Gently palpate the knee, thigh, and hip; any local tenderness is over the hip joint anteriorly and not in the knee. Next, determine the range of hip motion: The salient finding is loss of medial rotation, flexion and abduction of the hip. The degree of restriction of range of motion depends upon the severity of the slip. When the hip is flexed, it goes into lateral rotation and does not flex fully. This is a very suggestive physical finding of slipped capital femoral epiphysis (Fig 3–58B). In extension in prone position, medial rotation of the hip is limited; a lateral rotation contracture is present (Fig 3–58C). In uncomplicated slipped capital femoral epiphysis, there is an extension contracture, that is, increased extension and limitation of flexion of the hip. On the Thomas test the presence of a flexion deformity of the hip suggests an intra-articular inflammatory process such as chondrolysis of the hip. Measure actual and apparent lower limb lengths and the circumference of the proximal thighs; in moderate or severe slips ¼ to ½ inch shortening of the involved limb and disuse atrophy of the upper thigh are present.

In *acute slipped capital femoral epiphysis* the clinical picture is different; the onset of pain is sudden, and the pain is sharp, severe, and persistent. The patient is unable to bear weight on the affected lower limb. In acute-on-chronic slip a sudden increased displacement takes place in a previously minimal slip. On inquiry, a history of prior limp and/or pain may be obtained. *Acute traumatic slip* occurs following a major trauma such as a fall from a height or an automobile accident, similar to fracture of the neck of the femur.

In infants and children the slip may result from child abuse. The slip takes place through the normal growth plate. There is no history of previous pain.

Examination of an acute slip should be *very gentle.* Do not ask the patient to walk, and do not force the hip through range of motion. The hip is excruciatingly painful. There is hemarthrosis in the hip, and all range of hip motion is guarded. The femoral head–neck junction is very unstable; forceful motions may cause further displacement of the epiphysis. Place the patient immediately in a wheelchair. Instruct the x-ray technician to be gentle and to support the

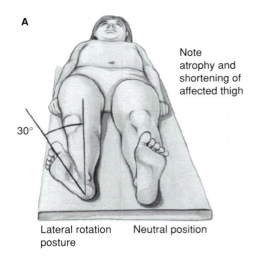

Note atrophy and shortening of affected thigh

30°

Lateral rotation posture   Neutral position

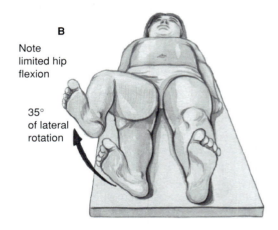

Note limited hip flexion

35° of lateral rotation

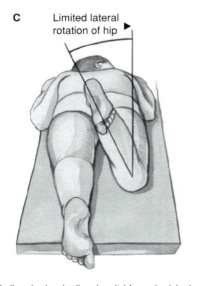

Limited lateral rotation of hip ▶

Figure 3–58. Physical findings in chronic slipped capital femoral epiphysis. **A.** Note the posture of the affected lower limb—it is held in lateral rotation. **B.** On flexion of the hip, the thigh rides further laterally. Normal hip flexion is limited. There is an extension deformity of the hip. **C.** In prone position, note the limitation of medial rotation of the hip.

limbs when transferring the patient to the x-ray table. The patient is admitted to the hospital on an emergency basis and placed in counterpoised traction.

Definition and Classification.

In this affliction there is spontaneous lysis of the capital femoral epiphysis, and the femoral neck displaces anteriorly and upward on the femoral head at the growth plate. The femoral head–neck shaft angle is that of varus angulation—coxa vara. Slipped capital femoral epiphysis is a misnomer because the femoral head is not displaced; its anatomic relationship in the acetabulum is normal. Tradition, however, dictates use of the term "slipped capital femoral epiphysis." An alternate term is adolescent coxa vara.

The displacement may be gradual (chronic) or sudden—acute-on-chronic or acute traumatic. The chronic slip is rather *stable*, whereas the acute slip is *unstable*.

Occasionally the femoral neck is displaced downward and anteriorly in relation to the femoral head. The femoral head–neck-shaft angle is that of valgus angulation—coxa valga. This rare type of slipped capital femoral epiphysis occurs in tall, slender adolescents. The physical findings of a valgus slip differ from those of a varus slip. The affected limb is longer than the contralateral normal limb. Adduction of the valgus slipped hip is restricted; that is, there is an abduction contracture. A common pitfall when one examines a hip is to test the range of abduction and not adduction. Avoid it! Because of the longer lower limb and hip abduction contracture, there is an infrapelvic pelvic obliquity with postural scoliosis. The gait is awkward: The patient has to circumduct the abducted longer involved hip to clear the leg in the swing phase of gait. Hip flexion is restricted and hip extension is increased as the femoral neck is displaced anteriorly in relation to the femoral neck. The distribution of pain is anteromedial in the thigh–knee, similar to that with a varus slip. Often the diagnosis is not made because of the rarity of valgus slip and the lack of experience of the orthopedic surgeon.

Posterior displacement of the femoral neck, that is, anterior slipped capital femoral epiphysis, is very rare. It is post-traumatic, sustained during a severe injury such as a car accident or fall from a height.

There is bilateral involvement in 25 percent of the cases; when slipped capital femoral epiphysis is associated with an endocrine disorder, bilateral involvement occurs in 50 to 75 percent of the patients.

Once the pathologic process of slipping has started, its *course* is variable. In some cases the femoral neck keeps steadily displacing forward and upward, whereas in others no apparent or minimal further displacement takes place. The degree of displacement is best measured in the lateral radiographic projection. The severity of slipping is classified into four grades: *grade I* or *preslip*, which is charac-terized by widening and rarefaction of the growth plate, but the capital femoral epiphysis is not displaced; *grade II* or *minimal slip*, in which the extent of displacement is less than one third of the upper metaphyseal width of the femoral neck; *grade III* or *moderate*, which is greater than one third but less than one half; and *grade IV* or *severe*, in which displacement is greater than 50 percent.

Incidence, Race, Age, and Gender.

Slipped capital femoral epiphysis is more common in the black and the male, with a male to female ratio of 2:1 or 3:1.

Most cases of slipped capital femoral epiphysis occur between 11 and 15 years of age (females 11 to 13 years and males 13 to 15 years), a period of rapid and marked bone growth. The upper age limit coincides with closure of the physis; in girls it is rarely seen after the onset of menarche. Slipped capital femoral epiphysis can occur in the juvenile (less than 10 years of age). In these cases endocrine dysfunction should be suspected and ruled out.

Pathogenesis.

The capital femoral epiphysis slips when the shearing stress exerted on the femoral head is greater than the resistance provided by the mechanical stability of the growth plate. Anatomic structures that provide stability to the physis are (1) the *perichondral ring*, a fibrous collagenous band that encircles the growth plate, acting as a limiting membrane. The perichondral ring, thick and strong in childhood, thins and stretches out in adolescence; (2) transphyseal collagen fibers; (3) the mammillary processes at the epiphyseal–metaphyseal interface (the growth plate is stabilized by the interdigitating reciprocal pegs of bone and cartilage); (4) the contour of the growth plate, which is convex toward the epiphysis, thereby resisting linear and torque shear forces; (5) the inclination angle of the physis, which changes from horizontal position in childhood to oblique in adolescence, making the growth plate more vulnerable to shearing forces; and (6) the thickness of the growth plate.

Displacement between the femoral epiphysis and neck takes place primarily at the hypertrophied cartilage cell layer. Increase in the thickness of this cell layer decreases its shear strength. Growth hormone widens the hypertrophied cartilage cell layer of the growth plate by stimulation of cartilage cell metabolism due to increased synthesis of somadelin. Estrogens and androgens decrease the thickness of the growth plate by depressing proliferation of cartilage cells.[584] In his experiments in rats, Harris demonstrated that pituitary growth hormone decreases the shearing strength of the physis whereas sex hormones increase it.[556]

Clinically the obese adolescent with underdeveloped genitalia has a deficiency of sex hormones, whereas the tall thin adolescent has an excess of growth hormones.[557]

Slipped capital femoral epiphysis occurs during administration of growth hormone for treatment of short stature. Also, when treating hypothyroidism and restoring thyroid function, acidophilic cells in the pituitary regenerate and a surge of growth hormone secretion occurs; as a result the physis widens, its shear strength decreases, and slipped capital femoral epiphysis develops. Patients with craniopharyngioma and those receiving chorionic gonadotropin are predisposed to slipped capital femoral epiphysis.

In hypothyroidism (cretinism or juvenile myxedema), the physis is weakened because of the deficiency in the matrix of the cartilage of the growth plate. A list of endocrinopathies in which the patient is at risk to develop slipped capital femoral epiphysis is given in Table 3–6. Caution! Rule out endocrine or metabolic disorders when a patient under 10 years of age or over 15 to 16 years of age presents with slipped capital femoral epiphysis. Also, patients with endocrinopathy, particularly those with hypothyroidism and those patients receiving growth hormone therapy, should have their hips thoroughly and repeatedly examined because they are at risk for slipped capital femoral epiphysis.

Imaging Findings. These depend upon the degree of slip and whether it is chronic or acute. The displacement of the femoral epiphysis is best visualized in the lateral projection (frog-leg or Lowenstein or true lateral). When there is restriction of medial rotation of the hips (which is the usual deformity), the x-ray tube should be tilted laterally so that the x-ray beam is in the same plane as the proximal femoral growth plate. The lateral projection shows the posterior slip.

In the *preslip or grade I,* the physis is widened and irregular, with patchy porosis on its metaphyseal side. There

is no anterior or superior displacement of the femoral neck on the epiphysis.

When displacement takes place, the femoral epiphysis is posterior in its relation to the femoral neck. In the normal hip in the true lateral projection, the physis and femoral neck are at right angles (90 degrees) to each other, with a lower limit of 87 degrees (Fig 3–59A). With slipping of the capital epiphysis the physeal–femoral neck angle decreases (Fig 3–59B).

In the frog-leg lateral radiogram, Southwick measures the degree of slipping by the femoral head-shaft angle. First, draw the physeal line between the upper and lower limits of the metaphyseal surface of the growth plate; second, draw the neck line (N1) perpendicular to the physeal line (P1); third, draw the diaphyseal line (D1) parallel to the femoral shaft. The femoral head-shaft angle is the angle formed between the lines N1 and P1 (Fig 3–60).

In the AP projection, when the capital epiphysis is positioned medially, a line drawn on the superior border of the femoral neck does cut across the head. This is referred to in the literature by various names—Perkins' sign, Trethovan's sign, or Kline's sign. In the normal hip the ossified epiphysis overhangs the neck: A line drawn along the upper margin of the femoral neck transects the femoral head (Fig 3–61).

In the skeletally immature child, the ossified part of the femoral head is smaller than the diameter of the femoral neck at the physis. At 10 years the two are of the same diameter and at 12 years the ossified femoral epiphysis

TABLE 3–6. ENDOCRINE AND METABOLIC DISORDERS AS A PREDISPOSING CAUSE OF SLIPPED CAPITAL FEMORAL EPIPHYSIS

1. Increased growth hormone activity
   Exogenous—growth hormone therapy for treatment of short stature
   Chorionic gonadotropin therapy
   Pituitary adenoma
   Gigantism
2. Acromegaly
3. Craniopharyngioma
4. Hypopituitarism
5. Hypothyroidism
6. Hyperthyroidism (transient)
7. Hyperparathyroidism
8. Hypogonadism
9. Kleinfelter's syndrome
10. Renal osteodystrophy
11. Decreased vitamin D function
    Dietary deficiency
    Vitamin D–refractory hypothyroidism
12. Vascular ischemia of metaphysis following surgery
13. Following radiation of pelvic bones

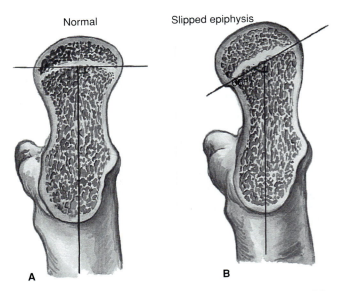

Figure 3–59. The capital physeal–femoral neck angle. First, draw a horizontal line between the anterior and posterior borders of the growth plate; second, draw a longitudinal line in the center of the femoral neck. The angle subtended between the lines on the posterior side is the physeal–femoral neck angle. **A.** In the normal hip it is 90 degrees (lower limit 87 degrees). **B.** In slipped capital femoral epiphysis it is decreased, in this drawing to 65 degrees.

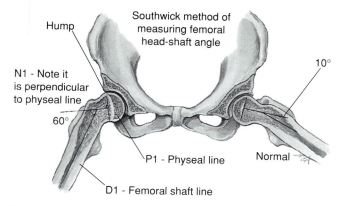

Figure 3–60. Measurement of femoral head-shaft angle in the frog-leg radiogram according to Southwick. P1 is the physeal line between the superior and inferior margins of the capital physis. N1 is the line drawn perpendicular to the physeal line P1. D1 is the line drawn parallel to the femoral shaft. The angle formed between the lines N1 and D1 is the femoral head-shaft angle. Note that in the normal left hip it is 10 degrees, whereas in the slipped right capital femoral epiphysis it is 60 degrees.

overhangs the femoral neck; if it does not—that is, the ossified nucleus is smaller—delayed bone maturation and hypothyroidism should be suspected.[545]

In the AP radiogram of the hips, look for the metaphyseal blanch sign of Steel, a crescent-shaped area of increased density (radiopacity) (Fig 3–62).[598] It is produced by the superimposition of the posteriorly displaced epiphysis on the area of increased metaphyseal density.

Consequent to healing in chronic slipped capital femoral epiphysis radiographic changes are seen in the femoral neck. Callus forms at the inferior and posterior junction of the head and neck, and the anterosuperiorly displaced protruded portion of the juxtaphyseal femoral neck molds to form a "hump." This bony protuberance of the femoral neck blocks abduction and medial rotation (Fig 3–63). In acute slip the radiographic findings of callus are not present because healing has not taken place. The degree of displacement is more severe than in chronic slip and it may be complete.

Posterior displacement of the femoral head is best demonstrated by CT, which is made in uncertain cases when physical findings suggest slipped capital femoral epiphysis but plain radiograms appear normal; not infrequently adequate radiograms are difficult to make in the obese patient. Following internal fixation with a screw, when there is a question of whether the tip of the screw has penetrated the joint, CT imaging will rule it out.

Bone imaging with technetium-99m shows increased uptake in the involved capital physis, and in uncomplicated slipped capital femoral epiphysis this may be of some diagnostic value only in unilateral cases. Bone scintigraphy, however, detects avascular necrosis and chondrolysis.

Ultrasonography is of definite value in detecting effusion in the hip joint. This assists in decision-making as to whether or not to aspirate or not aspirate the hip joint in acute slipped capital femoral epiphysis, in order to prevent tamponade of blood vessels. Ultrasonograms also depict the slip and postoperatively, following internal fixation, whether the screw is in the joint.

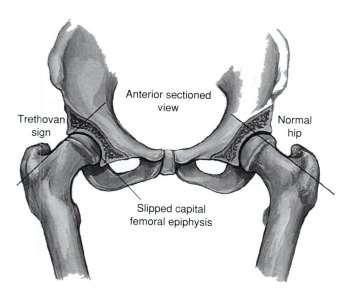

Figure 3–61. Radiographic sign of medial slip of the epiphysis in the AP projection in the slipped right hip. A line drawn along the superior border of the femoral neck does not pass through the femoral head. The epiphysis does not overhang the neck. (Trethovan's sign, Kline's sign, or Perkins' sign). In the normal hip a line drawn along the superior neck transects the capital epiphysis.

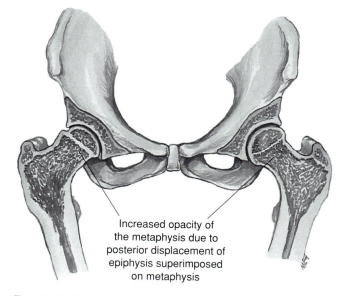

Figure 3–62. Steel's metaphyseal blanch sign. Note the crescent-shaped area of increased density in the metaphysis immediately adjacent to the physis. This image is given by the superimposition of the posteriorly displaced epiphysis in the metaphysis—"double density."

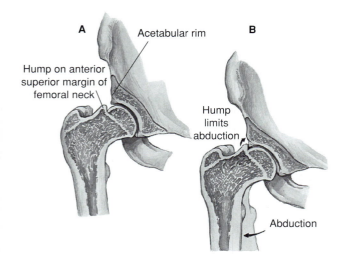

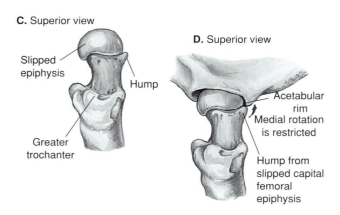

Figure 3–63. Bony deformity in slipped capital femoral epiphysis blocking range of motion. **A.** Note the bony "hump" in the metaphysis blocking hip abduction, flexion, and medial rotation formed by the protuberance of the anterior and superior parts of the displaced femoral neck. **B.** Impingement of this "hump" against the margin of the acetabulum blocks hip abduction, medial rotation, and flexion. **C, D.** Superior views showing the bump in the metaphysis of the femoral neck and how it restricts medial rotation of the hip.

Treatment. When diagnosis of chronic slipped capital femoral epiphysis is made, the patient must be taken off his feet. Weight-bearing is forbidden. Place the patient in a wheelchair and admit him to the hospital on an emergency basis. Do not yield to the economic pressures of health maintenance organizations and insurance companies! Minor trauma may cause acute displacement on chronic slip and markedly increase the risk of avascular necrosis. Acute slip unquestionably demands immediate emergency admission to the hospital and treatment.

The treatment of slipped capital femoral epiphysis is operative. The chronic slipped epiphysis is fixed with one cannulated screw inserted perpendicular to the physis and in the center of the epiphysis. The objective is to transfix the epiphysis in place, prevent further slipping, and enhance physeal closure and bony fusion (Fig 3–64). With the mod-

ern image intensification radiography and surgical technique of fixation with a cannulated screw, this has become a simple procedure. In the past, when more than a quarter of the neck was slipped, osteotomy to correct the deformity was recommended. Because of the serious complication of avascular necrosis, femoral neck osteotomy to correct the deformity is no longer performed. Even in moderate or severe chronic slips the epiphysis is fixed with one cannulated screw, and the lateral rotation-extension-varus deformity is corrected at the intertrochanteric or subtrochanteric level after healing has taken place. Some surgeons prefer basal neck osteotomy, which is near the deformity but has increased probability of injury to the blood supply of the femoral head.[531,533,569]

The literature contains several reports of good results by nonsurgical management.[537,565] Such conservative treatment is tedious and prolonged, and further slip can occur during treatment. Sex hormone therapy induces closure of the physis; it may be indicated in the poor surgical risk patient, but the drawbacks of endocrine therapy versus the surgical risk should be carefully weighed.

Open epiphyseodesis with autogenous bone grafting avoids the problem of pin penetration and provides direct visualization and approach to the pathology of the femoral head, enabling the surgeon to resect the bony prominence (hump) blocking hip motion. It has the lowest complication rate of chondrolysis and avascular necrosis, and bone grafting accelerates closure of the physis and provides an additional avenue for new blood supply to the femoral head, a definite advantage in moderate or severe displaced acute slip, which has a high incidence of avascular necrosis.[544,558,559,605] Its disadvantages are a longer and more complex operation with greater pain and morbidity postoperatively and prolonged convalescence. Resorption and/or fracture of the graft with further slipping can occur. Internal fixation with a single cannulated screw provides immediate stabilization of the epiphysis, and the percutaneous technique has made it a very simple and effective procedure. It is the method of choice in the treatment of slipped capital femoral epiphysis. Open epiphyseodesis is indicated when adequate visualization control cannot be obtained in the operating room because of a very obese patient; it is safer than inserting pins blindly and having their tips protrude into the hip joint. It is also indicated in severe valgus slips, which are very difficult to pin. Open epiphyseodesis with simultaneous internal fixation with one cannulated AO screw is also indicated when bone scan with technetium-99m shows the femoral head is avascular after decompression of the hip.

Acute-on-Chronic Slip. These patients give a history of pain in the anteromedial thigh and knee of several weeks' duration. Following minimal or moderate trauma, they experience acute sudden pain and are unable to walk and bear weight on the affected lower limb.

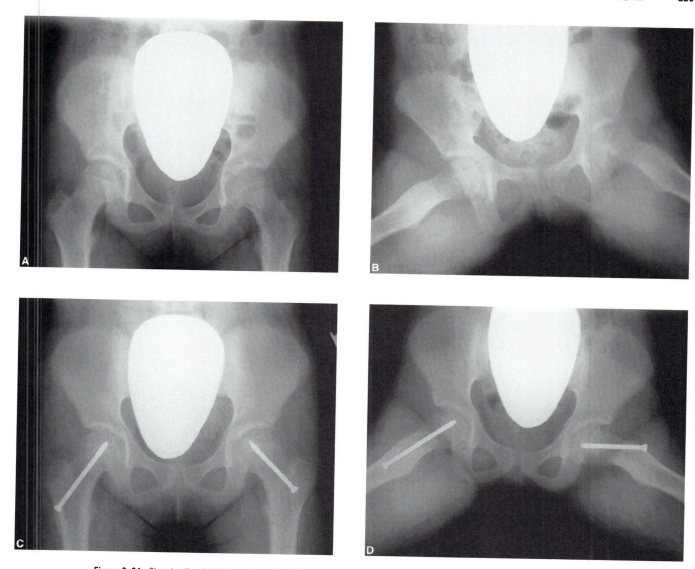

Figure 3–64. Chronic slip of left hip and preslip of the right hip. **A, B.** Preoperative AP and frog lateral views. **C, D.** Postoperative bilateral pinning with one AO cannulated screw.

The radiograms of the hip show the marked slip and signs of previous chronic slip by the presence of callus at the inferior-posterior junction of the femoral neck and head and by the rounded protuberance—"the hump"—on the anterior and superior margin of the femoral neck (Fig 3–65A, B). The degree of slip is usually less and avascular necrosis less frequent than in the acute traumatic type.

Ultrasonography of the hip is performed when the capsule is distended and decompression of the hip by aspiration is being considered. Perform ultrasonography of the hip; when the capsule is distended, aspirate and decompress the hip to prevent tamponade of the blood supply and avascular necrosis.

If there is less than a 30 percent slip, pin in situ; if more than 30 percent slip, it is best to reduce the slip but only to the pre-acute slip position. Do not stretch and fur-

ther injure the blood supply to the femoral head. Some surgeons prefer gradual reduction by traction, slowly abducting and medially rotating and flexing the hip. Because of the risk of further slip in traction, such as while getting on and off the bed pan, and noncompliance with traction, I recommend immediate reduction of the slip under general anesthesia. Gently transfer the patient on the fracture table and first attempt reduction by simple medial rotation of the hip while applying longitudinal traction with the hip in extension. If unable to achieve replacement of the femoral epiphysis, flex the hip to 90 degrees and do not permit the hip to laterally rotate; while maintaining the hip in neutral rotation, extend and abduct the hip. Internally fix with two cannulated screws (some surgeons prefer one screw). The screw should be perpendicular to the capital physis in the center of the femoral head. Do not place screws on the superoposterior quadrant because they injure the lateral

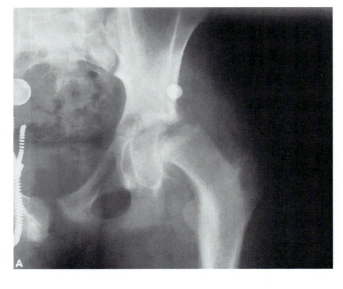

A

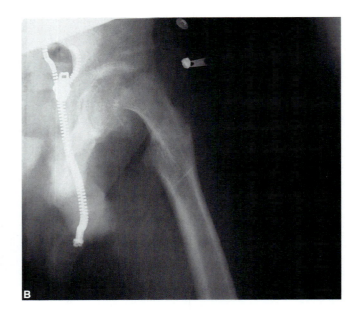

B

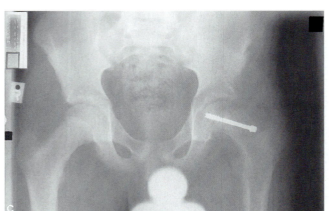

C

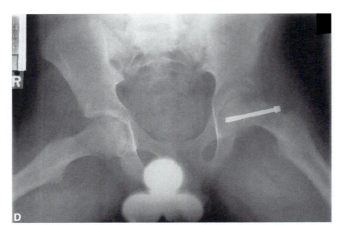

D

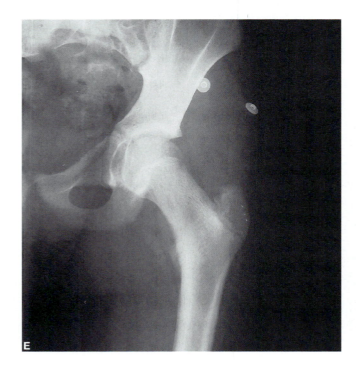

E

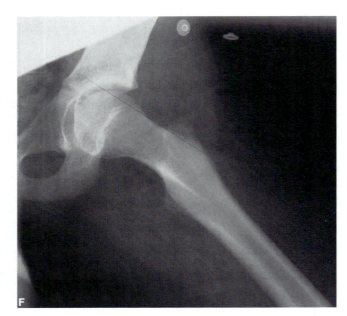

F

epiphyseal vessel of Brodetti and result in segmental avascular necrosis.

When the degree of slip is greater than three fourths of the diameter of the femoral neck, it is best to perform open epiphyseodesis with simultaneous internal fixation with one AO screw (Fig 3–65C, D). In my experience, this method of fixation offers the best chance of providing a congruent and functional hip. The hip is immobilized in a spica cast for 3 to 4 weeks.

A common pitfall when avascular necrosis develops is to maintain the pins or screws in the necrotic femoral head because the physis is not closed. The femoral head collapses and the screws penetrate the joint and cause chondrolysis of the hip. Take the screws out as soon as possible; do not leave them penetrating the joint.

Postoperative bone scan with technetium-99m detects avascular necrosis early, before the plain radiograms. Perform it immediately after surgery and then 2 months later. When the femoral head remains cold, it is very probable that avascular necrosis is present.

Acute Traumatic Slip.   Perform ultrasonography of the hip. When there is marked distention of the hip joint capsule; decompress the hip by immediate aspiration in order to prevent tamponade of the blood supply to the hip. When the degree of slip is 30 percent or less, do not reduce the fracture. In the young child, immobilize the hip in abduction-medial rotation, whereas the older child and adolescent require internal fixation with two cannulated screws. If over 30 percent of the capital epiphysis is slipped, it requires reduction, always gently, either gradually by traction or acutely by gentle manipulation and internal fixation with two cannulated screws. The prognosis is poor because of the high incidence of avascular necrosis, especially in the older child and adolescent.

Avascular Necrosis.   This serious complication may be segmental or total. In *untreated chronic slips,* avascular necrosis does not occur. During internal fixation of the chronic slip with a cannulated screw one may damage the lateral epiphyseal artery which supplies the superior weight-bearing portion of the femoral head. Brodetti, in his injection studies, showed that the lateral epiphyseal artery constantly traverses the superior and posterior part of the femoral head.[539] Guide pins, drills, and screws placed in the superior part of the femoral head damage the lateral epiphyseal artery and cause segmental avascular necrosis. Do not insert

the screw in a valgus position into the superior part of the femoral head.

In the past open reduction of chronic slipped capital femoral epiphysis by cuneiform osteotomy of the femoral neck was commonly performed and was a major cause of avascular necrosis. This procedure has been abandoned, and occasionally a few surgeons carry out compensatory osteotomy at the base of the femoral neck.[531,533,569] Varus extension lateral rotation deformity is corrected by intertrochanteric or subtrochanteric valgus-flexion medial rotation osteotomy after healing of the slip. Most surgeons prefer this method.

The problem is avascular necrosis in acute slipped capital femoral epiphysis in severe slips, when the extraosseous blood vessels in the retinaculum are either kinked or disrupted and/or are compressed by tamponade from the intra-articular hemorrhage. Over-reduction of the acute-on-chronic slip further disrupts the vessels. As outlined in the treatment of acute slip, I recommend decompression of the hip by aspiration, immediate gentle reduction on an emergency basis, and never over-reducing beyond the pre-acute chronic slip position.

Clinically, following reduction and pinning of the acute slipped capital femoral epiphysis, when the patient complains of persisting pain and stiffness of the hip, avascular necrosis should be suspected. Perform bone scan with technetium-99m; it shows a cold femoral head and confirms the diagnosis of avascular necrosis. The following vicious events follow: The femoral head collapses, the pins penetrate into the hip joint, and chondrolysis develops. How should you manage this complex problem? Remove the pins before they penetrate into the hip joint. Should you perform open epiphyseodesis if the capital femoral physis is still open, with iliac or fibular graft, preferably with its vascular supply intact? I recommend the autogenous bone graft when *avascular necrosis is total* because it makes biologic sense. Long-term results are not available at present. The alternative of management of total necrosis is prolonged weight relief with extensive physical therapy to restore functional range of motion. The best result that one can hope for from such conservative management is a deformed collapsed femoral head with minimal to moderate pain and functional range of hip flexion-extension but marked restriction of hip rotation and abduction-adduction. The prognosis is poor in total head involvement. Most of these cases develop progressive osteoarthritis and require total joint arthroplasty or hip arthrodesis.

Segmental avascular necrosis has a better prognosis. It can be managed by valgus rotation intertrochanteric

Figure 3–65. Acute-on-chronic slip in a 14-year-old male. **A, B.** AP and lateral radiograms showing the severe slip of the left hip. **C, D.** AP and frog lateral views showing pinning with an AO cannulated screw after reduction. The hip joint was decompressed and an open epiphyseodesis was performed because the head was avascular on the bone scan with technetium-99m. **E, F.** Postoperative AP and lateral radiograms view after removal of pins.

osteotomy, relieving weight-bearing stress on the necrotic fragment and bringing viable bone into the weight-bearing area. Accurate preoperative planning by CT and torsion studies and MRI is crucial for success. Vascularized fibular bone graft and curettage of the dead bone are another option.

Chondrolysis

This is a serious problem and complication of slipped capital femoral epiphysis. Clinically it presents with flexion deformity of the hip with restriction of range of hip motion in all planes. Stiffness of the hip increases with muscle spasm and pain. Chondrolysis of the hip may follow treatment of slipped capital femoral epiphysis, or it may be present preoperatively. When hip flexion deformity is present, be suspicious of chondrolysis.

Radiograms show regional osteoporosis due to hyperemia of the synovium. This is a nonspecific finding. It is followed by narrowing of the articular cartilage space by at least 50 percent of its normal width. Consequent to the hypervascularity, premature closure of the growth plate of the femur and intrapelvic protrusion (Otto pelvis) develops. On the radiogram, eventually the subchondral bony plate appears to be moth-eaten and then disappears with destruction of the articular cartilage.

Bone scan with technetium-99m shows increased uptake in both the acetabulum and the femoral head. MRI demonstrates the narrowing of the joint space and irregularity of the articular cartilage.

The exact cause of chondrolysis is unknown. Autolysis of articular cartilage appears to be an autoimmune disease in genetically susceptible individuals. Lysosomal enzymes interfere with synthetic production of hyaline cartilage. Lack or paucity of synovial fluid production has been proposed as another possible cause of chondrolysis.[546,603]

The prevalence of chondrolysis varies. Predisposing factors are (1) gender—it is twice as common in girls as in boys, whereas slipped capital femoral epiphysis is four times more common in boys than in girls; (2) race—the incidence of chondrolysis is high in blacks and Hawaiians; (3) penetration of the pins into the joint; (4) prolonged immobilization in cast or in heavy skeletal traction with pins through the distal femur; (5) valgus osteotomy of the proximal femur and increased articular cartilage compression; and (6) marked incongruity of the hip joint due to severe slip.

The *course* of chondrolysis is divided into three stages: (1) *acute*—1 to 6 weeks after onset of symptoms, (2) *subacute*—6 weeks to 6 months, and (3) *chronic*—6 months from onset of symptoms.

Chondrolysis exhibits a wide spectrum of severity. Its natural history may follow a benign or a recalcitrant moderate or recalcitrant fulminating course. In the *benign form,* the pain, hip stiffness, muscle spasm, and articular cartilage space narrowing are transient. There is spontaneous restitution of articular cartilage space, with almost normal return of range of hip motion.[576] In the *recalcitrant moderate form,* initially there is progressive loss of joint space, but after 6 months there is some, but not full recovery. The end result is a relatively painless hip with functional range of hip motion and moderate narrowing of the articular cartilage space. In the *recalcitrant fulminating form,* there is rapid progressive destruction of articular cartilage with fibrosis and ankylosis of the hip joint in 6 to 12 months.

Treatment. It is individualized according to the stage of the disease and the severity of chondrolysis. In the acute stage, when the hip is stiff with marked restriction of motion in all planes and a flexion-adduction deformity is present, both lower limbs are placed in counterpoised, split Russell's traction with more weight on the affected hip. Active and passive exercises are performed several times a day to increase range of motion of the hip and to develop motor strength of muscles around the hip joint. Nonsteroidal anti-inflammatory drugs such as naproxen sodium and tolmetin sodium are given. The patient is allowed to be ambulatory part of the day with three-point crutch gait and partial weight-bearing on the affected limb.

In the benign form of chondrolysis, range of motion of the hip gradually improves. Radiograms are repeated every 6 to 8 weeks to assess restoration of the articular cartilage space.

In the moderate or severe form of chondrolysis, when there is no response to conservative forms of therapy, the patient is taken to the operating room and range of motion of the hip is determined under general anesthesia. If the hip moves normally, the patient is awakened and the above modalities of conservative management (traction, exercises, partial weight-bearing, and nonsteroidal anti-inflammatory drugs) are continued. It is not uncommon that the stiffness of the hip recurs because of pain and muscle spasm. In such a case, temporary use of an epidural anesthesia is appropriate. If the hip is stiff with marked restriction of range of motion under general anesthesia, myotomy of the adductors and iliopsoas tenotomy are performed with subtotal capsulectomy of the hip. It is crucial to relieve the femoral head from the constriction of the fibrosed capsule. Then the patient is placed in a continuous passive motion machine and prescribed physical therapy. Use epidural anesthesia for 5 to 7 days if the pain and stiffness of the hip recur. The preliminary results of such aggressive therapy in recalcitrant fulminating chondrolysis are promising.

Recently, arthrodiastasis of the hip joint has been employed—that is, distraction by skeletal traction with a special Orthofix apparatus and Orthofix screws in the pelvis and femur in conjunction with the continuous passive motion machine. Experience with this method is limited.

Lateral rotation-extension deformity of the hip is common in moderate and severe cases of chronic slipped capital femoral epiphysis treated by in situ screw fixation. The patient walks with marked out-toeing gait. These cases are treated by medial rotation/flexion intertrochanteric osteotomy after closure of the growth plate and healing of the slip.

■ IDIOPATHIC CHONDROLYSIS[609-620]

The presenting complaint is diffuse pain in the anterior aspect of the hip and the anteromedial thigh. The patient walks with a bizarre gait, circumducting the affected lower limb. There is no history of trauma or systemic signs to suggest infection.

Examination reveals an abduction contracture of the affected hip, in contrast to chondrolysis of slipped capital femoral epiphysis, in which there is an adduction contracture of the hip. Because of infrapelvic obliquity, mild postural scoliosis is present. Range of motion of the affected hip is restricted in all planes with a hip flexion deformity of moderate degree on the Thomas test. Bone scan with technetium-99m shows increased, diffuse uptake in both the acetabulum and femoral head.

In the differential diagnosis one should consider rheumatoid arthritis and tumorous lesions of the hip, such as synovial chondromatosis.

MRI assists in making the definitive diagnosis, and appropriate immunologic tests are performed to rule out rheumatoid arthritis.

Treatment follows the same principles as outlined for chondrolysis of the hip associated with slipped capital femoral epiphysis.

■ MERALGIA PARESTHETICA[621]

The presenting complaint is pain and/or numbness on the lateral aspect of the upper half of the thigh caused by compression and neuritis of the lateral femoral cutaneous nerve. It causes restriction of physical activities.

The diagnosis is made by the physical finding and local injection of xylocaine, which temporarily relieves the symptoms. Treatment consists of open decompression of the nerve as an outpatient procedure. The results are excellent.

■ LOWER LIMB LENGTH DISCREPANCY

The presenting complaint varies with the severity of the limb length disparity. Minor differences (0.5 to 1.5 cm) of limb length between the right and left sides are very common. Often the parents and patient are unaware of such minimal mismatching of sides; such slight lower limb length disparity (LLD) is of no clinical significance.

When the limb length discrepancy is greater than 2 to 2.5 cm (3/4 to 1 inch), the patient may present with a short leg limp, toe-walking on the short side, flexed knee on the long side, or postural scoliosis. When a major shortening is present due to longitudinal deficiency of the long bones such as the tibia or femur, the presenting complaint is "a short leg"; the deformity of proximal femoral focal deficiency or absence of the fibula is obvious.

History. Determine the cause of lower limb length disparity (Table 3–7). Was there a fracture of the femur or tibia which healed with shortening due to overriding or angulation? In such a case, there is a sudden change in the length of the femur or the tibia. Did the fracture involve the growth plates of the femur or tibia? In such an instance, growth inhibition is due to osseous bridging across the growth plate and shortening of the lower limb. The short-

---

TABLE 3–7. ETIOLOGY OF LOWER LIMB LENGTH DISPARITY

I. Caused by shortening
   A. Congenital (aplasia-hypoplasia-longitudinal deficiency)
      1. Proximal femoral focal deficiency
      2. Distal focal femoral deficiency
      3. Congenital short femur
      4. Developmental or infantile coxa vara
      5. Longitudinal deficiency of the fibula (fibular hemimelia)
      6. Longitudinal deficiency of the tibia (tibial hemimelia)
      7. Developmental hip dysplasia
      8. Severe malformation of the foot
      9. Congenital hemiatrophy
   B. Bone dysplasia—developmental (Ollier's disease [multiple enchondromatosis], fibrous dysplasia, dysplasia epiphysealis hemimelia [Trevor's disease], multiple epiphyseal dysplasia, neurofibromatosis
   C. Growth plate arrest—damage or interruption of blood supply
      1. Trauma to physis resulting in premature fusion
      2. Infection—osteomyelitis, septic or tuberculous arthritis
      3. Interruption of blood supply such as in Legg-Calvé-Perthes disease or slipped capital femoral epiphysis
      4. Radiation therapy
      5. Prolonged immobilization in hip spica cast
      6. Severe burns
   D. Paralysis—neuromuscular atrophy such as myelomeningocele, spastic hemiplegia, poliomyelitis, spinal cord lesions, injury to peripheral nerves—sciatic, femoral, or peroneal
   E. Fracture of femur and tibia resulting in overlapping or angulation and shortening

II. Caused by overgrowth
   A. Congenital hemihypertrophy
   B. Hemangiomatosis of soft tissues or arteriovenous fistulas
   C. Neurofibromatosis
   D. Localized gigantism
   E. Inflammatory affections producing increased blood supply to the growth plate such as rheumatoid arthritis, metaphyseal osteomyelitis, or hemarthrosis in hemophilia
   F. Increased blood supply to growth plate caused by trauma such as metaphyseal or diaphyseal fractures, osteotomies, or harvesting of bone graft

ening is insidious and gradually progressive. In the history ask for other causes of growth plate injury such as infection in the neonatal period or infancy.

Have the parents noted an atrophy or hypertrophy of the lower or upper limbs? Is there any atrophy of the face? Is there any difference in foot size? Does the child wear the same size shoes on both feet? How is the shoe wear? The patient with a limb length disparity has a toe-heel gait on the short side, and the shoe wear is greater at the toes than at the heel. Have they noted any skin abnormality such as hemangioma or café-au-lait spots? Is there any temperature difference between the right and left sides? Is there any history of chronic inflammation around the knee such as in juvenile rheumatoid arthritis? Inflammation stimulates growth through increased blood supply to the physis. Is there any history of dislocation of the hip or foot deformity such as club foot?

It is important to determine if the disparity in the lower limb lengths is progressive or static. Ask the parents if the leg is becoming progressively shorter. The various patterns of growth disparity between limbs are given by Shapiro and illustrated in Figure 3–66.[680] Try to determine the pattern of growth. For example, in rheumatoid arthritis, initially the growth is stimulated, but later the growth is retarded due to early closure of the physis.

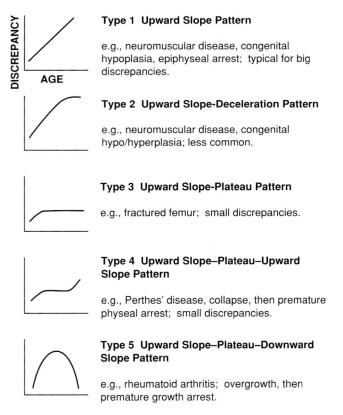

Type 1 Upward Slope Pattern

e.g., neuromuscular disease, congenital hypoplasia, epiphyseal arrest; typical for big discrepancies.

Type 2 Upward Slope-Deceleration Pattern

e.g., neuromuscular disease, congenital hypo/hyperplasia; less common.

Type 3 Upward Slope-Plateau Pattern

e.g., fractured femur; small discrepancies.

Type 4 Upward Slope–Plateau–Upward Slope Pattern

e.g., Perthes' disease, collapse, then premature physeal arrest; small discrepancies.

Type 5 Upward Slope–Plateau–Downward Slope Pattern

e.g., rheumatoid arthritis; overgrowth, then premature growth arrest.

Figure 3–66. Growth patterns in lower limb length disparity. (Drawn after Shapiro F: Developmental patterns in lower extremity length discrepancies. *J Bone Joint Surg* 64A:639, 1982.)

Is there any low back pain or cramps in the calf muscle? Is there any gait abnormality? Is the patient walking on his or her toes? Is there any joint instability or deformity of the knee, ankle, or hip? Does the knee give way? Is there any history of frequent ankle sprains? Is the ankle stiff or is the patient wearing a brace? In such an instance, the patient requires a short leg to clear the foot during ambulation. Is the patient self-conscious because of the marked shortening of his or her lower limb? Is there any difficulty with body image? Psychosocial factors should always be considered. The total child should be assessed as an individual.

Inquire as to previous treatment such as a shoe lift or previous surgery such as epiphyseal arrest or excision of a bony bridge. Then ask if the child has had a recent growth spurt and is developing secondary sex characteristics. In a girl, ask if she has begun her menarche. If yes, then ask how long ago. In boys, ask whether the voice has changed or facial hair is developing. Ask the parents about their height and stature and that of siblings and other members of the immediate family.

Physical Examination. Inspect the shoes for the size of lifts (raise) and for any abnormal wear and orthosis, if any. Then measure the patient's standing and sitting heights. In what percentile does his or her stature fall? This has bearing in consideration for future treatment. Inspect the patient while properly undraped, standing with the heels on the ground, both feet together, and the knees and hips in complete extension and neutral rotation with the feet pointing straight forward. Are the popliteal and gluteal creases, pelvis, dimples of the posterior iliac spines, and shoulders level? Observe the patient from the front and back. From the posterior view, place the radial border of your index fingers on the superior border of the iliac crests and compare the height of the pelvis on each side—is it level? Anteriorly place your thumbs on the anterosuperior iliac spines and compare their height. Drop a plumb line from the spinous process of C7 or the center of the base of the skull. Does it fall in the intergluteal cleft or is it shifted to the short leg side? Measure the lateral decompensation of the spine in centimeters—the distance of the plumb line from the intergluteal cleft.

Next place blocks of wood of various thicknesses (they come in increments of 1/8 inch up to 1/2 inch and then in increments of 1/4 inch) under the foot of the short limb and determine the height of the wood block(s) that makes the iliac crests horizontally level. This block method of measuring limb length includes the height of the foot and pelvis. It is more accurate than measuring the lower limb length from the anterosuperior iliac spines to the tip of the medial malleolus. However, it has its flaws; suprapelvic obliquity due to structural scoliosis tilts the pelvis horizontally.

Ask the patient to bend forward with and without the block under the foot of the short leg for detection of the scoliosis. On inspection of the spine posteriorly when a structural scoliosis is present, the rotation of the vertebrae is on the convex side, and the iliac crest on the concave side of the curve is high. If the scoliosis is due to leg length disparity and is postural, when the patient stands on the short leg without a lift, the rotation is to the concavity and leveling the pelvis with a block eliminates the scoliosis.

Is there mechanical axis deviation in the form of varus or valgus angulation of the tibia or femur? An asymmetric bowed leg or knock-knee apparently shortens the lower limb. While the patient is standing, be sure to inspect the legs from the front, back, and sides. Any genu recurvatum causes functional shortening of the lower limb.

While the patient is standing, inspect for any contractural deformity of the joints. Functionally, the lower limb on the side of the adducted hip is short, whereas on the side of the abducted hip it is long (Fig 3–67A, C). Is there any flexion deformity of the knee or genu recurvatum which makes the leg shorter? Is there equinus deformity of the foot and ankle which increases the functional length of the lower limb?

Next, assess the stability of the hip joint by performing a standing Trendelenburg test. The hip on the long limb side becomes progressively uncovered and causes instability and subluxation of the hip joint. When the patient is supine, check the stability of the hip by the Ortolani and Barlow tests and, when sitting, stability of the knee by the drawer and Lachman tests.

Ask the patient to walk and assess the gait for any abnormality. In the weight-bearing phase on the short limb, the shoulder on the side of the short limb dips down vertically a greater distance than normal. The knee of the long limb is in varying degrees of flexion and the hips circumduct to clear the foot. On the short side, the stance stride is shorter, and push-off is reduced.

With the patient in supine position, both hips and knees in complete extension and neutral rotation, and the feet and ankles in neutral position, clinically measure the actual and apparent limb lengths. Actual leg lengths are measured from the inferior margin of the anterosuperior iliac spine to the tip of the medial malleolus or to the sole of the heel with the foot and ankle in neutral position. Apparent leg lengths are measured from the umbilicus or the xiphoid process of the sternum to the tip of the medial or lateral malleolus or to the sole of the heel with the foot and ankle in neutral position (Fig 3–67A-C). A wiggly and ticklish child may pose a challenge for mensuration from the anterosuperior iliac spine or the umbilicus. An alternative method of measuring limb lengths is to place the patient in prone position with the hips and knees fully extended and the ankles and feet in neutral position. The actual leg length is measured from the ischial tuberosity to the tip of the medial or lateral malleolus or to the sole of the heel (Fig 3–67D, E).

Determine the *site of the discrepancy*. Is it in the femur or tibia or both? Is the foot small or short in height or is the problem at the hip and pelvis? First, determine the level of the knees and ankles. In the *Galeazzi test* both hips are flexed 90 degrees, with the hips in neutral position as to abduction and adduction. The level of the knees is then inspected. When the femur is short, the knee of the short leg is at a lower level than the long side. It is vital that you do not abduct or adduct the hips because adducting the hip and tilting the pelvis produce a positive Galeazzi sign on the adducted apparent short side (Fig 3–68).

The length of the tibia is determined by the *Ellis test*. This can be done with the patient in supine position. The knees are flexed 90 degrees and the feet are flat on a firm examination table. The knee on the short tibia side is at a lower level than the long side. A better way to perform the Ellis test is to ask the patient to lie in the prone position and flex the knees 90 degrees with the feet and ankles in neutral position. Then determine the level of the soles of the heels (Fig 3–69). Measure the *height of the foot* from the tip of the medial malleolus to the sole of the heel. Then measure the length of the foot from the posterior tip of the heel to the tip of the great toe. In congenital shortening and in hemiatrophy the foot is smaller on the short side.

Measure the circumferences of the calves at their maximal girth and the circumferences of the thighs at identical levels. Using the superior border of the patella as a reference point has its pitfall when a high-riding patella or other knee pathology is present. Therefore, it is best to measure a set distance proximal to the knee joint line or a set distance distal to the anterosuperior iliac spine. When hemiatrophy or hemihypertrophy is present, measure the circumferences and lengths of the upper limbs (arms and forearms).

Assess the hip, knee, and ankle for any joint deformity. What is the range of dorsiflexion of the ankle? Rule out equinus deformity. Determine the range of extension of the knee. Is there a flexion or hyperextension deformity of the knee? Perform a *Thomas test* to rule out a flexion deformity of the hip. A flexion deformity of the knee or hip apparently shortens the lower limb whereas an equinus deformity of the foot and ankle functionally lengthens the lower limb.

Next determine the range of hip abduction with the hips and knees in full extension and the pelvis level to rule out an adduction contracture of the hip, which causes apparent shortening of the lower limb. Also perform an *Ober test* to rule out abduction contracture of the hip, which causes apparent lengthening of the lower limb.

While the patient is in the supine position, assess the stability of the knee for absence of the cruciate ligaments by performing the drawer and Lachman tests. The stability of the hips should be checked by performing a Barlow and Ortolani maneuver.

Carefully inspect the skin for previous operative scars, hemangioma, or café-au-lait spots. Palpate with the dorsum

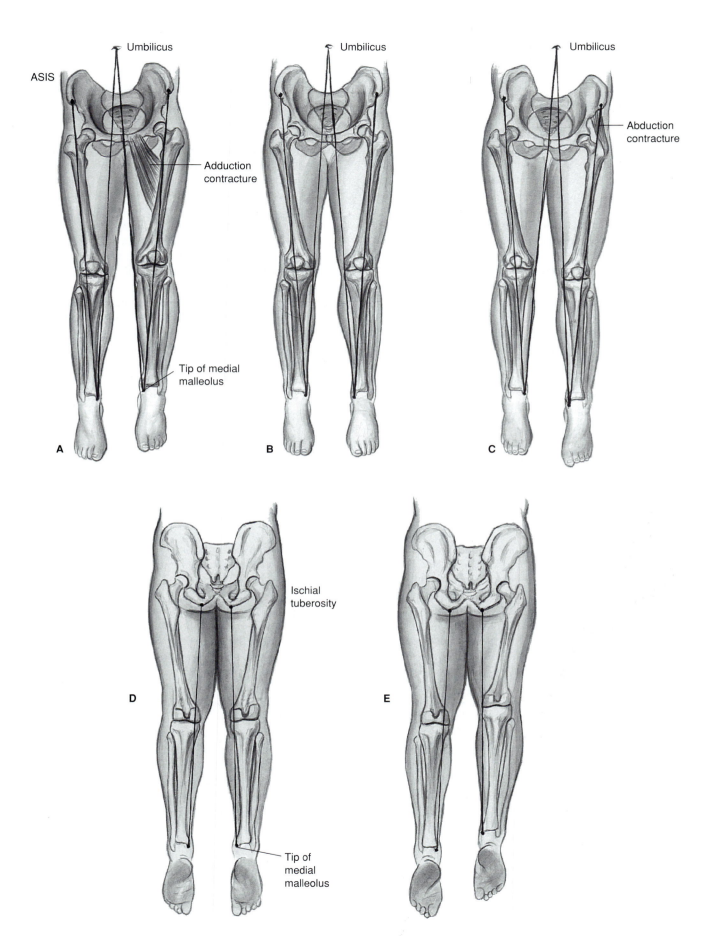

Umbilicus

ASIS

Adduction
contracture

Tip of medial
malleolus

A

Umbilicus

B

Umbilicus

Abduction
contracture

C

Ischial
tuberosity

Tip of
medial
malleolus

D

E

Figure 3–67. Mensuration of actual and apparent limb lengths. **A-C.** Actual limb lengths are measured from the inferior margin of the anterosuperior iliac spine to the tip of the medial malleolus. Apparent limb lengths are measured from the umbilicus to the tip of the medial malleolus. It is vital that both hips and knees be fully extended, in symmetric posture and in neutral rotation. In **A** there is an adduction contracture of the left hip. The actual limb lengths are even, but the apparent limb length on the left is short. In **B** there is no contractural deformity of the hips, and apparent and actual limb lengths are even. In **C** there is an abduction contracture of the left hip; the pelvis is tilted inferiorly on the side of the abduction contracture, and the apparent limb length is long on the left side. **D, E.** An alternate method of measuring limb lengths is to place the patient in prone position with the hips and knees fully extended and the ankles and feet in symmetric position. The actual leg length is measured from the ischial tuberosity to the tip of the medial malleolus. In **D** the limb lengths are even, whereas in **E** the right lower limb is short.

←———

of the proximal phalanges of your hand and determine the temperature of the skin. If there is circulatory insufficiency, the limb feels cold. Hypervascularity due to hemangiomatosis causes the limb to feel warm. If an arteriovenous fistula or aneurysm is suspected, use a stethoscope to detect bruit.

With the patient in prone position, examine the spine for scoliosis. Postural scoliosis disappears in the prone position. In prone posture tilt the pelvis to the right and left on the lumbar spine to rule out the presence of suprapelvic contractural deformity.

In congenital shortening and hemiatrophy, it is best to measure the length of the upper limbs from the posterior tip of the acromion process to the tip of the long finger with the elbow in complete extension. Measure the circumference of the arms and forearms for any atrophy. The steps in clinical assessment of a lower limb length disparity are summarized in Table 3–8.

Imaging Methods for Measuring Limb Lengths. The length of the femur is measured from the superior border of the subchondral bony plate of the capital femoral epiphysis to the

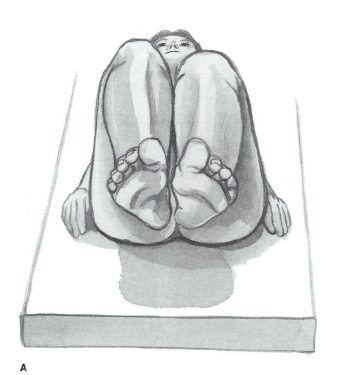

A

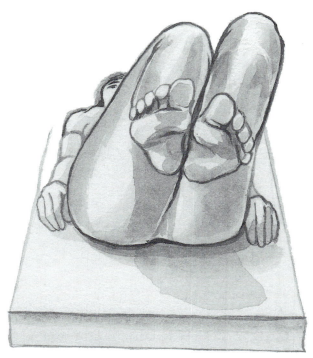

B

Figure 3–68. Galeazzi test. **A.** Note that both hips are flexed 90 degrees and in neutral position as to abduction and adduction. The knee on the short femur is at a lower level than the contralateral normal side. **B.** A pitfall to avoid is adducting or abducting the hips.

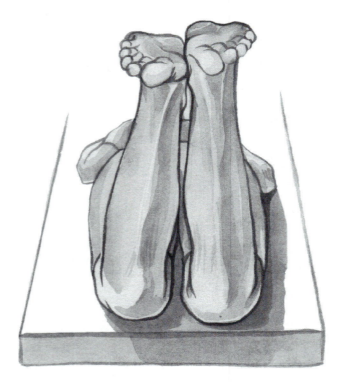

A

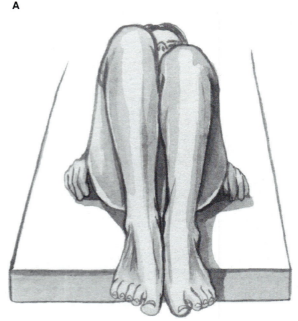

B

Figure 3–69. Ellis test determines the lengths of the tibiae. This can be performed with the patient in supine or prone position. **A.** In prone position the knees are flexed 90 degrees and the feet and ankles are in neutral position. Note the level of the soles of the heels. On the short leg they are at a lower level than on the opposite long leg. **B.** In supine posture the knees are flexed at a right angle and the feet are placed flat on a firm examination table. Note the level of the knees. On the short tibia side the knee level is lower than on the opposite long leg.

TABLE 3–8. STEPS IN CLINICAL ASSESSMENT OF A CHILD WITH LOWER LIMB LENGTH DISPARITY

1. Shoes—any raise or abnormal wear. Orthosis?
2. Standing and sitting heights—percentile of stature.
3. Inspection in stance—front and back. Level of iliac crests and popliteal and gluteal creases.
4. Plumb line test—drop it from C7 or base of skull. Does it fall in intergluteal cleft or is it shifted laterally?
5. Block test—height of wood block that makes the iliac crests horizontally level.
6. Adam's forward bending test—with and without block under the foot of the short leg.
   Postural scoliosis—rotation to concavity: with pelvis level and in supine position, scoliosis disappears.
   Structural scoliosis—rotation to convexity. Does leveling the pelvis aggravate scoliosis and increase decompensation of spine?
7. Mechanical axis deviation of the lower limb.
   Varus or valgus angulation when asymmetric causes apparent shortening. Genu recurvatum or knee flexion deformity?
8. Determination of contractural deformity of hip, knee, and ankle—on inspection in stance and range of motion lying down.
   A. Determine range of hip abduction in extension and flexion—adduction contracture of hip causes apparent shortening.
   B. Perform Ober test for abduction contracture—abduction of hip causes apparent lengthening.
   C. Perform Thomas test—flexion contracture of hip causes apparent shortening.
   D. Determine range of knee extension and flexion—knee flexion deformity causes apparent shortening.
   E. Severe recurvatum causes apparent shortening.
   F. Determine range of motion of ankle and foot—equinus deformity causes apparent lengthening.
9. Determination of stability of hip and knee.
   A. Standing Trendelenburg test—rule out long leg hip dysplasia.
   B. Drawer test and Lachman test for knee joint stability. Rule out absence of cruciate ligaments in the congenitally short femur and tibia.
10. Gait abnormality
    Short leg
    A. Shoulder dips down in stance phase.
    B. Look for equinus posture of foot and ankle, toe-heel, toe-toe, or plantigrade gait.
    C. Stride shortened.
    D. Push-off reduced.
    Long leg
    A. Flexed posture of knee.
    B. Circumduction of hip to clear lower limb.
11. Mensuration of lower limb lengths.
    A. Actual
       1. Anteror superior iliac spine (ASIS) to tip of medial malleolus.
       2. ASIS to sole of heel with ankle and foot in neutral.
    B. Apparent—umbilicus or xiphoid process to tip of medial or lateral malleolus or to sole of heel (foot and ankle in neutral).
    C. Prone actural limb length—from ischium to tip of medial or lateral malleolus or to sole of heel (foot and ankle in neutral).
12. Determination of site of discrepancy—femur, tibia, foot, or pelvis?
    A. Galeazzi test.
    B. Ellis test—supine and prone.
    C. Foot height—tip of medial malleolus to sole of heel.
13. Length of foot—posterior tip of heel to tip of great toe.
14. Mensuration of circumferences of calves (maximal girth) and thigh (at identical levels).
15. Skin and soft tissues.
    A. Inspect and rule out hemangioma, café-au-lait spots, operative scars.
    B. Temperature difference—Cold? Hot? Dorsum of phalanx. Arteriovenous fistula? Any bruit?

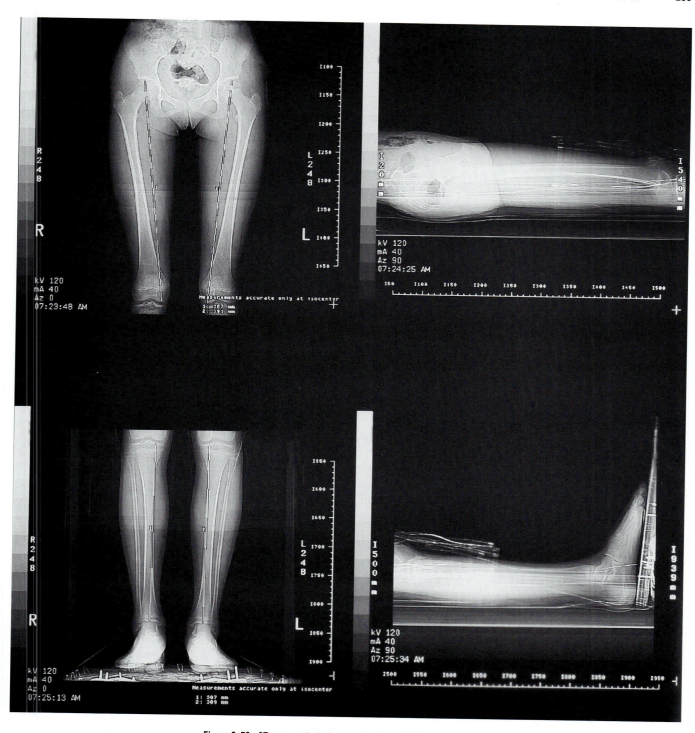

Figure 3–70. CT scan method of measuring lower limb lengths. See text.

inferior margin of the subchondral bony plate of the medial femoral condyle. The length of the tibia is measured from the top of the subchondral bony plate of the medial tibial plateau to the lower margin of the subchondral bony plate of the distal tibial epiphysis at the center of the ankle joint.

Regardless of the radiographic method employed, the hips and knees should be in full extension and neutral rotation. Lateral projections of the femur and tibia are made in the presence of fixed hip or knee flexion contracture. The child should not move during exposures.

CT Scan (Fig 3–70).   This is the method of choice because (1) it is accurate (the x-ray beam is perpendicular to the limb); (2) it visualizes the entire lower limbs and pelvis, thereby depicting associated bone and joint deformities; (3) it is easy to store; and (4) measurements of bone lengths are made on the console; you do not have to measure radiographs. Despite its minor drawbacks of availability in office practice and cost, CT has become the method of choice.

Teleroentgenography.   This technique is employed in infants and young children; a single exposure of the entire lower limbs including the pelvis is made on one film of appropriate size with the x-ray tube 6 feet away from the x-ray table (Fig 3–71). The magnification is almost 15 percent. Radiation to the patient is minimal, as it requires only one x-ray exposure.

Orthoroentgenography.   Complete cooperation and immobility of the patient are vital. Three successive exposures are made centered exactly over the hips, knees, and ankles with the patient lying supine on a single long film with the x-ray tube 6 feet away from the target (Fig 3–72). Direct measurements are made on the x-ray film; one may include a special ruler to facilitate mensuration. The radiation dosage is about the same or slightly less than for a CT scan. Its only advantage is its availability, particularly in an office practice.

These imaging methods do not include the height of the foot and the disparity between the right and left sides of the pelvis. Determine foot height by making a standing lateral radiogram of both feet. Also, it is vital to make standing radiograms of the entire spine, including the pelvis, with and without blocks under the short leg to detect pelvic obliquity, discrepancy, and scoliosis.

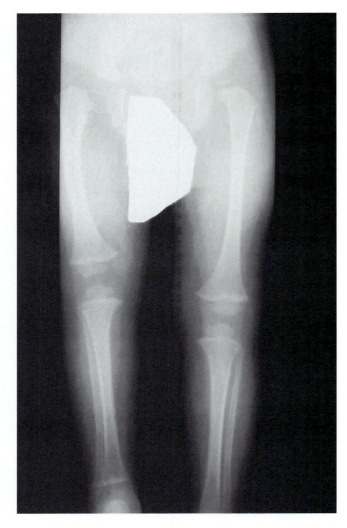

Figure 3–71. Teleroentgenography of lower limbs in proximal femoral focal deficiency on the patient's right.

Prediction of Lower Limb Disparity at Skeletal Maturity

Three methods are available.

The White-Menelaus "Rule of Thumb."   This is a simple method; it is easy to calculate and provides a rough estimate as to timing of growth arrest. The system, popularized by Menelaus, is based on two observations made by White: (1) The distal femoral physis grows 10 mm (3/8 inch) and the proximal tibial physis grows 6 mm (1/4 inch) per year during adolescence; (2) growth of the distal femoral and proximal tibial physes stops at 14 years in girls and 16 years in boys (Fig 3–73).[693]

This method has the following drawbacks: (1) calculations are made on chronologic and not skeletal age; (2) the assumption that the relationship between the rate of growth and the age is a straight line is not always true; and (3) it does not consider the actual length of the femur and tibia; the amount of growth remaining varies directly according to the length of the long bone.

Method of Growth Remaining (Green-Anderson).   The growth prediction chart of Green and Anderson is used to calculate the growth remaining for the distal femur and proximal tibia according to the skeletal age of the patient (Fig 3–74). To calculate the amount, the following data are required: (1) skeletal age, (2) length of femur and tibia of both lower limbs, (3) chronologic age, and (4) percentage of growth inhibition.

To calculate the percentage of growth inhibition: the growth of the long bone minus the growth of the short long bone divided by the growth of the normal long bone.

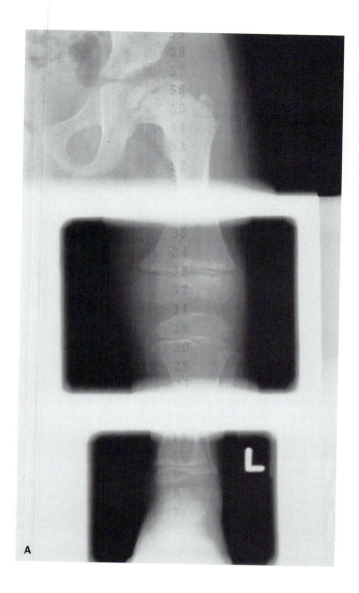

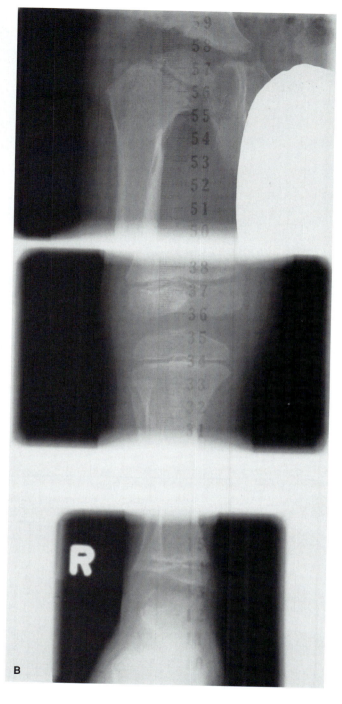

Figure 3–72. Orthoroentgenography. See text.

A period of observation for at least 3 years is desirable for proper computation. For example, a boy of 13 years skeletal age and of average percentile in tibia length has 2 cm of growth remaining from the proximal tibia. If there is inhibition of 20 percent, then, because the short leg will not grow at the same rate as the long leg and correction is achieved by the growth of the short leg, the amount of correction is 2 cm × 20 percent, which is 1.6 cm.

Moseley Straight Line Graph. In this method it is assumed that the longitudinal growth line of the long and short lower limb is a straight line. The graph is constructed by calculations based on the Green-Anderson data. The Moseley straight line method is simple, and it is the one most commonly used (Fig 3–75).

The following data are obtained and plotted on the chart: (1) bone age as determined by an AP radiogram

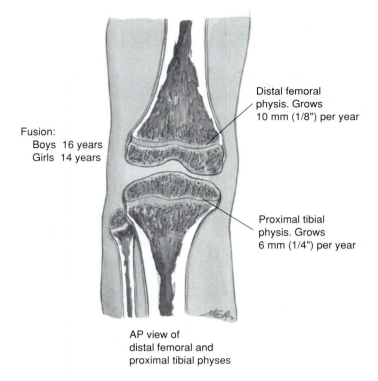

Figure 3–73. White-Menelaus rule of thumb for prediction of lower limb disparity at skeletal maturity. The distal femur grows 3/8 inch per year (10 mm) and the proximal tibia grows 1/4 inch per year (6 mm). The growth of the distal femoral and proximal tibial physis stops at 14 years in girls and 16 years in boys.

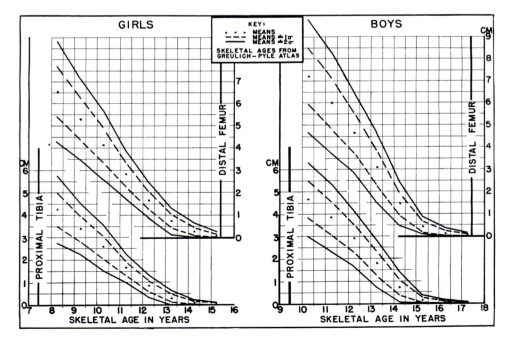

Figure 3–74. Growth remaining in normal distal femur and proximal tibia following consecutive skeletal age levels. Means and standard deviations derived from longitudinal series 50 girls and 50 boys. Growth chart may be used as a guide in estimating the amounts of growth which may be inhibited in the distal end of the normal femur or the proximal end of the normal tibia by epiphyseal arrest at the skeletal ages indicated on the base line. (Used with permission of the Children's Medical Center, Boston, Massachusetts.)

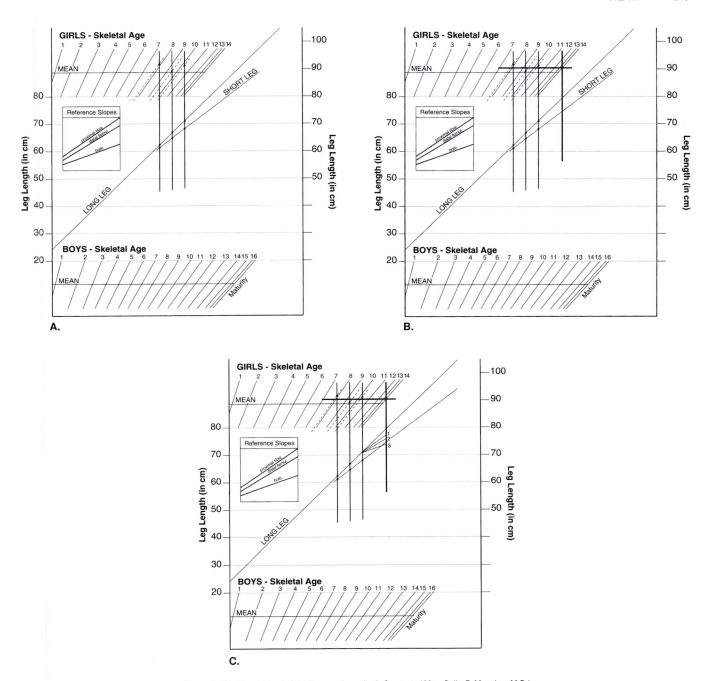

Figure 3–75. Moseley's straight line graph method. See text. (After Colin F. Moseley, M.D.)

of the left hand, (2) length of the long lower limb, and (3) length of the short lower limb as measured on a CT scan or orthoroentgenography. The length of the lower limbs is measured from the top of the femoral head to the middle of the subchondral bony plate of the distal tibia at the ankle.

STEP A. (1) Plot the length of the long lower limb on the line for the long limb and draw a vertical line (upward for

girls and downward for boys) through the skeletal age. This vertical line represents the current bone age. All points at this visit are plotted on the vertical line. (2) Next plot the length of the short limb on this vertical line and plot the point for current bone age, which lies in the same vertical line, placed in reference to the sloping line for skeletal age. Interpolate as necessary.

At subsequent visits repeat these steps. Each vertical line represents an office visit.

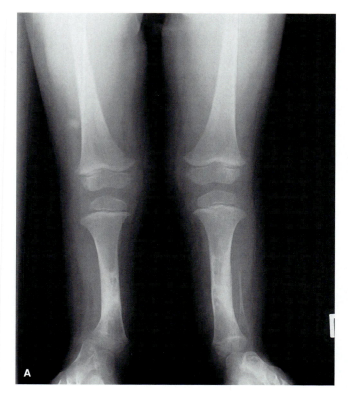

Figure 3–76. Ilizarov technique of tibial lengthening for a short tibia with congenital longitudinal deficiency of the fibula. **A.** Preoperative AP view of both lower limbs. **B to D.** AP, oblique, and lateral views of right tibia showing the Ilizarov-ring 1/2 pins and apparatus elongating the tibia.

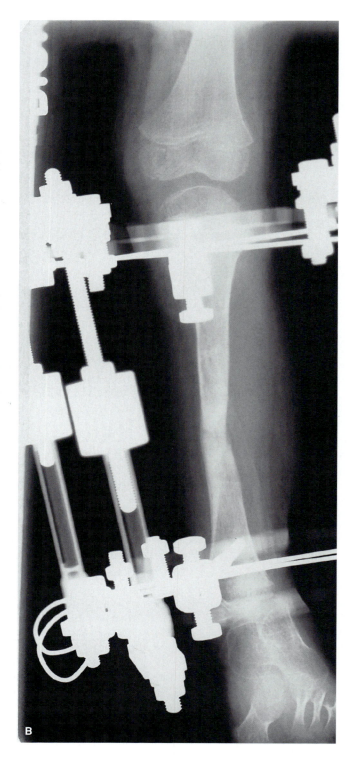

STEP B.   Predict the future growth of the lower limbs as follows: (1) Extend the growth line of the short limb to the right by drawing a straight line. Repeat the same for the long lower limb. (2) The limb length disparity is the distance in centimeters between the growth line of the long limb and that of the short limb. The short limb growth line lies inferior to that of the long limb. The percentage of inhibition is shown by the difference of the slope between the two growth lines. (3) Next draw a horizontal straight line through the points plotted in the skeletal age area. The intersection of this horizontal straight line with the scales in the skeletal age area represent the *skeletal age scale.* (4) Then drop a vertical straight line inferiorly through the maturity point to intersect the growth lines of the long lower limb. The difference between the two growth lines represents the lower limb length disparity at skeletal maturity.

STEP C.   The effect of epiphyseodesis is determined. (1) Chart the length of the long limb on the long leg growth line. (2) Draw a line parallel to the reference slope for the specific epiphyseodesis sites—the proximal tibia, the distal femur, or both. This new line is the growth line of the long

leg. When the slope of the long leg intersects the growth line of the short leg, the limb lengths are equalized.

Treatment.   One to 2 cm of disparity of limb lengths ordinarily does not require any treatment unless associated with an angular or rotational deformity. With 2 cm of short-

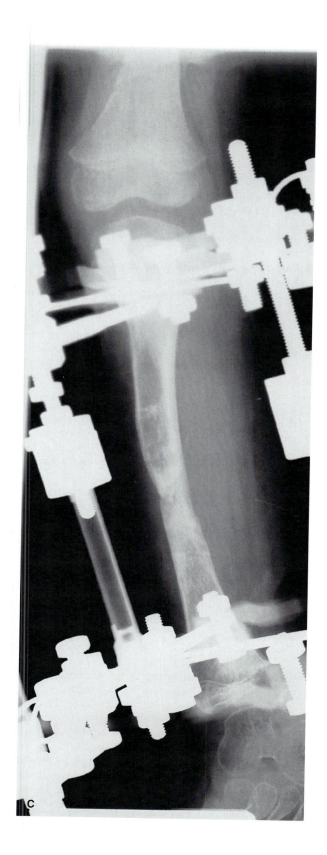

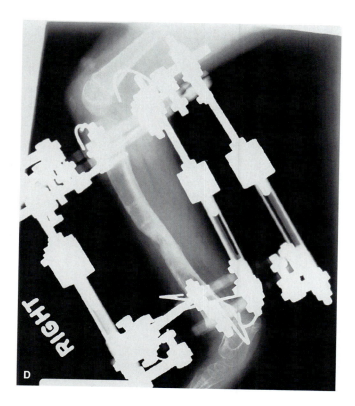

ening, if the spine is decompensated in the growing child, an appropriate lift (raise) to the shoe is given to compensate the spine.

Two to 5 cm of disparity is treated with a shoe lift until appropriate skeletal age, at which time an *epiphyseodesis* of the distal femur or proximal tibia is performed on the long leg to equalize limb lengths. The purpose of limb length equalization is not to make the limbs even in length, but to compensate the head, neck, and shoulders over the pelvis and provide symmetry to the trunk and the lower limbs. The technique applied is either the Phemister-Green technique, in which a rectangular piece of bone is removed, the growth plate curetted, and the block of bone turned 180 degrees and replaced, or the percutaneous epiphyseodesis, either the Canale-Bowen or the Macnicol technique.[632,634] It is crucial to follow a patient after an epiphyseodesis to ensure that overcorrection or undercorrection does not become a complication.

Limb lengthening, either femoral or tibial, is indicated when there is extreme shortening—more than 5 to 7 cm. Distraction osteogenesis can be performed by either the Ilizarov or Orthofix callotasis technique (Figs 3–76 and 3–77). Such procedures are fraught with complications such as pin tract infection, soft tissue contracture, knee or hip joint subluxation or dislocation, delayed consolidation, nerve or vessel injury, fracture, articular cartilage compression and injury, and psychosocial depression. These problems should be made very clear to the family before undertaking limb lengthening.

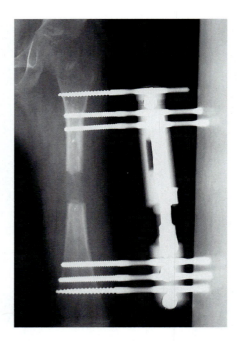

Figure 3–77. Orthofix technique of femoral lengthening as shown by the AP radiogram of the femur. Note the three Orthofix screws proximally and three distally and the elongated segment.

In the skeletally mature patient, limb equalization can be achieved by femoral shortening with intramedullary rod fixation. Tibial shortening is ordinarily not performed because of great potential of neurovascular injury and compartment syndrome. It is beyond the scope of this textbook to discuss surgical details.

REFERENCES

Congenital Dislocation of the Hip

1. Albee FH: The bone graft wedge. Its use in the treatment of relapsing, acquired, and congenital dislocation of hip. *NY Med J* 102:433, 1915
2. Albinana J, Quesada JA, Certucha JA: Children at high risk for congenital dislocation of the hip: Late presentation. *J Pediatr Orthop* 13:268, 1993
3. Ando M, Gotoh E: Significance of inguinal folds for diagnosis of congenital dislocation of the hip in infants aged three to four months. *J Pediatr Orthop* 10:331, 1990
4. Ando M, Gotoh E, Matsuura J: Tangential view arthrogram at closed reduction in congenital dislocation of the hip. *J Pediatr Orthop* 12:390, 1992
5. Andren L: Aetiology and diagnosis of congenital dislocation of the hip in newborns. *Radiology* 1:89, 1961
6. Andren L: Frequency and sex distribution of congenital dislocation of the hip among breech presentations. *Acta Orthop Scand* 31:152, 1961
7. Andren L, Borglin NE: A disorder of oestrogen metabolism as a causal factor of congenital dislocation of the hip. *Acta Orthop Scand* 30:169, 1961
8. Andren L, Borglin NE: Disturbed urinary excretion pattern of oestrogens in newborns with congenital dislocation of the hip. *Acta Endocrinol* 37:423, 1961
9. Ashley RK, Larsen LT, James PM: Reduction of dislocation of the hip in older children. *J Bone Joint Surg* 54A:545, 1972
10. Asplund S, Hjelmstedt A: Experimentally induced hip dislocation in vitro and in vivo. A study in newborn rabbits. *Acta Orthop Scand* (Suppl) 199, 1983
11. Atar D, Lehman WB, Tenenbaum Y, Grant AD: Pavlik harness versus Frejka splint in treatment of developmental dysplasia of the hip: Bicenter study. *J Pediatr Orthop* 13:311, 1993
12. Barlow TG: Early diagnosis and treatment of congenital dislocation of the hip. *J Bone Joint Surg* 44B:292, 1962
13. Barlow TG: Early diagnosis and treatment of congenital dislocation of the hip in the newborn. *Proc R Soc Med* 59:1103, 1966
14. Beddow FH: Facial paralysis complicating splintage for congenital dislocation of the hip in the newborn. *J Bone Joint Surg* 51B:714, 1969
15. Bennet GC: Screening for congenital dislocation of the hip. *J Bone Joint Surg* 74B:643, 1992
16. Berkley MF, Dickson JH, Cain TE, Donovan MM: Surgical therapy for congenital dislocation of the hip in patients who are 12 to 36 months old. *J Bone Joint Surg* 66A:412, 1984
17. Bertol P, Macnicol MF, Mitchell GP: Radiographic feature of neonatal congenital dislocation of the hip. *J Bone Joint Surg* 64B:176, 1982
18. Blockey NJ: Derotation osteotomy in the management of congenital dislocation of the hip. *J Bone Joint Surg* 66B:485, 1984
19. Bolton-Maggs BG, Crabtree SD: The opposite hip in congenital dislocation of the hip. *J Bone Joint Surg* 65B:279, 1983
20. Brashear HR: Epiphyseal avascular necrosis and its relation to longitudinal bone growth. *J Bone Joint Surg* 45A:1423, 1963
21. Browne D: Congenital deformities of mechanical origin. *Arch Dis Child* 30:37, 1955
22. Browne D: Treatment of congenital dislocation of the hip. *Proc R Soc Med* 41:388, 1948
23. Browne RS: The management of late diagnosed congenital dislocation and subluxation of the hip—with special reference to femoral shortening. *J Bone Joint Surg* 61B:27, 1982
24. Browning WH, Rosenkrantz H, Tarquinio T: Computed tomography in congenital hip dislocation. The role of acetabular anteversion. *J Bone Joint Surg* 64A:27, 1982
25. Bucholz RW, Ogden JA: Patterns of ischemic necrosis of the proximal femur in nonoperatively treated congenital hip disease, in *Proceedings of the Sixth Open Scientific Meeting of the Hip Society.* St. Louis, CV Mosby, 1978, pp 43–63
26. Butel J, Francois M, Charignon G, Garrel JF, Faure C: Effets de la résection du limbus sur le développement ulterieur du toit cotyloidien. *Acta Orthop Belg* 39:598, 1973
27. Camp J, Herring JA, Dworezynski C: Comparison of inpatient and outpatient traction in developmental dislocation of the hip. *J Pediatr Orthop* 14:9, 1994

28. Carter CO, Wilkinson JA: Genetic and environmental factors in the etiology of congenital dislocation. *Clin Orthop* 33: 119, 1964

29. Castelein RM, Sauter AJM, de Vlieger M, van Linge B: Natural history of ultrasound hip abnormalities in clinically normal newborns. *J Pediatr Orthop* 12:423, 1992

30. Clarke NMP, Clegg J, Al-Chalabi AN: Ultrasound screening of the hips at risk for CDH. *J Bone Joint Surg* 71B:9, 1989

31. Coleman SS: *Congenital Dysplasia and Dislocation of the Hip.* St. Louis, CV Mosby, 1976

32. Dega W: Transiliac osteotomy in the treatment of congenital hip dysplasia. *Chir Narzadow Ruchu Orthop Pol* 39:601, 1974

33. Dias JJ, Thomas IH, Lamont AC, Mody BS, Thompson JR: The reliability of ultrasonographic assessment of neonatal hips. *J Bone Joint Surg* 75B:479, 1993

34. D'Souza L, Jagannathan S, McManus F: The subcostal nerve (ouch!): Anatomical awareness in Salter's innominate osteotomy. *J Pediatr Orthop* 14:660, 1994

35. Engeseater LB, Wilson DJ, Nag D, Benson MKD: Ultrasound and congenital dislocation of the hip. *J Bone Joint Surg* 72B:197, 1990

36. Faciszewski T, Kiefer GN, Coleman SS: Pemberton osteotomy for residual acetabular dysplasia in children who have congenital dislocation of the hip. *J Bone Joint Surg* 75A: 643, 1993

37. Fiddian NJ, Gardiner JC: Screening for congenital dislocation of the hip by physiotherapists. *J Bone Joint Surg* 76B: 458, 1994

38. Fish DN, Herzenberg JE, Hensinger RN: Current practice in use of prereduction traction for congenital dislocation of the hip. *J Pediatr Orthop* 11:149, 1991

39. Fleissner PR, Ciccarelli CJ, Eilert RE, Chang FM, Glancy GL: The success of closed reduction in the treatment of complex developmental dislocation of the hip. *J Pediatr Orthop* 14:631, 1994

40. Forlin E, Choi IH, Guille JT, Bowen JR, Glutting J: Prognostic factors in congenital dislocation of the hip treated with closed reduction. *J Bone Joint Surg* 74A:1140, 1992

41. Gabuzda GM, Renshaw TS: Current concepts review: Reduction of congenital dislocation of the hip. *J Bone Joint Surg* 74A:625, 1992

42. Gaenslen FJ: The Schanz subtrochanteric osteotomy for irreducible dislocation of the hip. *J Bone Joint Surg* 17:76, 1935

43. Gage JR, Winter RB: Avascular necrosis of the capital femoral epiphysis as a complication of closed reduction of congenital dislocation of the hip. *J Bone Joint Surg* 54A:373, 1972

44. Gardner E, Gray DJ: Prenatal development of the human hip joint. *Am J Anat,* 87:163, 1950

45. Garvey M, Donoghue VB, O'Brien N, Murphy JFA: Radiographic screening at four months of infants at risk for congenital hip dislocation. *J Bone Joint Surg* 74B:704, 1992

46. Gill AB: Plastic construction of an acetabulum in congenital dislocation of the hip—the shelf operation. *J Bone Joint Surg* 17:48, 1935

47. Gillespie R, Torode I: Classification and management of congenital abnormalities of the femur. *J Bone Joint Surg* 65B:447, 1983

48. Good C, Walker G: The hip in the molded baby syndrome. *J Bone Joint Surg* 66B:491, 1984

49. Graf R: New possibilities for the diagnosis of congenital hip joint dislocation by ultrasonography. *J Pediatr Orthop* 3: 354, 1983

50. Grech P: *Hip Arthrography.* London, Chapman & Bell, 1977

51. Green NE, Griffin PP: Hip dysplasia associated with abduction contracture of the contralateral hip. *J Bone Joint Surg* 64A:1273, 1982

52. Greenhill BJ, Hugosson C, Jacobsson B, Ellis RD: Magnetic resonance imaging study of acetabular morphology in developmental dysplasia of the hip. *J Pediatr Orthop* 13:314, 1993

53. Gregosiewicz A, Wosko I: Risk factors of avascular necrosis in the treatment of congenital dislocation of the hip. *J Pediatr Orthop* 8:17, 1988

54. Grill F, Bensahel H, Canadell I, Dungl P, Matasovic T, Vizkelety T: The Pavlik harness in the treatment of the congenital dislocating hip: Report on a multicenter study of the European Paediatric Orthopaedic Society. *J Pediatr Orthop* 8:1, 1988

55. Guille JT, Forlin E, Kumar SJ, MacEwen GD: Triple osteotomy of the innominate bone in treatment of developmental dysplasia of the hip. *J Pediatr Orthop* 12:718, 1992

56. Harcke HT, Kumar SJ: Current concepts review. The role of ultrasound in the diagnosis and management of congenital dislocation and dysplasia of the hip. *J Bone Joint Surg* 73A: 622, 1991

57. Harris NH, Lloyd-Roberts GC, Gallien R: Acetabular development in congenital dislocation of the hip. *J Bone Joint Surg* 57B:46, 1975

58. Hass J: *Congenital Dislocation of the Hip.* Springfield, IL, Charles C Thomas, 1951

59. Hensinger RN: Congenital dislocation of the hip. *CIBA Clin Symp* 31:3, 1979

60. Hernandez RJ, Tachdjian MO, Poznanski AK, and Dias LS: CT determination of femoral torsion. *AJR,* 137:97, 1981.

61. Herndon WA, Bolano L, Sullivan JA: Hip stabilization in severely involved cerebral palsy patients. *J Pediatr Orthop* 12:68, 1992

62. Herold HZ: Avascular necrosis of the femoral head due to malposition in untreated congenital dislocation of the hip. *Int Orthop* 2:293, 1979

63. Hilgenreiner H: Zur Fruhdiagnose und Frhubehandlung der angeborenen Huftgelenkverrenkung. *Med Klin* 21:1385, 1952

64. Hogh J, Macnicol MF: The Chiari pelvic osteotomy. A longterm review of clinical and radiographic results. *J Bone Joint Surg* 69B:365, 1987

65. Holen KJ, Terjesen T, Tegnander A, Bredland T, Saether OD, Eik-Nes SH: Ultrasound screening for hip dysplasia in newborns. *J Pediatr Orthop* 14:667, 1994

66. Hughes JR: Acetabular dysplasia and acetabuloplasty, in Tachdjian MO (ed): *Congenital Dislocation of the Hip.* New York, Churchill Livingstone, 1982, pp 665–693.

67. Hughes JR: Intrinsic obstructive factors in congenital dislocation of the hip: The role of arthrography, in Tachdjian MO (ed): *Congenital Dislocation of the Hip.* New York, Churchill Livingstone, 1982, pp 227–245

68. Hummer CD, MacEwen GD: Torticollis and congenital hip dysplasia. *J Bone Joint Surg* 55B:665, 1973

69. Ilfeld FW: The management of congenital dislocation and dysplasia of the hip by means of a special splint. *J Bone Joint Surg* 39A:99, 1957

70. Iwahara T, Ideda A: On the ipsilateral involvement of congenital muscular torticollis and congenital dislocation of the hip. *J Jpn Orthop Assoc* 35:1221, 1962

71. Jacobs JE: Metatarsus varus and hip dysplasia. *Clin Orthop* 16:203, 1960

72. Joachimsthal G: Die angeborene Huftverrenkung als Teilerscheinung anderer angeborener Anomalien. *Z Orthop* 22:31, 1908

73. Jomha NM, McIvor J, Sterling G: Ultrasonography in developmental hip dysplasia. *J Pediatr Orthop* 15:101, 1995

74. Jones GT, Schoenecker PL, Dias LS: Developmental dysplasia potentiated by inappropriate use of the Pavlik harness. *J Pediatr Orthop* 12:722, 1992

75. Kahle WK, Anderson MB, Alpert J, Stevens PM, Coleman SS: The value of preliminary traction in the treatment of congenital dislocation of the hip. *J Bone Joint Surg* 72A:1043, 1990

76. Kahle WK, Coleman SS: The value of the acetabular teardrop figure in assessing pediatric hip disorders. *J Pediatr Orthop* 12:586, 1992

77. Kalamchi A, MacEwen GD: Avascular necrosis following treatment of congenital dislocation of the hip. *J Bone Joint Surg* 62A:876, 1980

78. Kalamchi A, MacFarlane R: The Pavlik harness: Results in patients over three months of age. *J Pediatr Orthop* 2:3, 1982

79. Kawamura B, Hosono S, Yokogushi K: Dome osteotomy of the pelvis, in Tachdjian MO (ed): *Congenital Dislocation of the Hip.* New York, Churchill Livingstone, 1982, pp 609–623

80. Kershaw CJ, Ware HE, Pattinson R, Fixsen JA: Revision of failed open reduction of congenital dislocation of the hip. *J Bone Joint Surg* 75B:744, 1993

81. Klaue K, Sherman M, Perren SM, Wallin A, Looser C, Ganz R: Extra-articular augmentation for residual hip dysplasia. *J Bone Joint Surg* 75B:750, 1993

82. Klisiç P: Open reduction with femoral shortening and pelvic osteotomy, in Tachdjian MO (ed): *Congenital Dislocation of the Hip.* New York, Churchill Livingstone, 1982, pp 417–426

83. Krikler SJ, Dwyer NStJP: Comparison of results of two approaches to hip screening in infants. *J Bone Joint Surg* 74B:701, 1992

84. Langenskiöld A, Salenius P: Epiphyseodesis of the greater trochanter. *Acta Orthop Scand* 38:199, 1967

85. Langenskiöld A, Sarpio C, Michelsson JE: Experimental dislocation of the hip in the rabbit. *J Bone Joint Surg* 44B:209, 1962

86. Laurenson RD: The acetabular index—a critical review. *J Bone Joint Surg* 41B:702, 1959

87. LeCoeur P: Osteotomie isthmique de bascule, in Chapchal G (ed): *Beckenosteotomie—Pfannendachplastik.* Stuttgart, Georg Thieme, 1965

88. LeDamany P: Congenital luxation of the hip. *Am J Orthop Surg* 11:541, 1914

89. LeDamany P: La luxation congénitale de la hanche, in *Etudes d'Anatomie Comparée d'Anthropogenie Normale et Pathologique, Déductions Thérapeutique.* Paris, Felix Alcan, 1912

90. Lee DY, Choi IH, Lee CK, Cho TJ: Assessment of complex hip deformity using three-dimensional CT image. *J Pediatr Orthop* 11:13, 1991

91. Lejman T, Strong M, Michno P: Capsulorrhaphy versus capsulectomy in open reduction of the hip for developmental dysplasia. *J Pediatr Orthop* 15:98, 1995

92. Leveuf J: Primary congenital subluxation of the hip. *J Bone Joint Surg* 29:149, 1947

93. Leveuf J: Results of open reduction of "true" congenital dislocation of the hip. *J Bone Joint Surg* 30A:875, 1948

94. Lieberman JR, Altchek DW, Salvati EA: Recurrent dislocation of a hip with a labral lesion: Treatment with a modified Bankart-type repair. *J Bone Joint Surg* 75A:1524, 1993

95. Lloyd-Roberts GC, Swann M: Pitfalls in the management of congenital dislocation of the hip. *J Bone Joint Surg* 48B:666, 1966

96. Lorenz A: La riduzione della lussazione congenita dell' anca. *Arch Orthop* 14:1, 1897

97. Lorenz A: *Pathologie und Therapie der Angeborenun Huftvevrenkung auf Grundlage von Hundert Operatie Behandelten Fallen.* Vienna, Wein und Leipzig, 1895

98. Ludloff K: The open reduction of the congenital hip dislocation by an anterior incision. *Am J Orthop Surg* 10:438, 1913

99. Macnicol MF: Results of a 25-year screening program for neonatal hip instability. *J Bone Joint Surg* 72B:1057, 1990

100. Macnicol MF, Makris D: Distal transfer of the greater trochanter. *J Bone Joint Surg* 73B:838, 1991

101. McCauley RG, Wunderlich BK, Zimbler S: Air embolism as a complication of hip arthrography. *Skeletal Radiol* 6:11, 1981

102. McKibbin B: Anatomical factors in the stability of the hip joint in the newborn. *J Bone Joint Surg* 52B:148, 1970

103. Makin M: Closure of the epiphysis of the femoral head and of the triradiate cartilage of the acetabulum following surgery for congenital hip dislocation. *Isr J Med Sci,* 16:307, 1980

104. Mankey MG, Arntz CT, Staheli LT: Open reduction through a medial approach for congenital dislocation of the hip. *J Bone Joint Surg* 75A:1334, 1993

105. Marafioti RL, Westin GL: Factors influencing results of acetabuloplasty in children. *J Bone Joint Surg* 62A:765, 1980

106. Marchetti PG: Classification and treatment of hip subluxation in childhood and adolescence, in Tachdjian MO (ed): *Congenital Dislocation of the Hip.* New York, Churchill Livingstone, 1982, pp 321–337

107. Matsuno T, Ichioka Y, Kaneda K: Modified Chiari pelvic osteotomy: A long-term follow-up study. *J Bone Joint Surg* 74A:470, 1992

108. Mau H, Dorr WM, Henkel L, Lutsche J: Open reduction of congenital dislocation of the hip by Ludloff's method. *J Bone Joint Surg* 53A:1281, 1971

109. Mendez AA, Keret D, MacEwen GD: Obturator dislocation as a complication of closed reduction of the congenital dislocated hip: A report of two cases. *J Pediatr Orthop* 10:265, 1990

110. Michelsson J-E, Langenskiöld A: Dislocation or subluxation of the hip. Regular sequels of immobilization of the knee in extension in young rabbits. *J Bone Joint Surg* 54A:1177, 1972

111. Milgram JW, Tachdjian MO: Pathology of the limbus in un-treated teratologic congenital dislocation of the hip. A case report of a ten-month-old infant. *Clin Orthop* 119:107, 1976

112. Mitchell GP: Problems in the early diagnosis and management of congenital dislocation of the hip. *J Bone Joint Surg* 54B:4, 1972

113. Mitchell GP: The delayed Trendelenburg hip test. *Inter Congress Series,* No 291, SICOT, 1972

114. Moore FH: Examining infants' hips—can it do harm? *J Bone Joint Surg* 71B:4, 1989

115. Mooney JF, Kasser JR: Brachial plexus palsy as a complication of Pavlik harness use. *J Pediatr Orthop* 14:677, 1994

116. Mubarak S, Garfin S, Vance R, McKinnon B, Sutherland D: Pitfalls in the use of the Pavlik harness for treatment of congenital dysplasia, subluxation, and dislocation of the hip. *J Bone Joint Surg* 63A:1239, 1981

117. Noritake K, Yoshihashi Y, Hattori T, Miura T: Acetabular development after closed reduction of congenital dislocation of the hip. *J Bone Joint Surg* 75B:737, 1993

118. Novick G, Ghelman B, Schneider M: Sonography of the neonatal and infant hip. *AJR* 141:639, 1983

119. Ogden JA: Changing patterns of proximal femoral vascularity. *J Bone Joint Surg* 56A:941, 1974

120. Ogden JA, Southwick WO: A possible cause of avascular necrosis complicating the treatment of congenital dislocation of the hip. *J Bone Joint Surg* 55A:1770, 1973

121. Oh WH: Dislocation of the hip in birth defects. *Orthop Clin North Am* 7:315, 1976

122. Ombredanne L: *Précis Clinique et Opératoire de Chirurgie Infantile.* Paris, Masson, 1932

123. Ortolani M: *La Lussazione Congenital dell'Anca.* Bologna, Casa Editrice Licinio Cappelli, 1948

124. Ortolani M: Un segno poco noto e sue importanza per la diagnosi precoce di preussasione congenita dell'anca. *Pediatria* 45:129, 1937

125. O'Sullivan ME, O'Brien T: Acetabular dysplasia presenting as developmental dislocation of the hip. *J Pediatr Orthop* 14:13, 1994

126. Palmen K, Von Rosen S: Late diagnosis dislocation of the hip joint in children. *Acta Orthop Scand* 46:90, 1975

127. Papavasiliou VA, Piggott H: Acetabular floor thickening and femoral head enlargement in congenital dislocation of the hip: Lateral displacement of femoral head. *J Pediatr Orthop* 3:22, 1983

128. Paterson DC: The early diagnosis and screening of congenital dislocation of the hip, in Tachdjian MO (ed): *Congenital Dislocation of the Hip.* New York, Churchill Livingstone, 1982, pp 145–157

129. Pavlik A: Di funktionelle Behandlungsmethode mittels Reimenbugel als Prinzip der knoservativen Therapie bei angeborenen Huftgelenksverrenkungen der Sauglinge. *Z Orthop* 89:341, 1957

130. Pemberton PA: Osteotomy of the ilium with rotation of the acetabular roof for congenital dislocation of the hip. *J Bone Joint Surg* 40A:724, 1958

131. Pemberton PA: Pericapsular osteotomy of the ilium for congenital subluxation and dislocation of the hip. *J Bone Joint Surg* 47A:65, 1965

132. Perkins G: Signs by which to diagnose congenital dislocation of the hip. *Lancet* 1:648, 1928

133. Perlik PC, Westin GW, Marafioti RL: Combination pelvic osteotomy for acetabular dysplasia in children. *J Bone Joint Surg* 67A:842, 1985

134. Peterson HA, Klassen RA, McLeod RA, Hoffman AD: The use of computed tomography in dislocation of the hip and femoral neck antetorsion in children. *J Bone Joint Surg* 63B: 198, 1981

135. Ponseti IV: Growth and development of the acetabulum in the normal child. Anatomical, histological, and roentgenographic studies. *J Bone Joint Surg* 60A:575, 1978

136. Ponseti IV: Morphology of the acetabulum in congenital dislocation of the hip. Gross, histological, and roentgenographic studies. *J Bone Joint Surg* 600:586, 1978

137. Porat S, Robin GC, Howard CB: Cure of the limp in children with congenital dislocation of the hip and ischaemic necrosis. *J Bone Joint Surg* 76B:463, 1994

138. Portinaro NMA, Matthews SJE, Benson MKD: The acetabular notch in hip dysplasia. *J Bone Joint Surg* 76B:271, 1994

139. Quinn RH, Renshaw TS, DeLuca PA: Preliminary traction in the treatment of developmental dislocation of the hip. *J Pediatr Orthop* 14:636, 1994

140. Rab GT: Biomechanical aspects of Salter osteotomy. *Clin Orthop* 132:82, 1978

141. Ramsey PL, Hensinger RN: Congenital dislocation of the hip associated with central core disease. *J Bone Joint Surg* 57A:648, 1975

142. Ramsey PL, Lasser S, MacEwen GD: Congenital dislocafjtion of the hip: Use of the Pavlik harness in the child during the first 6 months of life. *J Bone Joint Surg* 58A:1000, 1976

143. Rombouts J-J, Kaelin A: Inferior (obturator) dislocation of the hip in neonates. *J Bone Joint Surg* 74B:708, 1992

144. Rungee JL, Reinker KA: Ossific nucleus eccentricity in congenital dislocation of the hip. *J Pediatr Orthop* 12:61, 1992

145. Ryder CT, Crane L: Measuring femoral anteversion: The problem and a method. *J Bone Joint Surg* 35A:321, 1953

146. Salter RB: Innominate osteotomy in the treatment of congenital dislocation and subluxation of the hip. *J Bone Joint Surg* 43B:518, 1961

147. Salter RB: Role of innominate osteotomy in the treatment of congenital dislocation and subluxation of the hip in the older child. *J Bone Joint Surg* 48A:1413, 1966

148. Salter RB, Kostiuk S, Dallas S: Avascular necrosis of the femoral head as a complication of treatment for congenital dislocation of the hip in young children: A clinical and experimental investigation. *Can J Surg,* 12:44, 1969

149. Salter RB, Kostiuk J, Schatzker J: Experimental dysplasia of the hip and its reversibility in newborn pigs. *J Bone Joint Surg* 45A:1781, 1963

150. Samuelson KM, Nixon GW, Morrow RE: Tomography for evaluation of congenital dislocation of the hip while in a spica cast. *J Bone Joint Surg* 56A:844, 1974

151. Schanz A: Zur Behandlung der veralteten angeborenen Huftverrenkung. *Munch Med Wochenschr* 69:930, 1922

152. Schoenecker PL, Strecker WB: Congenital dislocation of the hip in children. Comparison of the effects of femoral shortening and of skeletal traction in treatment. *J Bone Joint Surg* 66A:21, 1984

153. Schultiz K-P: Die Retrotorsion des Femur nach Derotations Varisierungosteotomien im Kindesalter. *Z Orthop* 107:241, 1970

154. Severin E: Congenital dislocation of the hip. Development of the joint after closed reduction. *J Bone Joint Surg* 32A: 507, 1950

155. Severin E: Contribution to the knowledge of congenital dislocation of the hip joint. Late results of closed reduction and arthrographic studies of recent cases. *Acta Chir Scand* (Suppl) 63:1941

156. Smith WS, Badgley CE, Orwig JB, Harper JM: Correlation of post-reduction roentgenograms and thirty-one year follow-up in congenital dislocation of the hip. *J Bone Joint Surg* 50A:1081, 1968

157. Smith WS, Coleman CR, Olix ML, Slager RF: Etiology of congenital dislocation of the hip. An experimental approach to the problem using young dogs. *J Bone Joint Surg* 45:491, 1963

158. Somerville EW: *Displacement of the Hip in Childhood.* New York, Springer-Verlag, 1982, p 41

159. Sommer J: Atypical hip click in the newborn. *Acta Orthop Scand* 42:353, 1971

160. Sosna A, Rejholec M: Ludloff's open reduction of the hip: Long-term results. *J Pediatr Orthop* 12:603, 1992

161. Staheli LT: Slotted acetabular augmentation. *J Pediatr Orthop* 1:321, 1981

162. Staheli LT, Chew DE: Slotted acetabular augmentation in childhood and adolescence. *J Pediatr Orthop* 12:569, 1992

163. Stanisavljevic S: *Diagnosis and Treatment of Congenital Hip Pathology in the Newborn.* Baltimore, Williams & Wilkins, 1964

164. Stanton RP, Capecci R: Computed tomography for early evaluation of developmental dysplasia of the hip. *J Pediatr Orthop* 12:727, 1992

165. Steel HH: Triple osteotomy of the innominate bone. *J Bone Joint Surg* 55A:343, 1973

166. Strayer LM Jr: Embryology of the human hip joint. *Clin Orthop* 74:221, 1971

167. Sutherland DH, Greenfield R: Double innominate osteotomy. *J Bone Joint Surg* 59A:1082, 1977

168. Suzuki R: Complications of the treatment of congenital dislocation of the hip by the Pavlik harness. *Int Orthop* 3:77, 1979

169. Suzuki S: Reduction of CDH by the Pavlik harness. *J Bone Joint Surg* 76B:460, 1994

170. Suzuki S: Ultrasound and the Pavlik harness in CDH. *J Bone Joint Surg* 75B:483, 1993

171. Suzuki S, Kasahara Y, Futami T, Ushikubo S, Tsuchiya T: Ultrasonography in congenital dislocation of the hip. *J Bone Joint Surg* 73B:879, 1991

172. Suzuki S, Yamamuro T: Avascular necrosis in patients treated with the Pavlik harness for congenital dislocation of the hip. *J Bone Joint Surg* 72A:1048, 1990

173. Synder M, Forlin E, Xin S, Bowen JR: Results of the Kalamchi modification of Salter osteotomy in the treatment of developmental dysplasia of the hip. *J Pediatr Orthop* 12: 449, 1992

174. Tachdjian MO: Salter's innominte osteotomy to derotate the maldirected acetabulum, in Tachdjian MO (ed): *Congenital Dislocation of the Hip.* New York, Churchill Livingstone, 1982, pp 525–541

175. Tachdjian MO, Edelstein D: Periacetabular osteotomy through the subinguinal medial adductor approach. Paper presented at the American Orthopedic Association Annual Meeting, 1985, San Diego. *Orthop Trans* Vol 9, No 2, Spring, 1985

176. Tasnavites A, Murray DW, Benson MKD'A: Improvement in acetabular index after reduction of hips with developmental dysplasia. *J Bone Joint Surg* 75B:755, 1993

177. Terjesen T: Closed reduction guided by dynamic ultrasound in late-diagnosed hip dislocation. *J Pediatr Orthop* 12:54, 1992

178. Thompson RC: A new physical test in dislocation of the hip. *J Bone Joint Surg* 54A:1326, 1972

179. Tönnis D: *Congenital Dysplasia and Dislocation of the Hip.* Berlin, Springer-Verlag, 1987, p 91

180. Trevor D, Johns DL, Fixsen JA: Acetabuloplasty in the treatment of congenital dislocation of the hip. *J Bone Joint Surg* 57B:167, 1975

181. Tucci JJ, Kumar SJ, Guille JT, Rubbo ER: Late acetabular dysplasia following early successful Pavlik harness treatment of congenital dislocation of the hip. *J Pediatr Orthop* 11:402, 1991

182. Viere RG, Birch JG, Herring JA, Roach JW, Johnston CE: Use of the Pavlik harness in congenital dislocation of the hip. *J Bone Joint Surg* 72A:238, 1990

183. Vizkelety T: Overdiagnosis and overtreatment of the congenital dislocation and dysplasia of the hip, in Vigliani F, Ortolani M Jr (eds): *Congenital Hip Dislocation: Today.* Rome, CIC Edizioni Internazionali, 1988, pp 169–176

184. Wagner H: Experiences with spherical acetabular osteotomy for the correction of the dysplastic acetabulum, in Weil UH (ed): *Progress in Orthopedic Surgery,* Vol 2. Heidelberg, Springer-Verlag, 1978, p 131

185. Wagner H: Osteotomies for congenital hip dislocation, in *The Hip: Proceedings of the Fourth Meeting of the Hip Society, 1976.* St. Louis, CV Mosby, 1976, pp 45–66

186. Watanabe RS: Embryology of the human hip. *Clin Orthop* 98:8, 1974

187. Weiner DS: Congenital dislocation of the hip associated with congenital muscular torticollis. *Clin Orthop* 121:163, 1976

188. Weiner DS, Hoyt WA, O'Dell HW: Congenital dislocation of the hip—the relationship of pre-manipulation traction and age to avascular necrosis of the femoral head. *J Bone Joint Surg* 59:306, 1977

189. Weiner LS, Kelley MA, Ulin RI, Wallach D: Development of the acetabulum and hip: Computed tomography analysis of the axial plane. *J Pediatr Orthop* 13:421, 1993

190. Westin GW: The stick femur. *J Bone Joint Surg* 52B:778, 1970

191. Westin GW, Dallas TG, Watanabe BM, Ilfeld FW: Skeletal traction vs. femoral shortening in treatment of older children with congenital hip dislocation. *Isr J Med Sci* 16:318, 1980

192. Wilkinson JA: Breech malposition and intrauterine dislocations. *Proc R Soc Med,* 59:1106, 1966

193. Wilkinson JA: *Congenital Displacement of the Hip Joint.* Berlin, Springer, 1985

194. Wilkinson JA: Prime factors in the etiology of congenital dislocation of the hip. *J Bone Joint Surg* 45B:268, 1963

195. Wynne-Davies R: Acetabular dysplasia and familial joint laxity: Two aetiological factors in congenital dislocation of the hip. A review of 589 patients and their families. *J Bone Joint Surg* 52B:704, 1970

196. Zionts LE, MacEwen GD: Treatment of congenital dislocation of the hip in children between the ages of one and three years. *J Bone Joint Surg* 68:829, 1986

197. Zsernaviczky J, Turk G: Two new radiological signs in the early diagnosis of congenital dysplasia of the hip joint. *Int Orthop* 2:223, 1978

Congenital Abduction Contracture of the Hip and Pelvic Obliquity

198. Green NE, Griffin PP: Hip dysplasia associated with abduction contracture of the contralateral hip. *J Bone Joint Surg* 64A:1273, 1982

Developmental Coxa Vara

199. Almond HG: Familial infantile coxa vara. *J Bone Joint Surg* 38B:539, 1956
200. Amstutz HC: Developmental (infantile) coxa vara—a distinct entity. Report of two patients with previously normal roentgenograms. *Clin Orthop* 72:242, 1970
201. Babb FS, Ghormley RK, Chatterton CC: Congenital coxa vara. *J Bone Joint Surg* 31A:115, 1949
202. Blockey NJ: Observations on infantile coxa vara. *J Bone Joint Surg* 51B:106, 1969
203. Golding, FC: Congenital coxa vara and the short femur. *Proc R Soc Med* 32:641, 1969
204. Haas SL: Lengthening of the femur with simultaneous correction of coxa vara. *J Bone Joint Surg* 15:219, 1933
205. Johanning K: Coxa vara infantum. II. Treatment and results of treatment. *Acta Orthop Scand* 22:100, 1952
206. Langenskiöld A, Salenius P: Epiphyseodesis of the greater trochanter. *Acta Orthop Scand* 38:199, 1967
207. Le Mesurier AB: Developmental coxa vara. *J Bone Joint Surg* 30B:595, 1948
208. Merle D'Aubigne R, Descamps L: L'ostéotomie plane oblique dans la correction des déformations des mêmbres. *Mem Acad Chir* 78:271, 1952
209. Merle D'Aubigne R, Vaillant JM: Correction simultanée des angles d'inclinasion et de torsion du col femoral par l'ostéotomie plane oblique. *Rev Chir Orthop* 47:94, 1961
210. Pauwels F: *Biomechanics of the Normal and Diseased Hip.* New York, Springer, 1976
211. Salenius P, Videman T: Growth disturbances of the proximal end of the femur—an animal experimental study with tetracycline. *Acta Orthop Scand* 41:199, 1970
212. Schanz A: Zur Behandlung der angeborenen coxa vara. *Z Orthop* 44:261, 1924
213. Von Lanz T, Wachsmuth W: *Praktische Anatomie.* Berlin, Springer, 1938, p 138
214. Weinstein JN, Kuo KN, Millar EA: Congenital coxa vara. A retrospective review. *J Pediatr Orthop* 4:70, 1984

Congenital Shortening or Hypoplasia of the Femur

215. Ring PA: Congenital short femur in simple femoral hypoplasia. *J Bone Joint Surg* 41B:73, 1959

Proximal Femoral Focal Deficiency

216. Aitken GT: Proximal femoral focal deficiency—definition, classification and management, in *Proximal Femoral Focal Deficiency: A Congenital Anomaly.* National Academy of Sciences, 1969, p 1
217. Amstutz HC: The morphology, natural history, and treatment of proximal femoral focal deficiency, in Aitken GT (ed): *Proximal Femoral Focal Deficiency: A Congenital Anomaly.* National Academy of Sciences, 1969, p 50
218. Bevan-Thomas WH, Millar EA: A review of proximal focal femoral deficiencies. *J Bone Joint Surg* 49A:1376, 1967
219. Eilert R: Congenital short femur, in Kalamchi A (ed): *Congenital Lower Limb Deficiencies.* New York, Springer-Verlag, 1989, pp 89–107
220. Epps CH Jr: Proximal femoral focal deficiency. *J Bone Joint Surg* 65A:867, 1983
221. Fixsen JA, Lloyd Roberts GC: The natural history and early treatment of proximal femoral dysplasia. *J Bone Joint Surg* 56B:1974
222. Gillespie R, Torode IP: Classification and management of congenital abnormalities of the femur. *J Bone Joint Surg* 65B:557, 1983
223. Gilsanz V: Distal focal femoral deficiency. *Radiology* 147:104, 1983
224. Grill F, Dungl P: Lengthening for congenital short femur. Results of different methods. *J Bone Joint Surg* 73:439, 1991
225. Grissom LE, Harcke HT: Sonography in congenital deficiency of the femur. *J Pediatr Orthop* 14:29, 1994
226. Gupta DKS, Gupta SK: Familial bilateral proximal femoral focal deficiency. Report of a kindred. *J Bone Joint Surg* 66A:1470, 1984
227. Hillmann JS, Mesgarzadeh M, Revesz G, Bonakdarpour A, Clancy M, Betz RR: Proximal femoral focal deficiency: Radiologic analysis of 49 cases. *Radiology* 165:769, 1987
228. Johansson E, Aparisi T: Missing cruciate ligament in congenital short femur. *J Bone Joint Surg* 65A:1109, 1985
229. King RE: Some concepts of proximal femoral focal deficiency. *J Bone Joint Surg* 49A:1470, 1967
230. Kostuik JP, Gillespie R, Hall JE, Hubbard S: Van Nes rotational osteotomy for treatment of proximal femoral focal deficiency and congenital short femur. *J Bone Joint Surg* 57A:1039, 1975
231. Krajbich J: Proximal femoral focal deficiency, in Kalamchi A (ed): *Congenital Lower Limb Deficiencies.* New York, Springer-Verlag, 1989, pp 108–127
232. Mital MA, Masalawalla KS, Desai MG: Bilateral congenital aplasia of the femur. *J Bone Joint Surg* 45B:561, 1963
233. Pappas AM: Congenital abnormalities of the femur and related lower extremity malformations: Classification and treatment. *J Pediatr Orthop* 3:45, 1983
234. Pirani S, Beauchamp RD, Li D, Sawatzky B: Soft tissue anatomy of proximal femoral focal deficiency. *J Pediatr Orthop* 11:563, 1991
235. Sanpera I, Sparks LT: Proximal femoral focal deficiency: Does a radiologic classification exist? *J Pediatr Orthop* 14:34, 1994
236. Torode IP, Gillespie R: Rotationplasty of the lower limb for congenital defects of the femur. *J Bone Joint Surg* 65B:569, 1983
237. Van Nes CP: Rotation-plasty for congenital defects of the femur. Making use of the ankle of the shortened limb to control the knee joint of a prosthesis. *J Bone Joint Surg* 32B:12, 1950

Acute Suppurative (or Septic) Arthritis of the Hip

238. Bobechko WP, Mandel L: Immunology of cartilage in septic arthritis. *Clin Orthop* 108:84, 1975

239. Borman TR, Johnson RA, Sherman FC: Gallium scintigraphy for diagnosis of septic arthritis and osteomyelitis in children. *J Pediatr Orthop* 6:317, 1986

240. Chung WK, Slater GL, Bates EH: Treatment of septic arthritis of the hip by arthroscopic lavage. *J Pediatr Orthop* 13:444, 1993

241. Curtiss PH Jr: Destruction of articular cartilage in septic arthritis. I. In vitro studies. *J Bone Joint Surg* 45A:797, 1963

242. Curtiss PH Jr: The pathophysiology of joint infections. *Clin Orthop* 96:129, 1973

243. Griffin PP: Bone and joint infections in children. *Pediatr Clin North Am* 14:533, 1967

244. Griffin PP, Green WT: Hip joint infections in infants and children. *Orthop Clin North Am* 9:123, 1978

245. Herndon WA, Knauer S, Sullivan A, Gross RH: Management of septic arthritis in children. *J Pediatr Orthop* 6:576, 1986

246. Ivey M, Clark R: Arthroscopic debridement of the knee for septic arthritis. *Clin Orthop* 199:201, 1985

247. Jackson A, Nelson JD: Etiology and management of acute suppurative bone and joint infections in pediatric patients. *J Pediatr Orthop* 2:313, 1982

248. Lloyd Roberts GC: Some aspects of orthopaedic surgery in childhood. *Ann R Coll Surg* 57:25, 1975

249. Mitchell GP: Management of acquired dislocation of the hip in septic arthritis. *Orthop Clin North Am* 11:51, 1980

250. Morrissy RT: Bone and joint sepsis in children. *AAOS Instr Course Lect* 31:49, 1982

251. Nade S: Acute septic arthritis in infancy and childhood. *J Bone Joint Surg* 65B:234, 1983

252. Porat S, Goitien K, Saperia BS, Liebergall M, Abu-Dalu K, Katz S: Complications of suppurative arthritis and osteomyelitis in children. *Int Orthop* 15:205, 1991

253. Smith T: On the acute arthritis of infants. *St Bart Hosp Rep* 10:189, 1874

254. Wilson NIL, DiPaola M: Acute septic arthritis in infancy and childhood. *J Bone Joint Surg* 68B:584, 1986

Pyomyositis of Adductor Muscles of the Hip

255. DeBoeck H, Haentjens P, Verhaven E: Osteomyelitis of the acetabulum. *Acta Orthop Belg* 56:621, 1990

256. Hall RL, Callaghan JJ, Moloney E, Martinez S, Harrelson JM: Pyomyositis in a temperate climate. Presentation, diagnosis, and treatment. *J Bone Joint Surg* 72A:1240, 1990

257. Hirano T, Srinivasan G, Janakiraman N, Pleviak D, Mukhopadhyay D: Gallium 67 citrate scintigraphy in pyomyositis. *J Pediatr* 97:596, 1980

258. Perry J, Barrack RL, Burke SW, Haddad RJ Jr: Psoas abscess mimicking a septic hip. Diagnosis by computed tomography. *J Bone Joint Surg* 67A:1281, 1985

259. Tucker RE, Winter WG Jr, Del Valle C, Uematsu A, Libke R: Pyomyositis mimicking malignant tumor. Three case reports. *J Bone Joint Surg* 60A:701, 1978

Psoas Abscess and Infected Iliopsoas Bursitis

260. Firor HV: Acute psoas abscess in children. *Clin Pediatr* 11:228, 1972

261. Malhotra R, Singh KD, Bhan S, Dave PK: Primary pyogenic abscess of the psoas muscle. *J Bone Joint Surg* 74A:278, 1992

262. Manueddu CA, Hoogewoud HM, Belague F, Waldeburger M: Infective iliopsoas bursitis. A case report. *Int Orthop* 15:135, 1991

263. Schwaitzberg SD, Pokorny WJ, Thurston RS, McGill CW, Athey PA, Harberg FJ: Psoas abscess in children. *J Pediatr Surg* 20:339, 1985

Osteomyelitis

264. Abernethy LJ, Lee YC, Cole WG: Ultrasound localization of subperiosteal abscesses in children with late-acute osteomyelitis. *J Pediatr Orthop* 13:766, 1993

265. Abril JC, Castillo F, Loewinsonh AF, Rivas C, Bernacer M: Chronic recurrent multifocal osteomyelitis after acute lymphoblastic leukaemia. *Review Int Orthop* 18:126, 1994

266. Beaupré A, Carroll N: The three syndromes of iliac osteomyelitis in children. *J Bone Joint Surg* 61A:1087, 1979

267. Berard J, Chauvot P, Michel CR: Negative bone scintigraphy in osteomyelitis in children. Difficulties in interpretation. *Rev Chir Orthop* 68:475, 1982

268. Berkowitz ID, Wenzel W: "Normal" technetium bone scans in patients with acute osteomyelitis. *Am J Dis Child* 134:828, 1980

269. Buithieu J, Marton D, Duhaime M, Danais S: Ostéomyelite aigue chez l'enfant. *Union Med Can* 115:8, 1986

270. Canale ST, Harkness RM, Thomas PA, Massie JD: Does aspiration of bones and joints affect results of later bone scanning? *J Pediatr Orthop* 5:23, 1985

271. Carr AJ, Cole WG, Roberton DM, Chow CW: Chronic multifocal osteomyelitis. *J Bone Joint Surg* 75B:582, 1993

272. Choma TJ, Davlin LB, Wagner JS: Iliac osteomyelitis in the newborn presenting as nonspecific musculoskeletal sepsis. *Orthopedics* 17:632, 1994

273. Chung SMK, Borns P: Acute osteomyelitis adjacent to the sacro-iliac joint in children. Report of two cases. *J Bone Joint Surg* 55A:630, 1973

274. Cole WG: The management of chronic osteomyelitis. *Rev Clin Orthop* 264:84, 1991

275. Cole WG, Dalziel RE, Leitl S: Treatment of acute osteomyelitis in childhood. *J Bone Joint Surg* 64A:218, 1982

276. Craigen MA, Watters J, Hackett JS: The changing epidemiology of osteomyelitis in children. *J Bone Joint Surg* 74B:541, 1992

277. Demoupolos GA, Bleck EE, McDougall IR: Role of radionuclide imaging in the diagnosis of acute osteomyelitis. *J Pediatr Orthop* 8:558, 1988

278. Dirschl DR: Acute pyogenic osteomyelitis in children. *Rev Orthop Rev* 23:305, 1994

279. Dormans JP, Drummond DS: Pediatric hematogenous osteomyelitis: New trends in presentation, diagnosis and treatment. *J Am Acad Orthop Surg* 2:333, 1994

280. Ebong WW: Bilateral pelvic osteomyelitis in children with sickle-cell anemia. Report of four cases. *J Bone Joint Surg* 64A:945, 1982

281. Edwards MS, Baker CJ, Granberry WM, Barrett FF: Pelvic osteomyelitis in children. *Pediatrics* 61:62, 1978

282. Ellefsen BK, Frierson MA, Raney EM, Ogden JA: Humerus varus: A complication of neonatal, infantile, and childhood injury and infection. *J Pediatr Orthop* 14:479, 1994

283. Epps CH Jr, Bryand DD, 3rd, Coles MJ, Castro O: Osteomyelitis in patients who have sickle-cell disease. Diagnosis and management. *J Bone Joint Surg* 73A:1281, 1991

284. Epremian BE, Perez LA: Imaging strategy in osteomyelitis. *Clin Nucl Med* 2:218, 1977

285. Frederiksen B, Christiansen P, Knudsen FU: Acute osteomyelitis and septic arthritis in the neonate, risk factors and outcome. *Eur J Pediatr* 152:577, 1993

286. Giedion A, Holthusen W, Masel LF, Vischer D: Subacute and chronic "symmetrical" osteomyelitis. *Ann Radiol (Paris)* 15:329, 1972

287. Gledhill RB: Subacute osteomyelitis in children. *Clin Orthop* 96:57, 1973

288. Green NE, Beauchamp RD, Griffin PP: Primary subacute epiphyseal osteomyelitis. *J Bone Joint Surg* 63A:107, 1981

289. Green WT, Shannon MA: Osteomyelitis of infants. A disease different from osteomyelitis of older children. *Arch Surg* 32:462, 1936

290. Hoffman EB, deBeer JDV, Keys G, Anderson P: Diaphyseal primary subacute osteomyelitis in children. *J Pediatr Orthop* 10:250, 1990

291. Howard CB, Einhorn M, Dagan R, Yagupski P, Porat S: Fine-needle bone biopsy to diagnose osteomyelitis. *J Bone Joint Surg* 76B:311, 1994

292. Howard CB, Einhorn M, Dagan R, and Nyska M: Ultrasound in diagnosis and management of acute haematogenous osteomyelitis in children. *J Bone Joint Surg* 75B:79, 1993

293. Howman-Giles R, Uren R: Multifocal osteomyelitis in childhood. Review by radionuclide bone scan. *Clin Nucl Med* 17:274, 1992

294. Kaiser S, Rosenborg M: Early detection of subperiosteal abscess by ultrasonography. *Pediatr Radiol* 24:336, 1994

295. King DM, Mayo KM: Subacute haematogenous osteomyelitis. *J Bone Joint Surg* 51B:458, 1969

296. Mader JT, Landon GC, Calhoun J: Antimicrobial treatment of osteomyelitis. *Clin Orthop* 295:87, 1993

297. Mah ET, LeQuesne GW, Gent RJ, Paterson DC: Ultrasonic features of acute osteomyelitis in children. *J Bone Joint Surg* 76B:969, 1994

298. Ogden JA, Lister G: The pathology of neonatal osteomyelitis. *Pediatrics* 55:474, 1975

299. Paley D, Moseley CF, Armstrong P, Prober CG: Primary osteomyelitis caused by coagulase-negative staphylococci. *J Pediatr Orthop* 6:622, 1986

300. Roberts JM, Drummond DS, Breed AL, Chesney J: Subacute hematogenous osteomyelitis in children: A retrospective study. *J Pediatr Orthop* 2:249, 1982

301. Ross ERS, Cole WG: Treatment of subacute osteomyelitis in childhood. *J Bone Joint Surg* 67B:443, 1985

302. Scoles PV, Hilty MD, Sfakianakis GN: Bone scan patterns in acute osteomyelitis. *Clin Orthop* 153:210, 1980

303. Scott RJ, Christofersen MR, Robertson WW, Davidson RS, Rankin L, Drummond DS: Acute osteomyelitis in children: A review of 116 cases. *J Pediatr Orthop* 10:649, 1990

304. Siffert RS: The effect of juxta-epiphyseal pyogenic infection on epiphyseal growth. *Clin Orthop* 10:131, 1957

305. Teates CD, Williamson BRJ: "Hot and cold" bone lesion in acute osteomyelitis. *AJR* 129:157, 1977

306. Trueta J: Acute hematogenous osteomyelitis: Its pathology and treatment. *Bull NY Acad Med* 35:25, 1959

307. Trueta J: The normal vascular anatomy of the human femoral head during growth. *J Bone Joint Surg* 39B:358, 1957

308. Trueta J: The three types of acute hematogenous osteomyelitis. A clinical and vascular study. *J Bone Joint Surg* 41B:671, 1959

309. Wegener WA, Alavi A: Diagnostic imaging of musculoskeletal infection. *Orthop Clin North Am* 22:401, 1991

Acute Transient Synovitis of the Hip

310. Adam R, Hendry GMA, Moss J, Wild SR, Gillespie I: Arthrosonography of the irritable hip in childhood: A review of 1 year's experience. *Br J Radiol* 59:205, 1986

311. Bickerstaff DR, Neal LM, Booth AJ, Brennan PO, Bell MJ: Ultrasound examination of the irritable hip. *J Bone Joint Surg* 72B:549, 1990

312. Brown I: A study of the "capsular" shadow in disorders of the hip in children. *J Bone Joint Surg* 57B:175, 1975

313. Egund N, Wingstrand H, Forsberg L, Petterson H, Sunden G: Computed tomography and ultrasonography for diagnosis of hip joint effusion in children. *Acta Orthop Scand* 57:211, 1986

314. Futami T, Kasahara Y, Suzuki S, Ushikubo S, Tsuchiya T: Ultrasonography in transient synovitis and early Perthes' disease. *J Bone Joint Surg* 73B:635, 1991

315. Gershuni DH, Axer A, Hendel D: Arthrographic findings in Legg-Calvé-Perthes disease and transient synovitis of the hip. *J Bone Joint Surg* 60A:457, 1978

316. Gershuni DH, Hargens AR, Lee YF, Greenberg EN, Zapf R, Akeson WH: The questionable significance of hip joint tamponade in producing osteonecrosis in Legg-Calvé-Perthes syndrome. *J Pediatr Orthop* 3:280, 1983

317. Harrison MHM, Blakemore ME: A study of the "normal" hip in children with unilateral Perthes' disease. *J Bone Joint Surg* 62B:31, 1980

318. Haueisen DC, Weiner DS, Weiner SD: The characterization of "transient synovitis of the hip" in children. *J Pediatr Orthop* 6:11, 1986

319. Jacobs BW: Synovitis of the hip in children and its significance. *Pediatrics* 47:558, 1974

320. Jappinen S, Kallio P, Siponmaa A-K: Ultrasound x-ray and articular puncture in the diagnosis of synovial fluid effusion in the hip of children. *Pediatr Radiol* 14:238, 1984

321. Kallio P, Ryoppy S: Hyperpressure in juvenile hip disease. *Acta Orthop Scand* 56:211, 1985

322. Kallio P, Ryoppy S, Jappinen S, Siponmaa A-K, Jaaskelainen J, Kunnamo I: Ultrasonography in hip disease in children. *Acta Orthop Scand* 56:367, 1985

323. Kallio P, Ryoppy S, Kunnamo I: Transient synovitis and Perthes' disease. *J Bone Joint Surg* 68B:898, 1986

324. Landin LA, Danielsson LG, Wattsgard C: Transient synovitis of the hip. *J Bone Joint Surg* 69B:238, 1987

325. Lovett RW, Morse JL: A transient or ephemeral form of hip-disease, with a report of cases. *Boston Med Surg J* 127:161, 1892

326. Marchal GJ, Van Holsbeeck MT, Raes M: Transient synovitis of the hip in children: Role of US. *Radiology* 162:825, 1987

327. Nachemson A, Scheller S: A clinical and radiological follow-up study of transient synovitis of the hip. *Acta Orthop Scand* 40:479, 1969

328. Sharwood PF: The irritable hip syndrome in children. A long-term follow-up. *Acta Orthop Scand* 52:633, 1981

329. Valderrama JAF de: The "observation hip" syndrome and its late sequelae. *J Bone Joint Surg* 45B:462, 1963

330. Vegter J: The influence of joint posture on intra-articular pressure: A study of transient synovitis and Perthes' disease. *J Bone Joint Surg* 69B:71, 1987

331. Wingstrand H, Egund N, Carlin NO, Forsberg L, Gustafson T, Sunden G: Intracapsular pressure in transient synovitis of the hip. *Acta Orthop Scand* 56:204, 1985

Legg-Calvé-Perthes Disease

332. Axer A, Gershuni DH, Hendel D, Mirovski Y: Indications for femoral osteotomy in Legg-Calvé-Perthes disease. *Clin Orthop* 150:78, 1980

333. Axer A, Schiller MG, Segal D, Rzetelny V, Gershuni-Gordon DH: Subtrochanteric osteotomy in the treatment of Legg-Calvé-Perthes syndrome (L.C.P.S.). *Acta Orthop Scand* 44:31, 1973

334. Barer M: Role of innominate osteotomy in the treatment of children with Legg-Perthes disease. *Clin Orthop* 135:82, 1978

335. Bennett JT, Mazurek RT, Cash JD: Chiari's osteotomy in the treatment of Perthes' disease. *J Bone Joint Surg* 73B:225, 1991

336. Bensahel H, Bok B, Cavailloles F, Csukonyi Z: Bone scintigraphy in Perthes' disease. *J Pediatr Orthop* 3:302, 1983

337. Bjerkreim I, Hauge MF: So-called recurrent Perthes' disease. *Acta Orthop Scand* 47:181, 1976

338. Blakemore ME, Harrison MHM: A prospective study of children with untreated Catterall Group I Perthes' disease. *J Bone Joint Surg,* 61B:329, 1979

339. Bluemm RG, Falke THM, Ziedees des Plantes BGJ, Steiner RM: Early Legg-Perthes' disease (ischemic necrosis of the femoral head) demonstrated by magnetic resonance imaging. *Skelet Radiol* 14:95, 1985

340. Bobechko WP: The Toronto brace for Legg-Perthes disease. *J Bone Joint Surg* 58B:115, 1976

341. Bos CFA, Bloem JL, Bloem RM: Sequential magnetic resonance imaging in Perthes' disease. *J Bone Joint Surg* 73B:219, 1991

342. Bowen JR, Foster BK, Hartzell CR: Legg-Calvé-Perthes disease. *Clin Orthop* 185:97, 1985

343. Brotherton BJ: The long-term results of the treatment of Perthes' disease by recumbency and femoral head containment. *J Bone Joint Surg* 58B:131, 1976

344. Brotherton BJ, McKibbin B: Perthes' disease treated by prolonged recumbency and femoral head containment: A long-term appraisal. *J Bone Joint Surg* 59B:8, 1977

345. Burwell RG, Dangerfield PH, Hall DJ, Vernon CL, Harrison MHM: Perthes' disease: An anthropometric study revealing impaired and disproportionate growth. *J Bone Joint Surg* 60B:461, 1978

346. Caffey J: The early roentgenographic changes in essential coxa plana: Their significance in pathogenesis. *Am J Roentgenol* 103:620, 1968

347. Caffey JP: *Pediatric X-ray Diagnosis.* 6th ed. Vol. II. Chicago, Year Book Medical Publishers, 1972, p 1150

348. Calvé J: Sur une forme particulière de coxalgie grefée. Sur des déformations caracteristique de l'extremité superieure du fémur. *Rev Chir (Paris)* 42:54, 1910

349. Calvér R, Benugopal V, Dorgan J, Bentley G, Gimlette T: Radionuclide scanning in the early diagnosis of Perthes' disease. *J Bone Joint Surg* 63B:379, 1981

350. Canario AT, Williams L, Weintroub S, Catterall A, Lloyd-Roberts GC: A controlled study of the results of femoral osteotomy in severe Perthes' disease. *J Bone Joint Surg* 62B:438, 1980

351. Catterall A: *Legg-Calvé-Perthes' Disease.* Edinburgh, Churchill Livingstone, 1982

352. Catterall A: The natural history of Perthes' disease. *J Bone Joint Surg* 53B:37, 1971

353. Catterall A, Lloyd-Robert GC, Wynne-Davies R: Association of Perthes' disease with congenital anomalies of genitourinary tract and inguinal region. *Lancet* 1:996, 1971

354. Catterall A, Pringle J, Byers PD, Fulford GE, Kemp HBS, Dolman CL, Bell HM, McKibbin B, Ralis Z, Jensen OM, Lauritzen J, Ponseti IV, Ogden J: A review of the morphology of Perthes' disease. *J Bone Joint Surg* 64B:269, 1982

355. Chiari K: Medial displacement osteotomy of the pelvis. *Clin Orthop* 98:55, 1974

356. Chiari K, Endler M, Hackel H: Die Behandlung der Coxa magna bei M. Perthes mit der Beckenosteotomie. *Arch Orth Traum Surg* 91:183, 1978

357. Christensen F, Soballe K, Ejsted R, Luxhoj T: The Catterall classification of Perthes' disease. An assessment of reliability. *J Bone Joint Surg* 68A:614, 1985

358. Clarke TE, Finnegan TL, Fisher RL, Bunch WH, Gossling HR: Legg-Perthes disease in children less than four years old. *J Bone Joint Surg* 60A:166, 1978

359. Coates CJ, Paterson JMH, Woods KR, Catterall A, Fixsen JA: Femoral osteotomy in Perthes' disease. *J Bone Joint Surg* 72B:581, 1990

360. Conway JJ: A scintigraphic evaluation of Legg-Calvé-Perthes disease. *Sem Nucl Med,* 23:274, 1993

361. Conway JJ: Radionuclide evaluation of Legg-Calvé-Perthes disease, in *Pediatric Nuclear Medicine.* 2nd ed. New York, Springer-Verlag, 1985, pp 302–315

362. Conway JJ: Radionuclide bone scintigraphy in pediatric orthopedics. *Pediatr Clin North Am* 33:1313, 1986

363. Craig WA, Kramer WG: Combined iliac and femoral osteotomies in Legg-Calvé-Perthes syndrome. *J Bone Joint Surg* 56A:1314, 1974

364. Crutcher JP, Staheli LT: Combined osteotomy as a salvage procedure for severe Legg-Calvé-Perthes disease. *J Bone Joint Surg* 12:151, 1992

365. Curtis BH, Gunther SF, Gossling HR, Paul SW: Treatment for Legg-Perthes disease with the Newington ambulation-abduction brace. *J Bone Joint Surg* 56A:1135, 1974

366. Dekker M, van Rens ThJG, Slooff TJJH: Salter's pelvic osteotomy in the treatment of Perthes' disease. *J Bone Joint Surg* 63B:282, 1981

367. Dickens DRV, Menelaus MB: The assessment of prognosis in Perthes' disease. *J Bone Joint Surg* 60B:189, 1978

368. Dolman CL, Bell HM: The pathology of Legg-Calvé-Perthes disease. A case report. *J Bone Joint Surg* 55A:187, 1973

369. Edsberg B, Rubenstein E, Reimers J: Containment of the femoral head in Perthes' disease and its prognostic significance. *Acta Orthop Scand* 50:191, 1979

370. Ellis W: Metaphysis in Perthes' disease: A method of assessment and selection for treatment. *J Pediatr Orthop* 4:731, 1984

371. Erken EHW, Katz K: Irritable hip and Perthes' disease. *J Pediatr Orthop* 10:322, 1990

372. Ferguson AB: Early roentgenographic changes in Perthes' disease. *Clin Orthop* 1:33, 1953

373. Ferguson AB Jr: The pathology of Legg-Perthes disease and its comparison with aseptic necrosis. *Clin Orthop* 106:7, 1975

374. Fisher RL: An epidemiological study of Legg-Perthes disease. *J Bone Joint Surg* 54A:769, 1972

375. Freehafer AA: Osteochondritis dissecans following Legg-Calvé-Perthes disease. A report of one case. *J Bone Joint Surg* 42A:777, 1960

376. Freeman MAR, England JPS: Experimental infarction of the immature canine femoral head. *Proc R Soc Med* 62:431, 1969

377. Futami T, Kasahara Y, Suzuki S, Ushikubo S, Tsuchiya T: Ultrasonography in transient synovitis and early Perthes' diseases. *J Bone Joint Surg* 73B:635, 1991

378. Fulford GE, Lunn PG, Macnicol MF: A prospective study of nonoperative and operative management of Perthes' disease. *J Pediatr Orthop* 13:281, 1993

379. Gage HC: A possible early sign of Perthes' disease. *Br J Radiol* 6:295, 1933

380. Garceau GJ: Surgical treatment of coxa plana. *J Bone Joint Surg* 46B:779, 1964

381. Genez BM, Wilson MR, Houk RW, et al: Early osteonecrosis of the femoral head: Detection in high-risk patients with MR imaging. *Radiology* 168:521, 1988

382. Gershuni DH, Axer A, Hendel D: Arthrographic findings in Legg-Calvé-Perthes' disease and transient synovitis of the hip. *J Bone Joint Surg* 60A:457, 1978

383. Gershuni DH, Hargens AR, Lee Y, Greenberg EN, Zapf R, Akeson WH: The questionable significance of hip joint tamponade in producing osteonecrosis in Legg-Calvé-Perthes syndrome. *J Pediatr Orthop* 3:280, 1983

384. Girdany BR, Osman MZ: Longitudinal growth and skeletal maturation in Perthes' disease. *Radiol Clin North Am* 6:245, 1968

385. Glass RBJ, Poznanski AK, Fisher MR, Rogers LF, Tachdjian MO, Dias L, Pachman LM: Magnetic resonance imaging of pediatric hip diseases. Personal communication.

386. Gledhill RB, McIntyre JM: Transient synovitis and Legg-Calvé-Perthes disease: A comparative study. *Can Med Assoc J* 100:311, 1969

387. Goff CW: *Legg-Calvé-Perthes Syndrome and Related Osteochondroses of Youth.* Springfield, IL, Charles C Thomas, 1954

388. Gold AM: Osteochondritis dissecans of the femoral head. *Bull Hosp Joint Dis* 1:30, 1940

389. Goldman AB, Hallel T, Salvati EM, Freiberger RH: Osteochondritis dissecans complicating Legg-Perthes disease. *Radiology* 121:561, 1976

390. Gossling HR: Legg-Perthes' disease. Part III. Analysis of poor results, in *AAOS Instruct Course Lect* 22:301–305, 1973

391. Green NE, Beauchamp RD, Griffin PP: Epiphyseal extrusion as a prognostic index in Legg-Calvé-Perthes disease. *J Bone Joint Surg* 63B:900, 1981

392. Green NE, Griffin PP: Intra-osseous venous pressure in Legg-Perthes disease. *J Bone Joint Surg* 64A:666, 1982

393. Griffin PP, Green NE, Beauchamp RD: Legg-Calvé-Perthes' disease: Treatment and prognosis. *Orthop Clin North Am* 11:127, 1980

394. Guilleminet M, Barbier JM: Osteochondritis dissecans of the hip. *J Bone Joint Surg* 39B:268, 1957

395. Haas A: Umbau von Perthes'schen Krankheit in Osteochondritis Dissecans. *Zbl Chir* 64:2873, 1937

396. Hall AJ, Barker DJP, Dangerfield PH, Osmond C, Taylor JF: Small feet and Perthes' disease. A survey in Liverpool. *J Bone Joint Surg* 70B:611, 1988

397. Hall DJ, Harrison MHM: An association between congenital abnormalities and Perthes' disease of the hip. *J Bone Joint Surg* 61B:18, 1979

398. Hall G: Some observations of Perthes' disease (Robert Jones prize essay of the British Orthopaedic Association 1981). *J Bone Joint Surg* 63B:631, 1981

399. Hallel T, Salvati EA: Osteochondritis dissecans following Legg-Calvé-Perthes disease. *J Bone Joint Surg* 58A:708, 1976

400. Haraldsson S: Derotation varization osteotomy of the femur in the treatment of Perthes' disease. *Acta Orthop Scand* 44:105, 1973

401. Harrison MHM, Bassett CAL: Use of pulsed electromagnetic fields in Perthes' disease: Report of a pilot study. *J Pediatr Orthop* 4:579, 1984

402. Harrison MHM, Blakemore ME: A study of the "normal" hip in children with unilateral Perthes' disease. *J Bone Joint Surg* 62B:31, 1980

403. Harrison MHM, Menon MPA: Legg-Calvé-Perthes disease. The value of roentgenographic measurement in clinical practice with specific reference to the broomstick plaster method. *J Bone Joint Surg* 48A:1301, 1966

404. Harrison MHM, Turner MH: Containment splintage for Perthes' disease of the hip. *J Bone Joint Surg* 56B:199, 1974

405. Harrison MHM, Turner MH, Jacobs P: Skeletal immaturity in Perthes' disease. *J Bone Joint Surg* 58B:37, 1976

406. Harry JD, Gross RH: A quantitative method for evaluating results of treating Legg-Perthes syndrome. *J Pediatr Orthop* 7:671, 1987

407. Haythorn SR: Pathological changes found in material removed at operation in Legg-Calvé-Perthes disease. *J Bone Joint Surg* 31A:599, 1949

408. Heikkinen E, Lanning P, Suramo I, Puranen J: The venous drainage of the femoral neck as a prognostic sign in Perthes' disease. *Acta Orthop Scand* 51:501, 1980

409. Heikkinen ES, Puranen J, Suramo I: The effect of intertrochanteric osteotomy on the venous drainage of the femoral neck in Perthes' disease. *Acta Orthop Scand* 47:89, 1976

410. Henderson RC, Renner JB, Sturdivant MC, Greene WB: Evaluation of magnetic resonance imaging in Legg-Perthes disease: A prospective, blinded study. *J Pediatr Orthop* 10:289, 1990

411. Herring JA, Williams JJ, Neustadt JN, Early JS: Evolution of femoral head deformity during healing phase of Legg-Calvé-Perthes disease. *J Pediatr Orthop* 13:41, 1993

412. Herring JA, Neustadt JB, Williams JJ, Early JS, Browne RH: The lateral pillar classification of Legg-Calvé-Perthes disease. *J Pediatr Orthop* 12:143, 1992

413. Hoffinger SA, Henderson RC, Renner JB, Dales MC, Rab GT: Magnetic resonance evaluation of "metaphyseal" changes in Legg-Calvé-Perthes disease. *J Pediatr Orthop* 13:602, 1993

414. Howorth MB: Coxa plana. *J Bone Joint Surg* 30A:601, 1948

415. Inoue A, Freeman MAR, Vernon-Roberts B, Mizuno S: The pathogenesis of Perthes' disease. *J Bone Joint Surg* 58B:453, 1976

416. Jensen OM, Lauritzen J: Legg-Calvé-Perthes' disease. *J Bone Joint Surg* 58B:332, 1976

417. Jonsater S: Coxa plana. A histopathologic and arthrographic study. *Acta Orthop Scand* (Suppl) 12, 1953

418. Joseph B: Morphological changes in the acetabulum in Perthes' disease. *J Bone Joint Surg* 71B:756, 1989

419. Kallio P, Ryoppi S, Jappinen S, Siponmaa A-K, Jaaskelainen J, Kunnamo I: Ultrasonography in hip disease in children. *Acta Orthop Scand* 56:367, 1985

420. Kamegaya M, Shinada Y, Moriya H, Tsuchiya K, Akita T, Someya M: Acetabular remodelling in Perthes' disease after primary healing. *J Pediatr Orthop* 12:308, 1992

421. Kamhi E, MacEwen GD: Treatment of Legg-Calvé-Perthes disease. Prognostic value of Catterall's classification. *J Bone Joint Surg* 57A:651, 1975

422. Kamhi E, MacEwen GD: Osteochondritis dissecans in Legg-Calvé-Perthes disease. *J Bone Joint Surg* 57A:506, 1975

423. Karpinski MRK, Newton G, Henry APJ: The results and morbidity of varus osteotomy for Perthes' disease. *Clin Orthop* 209:30, 1986

424. Katz JF: "Abortive" Legg-Calvé-Perthes disease or developmental variation in epiphyseogenesis of the upper femur. *J Mt Sinai Hosp* 32:651, 1965

425. Katz JF: Arthrography in Legg-Calvé-Perthes disease. *J Bone Joint Surg* 50A:467, 1968

426. Katz JF: Legg-Calvé-Perthes disease. The role of distortion of normal growth mechanisms in the production of deformity. *Clin Orthop* 71:193, 1970

427. Katz JF: Recurrent Legg-Calvé-Perthes disease. *J Bone Joint Surg* 55A:833, 1973

428. Kemp HBS: Perthes' disease—the influence of intracapsular tamponade on the circulation in the hip joint of the dog. *Clin Orthop* 156:105, 1981

429. Kemp HBS, Colmeley JA: Recurrent Perthes' disease. *Br J Radiol* 44:6754, 1971

430. Keret D, Harrison MHM, Clarke NMP, Hall DJ: Coxa plana—the fate of the physis. *J Bone Joint Surg* 66A:870, 1984

431. Kleinman RG, Bleck EE: Increased blood viscosity in patients with Legg-Perthes disease: A preliminary report. *J Pediatr Orthop* 1:131, 1981

432. Klisiç P, Bauer R, Bensahel H, Grill F: Chiari's pelvic osteotomy in the treatment of Legg-Calvé-Perthes disease. *Bull Hosp Joint Dis* 45:111, 1985

433. Klisiç P, Seferovic O, Blazevic U: Indications for treatment in coxa plana. *Int Orthop* 1:33, 1977

434. Konjetzny GE: Zur Pathologie und pathologischen Anatomie der Perthes-Calve'schen Krankheit (Osteochondritis coxae deformans juvenilis). *Acta Chir Scand* 74:361, 1934

435. Kruse RW, Guille JT, Bowen JR: Shelf arthroplasty in patients who have Legg-Calvé-Perthes disease. *J Bone Joint Surg* 73A:1338, 1991

436. Lang P, Jergesen HE, Moseley ME, Block JE, Chafetz NI, Genant HK: Avascular necrosis of the femoral head: High-field-strength MR imaging with histologic correlation. *Radiology* 162:717, 1987

437. Langenskiöld A: Changes on the capital growth plate and the proximal femoral metaphysis in Legg-Calvé-Perthes disease. *Clin Orthop* 150:110, 1980

438. Lee DY, Seong SC, Choi IH, Chung CY, Chang BS: Changes of blood flow of the femoral head after subtrochanteric osteotomy in Legg-Perthes' disease: A serial scintigraphic study. *J Pediatr Orthop* 12:731, 1992

439. Legg AT: An obscure affection of the hip joint. *Boston Med Surg J* 162:202, 1910

440. Legg AT: The end results of coxa plana. *J Bone Joint Surg* 9:26, 1927

441. Legg AT: The classic: An obscure affection of the hip joint. *Clin Orthop* 79:4, 1971

442. Lindholm TS, Laurent LE, Osterman K, Snellman O: Perthes disease of a severe type developing after satisfactory closed reduction of congenital dislocation of the hip. *J Bone Joint Surg* 60:15, 1978

443. Lloyd-Roberts GC: Editorials and annotations. The management of Perthes' disease. *J Bone Joint Surg* 64B:1, 1982

444. Loder RT, Farley FA, Herring JA, Schork MA, Shyr Y: Bone age determination in children with Legg-Calvé-Perthes disease: A comparison of two methods. *J Pediatr Orthop* 15:90, 1995

445. Loder RT, Schwartz EM, Hensinger RN: Behavioral characteristics of children with Legg-Calvé-Perthes disease. *J Pediatr Orthop* 13:598, 1993

446. Markisz JA, Knowles RJR, Altchek DW, Schneider R, Whalen JP, Cahill PT: Segmental patterns of avascular necrosis of the femoral heads: Early detection with MR imaging. *Radiology* 162:717, 1987

447. Martinez AG, Weinstein SL, Dietz FR: The weight-bearing abduction brace for the treatment of Legg-Perthes disease. *J Bone Joint Surg* 74A:12, 1992

448. McAndrew MP, Weinstein SL: A long-term follow-up of Legg-Calvé-Perthes disease. *J Bone Joint Surg* 66A:860, 1984

449. McElwain JP, Regan BF, Dowling F, Fogarty E: Derotational varus osteotomy in Perthes disease. *J Pediatr Orthop* 5:195, 1985

450. McKay D: Cheilectomy in Legg-Calvé-Perthes: Indications, technique and results. *Orthop Clin North Am* 11:141, 1980

451. McKibbin B, Ralis Z: Pathological changes in a case of Perthes' disease. *J Bone Joint Surg* 56B:438, 1974

452. Meehan PL, Angel D, Nelson JM: The Scottish Rite abduction orthosis for the treatment of Legg-Perthes disease. A radiographic analysis. *J Bone Joint Surg* 74A:2, 1992

453. Meyer J: Dysplasia epiphysealis capitis femoris. A clinical-radiological syndrome and its relationship to Legg-Calvé-Perthes disease. *Acta Orthop Scand* 34:183, 1964

454. Mirosky Y, Axer A, Hendel D: Residual shortening after osteotomy for Perthes' disease. *J Bone Joint Surg* 66B:184, 1984

455. Molloy MK, MacMahon B: Incidence of Legg-Perthes' disease (osteochondritis dissecans). *N Engl J Med* 275:988, 1966

456. Mose K: *Legg-Calvé-Perthes Disease.* Thesis. Aarhus, Denmark, Universitetsforlaget I Aarhus, 1964

457. Mose K, Hjorth L, Ulfeldt M, Christensen ER, Jensen A: Legg-Calvé-Perthes disease: The late occurrence of coxarthrosis. *Acta Orthop Scand* (Suppl) 169, 1977

458. Mukherjee A, Fabry G: Evaluation of the prognostic indices in Legg-Calvé-Perthes disease: Statistical analysis of 116 hips. *J Pediatr Orthop* 10:153, 1990

459. Neidel J, Boddenberg B, Zander D, Schicha H, Rutt J, Hackenbroch MH: Thyroid function in Legg-Calvé-Perthes disease: Cross-sectional and longitudinal study. *J Pediatr Orthop* 13:592, 1993

460. Neidel J, Zander D, Hackenbroch MH: Low plasma-levels of insulin-like growth factor I in Perthes' disease. *Acta Orthop Scand* 63:393, 1992

461. O'Garra JA: The radiographic changes in Perthes' disease. *J Bone Joint Surg* 41B:465, 1959

462. Olney BW, Asher MA: Combined innominate and femoral osteotomy for the treatment of severe Legg-Calvé-Perthes disease. *J Pediatr Orthop* 5:645, 1985

463. Paterson D, Savage JP: The nuclide bone scan in the diagnosis of Perthes' disease. *Clin Orthop* 209:23, 1986

464. Pauwels F: Des affections de la hanche d'origine mechanique et de leur traitement par l'ostéotomie d'adduction. *Rev Chir Orthop* 37:22, 1951

465. Perthes G: Ueber Ostéochondritis déformans juvénilis. *Arch Klin Chir* 101:779, 1913

466. Perthes GC: Uber arthritis déformans juvénilis. *Dtsch Z Chir* 107:111, 1910

467. Petrie JG, Bitenc I: The abduction weight-bearing treatment in Legg-Perthes disease. *J Bone Joint Surg* 53B:54, 1971

468. Petterson H, Wingstrand H, Thambert C, Nilsson IM, Jonsson K: Legg-Calvé-Perthes disease in hemophilia: Incidence and etiologic considerations. *J Pediatr Orthop* 10:28, 1990

469. Phemister DB: Operation for epiphysitis of the head of the femur (Perthes' disease). Findings and results. *Arch Surg* 2:221, 1921

470. Phemister DB: Repair of bone in the presence of aseptic necrosis resulting from fractures, transplantations and vascular obstruction. *J Bone Joint Surg* 12:769, 1930

471. Pinto MR, Peterson HA, Berquist TH: Magnetic resonance imaging in early diagnosis of Legg-Calvé-Perthes' disease. *J Pediatr Orthop* 9:19, 1989

472. Ponseti I: Legg-Perthes disease. Observations on pathological changes in two cases. *J Bone Joint Surg* 38A:739, 1956

473. Ponseti I, Cotton RL: Legg-Calvé-Perthes disease pathogenesis and evolution. Failure of treatment with L-triiodothyronine. *J Bone Joint Surg* 43A:261, 1961

474. Ponseti I, Maynard JA, Weinstein SL, Ippolito EO, Pous JG: Legg-Calvé-Perthes disease. Histochemical and ultrastructural observations of the epiphyseal cartilage and physis. *J Bone Joint Surg* 65A:797, 1983

475. Puranen J, Heikkinen E: Intertrochanteric osteotomy in the treatment of Perthes' disease. *Acta Orthop Scand* 47:79, 1976

476. Purvis JM, Dimon JH, Meehan PL, Lovell WW: Preliminary experience with the Scottish Rite Hospital abduction orthosis for Legg-Perthes disease. *Clin Orthop* 150:49, 1980

477. Quain S, Catterall A: Hinge abduction of the hip. *J Bone Joint Surg* 68B:61, 1986

478. Rab GT: Biomechanical aspects of Salter osteotomy. *Clin Orthop* 132:82, 1978

479. Rab GT, DeNatale JS, Herrman LR: Three-dimensional finite element analysis of Legg-Calvé-Perthes disease. *J Pediatr Orthop* 2:39, 1982

480. Rab GT, Wyatt M, Sutherland DH, Simon SR: A technique for determining femoral head containment during gait. *J Pediatr Orthop* 5:8, 1985

481. Ralston EL: Legg-Perthes disease and physical development. *J Bone Joint Surg* 37A:647, 1955

482. Ralston EL: Legg-Calvé-Perthes disease—factors in healing. *J Bone Joint Surg* 43A:249, 1961

483. Rayner PHW, Schwalbe SL, Hall DJ: An assessment of endocrine function in boys with Perthes' disease. *Clin Orthop* 209:124, 1986

484. Richards S, Coleman SS: Subluxation of the femoral head in coxa plana. *J Bone Joint Surg* 69:1312, 1987

485. Ritterbusch JF, Shantharam SS, Gelinas C: Comparison of lateral Pillar classification and Catterall classification of Legg-Calvé-Perthes' disease. *J Pediatr Orthop* 13:200, 1993

486. Robichon J, Desjardin JP, Koch M, Hooper CE: The femoral neck in Legg-Perthes disease, its relationship to epiphyseal change and its importance in early prognosis. *J Bone Joint Surg* 56B:62, 1974

487. Robinson HJ, Putter H, Sigmond MB, O'Connor S, Murray KR: Innominate osteotomy in Perthes' disease. *J Pediatr Orthop* 8:426, 1988

488. Salter RB: The scientific basis for innominate osteotomy in the treatment of Legg-Perthes' disease. *J Bone Joint Surg* 55B:216, 1973

489. Salter RB: Current concepts review. The present status of surgical treatment for Legg-Perthes' disease. *J Bone Joint Surg* 66A:961, 1984

490. Salter RB, Bell M: The pathogenesis of deformity of Legg-Perthes' disease: An experimental investigation. *J Bone Joint Surg* 50B:436, 1968

491. Salter RB, Rang M, Bell M: The scientific basis for innominate osteotomy in the treatment of Legg-Perthes' disease. *Ann R Coll Phys Surg Can* 5:62, 1972

492. Salter RB, Rang M, Blackstone IW, McArthur RC, Weighill FJ, Gygi AC, Stulberg SD: Perthes' disease: The scientific basis of methods of management and their indications, in Proceedings of the Orthopaedic Associations of the English-Speaking World. *J Bone Joint Surg* 59B:127, 1977

493. Salter RB, Thompson G: Legg-Calvé-Perthes disease. The prognostic significance of the subchondral fracture and a two-group classification of the femoral head involvement. *J Bone Joint Surg* 66A:479, 1984

494. Sanchis M, Zahir A, Freeman MAR: The experimental simulation of Perthes' disease by consecutive interruptions of the blood supply to the capital femoral epiphysis in the puppy. *J Bone Joint Surg* 55A:335, 1973

495. Schepers A, von Bormann PFB, Craig JJG: Coxa magna in Perthes' disease: Treatment by Chiari pelvic osteotomy. *J Bone Joint Surg* 60B:297, 1978

496. Shapiro F: Legg-Calvé-Perthes disease. A study of lower extremity length discrepancies and skeletal maturation. *Acta Orthop Scand* 53:437, 1982

497. Simmons ED, Graham HK, Szalai JP: Interobserver variability in grading Perthes' disease. *J Bone Joint Surg* 72B: 202, 1990

498. Sjovall H: Zur Frage der Behandlung der Coxa Plana. Mit besonderer Berucksichtigung der Frimarerfolge bei Konsenquenter Ruhigstellung. *Acta Orthop Scand* 13:324, 1942

499. Smith SR, Ions GK, Gregg PJ: The radiological features of the metaphysis in Perthes' disease. *J Pediatr Orthop* 2:401, 1982

500. Snow SW, Keret D, Scarangella S, Bowen JR: Anterior impingement of the femoral head: A late phenomenon of Legg-Calvé-Perthes' disease. *J Pediatr Orthop* 13:286, 1993

501. Snyder CH: A sling for use in Legg-Perthes' disease. *J Bone Joint Surg* 29:524, 1947

502. Somerville EW: Perthes' disease of the hip. *J Bone Joint Surg* 53B:639, 1971

503. Sponseller PD, Desai SS, Millis MB: Comparison of femoral and innominate osteotomies for the treatment of Legg-Calvé-Perthes disease. *J Bone Joint Surg* 70A:1131, 1988

504. Stevens PM, Williams P, Menelaus M: Innominate osteotomy for Perthes' disease. *J Pediatr Orthop* 1:47, 1981

505. Stillman BC: Osteochondritis dissecans and coxa plana. *J Bone Joint Surg* 48B:64, 1966

506. Stulbeg SD: Legg-Calvé-Perthes Disease: Update, in *The Hip: Proceedings of the Sixth Open Scientific Meeting of the Hip Society*. St. Louis, CV Mosby, 1978, pp 263–269

507. Stulberg SD, Cooperman DR, Wallenstein R: The natural history of Legg-Calvé-Perthes disease. *J Bone Joint Surg* 63A:1095, 1981

508. Suramo I, Puranen J, Heikkinen E, Vuorinen P: Disturbed patterns of venous drainage of the femoral neck in Perthes' disease. *J Bone Joint Surg* 56B:448, 1974

509. Suranen I, Puranan J, Heikkinen E, Vourinen P: Disturbed pattern of venous drainage of the femoral neck in Perthes' disease. *J Bone Joint Surg* 56:448, 1974

510. Suzuki S, Awaya G, Okada Y, Ikeda T, Tada H: Examination by ultrasound of Legg-Calvé-Perthes disease. *Clin Orthop* 220:130, 1987

511. Tachdjian MO, Jouett LD: Trilateral socket hip abduction orthosis for the tratment of Legg-Perthes disease. *J Bone Joint Surg* 50A:1271, 1968

512. Terjesen T: Ultrasonography in the primary evaluation of patients with Perthes' disease. *J Pediatr Orthop* 13:437, 1993

513. Terjesen T, Osthus P: Ultrasound in the diagnosis and follow-up of transient synovitis of the hip. *J Pediatr Orthop* 11:608, 1991

514. Thompson GH, Westin GW: Legg-Calvé-Perthes disease: Results of discontinuing treatment in the early reossification phase. *Clin Orthop* 139:70, 1979

515. Thompson SK, Woodrow JC: HLA antigens in Perthes' disease. *J Bone Joint Surg* 63B:278, 1981

516. Uttendaele D, DeKelver L, Croene PL, Fabry G: Conservative treatment in Perthes' disease: A comparison between containment and non-containment methods of treatment. *Acta Orthop Belg* 46:414, 1980

517. Valderrama JAF: The observation hip syndrome and its late sequalae. *J Bone Joint Surg* 45B:462, 1963

518. Van der Heyden AM, van Tongerloo RS: Shelf operation in Perthes' disease. *J Bone Joint Surg* 63B:282, 1981

519. Waldenström H: Die obere tuberculose Collumherd. *Z Orthop Chir* 24:487, 1909

520. Waldenström H: *Die Tuberculose des Collum Femoris im Kindesalter und ihre Beziehunger zur Huftgilenkenzundung.* Stockholm, 1910

521. Waldenström H: On coxa plana. *Acta Chir Scand* 55:577, 1923

522. Waldenström H: The definite form of the coxa plana. *Acta Radiol* 1:384, 1922

523. Waldenström H: The first stages of coxa plana. *J Bone Joint Surg* 20:559, 1938

524. Weiner SD, Weiner DS, Riley PM: Pitfalls in treatment of Legg-Calvé-Perthes disease using proximal femoral varus osteotomy. *J Pediatr Orthop* 11:20, 1991

525. Weinstein SL: Legg-Calvé-Perthes disease, in *AAOS Instructional Course Lectures*. St. Louis, CV Mosby, 1983, pp 272–291

526. Willett K, Hudson I, Catterall A: Lateral shelf acetabuloplasty: An operation for older children with Perthes' disease. *J Pediatr Orthop* 12:563, 1992

527. Woodward AH, Decker JS: Case report: Osteochondritis dissecans following Legg-Perthes' disease. *South Med J* 69:943, 1976

528. Wynne-Davies R, Gormley J: The aetiology of Perthes' disease. *J Bone Joint Surg* 60B:6, 1978

529. Yngve DA, Roberts JM: Acetabular hypertrophy in Legg-Calvé-Perthes disease. *J Pediatr Orthop* 5:416, 1985

530. Zahir A: Experimental stimulation of Perthes' disease in the puppy. *Proc R Soc Med* 64:641, 1971

Slipped Capital Femoral Epiphysis

531. Abraham E, Garst J, Barmada R: Treatment of moderate to severe slipped capital femoral epiphysis with extracapsular base-of-neck osteotomy. *J Pediatr Orthop,* 13:294, 1993

532. Aronson DD, Carlson WE: Slipped capital femoral epiphysis. *J Bone Joint Surg* 74A:810, 1992

533. Barmada R, Bruch RF, Gimbel JS, Ray RD: Base of the neck extracapsular osteotomy for correction of deformity in slipped capital femoral epiphysis. *Clin Orthop* 132:98, 1978

534. Bassett GS: Bone endoscopy: Direct visual confirmation of cannulated screw placement in slipped capital femoral epiphysis. *J Pediatr Orthop* 13:159, 1993

535. Baynham GC, Lucie RS, Cummings RJ: Femoral neck fracture secondary to in situ pinning of slipped capital femoral epiphysis: A previously unreported complication. *J Pediatr Orthop* 11:187, 1991

536. Bennet GC, Koreska J, Rang M: Pin placement in slipped capital femoral epiphysis. *J Pediatr Orthop* 4:574, 1984

537. Betz RR, Steel HH, Emper WD, Huss GK, Clancy M: Treatment of slipped capital femoral epiphysis. *J Bone Joint Surg* 72A:587, 1990

538. Boyer DW, Mickelson MR, Ponseti IV: Slipped capital femoral epiphysis. Long-term follow-up study of one hundred and twenty-one patients. *J Bone Joint Surg* 63A:83, 1981

539. Brodetti A: The blood supply of the femoral neck and head in relation to the damaging effects of nails and screws. *J Bone Joint Surg* 42B:794, 1960

540. Carlioz H, Vogt JC, Barba L, Doursounian L: Treatment of slipped upper femoral epiphysis: 80 cases operated on over 10 years (1968–1978). *J Pediatr Orthop* 4:153, 1984

541. Carney BT, Weinstein SL, Noble J: Long-term follow-up of slipped capital femoral epiphysis. *J Bone Joint Surg* 73:667, 1991

542. Chung SMK, Batterman SC, Brighton CT: Shear strength of the human femoral capital epiphyseal plate. *J Bone Joint Surg* 58A:94, 1976

543. Crandall DG, Gabriel KR, Akbarnia BA: Second operation for slipped capital femoral epiphysis: Pin removal. *J Pediatr Orthop* 12:434, 1992

544. Crawford AH: Current concepts review. Slipped capital femoral epiphysis. *J Bone Joint Surg* 70A:1422, 1988

545. Crawford AH, MacEwen GD, Fonte D: Slipped capital femoral epiphysis co-existent with hypothyroidism. *Clin Orthop* 122:135, 1977

546. Cruess RL: The pathology of acute necrosis of cartilage in slipping of the capital femoral epiphysis. A report of two cases with pathological sections. *J Bone Joint Surg* 45A:1013, 1963

547. Denton JR: Progression of a slipped capital femoral epiphysis after fixation with a single cannulated screw. *J Bone Joint Surg* 75A:425, 1993

548. Emery RJH, Todd RC, Dunn DM: Prophylactic pinning in slipped upper femoral epiphysis. Prevention of complications. *J Bone Joint Surg* 72B:217, 1990

549. Fahey JJ, O'Brien ET: Acute slipped capital femoral epiphysis. Review of the literature and report of ten cases. *J Bone Joint Surg* 47A:1105, 1965

550. Frymoyer J: Chondrolysis of the hip following Southwick osteotomy for severe slipped capital femoral epiphysis. *Clin Orthop* 99:120, 1974

551. Futami T, Kasahara Y, Suzuki S, Seto Y, Ushikubo S: Arthroscopy for slipped capital femoral epiphysis. *J Pediatr Orthop* 12:592, 1992

552. Gelberman RH, Cohen MS, Shaw BA, Kasser JR, Griffin PP, Wilkinson RH: The association of femoral retroversion with slipped capital femoral epiphysis. *J Bone Joint Surg* 68A:1000, 1986

553. Golding JSR: Chondrolysis of the hip. *J Bone Joint Surg* 55B(Abs.):214, 1973

554. Goldman A, Schneider R, Martel W: Acute chondrolysis complicating slipped capital femoral epiphysis. *Am J Roentgenol* 130:945, 1978

555. Hansson LI: Osteosynthesis with the hook-pin in slipped capital epiphysis. *Acta Orthop Scand* 53:87, 1982

556. Harris WR: The endocrine basis for slipping of the upper femoral epiphysis. An experimental study. *J Bone Joint Surg* 32B:5, 1950

557. Harris WR, Hobson KW: Histological changes in experimentally displaced upper femoral epiphysis in rabbits. *J Bone Joint Surg* 38B:914, 1956

558. Heyman CH, Herndon CH: Epiphyseodesis for early slipping of the upper femoral epiphysis. *J Bone Joint Surg* 36A:539, 1954

559. Howorth MB: The bone-pegging operation for slipping of the capital femoral epiphysis. *Clin Orthop* 48:79, 1966

560. Imhauser G: Three-dimensional correction osteotomy in severe epiphyseal dislocation. X. SICOT-Kongress, Paris, Les Publications. *Acta Med Belg* 532, 1967

561. Kallio PE, Foster BK, LeQuesne GW, Paterson DC: Remodeling in slipped capital femoral epiphysis: Sonographic assessment after pinning. *J Pediatr Orthop* 12:438, 1992

562. Kallio PE, LeQuesne GW, Paterson DC, Foster BK, Jones JR: Ultrasonography in slipped capital femoral epiphysis. *J Bone Joint Surg* 73B:884, 1991

563. Kampner SL, Wissinger HA: Anterior slipping of the capital femoral epiphysis. A case report. *J Bone Joint Surg* 54A:1531, 1972

564. Kibiloski LJ, Doane RM, Karol LA, Haut RC, Loder RT: Biomechanical analysis of single- versus double-screw fixation in slipped capital femoral epiphysis at physiological load levels. *J Pediatr* 14:627, 1994

565. King D: Slipping capital femoral epiphysis. *Clin Orthop* 48:71, 1966

566. Klein A, Joplin RJ, Reidy JA, Hanelin J: Roentgenographic changes in nailed slipped capital femoral epiphysis. *J Bone Joint Surg* 31A:1, 1949

567. Koval KJ, Lehman WB, Rose D, Koval RP, Grant A, Strongwater A: Treatment of slipped capital femoral epiphysis with a cannulated-screw technique. *J Bone Joint Surg* 71A:1370, 1989

568. Krahn TH, Canale ST, Beaty JH, Warner WC, Lourenco P: Long-term follow-up of patients with avascular necrosis after treatment of slipped capital femoral epiphysis. *J Pediatr Orthop* 13:154, 1993

569. Kramer WG, Craig WA, Noel S: Compensating osteotomy at the base of the femoral neck for slipped capital femoral epiphysis. *J Bone Joint Surg* 58A:796, 1976

570. LaCroix P, Verbrugge J: Slipping of upper femoral epiphysis: A pathological study. *J Bone Joint Surg* 33A:371, 1951

571. Lance D, Carlioz A: Acute chondrolysis following slipped capital femoral epiphysis. A study of 41 cases. *Rev Chir Orthop* 67:437, 1981

572. Lindaman LM, Canale ST, Beaty JH, Warner WC: A fluoroscopic technique for determining the incision site for percutaneous fixation of slipped capital femoral epiphysis. *J Pediatr Orthop* 11:397, 1991

573. Loder RT, Aronson DD, Greenfield ML: The epidemiology of bilateral slipped capital femoral epiphysis. *J Bone Joint Surg* 75A:1141, 1993

574. Loder RT, Farley FA, Herzenberg JE, Hensinger RN, Kuhn JL: Narrow window of bone age in children with slipped capital femoral epiphysis. *J Pediatr Orthop* 13:290, 1993

575. Lowe HG: Avascular necrosis after slipping of the upper femoral epiphysis. *J Bone Joint Surg* 43B:686, 1961

576. Lowe HG: Necrosis of articular cartilage after slipping of the capital femoral epiphysis. Report of six cases with recovery. *J Bone Joint Surg* 52B:108, 1970

577. Maletis GB, Bassett GS: Windshield-wiper loosening: A complication of in situ screw fixation of slipped capital femoral epiphysis. *J Pediatr Orthop* 13:607, 1993

578. Mandell GA, Keret D, Harcke HT, Bowen JR: Chondrolysis: Detection by bone scintigraphy. *J Pediatr Orthop* 12:80, 1992

579. Mankin HJ, Sledge CB, Rothschild S, Eisenstein A: Chondrolysis of the hip, in *The Hip: Proceedings of the Third Open Scientific Meeting of the Hip Society.* St. Louis, CV Mosby, 1975, pp 127–135

580. Mickelson MR, Ponseti IV, Cooper RR, Maynard JA: The ultrastructure of the growth plate in slipped capital femoral epiphysis. *J Bone Joint Surg* 59A:1076, 1977

581. Morrissy RT: Slipped capital femoral epiphysis: Natural history, etiology, and treatment. *AAOS Instr Course Lect* 29: 82, 1980

582. Nguyen D, Morrissy RT: Slipped capital femoral epiphysis: Rationale for the technique of percutaneous in situ fixation. *J Pediatr Orthop* 10:341, 1990

583. O'Brien ET, Fahey JJ: Remodeling of the femoral neck after in situ pinning for slipped capital femoral epiphysis. *J Bone Joint Surg* 59A:62, 1977

584. Ogden JA, Southwick WO: Endocrine dysfunction and slipped capital femoral epiphysis: The relationship to cartilage necrosis. *Yale J Biol Med* 50:1, 1977

585. Perkins G: Treatment of adolescent coxa vara. *Br Med J* 1: 55, 1932

586. Ponseti IV, McClintock R: The pathology of slipping of the upper femoral epiphysis. *J Bone Joint Surg* 38A:71, 1956

587. Pritchett JW, Kevin DP: Mechanical factors in slipped capital femoral epiphysis. *J Pediatr Orthop* 8:385, 1988

588. Ratliff AHC: Traumatic separation of the upper femoral epiphysis in young children. *J Bone Joint Surg* 50B:757, 1968

589. Rennie AM: The inheritance of slipped upper femoral epiphysis. *J Bone Joint Surg* 64B:180, 1982

590. Scham SM: The triangular sign in the early diagnosis of slipped capital femoral epiphysis. *Clin Orthop* 103:16, 1974

591. Schmidt R, Gregg JR: Subtrochanteric fractures complicating pin fixation of slipped capital femoral epiphysis. *Orthop Trans* 9:497, 1985

592. Segal LS, Davidson RS, Robertson WW, Drummond DS: Growth disturbances of the proximal femur after pinning of juvenile slipped capital femoral epiphysis. *J Pediatr Orthop* 11:631, 1991

593. Soeur R: Etiology and pathomechanics of slipped upper femoral epiphysis. *J Bone Joint Surg* 41B:618, 1959

594. Southwick WO: Compression fixation after biplane intertrochanteric osteotomy for slipped capital femoral epiphysis. A technical improvement. *J Bone Joint Surg* 55A:1218, 1973

595. Southwick WO: Osteotomy through the lesser trochanter for slipped capital femoral epiphysis. *J Bone Joint Surg* 49A: 807, 1967

596. Speer DP: Experimental epiphysiolysis: Etiologic models of slipped capital femoral epiphysis, in *The Hip: Proceedings of the Hip Society*. St. Louis, CV Mosby, 1982, pp 68–88

597. Spero CR, Masciale JP, Tornetta P, Star MJ, Tucci JJ: Slipped capital femoral epiphysis in black children: Incidence of chondrolysis. *J Pediatr Orthop* 12:444, 1992

598. Steel HH: The metaphyseal blanch sign of slipped capital femoral epiphysis. *J Bone Joint Surg* 68A:920, 1986

599. Sternlicht AL, Ehrlich MG, Armstrong AL, Zaleske DJ: Role of pin protrusion in the etiology of chondrolysis: A surgical model with radiographic, histologic, and biochemical analysis. *J Pediatr Orthop* 12:428, 1992

600. Szypryt EP, Clement DA, Colton CL: Open reduction or epiphyseodesis for slipped capital femoral epiphysis. A comparison of Dunn's operation and the Heyman-Herndon procedure. *J Bone Joint Surg* 69B:737, 1987

601. Tillema DA, Golding JSR: Chondrolysis following slipped capital femoral epiphysis in Jamaica. *J Bone Joint Surg* 53A: 1528, 1971

602. Towbin R, Crawford AH: Neonatal traumatic proximal femoral epiphysiolysis. *Pediatrics* 63:456, 1979

603. Waldenström CH: On necrosis of the joint cartilage by epiphyseolysis capitis femoris. *Acta Chir Scand* 67:936, 1930

604. Walters R, Simons S: Joint destruction—a sequel of unrecognized pin penetration in patients with slipped capital femoral epiphysis, in *The Hip: Proceedings of the Hip Society*. St. Louis, CV Mosby, 1980, pp 145–57

605. Weiner DS, Weiner S, Melby A, Hoyt WA: A 30-year experience with bone graft epiphyseodesis in the treatment of slipped capital femoral epiphysis. *J Pediatr Orthop* 4:145, 1984

606. Wells D, King JD, Roe TF, Kaufman FR: Review of slipped capital femoral epiphysis associated with endocrine disease. *J Pediatr Orthop* 13:610, 1993

607. Yoshioka Y, Schichikawa K: Autoimmunity and chondrolysis of the hip. A report of two cases. *Int Orthop* 11:289, 1987

608. Zionts LE, Simonian PT, Harvey JP Jr: Transient penetration of the hip joint during in situ cannulated-screw fixation of slipped capital femoral epiphysis. *J Bone Joint Surg* 73A: 1054, 1991

Idiopathic Chondrolysis

609. Bleck E: Idiopathic chondrolysis of the hip. *J Bone Joint Surg* 65A:1266, 1983

610. Duncan JW, Nasca R, Schrantz J: Idiopathic chondrolysis of the hip. *J Bone Joint Surg* 61A:1024, 1979

611. Duncan JW, Schrantz JL, Nasca RJ: The bizarre stiff hip, possible idiopathic chondrolysis. *JAMA* 231:382, 1975

612. Hughes AW: Idiopathic chondrolysis of the hip: A case report and review of the literature. *Ann Rheum Dis* 44:268, 1985

613. Ippolito E, Ricciardio-Pollini PT: Chondrolysis of the hip (idiopathic and secondary forms). *Ital J Orthop Traumatol* 7:335, 1981

614. Jones BS: Adolescent chondrolysis—diagnostic difficulties. Report of four cases. *Pediatr Radiol* 14:314, 1984

615. Kozlowski K, Scougall JL: Idiopathic chondrolysis diagnostic difficulties. Report of four cases. *Pediatr Radiol* 13:314, 1983

616. Moule N, Golding J: Idiopathic chondrolysis of the hip. *Clin Radiol* 25:247, 1974

617. Roy DR, Crawford AH: Idiopathic chondrolysis of the hip: Management by subtotal capsulectomy and aggressive rehabilitation. *J Pediatr Orthop* 8:203, 1988

618. Silvanantham M, Kannan-Kutty M: Idiopathic chondrolysis of the hip: Case report with a review of the literature. *Aust NZ J Surg* 47:229, 1977

619. Sparks LT, Dall G: Idiopathic chondrolysis of the hip in adolescents. Case reports. *S Afr Med J* 61:883, 1982

620. Wenger D, Mickelson M, Ponseti I: Idiopathic chondrolysis of the hip. *J Bone Joint Surg* 57A:268, 1975

Meralgia Paresthetica

621. Edelson R, Stevens P: Meralgia paresthetica in children. *J Bone Joint Surg* 76A:993, 1994

Lower Leg Length Discrepancy

622. Aldegheri R, Renzi-Brivio L, Agostini S: The callotasis method of limb lengthening. *Clin Orthop* 241:137, 1989

623. Anderson L, Westin GW, Oppenheim WL: Syme amputation in children: Indications, results and long-term follow-up. *J Pediatr Orthop* 4:550, 1984

624. Anderson M, Green WT, Messner MB: Growth and prediction of growth in the lower extremities. *J Bone Joint Surg* 45A:1, 1963

625. Anderson M, Messner MB, Green WT: Distribution of lengths of the normal femur and tibia in children from one to eighteen years of age. *J Bone Joint Surg* 46A:1197, 1964

626. Bayley N, Pinneau SR: Tables for predicting adult height from skeletal age. Revised for use with the Greulich-Pyle Hand Standards. *J Pediatr* 40:423, 1952

627. Beals RK: Hemihypertrophy and hemihypotrophy. *Clin Orthop* 166:199, 1982

628. Bianco AJ Jr: Femoral shortening. *Clin Orthop* 136:49, 1978

629. Blair VP, Schoenecker PL, Sheridan JJ, Capelli AM: Closed femoral shortening. *J Bone Joint Surg* 71A:1440, 1989

630. Blair VP III, Walker SJ, Sheridan JJ, Schoenecker PL: Epiphysiodesis: A problem of timing. *J Pediatr Orthop* 2:281, 1982

631. Blount WP, Clark GR: Control of bone growth by epiphyseal stapling. Preliminary report. *J Bone Joint Surg* 31A:464, 1949

632. Bowen RJ, Johnson WJ: Percutaneous epiphysiodesis. *Clin Orthop* 190:170, 1984

633. Brodin H: Longitudinal bone growth. The nutrition of the epiphyseal cartilages and the local blood supply. *Acta Orthop Scand* Suppl 20, 1955

634. Canale ST, Russell TA, Holcomb RL: Percutaneous pinning: Experimental study and clinical results. *J Pediatr Orthop* 6:150, 1986

635. Catagni MA, Bolano L, Cattaneo R: Management of fibular hemimelia using the Ilizarov methods. *Orthop Clin North Am* 22:715, 1991

636. Cattaneo A, Villa A, Catagni M, Tentori L: Traitement des inégalites du fémur par la méthode d'Ilizarov. *Rev Chir Orthop* 71:405, 1985

637. Chapman ME, Duwelius PJ, Bray TJ, Gordon JE: Closed intramedullary femoral osteotomy. Shortening and derotation procedures. *Clin Orthop* 287:245, 1993

638. Choi IH, Kumar SJ, Bowen JR: Amputation or limb lengthening to partial or total absence of the fibula. *J Bone Joint Surg* 72A:1391, 1990

639. DeBastiani G, Aldegheri R, Renzi-Brivio L, Trivella G: Chondrodiatasis—controlled symmetrical distraction of the epiphyseal plate. Limb lengthening in children. *J Bone Joint Surg* 68B:550, 1986

640. DeBastiani G, Aldegheri R, Renzi-Brivio L, Trivella G: Limb lengthening by callus distraction (callotasis). *J Pediatr Orthop* 7:129, 1987

641. DePablos J, Barrios C, Canadell J: Leg lengthening by distraction through the callus of an arthrodesis. *J Bone Joint Surg* 73B:458, 1991

642. Eyre-Brook AL: Bone shortening for inequality of leg lengths. *Br Med J*, 1:222, 1951

643. Galardi G, Comi G, Lozza L, Marchettini P, Novarina M, Facchini R, Paronzini A: Peripheral nerve damage during limb lengthening. *J Bone Joint Surg* 72B:121, 1990

644. Giles LG: Low-back pain associated with leg length inequality. *Spine* 6:510, 1991

645. Giles LG: Lumbar spine structural changes associated with leg length inequality. *Spine* 7:159, 1982

646. Green WT, Anderson M: Epiphyseal arrest for the correction of discrepancies in length of the lower extremities. *J Bone Joint Surg* 39A:353, 1957

647. Green WT, Anderson M: Experiences with epiphyseal arrest in correcting discrepancies in length of the lower extremities in infantile paralysis. *J Bone Joint Surg* 29:659, 1947

648. Greulich WW, Pyle SI: *Radiographic Atlas of Skeletal Development of the Hand and Wrist,* 2nd ed. Stanford, Stanford University Press, 1959

649. Hadlow AT, Nicol RO: A formula for diaphyseal limb lengthening. *J Bone Joint Surg* 72B:146, 1990

650. Helms CA, McCarthy S: CT scanograms for measuring leg length discrepancy. *Radiology* 151:802, 1984

651. Hootnick D, Boyd NA, Fixsen JA, Lloyd-Roberts GC: The natural history and management of congenital short tibia with dysplasia or absence of the fibula. *J Bone Joint Surg* 59B:267, 1977

652. Ilizarov GA: Clinical application of the tension/stress effect for limb lengthening. *Clin Orthop* 250:8, 1990

653. Ilizarov GA: The tension/stress effect on the genesis and growth of tissues. I. The influence of stability of fixation and soft tissue preservation. *Clin Orthop* 238:249, 1989

654. Ilizarov GA: The tension/stress effect on the genesis and growth of tissues. II. The influence of the rate and frequency of distraction. *Clin Orthop* 239:263, 1989

655. Jones DC, Moseley CF: Subluxation of the knee as a complication of femoral lengthening by the Wagner technique. *J Bone Joint Surg* 67B:33, 1985

656. Kalamchi A, Cowell HR, Kim KI: Congenital deficiency of the femur. *J Pediatr Orthop* 5:129, 1985

657. Kawamura B, Mosono S, Takahashi T, Yano T, Kobayashi Y, Shibata N, Shinoda Y: Limb lengthening by means of subcutaneous osteotomy: Experimental and clinical studies. *J Bone Joint Surg* 50A:851, 1986

658. Lampe HI, Swierstra BA, Diepstraten AF: Timing of physiodesis in limb length inequality. The Straight Line Graph applied in 30 patients. *Acta Orthop Scand* 63:672, 1992

659. Miller LS, Bell DF: Management of congenital fibular deficiency by Ilizarov technique. *J Pediatr Orthop* 12:651, 1992

660. Millis MB, Hall JE: Transiliac lengthening of the lower extremity. A modified innominate osteotomy for the treatment of postural imbalance. *J Bone Joint Surg* 61A:1182, 1979

661. Monticelli G, Spinelli R: Distraction epiphysiolysis as a method of limb lengthening. I. Experimental study. *Clin Orthop* 154:254, 1981

662. Moseley CF: A straight-line graph for leg-length discrepancies. *J Bone Joint Surg* 59A:174, 1977

663. Murray DW, Kambouroglou G, Kenwright J: One-stage lengthening for femoral shortening with associated deformity. *J Bone Joint Surg* 75B:566, 1993

664. Oppenheim WL, Namba R: Closed femoral shortening modification using an internal splint. *J Pediatr Orthop* 8:609, 1988

665. Osterman K, Merikanto J: Diaphyseal bone lengthening in children using Wagner device: Long-term results. *J Pediatr Orthop* 11:449, 1991

666. Paley D: Current techniques of limb lengthening. *J Pediatr Orthop* 8:73, 1988

667. Papaioannou T, Stokes I, Kenwright MA: Scoliosis associated with limb-length inequality. *J Bone Joint Surg* 64A:59, 1982

668. Pappas AM, Nehme M: Leg length discrepancy associated with hypertrophy. *Clin Orthop* 144:198, 1979

669. Park EA, Richter CP: Transverse lines in bone; mechanism of their development. *Bull Johns Hopkins Hosp* 93:234, 1953

670. Phemister DB: Operative arrestment of longitudinal growth of bones in the treatment of deformities. *J Bone Joint Surg* 15:1, 1933

671. Pouliquen JC, Beneux J, Judet R, Cogan D: Tibia lengthening in children. Results and complications. *Rev Chir Orthop* 62(Suppl 2):125, 1978

672. Pouliquen JC, Gorodischer S, Verneret C, Richard L: Allongement du femur chez l'enfant et l'adolescent. Etude comparative d'une serie de 82 cas. *Rev Chir Orthop* (in press)

673. Price CT: Metaphyseal and physeal lengthening. *AAOS Instr Course Lect* 38:331, 1989

674. Price CT, Mann JW: Experience with the Orthofix device for limb lengthening. *Orthop Clin North Am* 22:651, 1991

675. Pyle SL, Hoerr NL: *Radiographic Atlas of Skeletal Development of the Knee.* Springfield, IL, Charles C Thomas, 1955

676. Rigault P, Boucquay P, Padovani JP, Raux P, Findori G: Progressive femoral lengthening in children. A propos of 36 cases. *Rev Chir Orthop* 66:13, 1980

677. Rigault P, Dolz G, Padovani JP, Touzet P, Mallet JF, Finidori G, Raux P: Progressive tibial lengthening in children (author's transl). *Rev Chir Orthop* 67:461, 1981

678. Salai M, Chechick A, Ganel A, Blankstein A, Horoszowski H: Subluxation of the hip joint during femoral lengthening. *J Pediatr Orthop* 5:642, 1985

679. Saleh HM, Miln EA: Weightbearing parallel beam scanography for the measurement of leg length and joint alignment. *J Bone Joint Surg* 76B:156, 1994

680. Shapiro F: Developmental patterns in lower-extremity length discrepancies. *J Bone Joint Surg* 64A:639, 1982

681. Shapiro F: Legg-Calvé-Perthes' disease: A study of lower extremity length discrepancies and skeletal maturation. *Acta Orthop Scand* 53:437, 1982

682. Shapiro F: Longitudinal growth of the femur and tibia after diaphyseal lengthening. *J Bone Joint Surg* 69A:684, 1987

683. Stanitski DF, Bullard M, Armstrong P, Stanitski C: Results of femoral lengthening using the Ilizarov technique. *J Pediatr Orthop* 15:224, 1995

684. Stephens DC: Femoral and tibial lengthening. *J Pediatr Orthop* 3:424, 1983

685. Stephens DC, Herrick W, MacEwen GD: Epiphysiodesis for limb length inequality: Results and indications. *Clin Orthop* 136:41, 1978

686. Tanner JM, Whitehouse RH, Marshall WA, Healy NJR, Goldstein H: *Assessment of Skeletal Maturity and Prediction of Adult Height (TW2 Method).* London, Academic Press, 1975

687. Thompson TC, Straub LR, Campbell RD: An evaluation of femoral shortening with intramedullary nailing. *J Bone Joint Surg* 36A:43, 1954

688. Torode IP, Gillespie R: Anteroposterior instability of the knee: A sign of congenital limb deficiency. *J Pediatr Orthop* 3:467, 1983

689. Velazquez RJ, Bell DF, Armstrong PF, Babyn P, Tibshirani R: Complications of use of Ilizarov technique in the correction of limb deformities in children. *J Bone Joint Surg* 75A:1148, 1993

690. Wagner H: Operative lengthening of the femur. *Clin Orthop* 136:125, 1978

691. Wagner H: Surgical lengthening of the femur. Report of fifty-eight cases (author's transl). *Ann Chir* 43:263, 1980

692. Wasserstein I: Distraction compression method of elongation of the lower extremity with use of bone tubular homograft. *Ortop Travmatol Protez* 29:44, 1968

693. Westh RN, Menelaus MB: A simple calculation for the timing of epiphysial arrest: A further report. *J Bone Joint Surg* 63B:117, 1981

694. Winquist RA, Hansen ST Jr, Pearson RE: Closed intramedullary shortening of the femur. *Clin Orthop* 136:54, 1978

695. Yosipovitch ZH, Palti Y: Alterations in blood pressure during leg-lengthening. A clinical and experimental investigation. *J Bone Joint Surg* 49A:1352, 1967

THE NECK AND UPPER LIMB

The neck and upper limbs are interrelated. Pain in the shoulder and upper limb may be referred from the cervical spine. An examination of the upper limb without assessing the neck is incomplete, and vice versa. The deformities and affections of the neck and upper limb are therefore presented in the same chapter.

■ NECK

The presenting complaints of neck affections are deformity, pain, stiffness, and paralysis. The pathologic process may involve (1) the bones and joints of the cervical spine, (2) the muscles and soft tissues, (3) the spinal cord or brachial plexus, (4) subclavian and carotid vessels, especially in congenital heart disease and in Marfan's syndrome, and (5) the pharynx, trachea, or thyroid gland. Always examine the head, and do not forget the lymph nodes in the triangles of the neck. The abnormality may be congenital (present at birth) or developmental (manifesting prenatally, perinatally, or postnatally); it may be due to malposture in utero which, in essence, is a packaging problem, or it may be due to paralysis, infection, inflammation, trauma, or tumor. It is always best to think of systems and organs in working out a diagnostic problem. Also, each disease has a chronology; pay attention to the age of the patient, as there is a certain age specificity in the presentation of various disease entities.

EXAMINATION

It follows a definite order. Depending upon the age of the child, the symptoms, and the condition of the patient, deviations from this order may be required.

Inspection

First, inspect the resting posture of the neck and head, in stance in the older child or in the mother's lap in the young infant or the child with delayed motor development. Is the neck in the midline or tilted to one side and the chin rotated to the opposite side? This is a physical finding of torticollis. Are the eyes level in the horizontal plane or tilted? The neck may be tilted without rotation. What is the level of the ears? Inspect the shape of the skull—is there plagiocephaly with flattening of the face on the side of the torticollis?

Palpate the fontanelles—are they open? The posterior fontanelle closes at 2 months, whereas the anterior fontanelle closes at 18 months. In hydrocephalus the fontanelles bulge. In cleidocranial dysplasia the typical appearance is a large head, small face, eyes set wider than normal, drooping shoulders, and a narrow chest. Measure the circumference of the head when there is any clinical suggestion of hydrocephaly or microcephaly.

Are the ears set low? This finding is often associated with urinary tract anomalies. Is the palate high arched? Is

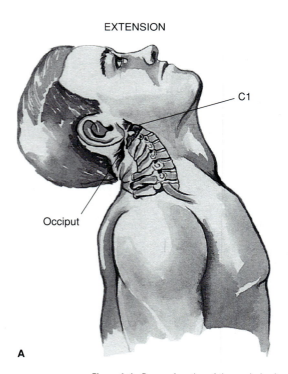

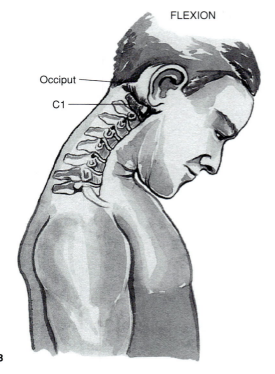

Figure 4–1. Range of motion of the cervical spine. **A.** Extension. **B.** Flexion. *(Continues)*

there a cleft palate? What is the dentition? How many teeth? A rule of thumb is that the first tooth appears at 6 months of age and then one tooth a month.

Inspect the nose and the hair of the child. Sparse, thin hair on the head, early balding, and a pear-shaped nose are findings of trichorhinophalangeal dysplasia, or Giedion syndrome. In hair-cartilage hypoplasia (metaphyseal chondrodysplasia), the hair is sparse, fine, and usually light in color.

Inspect the bridge of the nose. A depressed nasal bridge with flat facies, bulging forehead, and widespread eyes is the typical appearance of Larsen's syndrome (associated with multiple bilateral congenital dislocation of the radial heads, hips, knees, and clubfeet).

Are the eyes slanted with prominent epicanthal folds to suggest Down syndrome (trisomy 21)? When the facies has a mongoloid appearance, examine the hands. In Down syndrome, they are short and stubby with a single palmar crease with incurving of the little finger; look at the feet for increased space between the big and second toes. Atlantoaxial instability is common in Down syndrome.

Inspect the color of the sclerae—are they blue, suggesting osteogenesis imperfecta? The configuration of the skull in osteogenesis imperfecta resembles a soldier's helmet—the parietal and temporal bones are prominent, the occiput overhangs, the forehead is broad, and the face is triangular.

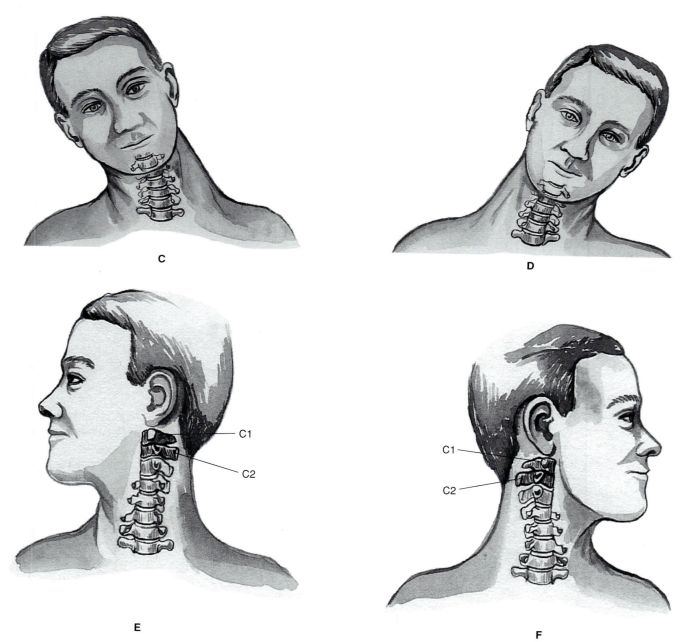

Figure 4–1 *(Continued)*. **C, D.** Lateral bending to the right and left. **E, F.** Rotation of the neck to the right and left.

Cauliflower-shaped ears are characteristic of diastrophic dysplasia, in which the hands are short and broad, the thumb metacarpals very short, and the metacarpophalangeal joints radially subluxated—resembling a hitchhiker's thumb.

These are a few examples of generalized syndromes and dysplasias to stress the importance of careful inspection of the head when examining the neck.

Range of Motion

The next step is to determine the active and passive range of motion of the cervical spine. The motions of the cervical spine are flexion and extension, lateral rotation, and lateral bending to the right and left (Fig 4–1).

Flexion-Extension

Ask the patient to touch his or her chin to the chest. Normally the child is able to touch the chin to the chest and then to bend the neck backward and look at the ceiling. About half of the range of flexion-extension movement takes place between the occiput and C1 and the remainder between C1 and C7. Sternocleidomastoid muscles are the primary flexors of the neck, and the paravertebral extensor muscle and trapezius are the primary extensors of the neck.

Rotation

Ask the child to twist the chin toward the right shoulder and then to the left shoulder. Half the rotation of the cervical spine takes place between C1 and C2 (atlantoaxial articulation); the remainder of rotation takes place between C3 and C7. The normal range of neck rotation is 60 to 80 degrees. The primary rotators of the neck are the sternocleidomastoids.

Lateral Bending

Ask the patient to touch the right ear to the right shoulder without elevating the shoulder. Repeat the same movement on the left side. Lateral bending occurs among all seven cervical vertebrae. The normal range of lateral tilting of the neck is about 45 degrees. The primary lateral benders of the neck are the scaleni anterior, medial, and posterior.

Passive range of motion of the neck is best determined with the patient supine, an assistant steadying both shoulders, and the examiner gently holding the head between his or her hands.

Palpation

Next, palpate the posterior, lateral, and anterior aspects of the neck. Posteriorly, feel the spinous process. Is there any local tenderness or enlargement of a spinous process or lamina? This is a common finding of involvement for an aneurysmal bone cyst, which presents as a painful, local mass. Next, feel the skull for any tumors, such as an os-

teoma. While examining the back of the neck, check for sensation in the posterior aspect of the head to rule out sensory deficit of the lesser and greater occipital nerves. Feel the paraspinal muscles for spasm. In the posterior triangle, rule out the presence of enlarged lymph nodes. Anteriorly and laterally, palpate the sternocleidomastoid muscle for contracture and the presence of a local mass; it is a common finding in congenital muscular torticollis. Feel the clavicles. Are there any defects in the mid- or lateral portions? Is there any local tenderness at the clavicle, acromion, or acromioclavicular joint? Feel the pulsations of the carotid and subclavian arteries.

Next feel the thyroid gland. Is it enlarged and tender on palpation? Feel the parotid glands. Palpate the mandibles for enlargement and tenderness—a common finding in Caffey's infantile cortical hyperostosis. Ask the patient to open and close his or her mouth to rule out temporomandibular derangement. Look at the pharynx for enlargement of lymph nodes and tonsils; a common cause of a stiff, painful neck is inflammatory subluxation of the upper cervical vertebrae, especially between C2 and C3. Look for a retropharyngeal mass; it is a very rare finding, but a retropharyngeal sarcoma may be the cause of pain in the neck.

Neurologic Assessment

Neurologic assessment is crucial in the examination of the neck. Carefully examine the motor strength of muscles in the upper limb; test for the presence or absence of deep tendon reflexes and perform a sensory examination to rule out anesthesia or hypesthesia. Neurologic examination is particularly important in brachial plexus paralysis and peripheral nerve injury and when spinal cord pathology is suspected.

C5 Neurologic Level. *Muscle Test.* The *deltoid muscle* is almost totally innervated by C5 (axillary nerve). Test motor strength by asking the patient to elevate his or her arm in 90 degrees of abduction, in flexion, and in extension (respectively testing the middle, anterior, and posterior parts of the deltoid) (Fig 4–2A). The *biceps brachii* muscle is innervated by the musculocutaneous nerve, having a dual level of innervation from C5 and C6. Test elbow flexion against gravity and resistance with the forearm in full supination (Fig 4–2B).

Reflex. Test the deep tendon biceps reflex. An absent or decreased biceps reflex indicates a neurologic deficit at the C5 and C6 level because the biceps brachii has a dual level of innervation at C5 and C6 (Fig 4–2C).

Sensation. Determine sensation on the skin covering the lateral aspect of the deltoid muscle in the upper arm (Fig 4–2D).

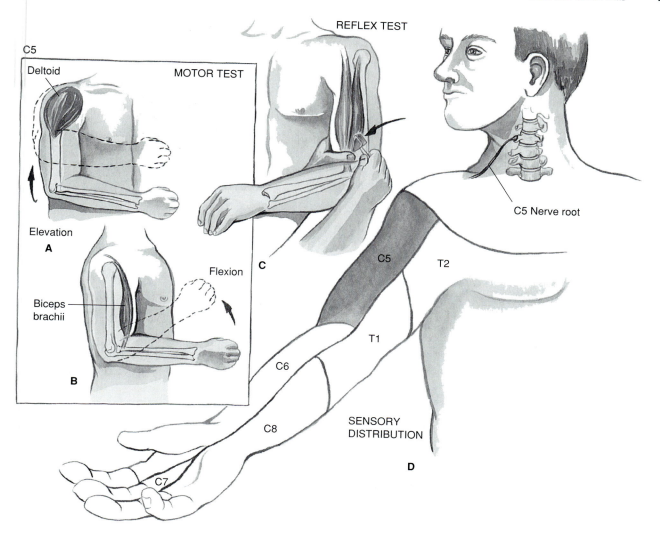

Figure 4–2. Determination of the integrity of C5 neurologic level. **A.** Testing the motor strength of the deltoid muscle. **B.** Testing the motor strength of the biceps brachii muscle. **C.** Biceps tendon reflex. **D.** Testing for sensory loss.

C6 Neurologic Level. *Muscle Test.* The muscles innervated by C6 are the biceps brachii, which are also innervated by the C5 level, and the wrist extensor group (radial nerve), which is also innervated by C7 (Fig 4–3A). This dual innervation of the wrist extensors ($C_6 + C_7$) and elbow flexors (C6 and C5) makes it difficult to assess muscle paralysis due to C6 level deficit.

Reflex. Determine the deep tendon reflexes of the brachioradialis and biceps brachii (Fig 4–3B). Their absence indicates a C6 level involvement.

Sensation. Loss of sensation of the lateral aspect of the forearm, the thumb, index, or radial half of the long finger indicates C6 level neurologic involvement (Fig 4–3C).

C7 Neurologic Level. *Muscle Test.* First, determine the motor strength of the triceps brachii by asking the patient to extend his or her elbow against gravity. The triceps brachii is innervated by the radial nerve at C7. Second, determine the motor strength of the wrist flexors—flexor carpi radialis and flexor carpi ulnaris—by asking the patient to flex the wrist against gravity, with the wrist first in radial deviation and then in ulnar deviation. Of the two wrist flexors, the flexor carpi radialis is the more important. Third, test the motor strength of the extensor digitorum communis and extensor indicis proprius by asking the patient to extend the fingers against gravity (Fig 4–4A).

Reflex. Test the triceps reflex by tapping the lower end of the triceps tendon with a reflex hammer with the elbow in flexion (Fig 4–4B).

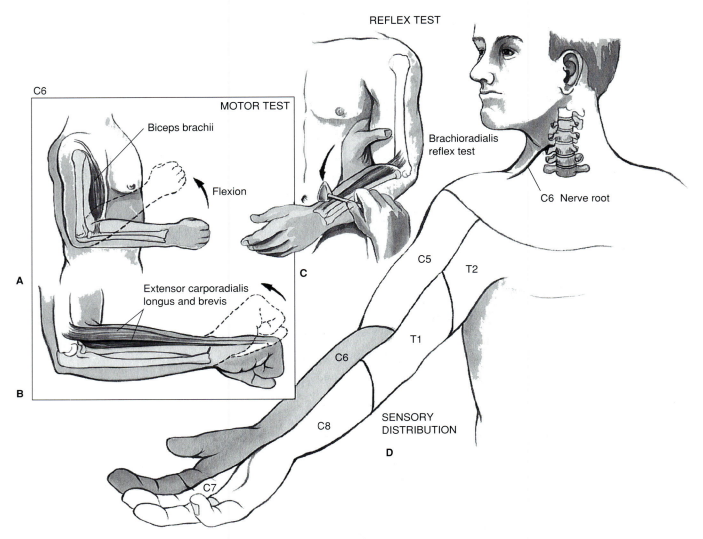

Figure 4–3. Determination of the integrity of C6 neurologic level. **A.** Testing the motor strength of the biceps brachi muscle. **B.** Testing the motor strength of the wrist dorsiflexors. **C.** Brachioradialis reflex. **D.** Testing for sensory loss.

Sensation. Absence of sensation of the volar and medial surface of the middle finger indicates C7 level neurologic involvement (Fig 4–4C).

C8 Neurologic Level. *Muscle Test..* Test the motor strength of the flexor digitorum superficialis (sublimus), which flexes the proximal interphalangeal joint, and the flexor digitorum profundis, which flexes the distal interphalangeal joint. Ask the patient to flex his or her fingers; inability to do so indicates C7 level neurologic deficit (Fig 4–5A). All of the palmar and dorsal interossei are supplied by the deep branch of the ulnar nerve (C8 + T1). To test their function, ask the patient to abduct the digits with the MP joints in full extension.

Reflex. Not present.

Sensation. Test sensation on the ulnar half of the distal forearm, the little finger, and the ulnar half of the ring finger (Fig 4–5B).

T1 Neurologic Level. *Muscle Test.* The dorsal interossei and abductor digiti quinti are tested by asking the patient to abduct the fingers with the metacarpophalangeal joint in full extension (Fig 4–6A).

Sensation. Test sensation on the medial side of the upper forearm and arm. Lack of sensation indicates T1 level neurologic involvement (Fig 4–6B).

CONGENITAL MUSCULAR TORTICOLLIS

In this asymmetric deformity of the head and neck, unilateral contracture and shortening of the sternocleidomastoid

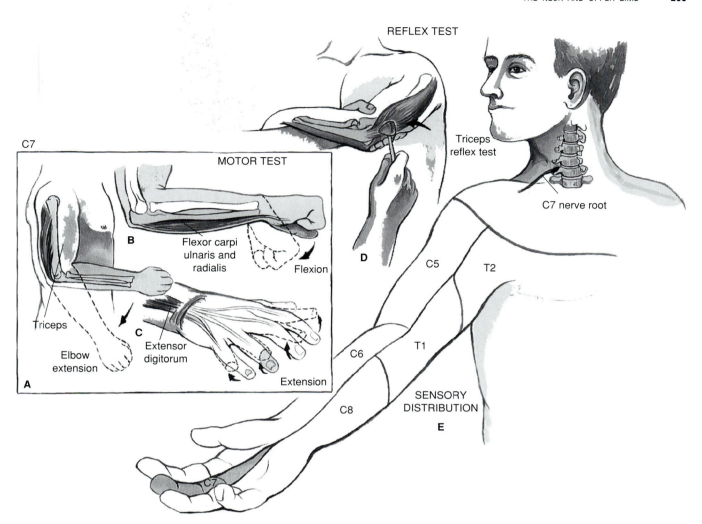

REFLEX TEST

Triceps reflex test

C7 nerve root

MOTOR TEST

C7

B

Flexor carpi ulnaris and radialis

Flexion

D

Triceps

C

Extensor digitorum

Elbow extension

A

Extension

C5

T2

T1

C6

C8

C7

SENSORY DISTRIBUTION

E

Figure 4–4. Determination of the integrity of C7 neurologic level. **A.** Testing the motor strength of the triceps brachii. **B.** Testing the motor strength of the wrist flexors. **C.** Testing the motor strength of the finger extensors. **D.** Triceps reflex. **E.** Testing for sensory loss. Note that C7 supplies the middle finger.

muscle causes the head to be tilted toward the involved side and the chin rotated toward the opposite shoulder (Fig 4–7A).

The deformity is more common in girls than in boys; the right side is involved in about 75 percent of the cases.[19] One out of five infants (20 percent) with congenital muscular torticollis have developmental dysplasia of the hip.[12] The condition is not genetic, and a family history is usually not present.

Etiology. The deformity is caused by fibrosis of the sternocleidomastoid muscle, which becomes contracted and shortened. The exact cause of muscle fibrosis in congenital muscular torticollis is not yet determined. Experimentally, in animals, venous occlusion produces edema, degeneration, acute inflammation, and eventually fibrosis of muscle fibers. Muscle fibrosis could not be produced experimentally by intramuscular hemorrhage, denervation, or occlu-

sion of the arterial supply.[2] Breech or difficult forceps deliveries are commonly present in the birth histories of infants with congenital muscular torticollis. Trauma and intramuscular hemorrhage have been proposed as etiologic factors; however, histologic examination of surgical specimens discloses no evidence of hemorrhage, hemosiderin, or reaction to trauma.[5] Congenital muscular torticollis is not caused by birth trauma. The deformity is present in infants born by normal delivery and by caesarean section.

The scientific and clinical evidence indicates that congenital muscular torticollis is most probably the result of local venous occlusion resulting from intrauterine malposition and compartment syndrome.[9]

Clinical Findings. The clinical appearance of the head tilted toward the contracted muscle and the chin rotated toward the contralateral shoulder is present at birth, or it may de-

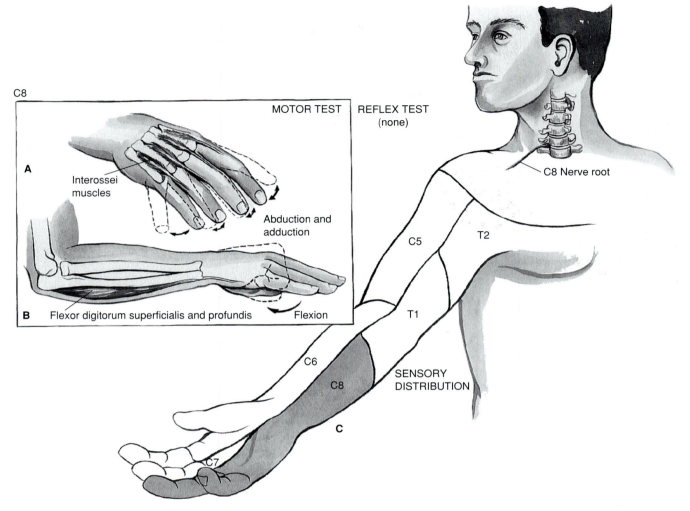

Figure 4–5. Determination of the integrity of C8 neurologic level. **A.** Testing the motor strength of the interossei. **B.** Testing the motor strength of the finger flexors. **C.** Testing for sensory loss. Note that C8 supplies the ring and little fingers of the hands and the lower half of the ulnar aspect of the forearm.

velop in the early neonatal period at about the second or third week of life. Lateral tilting of the head to the opposite side and rotation of the chin to the involved side are restricted.

During the first month of life, inspection and palpation of the involved sternocleidomastoid muscle disclose a fusiform swelling (or "tumor") in the sternal and clavicular heads. Ordinarily the superior portion of the muscle near its mastoid attachment is spared. The mass is nontender; it is initially semisoft but later becomes hard. It gradually enlarges during the following 2 to 4 weeks of life, attaining a maximum size of the distal phalanx of the adult thumb. Then it gradually regresses and disappears at 4 to 6 months of age. The mass may escape notice—a frequent occurrence (four out of five) in the series of congenital muscular torticollis reported by Coventry and Harris.[8]

In the 6-month and older infant the affected sternocleidomastoid muscle is contracted, cordlike, and shortened.

Secondary deformities of the face and head develop within the first year if the torticollis is left untreated. The face on the side of the contracted muscle becomes flattened—this is caused by external pressure on the facial bones due to position of the infant when sleeping in prone posture. In North America, most babies sleep prone; when placed face down, the infant spontaneously rotates the neck so that the affected side is down on the bed because that position is more comfortable. As a result, the face and ipsilateral skull flatten due to remodeling to conform to the bed. Asymmetry of the face increases with skeletal growth. The level of the eyes and ears becomes uneven. The child may complain of eyestrain. Cervicothoracic scoliosis with concavity to the affected side gradually develops in untreated cases.

Diagnosis. In taking the *history* of an infant with torticollis, ask the following specific questions: (1) The *birth order*—torticollis is more common in the first born. (2) The

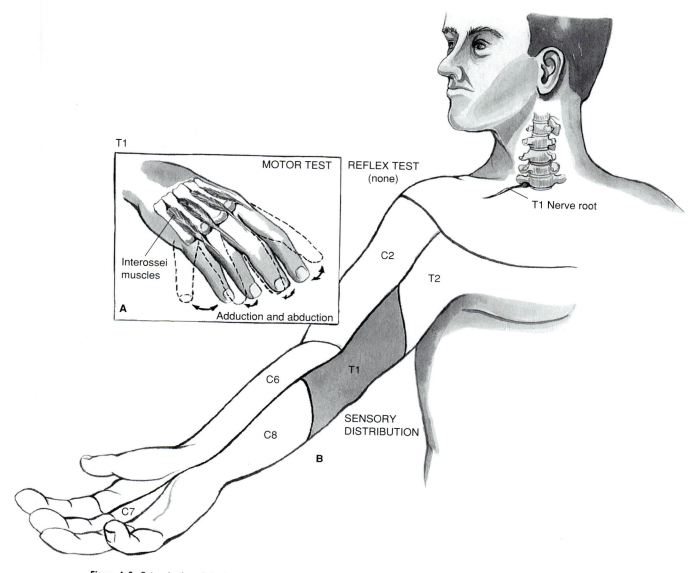

Figure 4–6. Determination of the integrity of T1 neurologic level. **A.** Interossei. **B.** Testing for sensory loss. Note that T1 supplies sensation to the medial aspect of the upper half of the forearm and arm.

presentation at birth—it is more frequent in breech and difficult forceps deliveries. (3) Were there any *injuries* or evidence of trauma? Was the clavicle fractured by compression of the shoulders during difficult delivery? When the clavicle is fractured, the tension on the sternocleidomastoid muscle tilts the head toward the affected side and rotates the chin toward the opposite side. In the neonate misdiagnosis of fracture of the clavicle as congenital muscular torticollis is not uncommon. (4) *Movements of the upper limbs,* spontaneous or by reflex stimulation—were they present or absent? In congenital muscular torticollis and fractured clavicle they are present, whereas in obstetrical brachial plexus paralysis the involved upper limb lies motionless at the side of the trunk with the elbow in extension. Did the baby move the fingers with a normal grasp

reflex? (5) Was there any obvious *deformity of the lower limbs?* Did the feet turn in (metatarsus varus) or turn out (calcaneovalgus or metatarsus valgus)? Did one lower limb appear longer than the other? This is seen in postural torticollis associated with congenital pelvic obliquity. During diaper changes, was one hip stiffer than the other? Hip adduction contracture is commonly present in postural torticollis. (6) Are there any *eye problems* such as vision deficits, ptosis, miosis, or enophthalmos? (7) The *deformity of the head and neck* observed by the parents. Is the head tilted to one side and the chin rotated to the opposite side, or is only the head tilted without rotatory deformity? Simple tilting of the head without rotation indicates a more diffuse problem such as inflammatory disease (cervical lymphadenitis or rheumatoid arthritis) or a painful bony

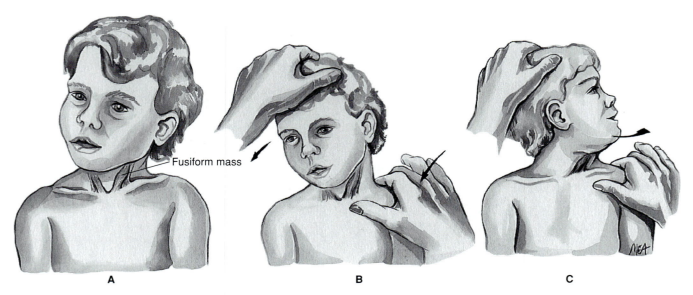

Figure 4–7. Congenital muscular torticollis. **A.** Congenital muscular torticollis on the left. Note that the head is tilted to the left and the chin rotated to the right. Note the contracted sternocleidomastoid muscle and the fusiform mass in its distal half. **B, C.** Passive stretching exercises. With one hand, steady the left shoulder gently but firmly. With the other hand, tilt the head to the right and then rotate it to the left. The neck is in neutral extension and not in flexion.

lesion such as osteoid osteoma or osteoblastoma. True torticollis (head-tilting and rotation) indicates a C1–C2 affliction or congenital muscular torticollis. (8) *Rigidity of the deformity*—is the deformity fixed or flexible? Does the infant voluntarily and actively rotate the chin from one side to the other? Is there any shifting torticollis—one day the left side and the next day the right side? Shifting torticollis suggests tumor of the spinal cord or brain (posterior fossa), hydromyelia, or syringomyelia. (9) Did the parents or pediatrician note any mass or "tumor" in the sternocleidomastoid muscle? Inquire about the age of the infant when the "tumor" was noted. Did it enlarge? How big? Is it regressing? When did it disappear? Was it tender? (10) Were there any events or findings at the birth or during the neonatal period to indicate brain damage? Inquire about the Apgar rating and appearance and color of the newborn. Was there any cyanosis or respiratory problems? How many minutes did it take for the infant's first breath or cry? Did he or she receive oxygen? Any seizures? Any jaundice? Was the muscle tone at birth normal, rigid, or flaccid? Were sucking and feeding normal? (11) Any gastroesophageal reflux? (12) Is the infant receiving any medication? Is there any evidence of drug intoxication?

The *examination* of an infant with torticollis should be methodical and thorough. A cardinal rule—do not begin your examination by twisting and stretching the neck! The infant begins to scream and becomes feisty. First, examine the lower limbs, feet first, and proceed cephalad through the leg, knee, hip, trunk, and neck. Babies, like adults, enjoy palpation of their feet; they smile and cooperate during the rest of the examination. Rule out talipes varus or metatarsus varus or valgus. Do the knees and hips have 5 to

15 degrees of flexion deformity? In the first 2 to 3 months of life, knee and hip flexion deformity is normal. Hyperextension of the knee and hip is abnormal, suggestive of hip dysplasia. The hips should be thoroughly examined to rule out hip subluxation or dislocation; because of intrauterine malposition and breech delivery these infants are at high risk for hip dysplasia.[12,24] If there is any hip abnormality, ultrasonograms of the hips should be made. Reexamine the hips of infants with congenital muscular torticollis at 6 weeks, 3 months, 6 months, and 1 year to rule out postnatal developmental hip subluxation or dislocation.

Congenital pelvic obliquity is ruled out by inspection of the popliteal, thigh, and inguinal creases with the lower limbs held parallel and determination of range of hip abduction in supine position and adduction with the infant prone to rule out abduction contracture. Are the anterosuperior and posterior iliac spines level?

Postural torticollis is due to shortening of the sternocleidomastoid muscle caused by intrauterine malposture. Because there is no true fibrotic contracture of the muscles, it responds quickly to passive manipulation exercises.

The spine is examined for scoliosis, especially in the cervicothoracic area. Look for rotation of the vertebrae. Are the shoulders level? Are there any external stigmata of vertebral column deficit, such as a tuft of hair or hemangioma? Is the neck short? Klippel-Feil syndrome is suggested by a low posterior hairline and short neck; it may be associated with torticollis due either to contracture of the sternocleidomastoid or to congenital vertebral bony deformities.

Finally, inspect the posture of the head and neck. Is the head simply tilted to one side, or is it tilted and the chin rotated to the opposite side? Look for ipsilateral flattening of the face and skull. Be cautious! Plagiocephaly is not always positional and acquired; it may be congenital, resulting from synostosis of the coronal sutures. Measure the head circumference. Is it small for the age of the patient? Palpate the calvarium. Are the anterior and/or posterior fontanelles open or closed? Make radiograms of the skull if congenital plagiocephaly due to craniostenosis is suspected.

The characteristic finding of congenital muscular torticollis is the fibrous, cordlike contracture of the sternocleidomastoid muscle. Extend the neck; palpate the muscle for contracture, and look for swelling ("tumor") on the distal half of the sternocleidomastoid muscle. Determine and record the range of neck motion. What is the degree of restriction of rotation of the neck to the side of the deformity and tilting of the head to the opposite side.

Not all torticollis is caused by contracture of the sternocleidomastoid. It may be due to shortening of the scaleneus anterior or omohyoid. Is the sternocleidomastoid muscle present? Unilateral congenital absence of the sternocleidomastoid may cause torticollis. Look for pterygium coli; the head may be tilted due to a contracted web of skin along the side of the neck. Palpate the clavicle for tenderness, crepitation, and local swelling. Is the ipsilateral shoulder drooping? Rule out fracture of the clavicle, which causes wry neck posture.

What is the level of the eyes and ears? Are they uneven? Is a visual or hearing disturbance causing the head tilt?

Palpate the neck for enlarged and tender lymph nodes. Cervical lymphadenitis causes pain and spasm of muscles along the side of the neck and results in wry neck posture. Inspect the throat. Is there any tumor or inflammation of the posterior pharynx, tonsillitis, or retropharyngeal abscess? Spontaneous hyperemic subluxation of the atlas causes torticollis.

Examine the peripheral joints for inflammatory disease. Rule out rheumatoid arthritis.

Is there spasm and tenderness of the posterior neck muscles? Pain is not a feature of congenital muscular torticollis. Acute calcification of a cervical disc may cause torticollis.

Tumors of the spinal cord or brain (posterior fossa) should be ruled out. The initial presenting deformity of a spinal cord tumor (if located in the cervical region) may be torticollis; muscle spasm is a common finding, particularly in the paravertebral muscles. Perform a thorough neurologic examination. Is there motor weakness—flaccid or spastic? Hemiparesis is suggested when the child uses one hand to the exclusion of the other when playing with toys. Rule out muscle atrophy. Check the deep tendon reflexes in the upper and lower limbs—are they diminished or absent? Are there abnormal reflexes such as a positive Babinski or Hoffmann sign?

Is there any sensory deficit, such as diminished awareness of pin prick? Check for presence of cremasteric reflex,

superficial abdominal skin reflex, and Beevor's sign. Is there dribbling of urine or a lax anal sphincter?

Every child with wry neck should have adequate radiograms of the cervical spine made to rule out osseous anomalies and skeletal torticollis. Congenital anomalies of the vertebrae that cause torticollis are hemivertebrae, Klippel-Feil syndrome, asymmetric facet joints or unilateral absence of C1 facet (hemiatlas), unilateral atlanto-occipital fusion, basilar impression, hypoplasia and asymmetry of the occipital condyles, occipital vertebrae, and anomalies of the odontoid such as absence or hypoplasia or os odontoideum.[10] Radiograms of the cervical spine also disclose acquired causes of torticollis, such as atlantoaxial rotary displacement (subluxation or dislocation) or fractures. Tumors of the vertebral column such as osteoblastoma, osteoid osteoma, and chordoma cause torticollis.

Other rare causes of intermittent torticollis in the child and adolescent are benign spasmodic torticollis, dystonia musculorum deformans, and hysterical or psychogenic wry neck. Gastroesophageal reflux may cause posturing of the neck and trunk in torticollis (Sandifer's syndrome).[23] The differential diagnosis of torticollis is given in Table 4–1.

Treatment. In the infant treatment consists of passive exercises to stretch the contracted sternocleidomastoid muscle. They are performed by the parents after adequate instruction.

The infant is placed supine on the mother's lap or the bed with the neck in comfortable extended position. Do not hyperextend the neck, as it will be painful!

Apply countertraction by holding the ipsilateral shoulder and chest with one hand and with the other hand tilting the head laterally away from the contracted muscle so that the opposite ear touches the contralateral shoulder; then rotate the chin toward the contracted muscle. Hold the muscle stretched to the count of 10. The exercises are performed 20 to 30 times each session, four to six sessions a day (Fig 4–7B, C).

Prone posture aggravates the flattening of the ipsilateral face and the contracture. Supine posture enhances the development of infantile scoliosis. When an infant is placed supine, wrapped in a blanket, he or she tends to roll to one side. This "side-lying" promotes the plastic deformation of the cartilaginous thoracic cage due to the influence of gravity and results in scoliosis. Therefore, parents are instructed to lay the infant part time supine and part time prone. The infant is stimulated to rotate his head to look toward the involved side, thereby actively stretching the muscle.

Ordinarily such conservative measures are successful in correcting the deformity in about 80 to 90 percent of the cases when passive stretching exercises are begun early in infancy and performed correctly every day. Occasionally a head-neck-chest orthosis is used in the older infant to maintain the head and neck in slightly overcorrected position.

TABLE 4–1. DIFFERENTIAL DIAGNOSIS OF TORTICOLLIS

Muscular
Congenital
    Postural torticollis—due to shortening of the sternocleidomastoid muscle caused
      by intrauterine malposture
    Muscular torticollis—due to fibrotic contracture of the sternocleidomastoid
      muscle
    Muscular torticollis—due to contracture of the scalenus anterior and/or
      omohyoid (very rare)
    Torticollis caused by unilateral congenital absence of the sternocleidomastoid
      muscle (very rare)
Acquired—unilateral inflammatory conditions
    causing irritation and spasm of ipsilateral sternocleidomastoid and other neck
    muscles (Note: the condition is painful.)
      Cervical lymphadenitis
      Tuberculosis
      Rheumatoid arthritis
      Retropharyngeal abscess
      Retropharyngeal tumors
Skin
    Pterygium coli—congenital skin web on the side of the neck
    Acquired unilateral skin contracture—on side of neck, postsurgical, burns
Skeletal
    Congenital anomalies
      Hemivertebrae
      Klippel-Feil syndrome
      Unilateral atlanto-occipital fusion
      Unilateral absence of C1 facet (hemiatlas)
      Asymmetric facet joints in cervical spine
      Basilar impression
      Hypoplasia and asymmetry of the occipital condyles
      Occipital vertebra
      Anomalies of the odontoid, such as absence or hyperplasia or os odontoideum
    Acquired
      Atlantoaxial rotary displacement, subluxation, dislocation
      Fracture
      Tumors of vertebral column such as osteoid osteoma, osteoblastoma
      Acute calcification of cervical disc
      Clavicle—fracture, osteomyelitis
Neurogenic
    Cervical spinal cord tumor
    Brain tumor—posterior fossa
    Syringomyelia
    Benign spasmodic torticollis
    Dystonia musculorum deformans
    Hysterical or psychogenic torticollis
Other
    Gastroesophageal reflux—Sandifer's syndrome

Surgical Treatment. In the child 12 to 18 months and older, it is unlikely that manipulation can adequately stretch the fibrous cord that replaces the sternocleidomastoid muscle. Surgical division of the sternocleidomastoid muscle is indicated, particularly if the restriction of range of rotation of the neck is greater than 30 degrees and there is facial deformity.[4] This author recommends distal release of the sternocleidomastoid muscle by partial excision of its clavicular attachment and Z-lengthening of the sternal attachment; the latter technique preserves the normal V contour of the neck provided by the sternocleidomastoid muscle and therefore

is esthetically more pleasing. In severe, neglected cases in the older patient, a bipolar release may have to be performed by sectioning the mastoid origin in addition to distal release. Injury to the spinal accessory nerve is a potential complication. Complete excision of the sternocleidomastoid muscle should not be performed. The end result of surgery is usually very satisfactory.

ACQUIRED CAUSES OF TORTICOLLIS

Atlantoaxial Rotary Displacement (Subluxation)

This is the most common cause of acquired torticollis in childhood. Following a minor injury or an upper respiratory infection, the child presents with the head tilted to one side and the chin rotated to the opposite side.

Initially the condition is painful, unlike congenital torticollis, which is not symptomatic. The pain and muscle spasm occur in the region of the sternocleidomastoid muscle on the side opposite the torticollis. The child resists any attempt to move the head. Inspect the child's face to rule out plagiocephaly. Palpate the neck and supraclavicular region for enlarged lymph nodes. Inspect the throat to rule out pharyngitis and enlarged tonsils. Upper respiratory infection causes hyperemia and ligamentous hyperlaxity, which causes the rotary displacement. Palpate the clavicle carefully to rule out osteomyelitis and tumors such as eosinophilic granuloma, osteoblastoma, or Ewing's sarcoma. A painful lesion on the clavicle causes torticollis.

Imaging Findings. Routine radiograms consist of open-mouth views and AP and lateral views with the lateral projection made with the neck in acute flexion and extension and in neutral position. Often it is difficult to interpret the open-mouth views because of unsatisfactory positioning of the neck. In the AP views, the lateral mass of C1 that is rotated anteriorly appears wider and closer to the midline, whereas the lateral mass that has rotated posteriorly appears narrower and away from the midline. These medial and lateral offsets of the lateral masses can also be produced in a normal neck with rotation of the head. Therefore, these findings are not diagnostic of rotary subluxation.

Flexion and extension views of the cervical spine show anterior or posterior shift with the rotary displacement. Instruct the radiologic technician to center the tube immediately distal to the mastoid process. Cineradiography is not recommended because of the high radiation doses. Dynamic CT depicts the subluxation, but I do not recommend it initially because of the high degree of radiation. The diagnosis is best made on clinical history and physical findings. Radiograms are made to rule out bone and joint pathology such as congenital malformations, tumors, infection, and invertebral disc calcification.

Treatment. In the acute stage, if the neck is flexible and the deformity is not fixed, a cervical collar is prescribed for support and comfort, and appropriate therapy is given to treat the upper respiratory infection, if present.

If the deformity is fixed or does not respond to the above conservative measures, it may be necessary to hospitalize the patient and place him in head-halter traction and prescribe analgesic agents and nonsteroidal anti-inflammatory medications. Ordinarily within a few days, full range of motion of the cervical spine can be restored and the patient is discharged with a cervical collar, which is worn for 2 to 4 weeks.

Hemiatlas

Hemiatlas with absence of the facet of C1 is a rare anomaly that may result in torticollis. In the infant and young child, ordinarily this deformity is not fixed and can be passively corrected by manipulation and stretching. As the child gets older, the deformity increases in severity and becomes rigid.[25]

The anomaly is difficult to detect in routine radiograms, but it is clearly depicted in a CT scan.

Treatment consists of traction to correct the torticollis and stabilization and fusion of the occiput to C2. Severe rigid torticollis requires gradual correction in a halo cast. Treatment with orthotic support is ineffective. It is best to perform arteriography prior to application of halo cast traction because the hemiatlas is often associated with vascular anomalies of the vertebral arteries. Traction may result in interruption of the blood supply to the mid-brain or spinal cord.

Inflammatory Torticollis

This may occur in juvenile rheumatoid arthritis. Diagnosis is readily made because most patients have involvement of multiple joints. It does not occur in the pauciarticular type of rheumatoid arthritis. If acute torticollis develops, one should rule out fracture of the odontoid process because of erosion by the hypertrophic synovium from the adjacent joints.[26-28]

Traumatic Acquired Torticollis

In children this is rare, occurring as a result of a fall or an auto accident. Often there is a fracture rather than a ligamentous injury. Traumatic tears of the transverse ligament of the atlas with atlantoaxial subluxation are rare but can occur, resulting in torticollis and even quadriparesis.[29-34] Treatment consists of posterior C1 and C2 fusion.

Neuromuscular Torticollis

This is seen in spinal cord tumors such as astrocytoma, which often are slow growing and clinically silent for some time. It presents with progressive stiffness and pain in the neck, which is held in flexion. The torticollis may shift from one side to the other, and there may be weakness and sensory disturbances in the upper or lower limbs. Check

Beevor's sign, superficial abdominal skin reflex, and the cremasteric reflex.[35-36]

Radiograms of the cervical spine show widening of the spinal canal. Magnetic resonance imaging (MRI) and myelography with metrizamide establish the diagnosis. Treatment is neurosurgical.

Torticollis Due to Bony Lesions of the Cervical Spine and Clavicle

Osteoblastoma, osteoid osteoma, eosinophilic granuloma, and Ewing's sarcoma are notorious for causing a painful lesion in the cervical spine or clavicle. Muscle spasm of the sternocleidomastoid muscle results in painful torticollis.

Treatment is individualized according to the nature of the lesion. Benign lesions are excised and bone grafted if indicated. Ewing's sarcoma is treated appropriately as described in the section on tumors.

Spondylolisthesis of the Cervical Spine

This condition is extremely rare. It presents clinically with stiffness and aching of the neck with slight restriction of range of motion. There is no history of injury. Ordinarily there are no signs or symptoms of spinal cord compression. Radiograms depict the slip. Treatment depends upon the degree of instability and the severity of symptoms. Stabilization of the cervical spine is indicated if the condition is symptomatic.

Atlantoaxial Instability[37-53]

Abnormal mobility between the first and second cervical vertebrae may be due to congenital anomalies of the odontoid process such as aplasia, hypoplasia, or a separate odontoid process (os odontoideum) (Fig 4–8). Occasionally the site of instability is the atlanto-occipital articulation.

It may also be due to ligamentous hyperlaxity or traumatic rupture of the ligaments or to developmental affections such as Down syndrome or Morquio's disease. In Down syndrome, in addition to ligamentous hyperlaxity, there is a higher incidence of congenital anomalies of the upper cervical vertebrae such as os odontoideum than in the normal population. Atlantoaxial instability may also be caused by inflammatory conditions such as rheumatoid arthritis.

Clinical Picture. Atlantoaxial instability may be totally asymptomatic and be accidently discovered in routine radiograms of the cervical spine. Symptoms vary from mild to severe neck pain and limitation of motion of the cervical spine to neurologic deficit resulting from impingement on the spinal cord by the anterior body of the axis and the base of the odontoid process. The physical signs include hyperreflexia, ankle clonus, a positive Babinski sign, motor weakness and difficulty in ambulation, sensory dysfunction, and torticollis. Bowel and bladder dysfunction may be the presenting complaint. Quadriplegia or even death may ensue following trauma.

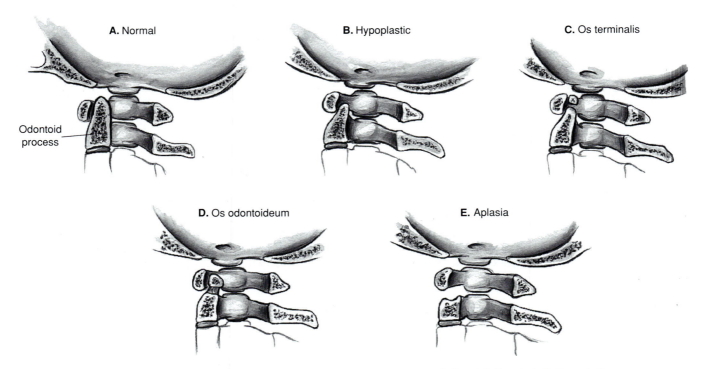

Figure 4–8. Atlantoaxial instability due to congenital anomalies of the odontoid process. **A.** Normal. **B.** Hypoplastic. **C.** Os terminalis. **D.** Os odontoideum. **E.** Aplasia.

In Down syndrome, atlantal instability is a manifestation of generalized ligamentous hyperlaxity. The reported incidence varies in the literature; it is approximately 15 percent. With increasing age the degree of instability increases. Most of the cases are asymptomatic, and in only a few patients does significant neurologic deficit develop which requires treatment.[35,40-41,45,48-50,53]

Imaging Findings. The following radiograms should be made: open-mouth, AP projections of the cervical spine, and lateral views with the neck in neutral, flexion, and extension.

Tomograms or three-dimensional computed tomography (CT) reconstructions are indicated when routine films do not show the pathologic anatomy. In the lateral projections, first determine the atlantodens interval (ADI). Measure the distance between the anterior border of the dens and the posterior ossified margin of the anterior ring of the atlas. In flexion, the interval between these two structures increases, whereas in extension it decreases. Measure the greatest distance. In children, the ADI in flexion normally should be 4 mm or less. In adults, normal ADI is less than 3 mm. The greater ADI in children is due to the cartilaginous state of the odontoid. The second determination in the radiograms is the space available for the spinal cord (SAC). This is the most important measurement (Fig 4–9A–C).

Measure the distance from the posterior aspect of the odontoid to the posterior ring of the atlas (sometimes the nearest posterior structure is the foramen magnum). Steel's rule of thirds is that one third of the space is for the odontoid, one third for the spinal cord, and one third for a safe zone. The space available for the spinal cord should normally be twice the diameter of the odontoid.[52] When there is less, the spinal cord is at risk for compression. An MRI scan is indicated when spinal cord compression is suspected and surgical intervention is to be carried out.

In atlantoaxial instability due to ligamentous hyperlaxity but with an intact odontoid, on flexion the ADI increases and the SAC decreases (Fig 4–9B). In extension, the ADI returns to normal and the SAC increases (Fig 4–9C).

When atlantoaxial instability is due to os odontoideum or a nonunion of a fracture of the odontoid process, ADI may be normal, but in flexion and/or extension, the SAC is markedly decreased.

Treatment. Treatment should be individualized. When there is neurologic deficit, cervical fusion is indicated. C1 and C2 vertebrae are fused in the reduced anatomic position. Whether the cervical spine should be stabilized by spinal fusion in Down syndrome depends upon the amount of space available for the spinal cord and not on absolute values of displacement.

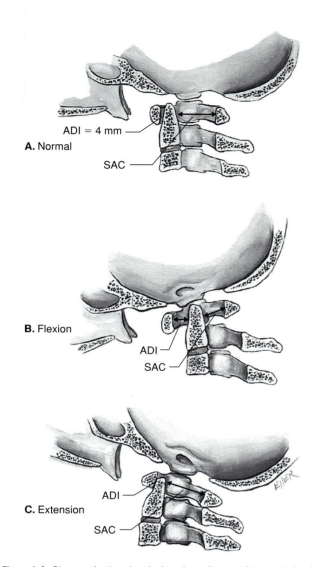

ADI = 4 mm

A. Normal

SAC

B. Flexion

ADI

SAC

ADI

C. Extension

SAC

Figure 4–9. Diagram of a lateral projection of a radiogram of the cervical spine illustrating the atlantodens interval (ADI) and the space available for spinal cord (SAC). **A.** Neck in neutral position. **B.** In flexion. **C.** In extension. Note that the normal ADI is 4 mm or less in a child.

Basilar Impression

In basilar impression or invagination there is a congenital or acquired deformity of the base of the skull with upward migration of the odontoid process into the foramen magnum causing spinal cord compression. There may also be blockage of the aqueduct of Sylvius and consequent increased intracranial pressure or hydrocephalus.

The vertebral anomalies in the congenital type may be abnormalities of the atlas, atlanto-occipital synostosis, and Klippel-Feil syndrome. In the acquired type the base of the skull is softened due to rickets or osteomalacia. The lack of bony support results in the upward invagination of the odontoid process into the foramen magnum.

Clinical Findings. These consist of motor and sensory deficits with weakness and paresthesia of the limbs. The child may present with an unsteady gait, dizziness, and nystagmus. Headache and pain in the upper posterior part of the neck are common.

Diagnosis. The diagnosis is made radiographically and by CT scan of the cervical spine and the base of the skull. In basilar impression, the tip of the odontoid is more than 4.5 mm above McGregor's line, which is a line drawn from the superior surface of the posterior edge of the hard palate to the most caudal point of the occipital curve of the skull.

Treatment. Treatment depends upon the symptoms and whether the basilar invagination is primary or acquired. Often the management of this problem falls in the realm of the neurosurgeon. If there is posterior impingement, a suboccipital craniotomy and decompression of the posterior ring of the atlas are performed, with posterior spinal fusion from the occiput to C2 or C3 (depending upon whether the posterior arch of C2 is decompressed). It is important to rule out a taut posterior dural band, which, if present, should be released. If the impingement is anterior and relieved with neck extension, an occipital-cervical fusion is performed with the neck in an extended position.

Klippel-Feil Syndrome

When an infant or child presents with a short neck and a low posterior hairline and stiffness of the neck with restriction of range of motion, synostosis of the cervical vertebrae or Klippel-Feil syndrome should be suspected.

This relatively uncommon deformity is caused by failure of segmentation of mesoderms of the vertebrae during the third to eighth week of fetal life. The degree of deformity depends upon the number of vertebrae involved. If only two to three vertebrae are fused, it may be clinically silent and accidently discovered in a radiogram made for another reason.

It is imperative to rule out associated anomalies, which can be more serious than the fusion of the vertebrae. One should remember that the original patient described by Klippel and Feil in 1912 died of renal failure.[62,63]

Examine the child for renal anomalies such as horseshoe kidney or absence of a kidney, hydronephrosis, and renal ectopia. In the reproductive and genital system, absence of the ovaries or vagina may occur. Cardiovascular system anomalies such as interventricular septal defect, patent ductus arteriosus, patent foramen ovale, or coarctation of the aorta can occur. An ectopic lung or agenesis of the lung may be encountered. Deafness is common. Spinal cord compression, facial nerve palsy, and synkinesia are some of the other anomalies involving the nervous system. Associated musculoskeletal anomalies such as torticollis, congenital high scapula, scoliosis, and pterygium colli should be noted.

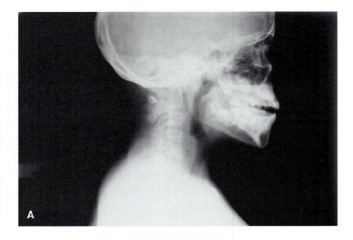

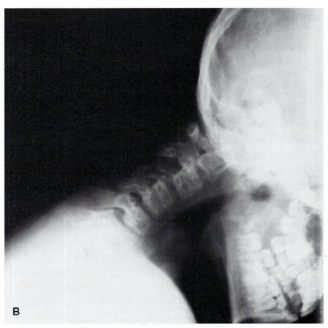

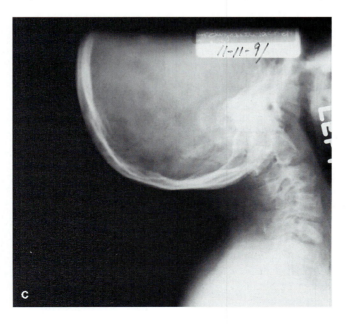

It behooves the surgeon to examine the child thoroughly to rule out these abnormalities when congenital synostosis of the cervical vertebrae is noted.

Imaging Findings. Routine radiographic studies should include lateral views of the cervical spine in neutral, flexion, and extension and AP and sometimes oblique views of the cervical spine (Fig 4–10). One may have to make laminagrams for proper visualization of the bony synostosis. The intervertebral disc spaces are narrow or obliterated, and the vertebral bodies are flattened and widened. The bony fusion may be posterior between the lamina or anterior between the vertebral bodies. Instability between the fused segments of the vertebrae may occur. Rule out spina bifida, hemivertebrae, cervical ribs, and platybasia.

A CT scan and MRI are performed when indicated to rule out intraspinal pathology. In early infancy, ultrasonography of the cervical spine depicts the cartilaginous synostosis. A chest radiogram and ultrasonogram of the abdomen should be made.

Treatment. Passive stretching exercises are performed to maintain range of motion. Correction of torticollis by orthotic devices may be attempted. There is no specific treatment. Cervical instability is treated by fusion if there is neurogenic deficit. Correction of torticollis and Sprengel's deformity greatly improves the physical appearance of the child.

Intervertebral Disc Calcification[68-74]

The child with intervertebral disc calcification presents with fever and a stiff and painful neck. There may be associated torticollis. Palpation reveals local tenderness over the affected disc interspace.

A thorough neuromuscular assessment should be carried out to rule out neurologic deficit; posterior or lateral extrusion of a calcified intervertebral disc can occur.[70] Examine the heart since there is a definite association between intervertebral disc calcification and congenital heart disease.

Ordinarily the pain and stiffness resolve spontaneously within 2 to 3 weeks after the onset of symptoms.

Calcification of intervertebral discs is rare in children. It is commonly located in the cervical spine; it does occur in the thoracic and lumbar regions, and more than one disc may be involved.

It is more preponderant in boys, with a 2:1 male-to-female ratio. The average age of clinical presentation and diagnosis is 7 years.

Figure 4–10. Klippel-Feil syndrome. Lateral view of the cervical spine showing synostosis between C2 and C3 and between C4 and C5. **A.** Neutral position. **B.** In flexion. **C.** In extension. There is no abnormal mobility between the fused and the unfused segments.

The exact cause is unknown; the condition is most probably a nonspecific inflammatory process. In children the intervertebral discs are supplied by blood vessels, whereas in the adult they are avascular. Pyogenic infection and trauma do not appear to be pathogenic factors.

Intervertebral disc calcification is not uncommon in the adult after the fifth decade of life. The lumbar and thoracic areas of the spine are the most common sites of affection. In the adult, intervertebral disc calcification is a degenerative process and may result from metabolic disease such as alkaptonuric ochronosis.

Imaging Findings. The radiographic appearance of calcification of an intervertebral disc is usually seen from 1 to 3 weeks after the onset of symptoms. Follow-up radiograms show gradual subsequent regression and disappearance of calcification. Occasionally calcification of the disc persists, with residual narrowing and irregularity of the disc space and osteophyte formation.[68]

Treatment. It is symptomatic, consisting of support to the cervical spine in the form of a soft collar and administration of nonsteroidal anti-inflammatory medication. The prognosis is excellent. Antibiotics, chelating agents, and radiation therapy should not be given.

■ SHOULDER

EXAMINATION

Inspect the shoulders from the front, back, and side. Is there any asymmetry? Is one shoulder higher than the other? Note the trapezius neck line. On the side of the elevated shoulder, it is shorter than on the opposite normal side. Are the scapulae winging? Is the winging symmetric or asymmetric? In Landouzy-Déjérine muscular dystrophy and other myopathies, the winging of the scapulae is symmetric, whereas in nerve palsy of the long thoracic nerve and paralysis of the serratus anterior or when there is an exostosis on the ventral surface of the scapula, the winging is asymmetric.

Note the inclination of the vertebral border of the scapulae and also the interscapular distance. Visually assess the vertical height of the scapula in relation to its width. The height should be greater; in Sprengel's deformity it is decreased. Ask the patient to elevate the shoulders and inspect the mobility of the scapulae on the thoracic cage.

From the anterior view, inspect the clavicles. Are they tilted superiorly, a finding in Sprengel's deformity? Are the shoulders drooping forward or downward? Look for congenital absence of the pectoral muscles or supernumerary nipples or mammary glands. From the lateral view, assess the relationship of the humeral head to the acromion. When there is inferior subluxation of the shoulder, a hollow is present immediately below the lateral margin of the acromion. In obstetrical brachial plexus palsy, the acromion

process is tilted downward and both it and the coracoid process are prominent. Both of these bony deformities block passive range of motion of the shoulders.

Next palpate the shoulders. Is there any local tenderness over the acromioclavicular joint, the rotator cuff, the attachment of the short head of the biceps, the spinous process of the scapulae, or the body and vertebral border of the scapulae? The scapula is not an uncommon site for Ewing's sarcoma or osteomyelitis. Feel for increased local temperature and diffuse enlargement of the infraspinal portion of the scapula.

Perform a quick assessment of active range of shoulder motion. Look for limitation, asymmetry, and a break in the rhythm of motion. Ask the patient to carry out the following movements of both shoulders: First ask the patient to elevate the arms completely above his or her head. Note that at 90 degrees of elevation, the patient rotates the shoulder laterally and supinates the forearms for maximal elevation (Fig 4–11A).

Then ask the patient to swing the upper limb across the front of his or her chest and touch the opposite shoulder. This tests medial rotation and adduction of the shoulders (Fig 4–11B).

Next ask the patient to elevate the arms and touch the back of his or her neck. This tests elevation, abduction, and lateral rotation of the shoulders (Fig 4–11C). Then ask the patient to bring each hand behind his or her back and touch the inferior angle of the scapula. This tests medial rotation, adduction, and extension of the shoulders (Fig 4–11D). Ask the patient to reach behind his or her neck and try to scratch the superomedial angle of the scapula. This tests abduction, lateral rotation, and elevation of the shoulders (Fig 4–11E). Then ask the patient to reach behind the back and touch the opposite buttock with the dorsum of his or her hand. This tests extension, adduction, and medial rotation (Fig 4–11F).

Motions of the shoulder are complex, taking place at the glenohumeral and scapulocostal joints. During examination one determines pure glenohumeral, pure scapulocostal, and combined glenohumeral and scapulocostal motion. The term *shoulder elevation* is used to describe upward vertical motion of the humerus in any plane.

To test pure glenohumeral motion, stand behind the patient, hold the inferior angle of the scapula, and stabilize it against the thoracic cage (Fig 4–12A). Ask the patient to raise the arm vertically (Fig 4–12B). With the scapula fixed, pure glenohumeral motion is about 90 degrees. In combined glenohumeral and scapulothoracic motion, the first 20 degrees are pure glenohumeral; then the scapula rotates upward and anteriorly over the chest wall with a glenohumeral and scapulothoracic joint ratio of 2:1; that is, for every 30 degrees of shoulder elevation, 20 degrees take place at the glenohumeral joint and 10 degrees at the scapulothoracic joint (Fig 4–12C, D). At about 120 degrees of shoulder elevation the shoulder rotates laterally to liberate the surgical neck of the humerus from abutting the acromion,

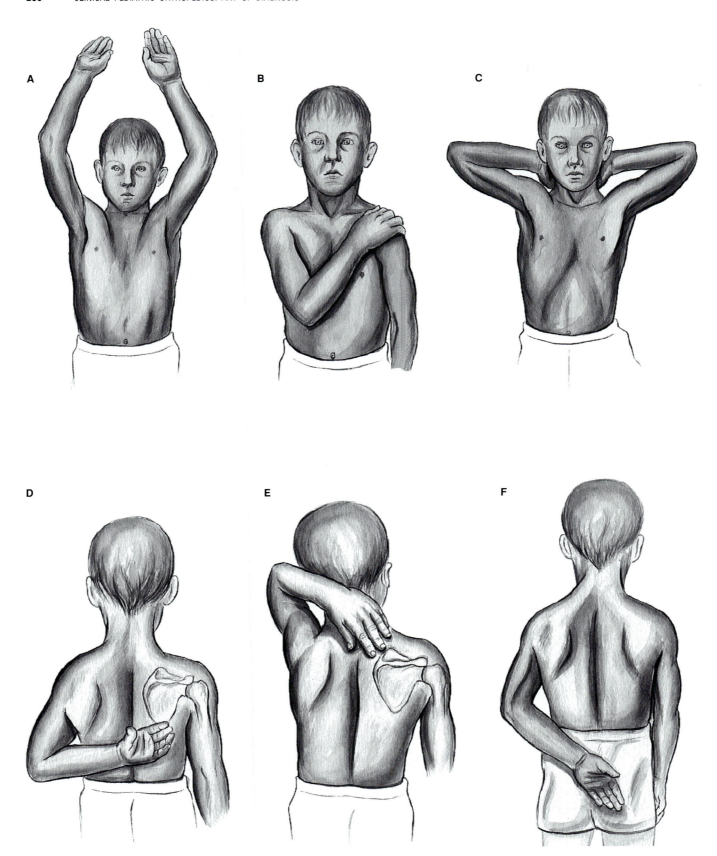

Figure 4–11. Rapid assessment of active range of shoulder motion. See text.

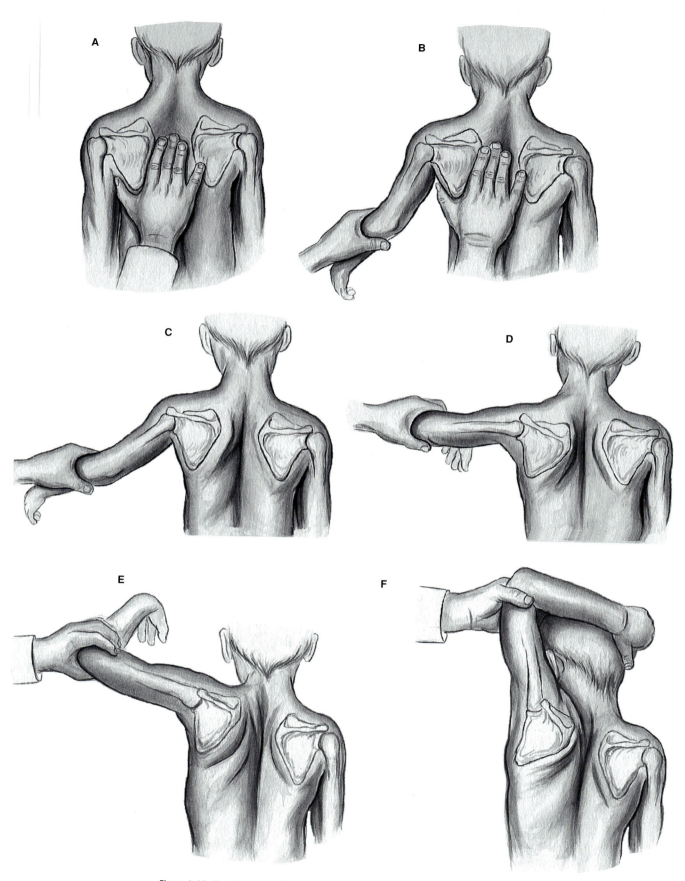

Figure 4–12. Elevation of shoulders—glenohumeral, scapulocostal, and combined. See text.

thereby allowing full elevation of the shoulder to 180 degrees (Fig 4–12E, F).

In the sagittal plane, backward motion is extension (normal range 45 degrees) and forward movement of the shoulder is flexion (normal range 90 degrees) (Fig 4–13A–C). In the horizontal plane, motions of the shoulder from the midsagittal zero position are termed adduction, moving toward the body, and abduction, moving away from the body (Fig 4–14A–D).

Range of rotation is determined with the shoulder in 90 degrees of abduction and the arm at the side of the chest (Fig 4–15A, B, D). With the surgeon standing in front of the patient, first with the patient's elbow and arm at the side of his chest and the elbow flexed 90 degrees, the forearm is moved away from the center of the body—lateral rotation (normal range 45 to 50 degrees) (Fig 4–15C). In medial rotation the forearm is moved toward the body with the arm stabilized at the side of the chest (normal range 90 degrees) (Fig 4–15E). The range of rotation of the shoulder is also tested with the shoulder in neutral "zero" rotation, elevated 90 degrees and abducted 90 degrees. In medial rotation the forearm is rotated downward, and in lateral rotation the forearm is rotated upward (Fig 4–15A).

CONGENITAL HIGH SCAPULA (SPRENGEL'S DEFORMITY)

The presenting complaint is asymmetry of the shoulders, with the affected scapula abnormally high in the neck. This rare congenital deformity of the shoulder girdle was first described by Eulenberg; however, it is commonly referred to as Sprengel's deformity.[86,96] The deformity is the result of failure of descent of the scapula from its fetal position in the neck to its normal position in the upper posterior thorax. The exact cause is unknown. The "bleb" theory has been proposed by Engel and supported by the observations of Bonnevie and Bagg.[75–77,81,85]

Congenital high scapula is four times more common in girls than in boys. It occurs sporadically; however, occasionally it has an apparent autosomal dominant pattern of inheritance.

The affected scapula is high in its location and small, with decrease in its vertical diameter and apparent increase in its horizontal width (Fig 4–16A, B; See p. 286). Its supraspinous portion is tilted forward. Often fibrous adhesions are found between the scapula and the rib cage (Fig 4–16C). An omovertebral bone may connect the upper vertebral border of the scapula to the spinous process, lamina, or transverse process of one of the lower cervical vertebra, limiting elevation of the shoulder (Fig 4–16A, D).

Congenital high scapula is often associated with numerous anomalies (Table 4–2). Because it is not an isolated deformity, it is vital to examine the child carefully. There are varying degrees of involvement of the *muscles* connecting the scapula to the thoracic cage and vertebral column (Fig 4–17A, B). The affected muscles may be absent, hypoplastic and weak, or fibrosed and contracted. Histopathologic studies suggest an arrest of differentiation of the muscle fibers in the myoblastic stage with consequent degeneration, necrosis, fibrosis, and contracture. The muscles most commonly involved are the trapezius, deltoids, rhomboids, and levator scapulae and serratus anterior.

In the *vertebral column,* Klippel-Feil syndrome, torticollis, congenital scoliosis with hemivertebrae, diastematomyelia, platybasia, and spina bifida in the cervical region are not uncommon (Fig 4–17C, E).

In the limbs, congenital short humerus or femur, longitudinal deficiency of the radius or tibia, absence of rays in the hands or feet, fusion of ribs, or cervical ribs can occur. The clavicle on the affected shoulder girdle is tilted markedly upward, or it may be hypoplastic and fail to articulate with the acromion.

In the viscera, kidney malformations such as absence, ectopia, and hypoplasia are not uncommon. Situs inversus and cardiac malformations such as atrial septal defect can occur (Fig 4–17D). In the central nervous system, syringomyelia, intraspinal lipoma, and paraplegia can be present.

Clinical Assessment.   The deformity is present at birth; its severity varies. The affected scapula may be 1 to 12 cm higher than the normal opposite scapula. Involvement is often unilateral and very rarely bilateral.

In *bilateral* cases the neck is very short and thick; the cervical lordosis is markedly exaggerated, and abduction of both shoulders is limited.

In *unilateral* involvement, on *inspection* the level of the shoulders is asymmetric due to the high scapula. The trapezius neckline is short on the affected side. The involved scapula is hypoplastic, with decrease in its vertical diameter. Its shape is distorted, with the supraspinous portion of the scapula tilted forward. The level of the involved and opposite normal scapula should be determined; normally the scapula extends from the second to the seventh or eighth thoracic vertebra. In Sprengel's deformity, the superior medial tip of the scapula may be as high as the fourth cervical and its lower medial angle opposite the second thoracic level.

Mobility of the scapula on the thoracic cage is often restricted; decrease or loss of motion of the scapula may be due to fibrous adhesions between the scapula and posterior chest wall, the presence of an omovertebral bone, or both. A large omovertebral bone may be palpable in the supraclavicular area. Passive range of combined abduction of the shoulder is restricted because of loss of scapulocostal motion; range of motion of the glenohumeral joint is normal. Active range of shoulder motion may be limited because of motor weakness of the deltoid, supraspinatus, and upper trapezius muscles.

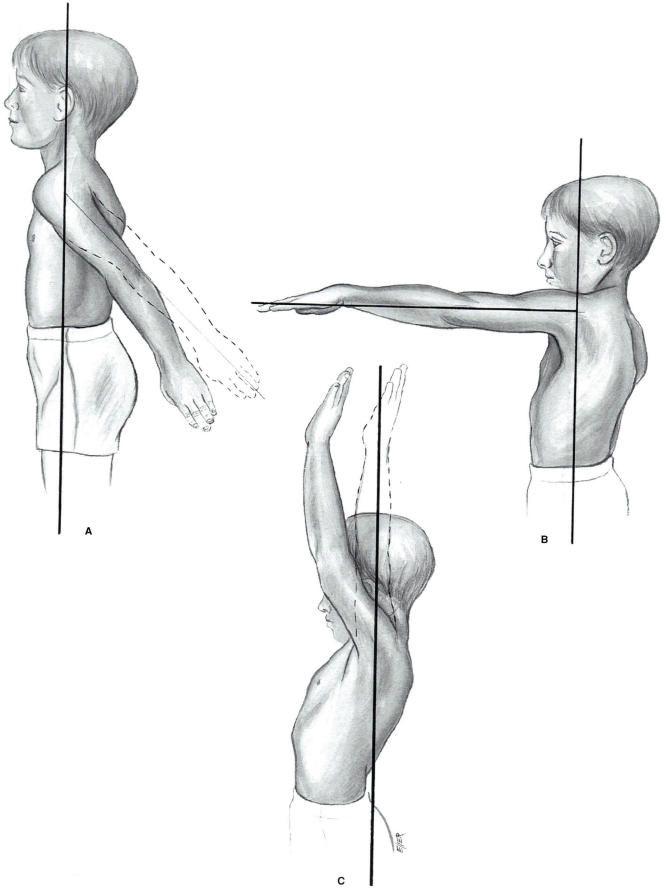

Figure 4–13. Motions of the shoulder in the sagittal plane. **A.** Extension of the shoulder. Normal range is 45 degrees. **B, C.** Flexion of the shoulder from 90 degrees to 180 degrees.

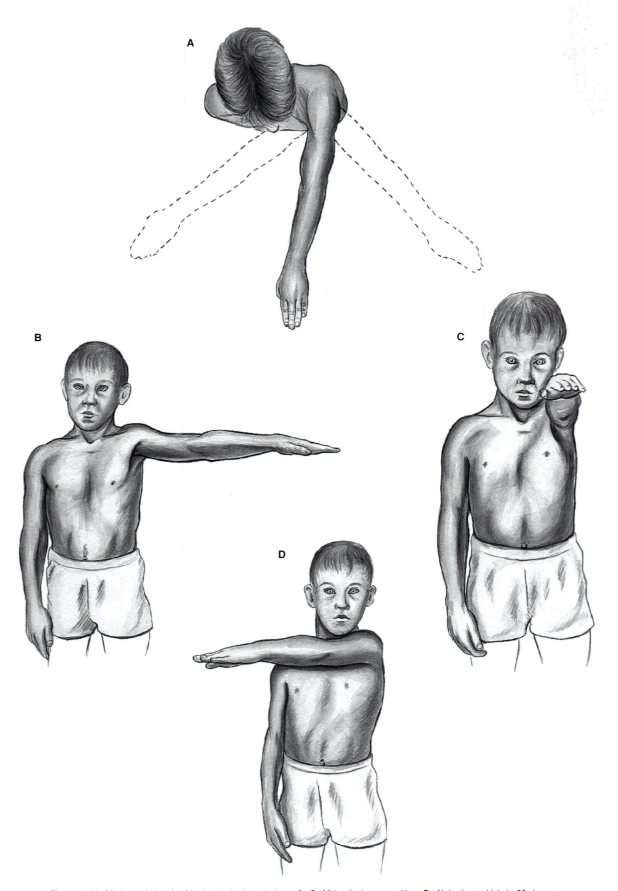

Figure 4–14. Motions of the shoulder in the horizontal plane. **A, C.** Midsagittal zero position. **B.** Abduction, which is 90 degrees. **D.** Adduction.

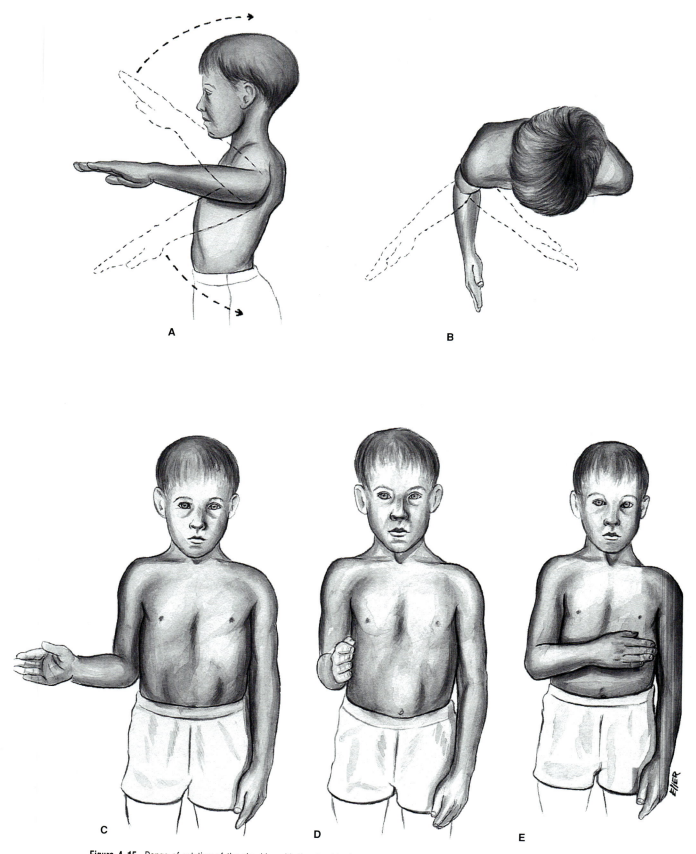

Figure 4–15. Range of rotation of the shoulder with the shoulder in neutral "zero" rotation, elevated 90 degrees, and abducted 90 degrees. See text for explanation.

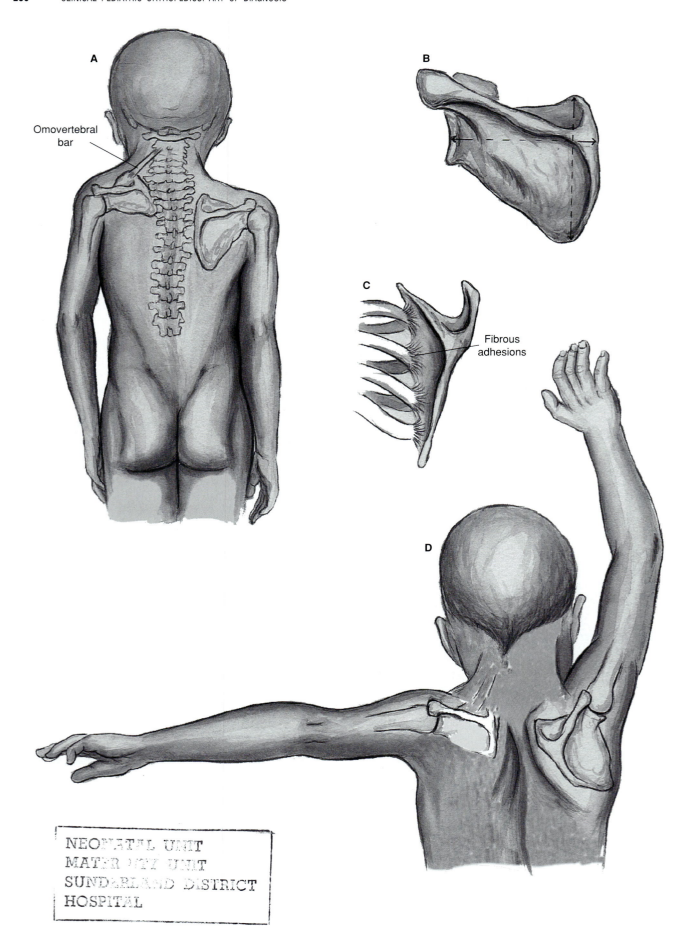

Omovertebral bar

Fibrous adhesions

TABLE 4–2. ANOMALIES ASSOCIATED WITH CONGENITAL HIGH SCAPULA (SPRENGEL'S DEFORMITY)

Muscles
  Aplasia, hypoplasia, fibrosis-contracture of trapezius, rhomboids, levator scapulae, serratus anterior, deltoid
Vertebral column
  Klippel-Feil syndrome
  Hemivertebrae—congenital scoliosis
  Spina bifida—cervical spine
  Diastematomyelia, platybasia
Upper limbs
  Clavicle—tilted upwards, hypoplastic
  Humerus—congenital shortening
  Longitudinal deficiency of radius
  Absence of rays of the hand
Lower limbs
  Congenital short femur
  Longitudinal deficiency of tibia
  Absence of rays of foot
Thoracic cage
  Fusion of ribs
  Supernumerary ribs—cervical ribs
Viscera
  Kidney—absence, hypoplasia, ectopia, polycystic
  Heart—atrial septal defect or other malformations
  Situs inversus
Central nervous system
  Intraspinal lipoma
  Syringomyelia

The lateral end of the clavicle on the affected side is tilted upward. There may be associated scoliosis, kyphosis, torticollis, and Klippel-Feil syndrome.

Diagnosis. When Sprengel's deformity is suspected, the following studies should be performed. First, *muscle testing* of the musculature of the shoulder girdle and both upper limbs. Palpate for absence or hypoplasia and fibrosis of the muscles. Grade their motor strength. It is best for a physical therapist to perform the muscle testing. Second, the following *radiograms* are made: (1) AP projection of both shoulders including cervical and thoracic spine, with arms at the side and both shoulders at normal abduction. (2) Lateral views of cervical and thoracic spine. (3) Oblique-lateral views of the scapula to demonstrate the omovertebral bone. *CT scan* of both shoulders demonstrates the omovertebral bone. *MRI* of the cervical spine is performed when intraspinal or spinal cord pathology is suspected. *Ultrasonography* of the abdomen, and, if necessary, intravenous pyelography are performed to rule out renal anomalies.

Asymmetry of shoulders is present in scoliosis, lower limb inequality, and obstetrical brachial plexus paralysis. Diagnosis of *lower limb length disparity* is readily made by the physical findings of short lower limb, uneven level of iliac crests in stance, and restoration of asymmetry of the levels of the shoulders and iliac crests to normal with appropriate lift under the foot of the short limb. In addition, in limb length disparity there are no deformities of the scapula and no restriction of range of motion of the involved shoulder joint.

Congenital scoliosis and Sprengel's deformity may coexist. Ask the patient to bend forward and inspect him or her for rotation of the vertebrae. Are there any abnormal hair patches or hemangioma or other stigmata of spinal dysraphism? The absence of deformity of the scapula, normal obliquity of the clavicle (it is not tilted cephalad), and radiography make the diagnosis of scoliosis.

In *obstetrical brachial plexus paralysis* the shoulder girdle on the paralyzed side may be high. Although the scapula is hypoplastic in both conditions, in obstetrical brachial plexus paralysis the lower medial border of the scapula is tilted laterally whereas in Sprengel's deformity it is tilted and tethered medially due to muscle fibrosis and contracture. The clinical history of difficult labor and paralysis at birth, the presence of flaccid paralysis of the elbow-forearm and hand, and a history of a varying degree of spontaneous recovery make the diagnosis of obstetrical brachial plexus paralysis.

Treatment. The modality of treatment varies according to the severity of deformity and degree of functional impairment. Other factors to consider are the age of the patient and association with other malformations such as Klippel-Feil syndrome, torticollis, congenital scoliosis, and kyphosis.

Cavendish has classified Sprengel's deformity into four grades of severity.[83] In grade I (very mild), the scapula is almost level and the deformity is not detectable when the patient is clothed. In grade II (mild), the shoulders are uneven, with the affected scapula 1 to 2 cm higher than the normal opposite scapula. Inspection reveals an obvious lump in the web of the neck which represents the superomedial part of the high scapula. When the "lump" is disfiguring, the supraspinous portion of the scapula is excised extraperiosteally. In grade III (moderate), the affected shoulder is 2 to 5 cm higher than the normal shoulder. The deformity is unsightly and easily detected. In such an

Figure 4–16. Sprengel's deformity (congenital high scapula). **A.** Note the high scapula with the omovertebral bar connecting the superomedial angle of the scapula to the cervical vertebra. **B.** The small scapula, with decrease in its vertebral height in relation to its horizontal diameter. **C.** Fibrous adhesions tethering the scapula to the rib cage. **D.** Limitation of elevation of the left shoulder. This is due to the omovertebral bar, to the fibrous adhesions between the scapula and the rib cage restricting scapulocostal motion, and to weakness of the deltoid and supraspinatus muscles.

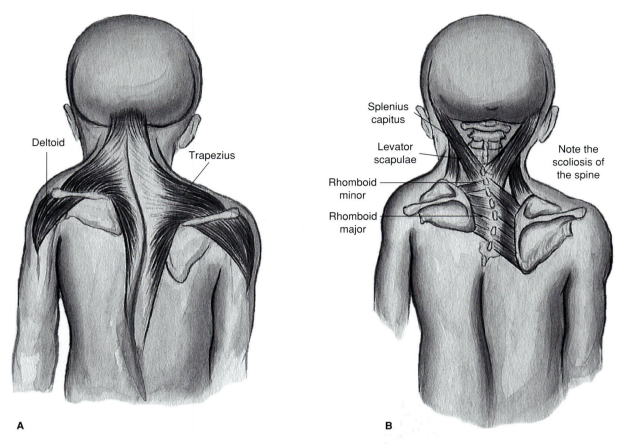

A

B

Figure 4–17. Anomalies associated with congenital high scapula. **A, B.** Fibrosis and hypoplasia of the trapezius, deltoids, rhomboids, levator scapulae, and serratus anterior. Always perform motor strength testing of the muscle in a patient with Sprengel's deformity. *(Continues)*

instance, lowering the scapula to a normal level markedly improves appearance. In grade IV (severe), the scapula is elevated greater than 5 cm. In some cases the superior angle of the scapula may be near the occiput, with marked webbing of the neck. In such a severe deformity, surgery improves appearance but a residual deformity remains.

The primary goals of treatment are to improve function and cosmetic appearance. Surgical intervention is not indicated when the range of passive abduction of the shoulder is full, the deformity is mild, the elevation of the affected scapula is less than two cm, and the shoulders are almost even. These cases are observed and reassessed once a year to ensure that the deformity is not increasing with skeletal growth.

When the deformity is moderate or severe and the function of the shoulder is impaired, surgery should be considered. Passive range of shoulder joint abduction is limited by the presence of an omovertebral bar or fibrous adhesions between the scapula and the thoracic cage. The deformity can be corrected either by the Green or Woodward procedure or the Klisiç modification.[88,91,97] All three procedures excise the omovertebral bar and release scapulocostal fibrous adhesions to restore passive range of shoulder abduction to normal. In the Woodward operation the trapezius

and rhomboid muscles are detached from their origins from the spinous processes and transferred distally. The omovertebral bone, if present, is resected. Fibrous bands binding the scapula to the rib cage are divided, and the supraspinous portion of the scapula is excised extraperiosteally. The procedure is relatively simple and is preferred by some surgeons when the deformity is moderate.

This author recommends a modification of Green's scapuloplasty; it consists first of osteotomy of the clavicle, which facilitates lowering of the scapula and prevents neurovascular traction injury. Then the patient is turned from supine to prone position. Through a midline incision the muscles connecting the scapula to the trunk are sectioned at their scapular insertion, and the omovertebral bone and supraspinous portion of the scapula are excised extraperiosteally (along with the periosteum to prevent regeneration). The scapula is transferred distally to normal level and anchored to the rib cage with sutures, and the muscles are reattached to the scapula in its new position. Green's procedure provides effective motor control of the scapula and checkreins winging of the scapula.

In the past, surgical correction of Sprengel's deformity was postponed until 3 to 4 years of age because of the complexity of the operation and the potential for neurovas-

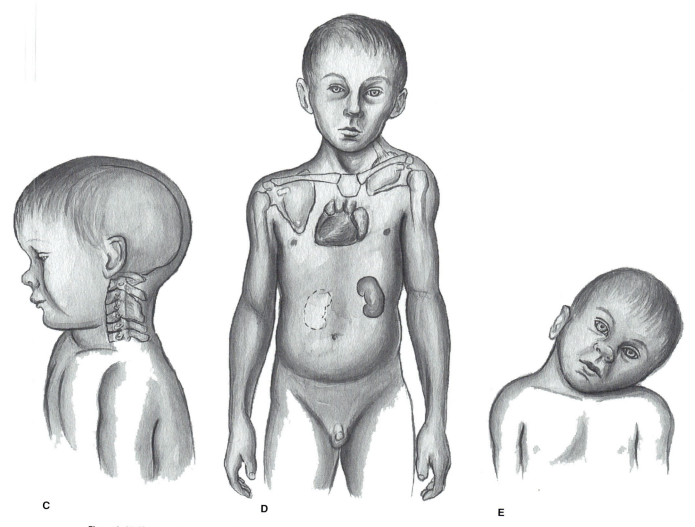

Figure 4–17 *(Continued).* **C.** Klippel-Feil syndrome in the cervical spine. **D.** Visceral anomalies. Note the absent kidney and dextrocardia. **E.** Torticollis.

cular injury. At present this author recommends surgery at 9 to 18 months of age, depending upon the severity of the deformity. With modern anesthesia and surgical techniques and in experienced hands, the operation has become relatively simple and not dangerous.

Following surgery, follow-up is important. These patients may develop scoliosis, and the scapula may migrate cephalad with skeletal growth of the spine.

CONGENITAL PSEUDARTHROSIS OF THE CLAVICLE

This rare anomaly presents immediately at birth or in early infancy as a firm swelling immediately lateral to the middle of the clavicle. On palpation it is not tender, and on passive movement a variable degree of painless motion is present at the pseudarthrosis site. The opposing ends of the clavicular fragments are enlarged. The longer sternal fragment is pulled upward by the sternocleidomastoid muscle and lies slightly superior and anterior to the shorter acromial fragment, which is tilted inferiorly by the weight of the upper limb. The shoulder droops and is rotated forward.

The right side is almost always involved; in the occasional case when the left side is affected, the heart is on the right side—dextrocardia. Very occasionally both clavicles are affected.

Etiology. The clavicle is the first osseous mass to form in the embryo; it develops from two centers of enchondral ossification. At the fourth week (0.11 mm stage) it appears as a mesenchymal bar in the neck inferior to the precoracoid area. At the seventh week of life the two precartilaginous masses fuse.[99] Congenital pseudarthrosis of the clavicle is due to failure of amalgamation of these two cartilaginous masses or defective normal ossification of the precartilaginous bridge connecting the acromial and sternal ossification centers of the clavicle.[100]

With the heart on the left, the subclavian artery is at a high level on the right side. In dextrocardia the high position of the subclavian artery is reversed to the left. Congenital pseudarthrosis of the clavicle occurs on the side with the high subclavian artery—the right side when the heart is on the left and the left side when the heart is on the right. It is proposed that the pseudarthrosis is caused by the exaggerated arterial pulsation and pressure on the clavicle by the high subclavian artery.[102]

In congenital pseudarthrosis of the clavicle, the first and second ribs are vertically oriented and abnormally high, causing the subclavian artery to be elevated. Additional etiologic factors account for the occurrence of the very rare bilateral case.

Trauma and nonunion of a birth fracture are not the cause of congenital pseudarthrosis of the clavicle. Familial incidence is reported; there is no genetic pattern.

Diagnosis. When an infant is seen with a swelling in the middle third of the clavicle, the following queries should be made: (1) birth history, specifically shoulder dystocia at delivery, (2) trauma at birth or during infancy, (3) lack of movement of the upper limb (pseudoparalysis), (4) pain on passive and active motion, (5) local tenderness, (6) size of the swelling increasing or decreasing, and (7) history of café-au-lait spots or other stigmata of neurofibromatosis in the patient or family?

Congenital pseudarthrosis of the clavicle in the newborn should be distinguished from fracture of the clavicle; in the latter there is a history of injury and pseudoparalysis of the upper limb, with lack of voluntary motion of the arm and local tenderness. In fracture, the swelling (the callus) remodels and disappears within 3 to 6 months. Abnormal mobility at the swelling site is present. In congenital pseudarthrosis of the clavicle these symptoms and signs are absent; also in pseudarthrosis of the clavicle, evidence of healing is absent, and radiolucent fibrous tissue is present at the pseudarthrosis site with enlargement of the bone ends and abnormal mobility (Fig 4–18).

In neurofibromatosis, the bone ends are attenuated and other stigmata of neurofibromatosis, such as café-au-lait spots and axillary or inguinal freckling, are present.

Congenital pseudarthrosis of the clavicle should not be misdiagnosed as cleidocranial dysostosis; in the latter, part or all of the clavicle is absent, local swelling is absent, and involvement is often bilateral, in contrast to congenital pseudarthrosis, in which involvement is almost always unilateral. Also found in cleidocranial dysostosis are other associated skeletal deformities such as bossing of the skull, small facial bones, scoliosis, abnormal epiphyses of the hands and feet, and defects and widening of the symphysis pubis.

Treatment. The pseudarthrosis mass is excised, and the bone ends are curetted and internally fixed with a threaded Kirschner wire and grafted with autogenous iliac cancellous onlay bone. Results are excellent. Bony union is readily achieved, the appearance is improved, and the strength of the shoulder girdle is increased. Opinions vary as to the appropriate age for surgery. This author recommends surgery at 1 year, whereas others recommend 3 years of age because of the need for intramedullary pin fixation.

In untreated cases, with skeletal growth, the "lump" and instability at the pseudarthrosis site increase, overlying skin becomes atrophic, and the deformity becomes cosmetically unsightly. The affected shoulder droops, and the patient may complain of mild pain and weakness of the shoulder.[106,107]

CLEIDOCRANIAL DYSPLASIA

Cleidocranial dysplasia is a developmental affection of the skeleton in which there is deficient ossification of bones formed in membrane. The clavicle may be absent laterally, in its middle third, occasionally in its sternal third, or very rarely in its entirety.

The condition affects not only the clavicle, but the cranium and pelvis as well. Bone preformed in cartilage, specifically the short tubular bones of the hands and feet, are also involved. The dysplasia is inherited as an autosomal dominant trait; the exact cause is unknown.[108–110]

Clinical Picture. The diagnosis may be made in infancy or in childhood. The presenting complaint is marked forward drooping and excessive forward mobility of the shoulders. In complete bilateral absence of the clavicles, the shoulders may be brought nearly together anteriorly. The chest is narrow. The sternocleidomastoid muscle and the anterior fibers of the deltoid are often hypoplastic. Impingement of the brachial plexus nerve is rare, but irritation and radiating pain and varying degrees of neurologic deficit may occur.

Examine the child's head, pelvis, hands, and feet. The head is large and brachycephalic, with widening of the interparietal diameter and bossing of the frontal, parietal, and occipital bones. The face is small with wide-set eyes. The chin is recessed (retrognathia), and the palate is narrow with a high arch. The permanent teeth are delayed in eruption and are maldeveloped. On palpation of the pelvis, the symphysis pubis is defective, with abnormal space between the pubic bones. The child's gait may be waddling with varying degrees of out-toeing. When associated coxa vara deformity is present, the Trendelenburg test is positive. The tips of the fingers and toes are pointed and short. The second metacarpal is abnormally long.

Imaging Findings. Radiograms show deficiency of one or both clavicles. The membranous bones of the skull are de-

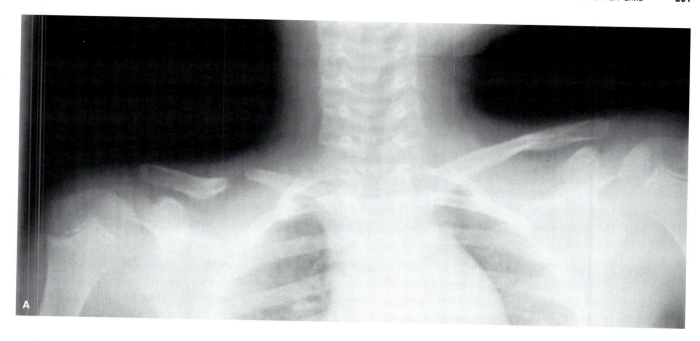

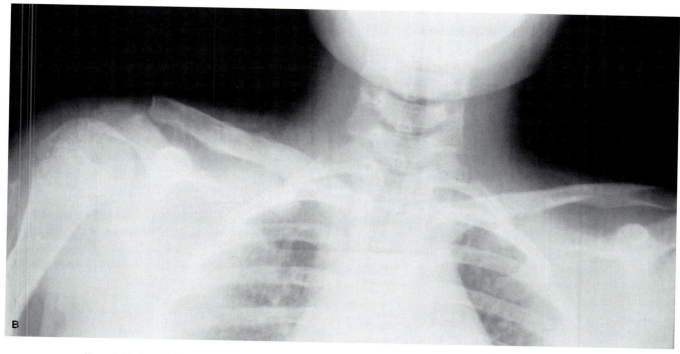

Figure 4–18. Congenital pseudarthrosis of the clavicle on the right. **A.** AP view of both clavicles. Note the pseudarthrosis on the right. **B.** Postoperative radiogram showing the healed pseudarthrosis. This was treated by bone grafting and internal fixation with a threaded Steinmann pin. The pin has been removed.

layed in development, with multiple wormian bones and delayed closure of the sutures. The anterior fontanelle is enlarged.

The symphysis pubis is wide, with delayed ossification of the innominate bones. Associated coxa vara may be present. Spina bifida occulta due to failure of ossification and closure of the lamina in the lumbar and thoracic region is commonly present. The manubrium of the sternum is poorly developed.

Ossification of the tarsal and carpal bones is delayed. In the hands and feet the phalanges are short and the distal phalanges tapered. The second to fifth metacarpals and metatarsals may have extra epiphyses proximally. The second metacarpal is relatively long.

Treatment. Ordinarily disability is minimal, if any, and no specific treatment is required.

CONGENITAL ABSENCE OF PECTORAL MUSCLES

Partial or complete absence of pectoral muscles is common. It is often unilateral. It is readily detected at birth or soon afterward. When associated with syndactyly and microdactyly, it is referred to as Poland's syndrome.[111–119]

The nipple over the absent pectoral muscle is often atrophic. Functional disability is ordinarily minimal, although there may be some weakness of adduction and medial rotation of the arm.

Treatment is not indicated for an absent pectoral muscle.

WINGING AND OTHER DISORDERS OF THE SCAPULA

Winging may be caused by paralysis of the serratus anterior muscle due to injury to the long thoracic nerve or congenital absence or hypoplasia of the serratus anterior. The scapula may also "wing" in obstetrical brachial plexus palsy. Bilateral cases are seen in fascio-scapulo-humeral muscular dystrophy (Landouzy-Déjérine).

A tumor such as an exostosis on the costal surface of the scapula can cause winging. This can be easily detected on routine radiograms. Sometimes one must resort to MRI or CT scan. Diagnosis is readily made by clinical examination and by imaging. Ask the patient to push against a wall to see if one or both scapulae wing. Palpate the deep surface of the scapula for the presence of an exostosis. Crepitation on abduction and adduction of the shoulder suggests the presence of an exostosis.

When muscle weakness is due to paralysis or congenital absence, shoulder abduction is limited. In paralysis of the serratus anterior, the patient has difficulty in raising his or her arms and in pushing movements.

Treatment. When winging of the scapula is due to an exostosis, it is excised. In muscular dystrophy, scapulocostal stabilization is indicated. In congenital absence or hypoplasia, transfers of muscles such as the latissimus dorsi are carried out.

Snapping or grating of the scapula may be caused by increased anterior inclination of the superior angle of the scapula. It varies from a fine grating noise to a coarse, audible popping. It develops gradually and occasionally is painful. Radiograms should always include an oblique scapular view.

Snapping shoulder is due to the catching of the lesser tuberosity of the humerus by the coracoid-brachialis muscle and the short head of the biceps. It may be painful. Snapping shoulder may also be caused by displacement of the long tendon of the head of the biceps from the bicipital groove.

OBSTETRICAL BRACHIAL PLEXUS PARALYSIS

The paralysis is evident at birth. The level and severity of nerve injury determine the extent of motor and sensory loss. In the whole-arm type, the affected upper limb lies motionless at the side of the trunk with the elbow in extension, the wrist in flexion, and the fingers in semiextension. On stimulation, there is no active movement. The grasp, asymmetric, tonic, and Moro reflexes are absent on the involved side.

Etiology. Paralysis is caused by forced stretching of one or more components of the brachial plexus by traction. The tensile strength of the lower plexus components is one half of that of the upper plexus components. Often the disruption occurs at the foramen or within the groove of the transverse processes; occasionally the nerve roots avulse from the spinal cord.

Obstetrical risk factors for injury to the brachial plexus at birth are (1) high birth weight, (2) cephalopelvic disproportion, (3) breech position, (4) shoulder dystocia, and (5) prolonged labor. In vertex presentation, traction forces are applied on the brachial plexus when one shoulder is trapped behind the symphysis pubis and it is freed and extracted by forced lateral flexion of the head and neck. In contrast, in breech presentation, traction forces on the brachial plexus are applied when the head is delivered by strong lateral flexion of the neck by pulling the trunk. Direct contusion of the brachial plexus by forceps can occur during delivery. Brachial plexus paralysis can occur during cesarean section when stretching forces are applied on the brachial plexus when the fetus, in breech position, is extracted by traction on the head and neck.

Incidence. Obstetrical brachial plexus paralysis occurs in 0.4 to 2.5 of every 1000 live births. Preventive measures and improved obstetrical care have not eliminated paralysis of the brachial plexus at birth; however, the severity and extent of paralysis have markedly decreased. It should be noted that fetal or maternal distress may demand rapid delivery and increase the risk of injury to the brachial plexus. In the modern medicolegal era, it is wise for the obstetrician to document details and factors in decision-making and communicate frankly with the mother and father of the baby.

Classification. According to the components of the plexus that are injured, obstetrical brachial plexus paralysis is grouped into three main types: (1) *Upper arm type—Erb-Duchenne.* Injury occurs to the upper trunk at the junction of the fifth and sixth nerve roots—Erb's point.[125] The result is varying degrees of paralysis of the fifth and sixth nerve roots or their derivation. (2) *Lower arm paralysis of Klumpke.* The eighth cervical and first thoracic roots are paralyzed. (3) *Paralysis of the entire arm.* All components of the brachial plexus are affected.

The degree of nerve injury may be classified into *mild, moderate, and severe.* With *mild* lesions, nerve fibers are simply stretched, with perineural edema and hemorrhage. The prognosis in this type of injury is good; with absorption of the edema and hemorrhage complete, early recovery takes place within 3 months. In *moderate* lesions due to forced traction, some of the nerve fibers are torn and others are stretched. Both intraneural and extraneural bleeding occurs. Recovery is slow and incomplete, with maximal return of function taking place up to 2 years of age. In the *severe* form, the trunks of the plexus are completely ruptured or avulsed. The prognosis is very poor, with almost no recovery of function.

Diagnosis. Thoroughly inspect the neonate. Has forceps injury caused cephalohematoma? Is there supraclavicular swelling or ecchymosis? Look at the eyes—enophthalmos, miosis, and ptosis (Horner's syndrome) may be present due to injury of the sympathetic fibers in the first dorsal root. Inspect the breathing—is the diaphragm moving? Rule out phrenic nerve palsy and paralysis of the diaphragm. When the diaphragm is paralyzed and respiratory stridor is present, fluoroscopic or ultrasonographic examination of the diaphragmatic motion and pediatric surgical consultation are appropriate.

Next rule out *associated injuries.* Initially do not perform a muscle test to determine the distribution and severity of paralysis. Stimulation and motion of a broken arm will be painful to the poor baby. Be gentle! *Fracture of the ipsilateral clavicle* is not uncommon in obstetrical brachial plexus paralysis. A broken clavicle is accompanied by local swelling and tenderness at the fracture site, whereas in simple brachial plexus injury the swelling, ecchymosis, and tenderness are supraclavicular. There may be *fracture-separation of the upper humeral physis or fractures of the humeral shaft.* Radiograms of the shoulder and upper arm settle the diagnosis. Make comparison views of the contralateral limb.

Traumatic shoulder dislocation, usually posterior or inferior, can occur at birth or soon afterward. Fortunately it is rare. Often diagnosis is delayed for months. *Gently* determine the range of motion of the affected shoulder and palpate the position of the humeral head. Dislocation of the shoulder should be suspected when there is restriction of range of glenohumeral motion. Caution! Do not be misled

by the normal range of scapulocostal motion. Abduction contracture of the shoulder is another suggestive sign. Routine radiograms in AP and axillary views are made, but often they are inconclusive. Ultrasonography shows the cartilaginous humeral head and glenoid of the scapula and assists in making the diagnosis. CT scan makes the definitive diagnosis of shoulder dislocation.

Assess the opposite upper limb and the lower limbs for *spasticity.* Transient paresis may result from hematomyelia produced by avulsion of the nerve roots from the spinal cord; anoxia at birth may cause central nervous system damage and cerebral palsy.

The infant with obstetrical brachial plexus paralysis is at high risk for *hip dysplasia* because of intrauterine malposition and breech presentation. Examine the hips by means of the Barlow and Ortolani tests. Perform ultrasonographic examination of the hips if any suggestion of hip instability is present. Dislocation of the hips may develop postnatally. Re-examine the hips at 6 weeks and again at 12 weeks and 6 months of age.

Probable associated injuries and deformities in obstetrical brachial plexus paralysis are summarized in Table 4–3.

Next, perform *muscle strength testing* to determine the distribution and severity of motor paralysis. It is best to have a pediatric physical therapist or occupational therapist assist you in muscle strength testing. Electric stimulation may be employed, particularly when testing parascapular muscles. Muscle testing is repeated at 3 months, 6 months, 1 year, 1½ years, and 2 years of age. In the neonate, paralysis ordinarily is more diffuse, with some involvement of most of the components of the plexus; however, recovery takes place rapidly and continues up to 18 to 24 months of age.

Finally, *sensation* to pin prick and touch is tested and the extent of sensory loss is recorded.

Differential Diagnosis. In the neonate, pseudoparalysis due to fracture of the clavicle, upper humeral physis, or humeral shaft, to osteomyelitis of the humerus or the clavicle, or to septic arthritis of the shoulder should be considered.

TABLE 4–3. INJURIES AND DEFORMITIES THAT MAY BE ASSOCIATED WITH OBSTETRICAL BRACHIAL PLEXUS PALSY

Horner syndrome—enophthalmos, miosis, ptosis

Paralysis of diaphragm—phrenic nerve palsy

Fracture of the ipsilateral clavicle

Fracture-separation of the proximal humeral growth plate

Fracture of the shaft of the humerus

Traumatic dislocation of the shoulder

Spasticity of the lower limbs or opposite upper limb due to hematomyelia or anoxia of the central nervous system

Hip dysplasia-dislocation

Pseudoparalysis is characterized by lack of spontaneous movement due to pain on motion. In brachial plexus paralysis, the Moro reflex and asymmetric tonic neck reflexes are absent, whereas in pseudoparalysis these reflexes are present. Also, careful inspection and palpation reveal local swelling, tenderness, and crepitation at the fracture site. Brachial plexus paralysis and fractures of the shoulder girdle may coexist. Local swelling occurs in the arm in acute osteomyelitis, whereas in septic arthritis the shoulder is swollen. On testing, range of motion of the shoulder is restricted and painful. It behooves the surgeon to remember that in septicemia in the neonate, systemic signs are absent; there may be no fever or elevation of the erythrocyte sedimentation rate or white blood count.

Spinal cord tumor or injury may mimic brachial plexus paralysis. Be suspicious when involvement is bilateral and in the presence of spasm and rigidity of the neck. Appropriate neurologic diagnostic studies, including MRI of the cervical spine, confirm the diagnosis of spinal cord tumor.

All patients with obstetrical brachial plexus paralysis should routinely have radiograms made of the clavicle, upper limb, and cervical spine—AP, lateral, oblique, and open-mouth views. Routine MRI is not recommended because the newborn must be deeply sedated or anesthetized. A cervical myelogram is not indicated because it is an invasive procedure. It is performed only when no return of function is seen in 3 to 6 months and microsurgical repair and nerve grafting of the brachial plexus are contemplated, or when there is a possibility of a spinal cord tumor. Request a neurosurgical consultation.

Prognosis for Spontaneous Recovery. This varies with the severity and type of paralysis. As a rule, maximum spontaneous recovery takes place within 18 to 24 months. Poor prognostic signs are (1) complete paralysis of the entire plexus, (2) the presence of Horner's syndrome, (3) paralysis of the parascapular muscles, and (4) paralysis of the phrenic nerve.

Residual Deformities. *Shoulder.* Pathogenic factors are muscle imbalance, asynergy of muscles controlling the shoulder, muscle contracture and fibrosis and contracture of ligamentous tissue and capsule. Zancolli has divided residual deformities of the shoulder into two groups. In group I there is joint contracture, and in group II there is pure flaccid paralysis without muscular contracture, joint deformity, or dislocation.[144] The two groups can be distinguished by Putti's scapular elevation sign (Fig 4–19).[139] The test is performed as follows: The elbow is flexed to 90 degrees with the arm held at the side of the trunk. When the shoulder deformity is medial rotation and adduction, the shoulder is adducted and laterally rotated; the upper medial corner of the scapula elevates when there is incongruity and subluxation of the glenohumeral joint. When the deformity is abduction and lateral rotation contracture, the shoulder is rotated medially and adducted and the superomedial border of the scapula elevates. When there is pure abduction contracture of the glenohumeral joint, the shoulder is simply adducted. When the Putti's sign is positive, the upper medial angle of the scapula elevates.

GROUP I. A common deformity is *fixed medial rotation-adduction contracture* of the shoulder with limitation of active and passive abduction and lateral rotation of the shoulder. It is caused by paralysis of the supraspinatus, infraspinatus, teres minor, and posterior and middle deltoid muscles with normal function of their antagonist muscles—pectoralis major, subscapularis, teres major, and latissimus dorsi. Secondary deformities of the glenoid fossa develop. It becomes broad and flattened, and, with the persistent medially rotated and adducted posture of the shoulder and fixed contracture of the subscapularis and pectorals, the shoulder tends to displace posteriorly (Fig 4–20). Bony deformities develop. The coracoid process becomes elongated, hooks downward, and laterally pushes the humeral head posteriorly. The acromion beaks downward; the shaft and upper end of the humerus develop retrotorsion; the scapula becomes smaller and higher in position. The bony deformities of the acromion and coracoid further limit lateral rotation and abduction of the shoulder. Limited abduction–lateral rotation and extension of the shoulder hamper the function in the upper limb, making it difficult for the patient to bring his hand to the top of his head or back of the neck. Function is further diminished by paralysis of the muscles of the hand and forearm.

Abduction–lateral rotation contracture is often caused by inferior subluxation or dislocation of the glenohumeral joint. Other etiologic factors are fibrosis and contracture of denervated supraspinatus, infraspinatus, and teres minor and previous operations, such as lateral transfer of medial rotators of the shoulder, excessive lateral rotation osteotomy of the humerus, and anteroinferior capsulotomy of the glenohumeral joint. Abduction–lateral rotation contracture of

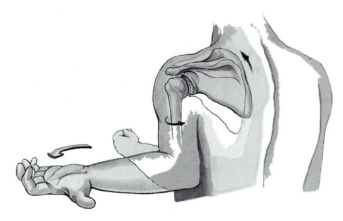

Figure 4–19. Putti's scapular elevation sign. Note that on lateral rotation of the shoulder the superomedial border of the scapula elevates as a result of incongruity and contracture of the glenohumeral joint.

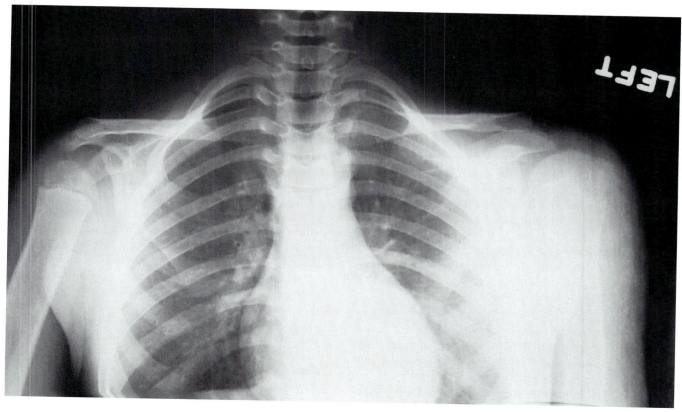

Figure 4–20. Radiogram of the shoulders in obstetrical brachial plexus palsy. Note the flattened dysplastic glenoid of the scapula on the right.

the shoulder is manifested clinically by winging of the scapula when the arm is postured at the side of the trunk. The glenohumeral joint is stiff and markedly limited in range of motion, especially abduction-adduction and medial and lateral rotation. When the glenohumeral joint is dislocated, one may feel the humeral head inferiorly and anteriorly or posteriorly. Functionally, the child is unable to bring his or her hand to the mouth or the front of the body. Radiograms demonstrate joint incongruity, with flattening of the glenoid fossa and anterior and inferior displacement of the humeral head. Computed tomography demonstrates subluxation.

Pure abduction contracture of the shoulder is caused by contracture of the supraspinatus muscle. When the arm is at the side, only the superomedial part of the scapula protrudes.

GROUP II. In *total flaccid paralysis of the shoulder,* the shoulder is flail and no contractural deformity is present.

Elbow. Deformities are flexion contracture and posterior dislocation of the radial head. Flexion deformity of the elbow is caused by strong pull of the biceps brachii and brachialis muscles as opposed to the weak triceps brachii and the use of the elbow in hyperflexed position to compensate

for limited abduction of the shoulder. The olecranon and coronoid process hypertrophy and further block extension of the elbow. In severe, neglected cases, elbow flexion deformity can be as much as 70 to 100 degrees.

Posterior dislocation of the radial head is caused by muscle imbalance with hyperactivity of the pronators and weak supinators of the forearm and improper, rigid splinting. This is a common deformity that is often missed.

Forearm and Hand. Paralysis and deformity are frequent in the lower-arm and whole-arm types of obstetrical brachial plexus paralysis. Supination contracture of the forearm and extension deformity of the wrist are very disabling.

Treatment. In the neonate and infant treatment consists of gentle, passive exercises to maintain range of motion of the shoulder, elbow, forearm, and wrist and to prevent development of contractural deformities. The physical therapist instructs the parents and supervises the therapy program. Guided active exercises using stimulation technique assist in the development of normal cerebral motor patterns. Rigid splinting should not be used, and the custom of pinning the arm in abduction and lateral rotation with the help of a diaper should be condemned; it is archaic and may cause dislocation of the shoulder and/or elbow joint. In the total flail upper limb type, the hand and wrist may be splinted part-time in functional position when the infant is several months old.

Neurosurgical repair of brachial plexus palsy by microsurgical techniques is controversial. Gilbert recommends repair of the brachial plexus with appropriate intercostal nerve grafts when there is no return of elbow flexion or shoulder abduction at 3 months of age.[128–130] This practice is not widely utilized in North America. This author does not recommend microsurgical intervention when paralysis is partial. However, when severe paralysis with a nearly flail upper limb persists in a child 3 to 6 months of age, this author recommends that the parents seek consultation with a competent neurosurgeon for possible repair of the brachial plexus. The indications, results, and drawbacks should be thoroughly discussed with the family, and appropriate imaging work-up in the form of cervical myelogram and MRI should be performed to delineate the exact pathology and the level of injury.

Management of Residual Deformities. Lateral rotation osteotomy of the humerus is performed when there is fixed medial rotation-adduction deformity of the shoulder with paralysis of the teres major and the latissimus dorsi muscles are not strong enough to transfer as lateral rotators of the shoulder. Other indications are marked retrotorsion of the humerus, as demonstrated by CT scan, and structural deformity of the glenohumeral joint with incongruity and some posterior displacement. The Putti sign is positive. The objective of surgery is to improve posture and function of the arm. It increases range of lateral rotation and abduction of the shoulder.

For simple medial rotation contracture of the shoulder, subscapularis recession at its origin is effective to correct the deformity.[123] When medial rotation contracture of the shoulder is associated with weakness of the lateral rotators of the shoulder, latissimus dorsi and teres major muscles are transferred to the rotator cuff.[134]

Flail shoulder is treated by arthrodesis near skeletal maturity. It is important, however, that the hand be functional and that the trapezius, scapulocostal muscles, and scapular elevators are normal or good in motor strength.

■ ELBOW

EXAMINATION

The elbow is a hinge joint consisting of the humeroradial and humeroulnar joints. Begin by inspecting the resting posture of the elbow joint in stance and in gait. Is it held in flexion or extension? Does the degree of elbow flexion increase abnormally during ambulation, indicating spasticity? Next, look for scars (surgical or traumatic) and needle punctures. Is there diffuse soft tissue swelling of the elbow joint due to synovitis? Is there effusion? Rule out localized

soft tissue swelling such as that seen in olecranon bursitis. In the Little League elbow, the swelling is lateral in the region of the humeroradial joint. Is there any abnormal bony prominence as in subluxation or dislocation of the radial head? Is the medial or lateral epicondyle of the distal humerus of one side more prominent than that of the contralateral side?

Next, determine the *carrying angle* of the elbow joint, which is the angle formed between the longitudinal axis of the arm and forearm with the elbow in neutral extension and the forearm in complete supination (Fig 4–21A). *Cubitus varus* denotes medial deviation of the forearm in relation to the arm, whereas *cubitus valgus* denotes lateral deviation. The normal carrying angle varies; it is greater in the female (10 to 15 degrees) than in the male (5 degrees). Assess the carrying angle from the front. When the forearm is pronated the carrying angle disappears, and on progressive flexion of the elbow it decreases. The importance of full supination of the forearm and neutral extension of the elbow cannot be overemphasized.

Ask the patient to acutely flex the elbow. In the normal elbow the tip of the long finger touches the lateral end of the clavicle. In cubitus varus deformity the fingertips point lateral to the shoulder (Fig 4–21B). In cubitus valgus deformity the fingers point medial to the shoulder, toward the patient's mouth (Fig 4–21C, D). Cubitus valgus deformity occurs in radial head dislocation, in malunion of supracondylar fractures of the humerus, and in malunion and growth arrest of the lateral condyle of the humerus. Cubitus varus deformity commonly occurs as a complication of nonunion of a supracondylar fracture of the humerus, physeal injury of the medial part of the trochlea of the distal humerus, and asymmetric growth arrest.

Inspect and palpate the *bony prominences* of the posterior aspect of the elbow joint: (1) the medial epicondyle, (2) the olecranon process, and (3) the lateral epicondyle. With the elbow flexed 90 degrees these three bony landmarks form an equilateral triangle, lying in a plane parallel to the plane of the posterior surface of the upper arm (Fig 4–22A). When the elbow is completely extended these bony points form a straight line (Fig 4–22B). Changes in the carrying angle of the elbow when examined posteriorly with the elbow flexed 90 degrees are readily detected by the medial tilting (cubitus varus) or lateral tilting (cubitis valgus) of the lower end of the humerus.

Range of Motion. Determine both the active and passive ranges. The plane of motion at the elbow (a hinge joint) is in only one plane—flexion and extension (Fig 4–23). The zero starting position is the extended straight elbow. *Flexion* is the movement of bending the elbow away from the zero starting position. Ask the child to touch his fingers to the front of his shoulder. With a normal elbow, he should be able to do so. Soft tissue on the anterior aspect of the upper arm limits elbow flexion. The biceps brachii, brachialis, and brachioradialis are the primary flexors of the

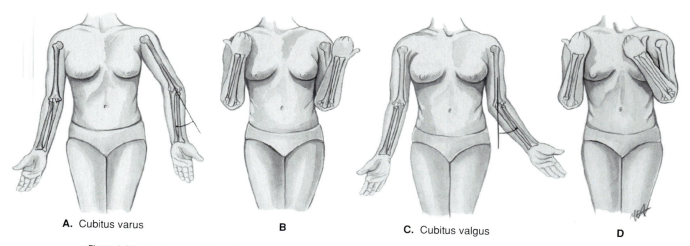

A. Cubitus varus   **B**   **C.** Cubitus valgus   **D**

Figure 4–21. Carrying angle of the elbow. **A.** Cubitus varus on the left. Note that the longitudinal axis of the forearm is tilted medially in relation to the longitudinal axis of the arm. The right elbow is normal. **B.** In cubitus varus (left) on acute flexion of the elbow, the fingers point laterally to the lateral end of the clavicle. In the normal elbow (right) the fingers point to the shoulder. **C.** Cubitus valgus (left). Note that the longitudinal axis of the forearm is tilted laterally in relation to the longitudinal axis of the arm. **D.** In acute flexion of the elbow, the hand points medially toward the sternum.

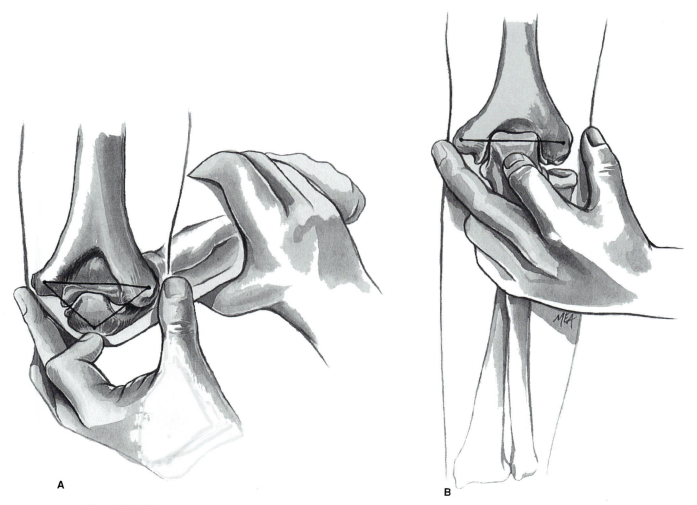

A   **B**

Figure 4–22. Relationship of the bony prominence of the posterior aspect of the elbow joint. **A.** In 90 degrees of flexion, note that the medial epicondyle, olecranon process, and lateral epicondyle form an equilateral triangle. **B.** When the elbow is in complete extension, they form a straight line.

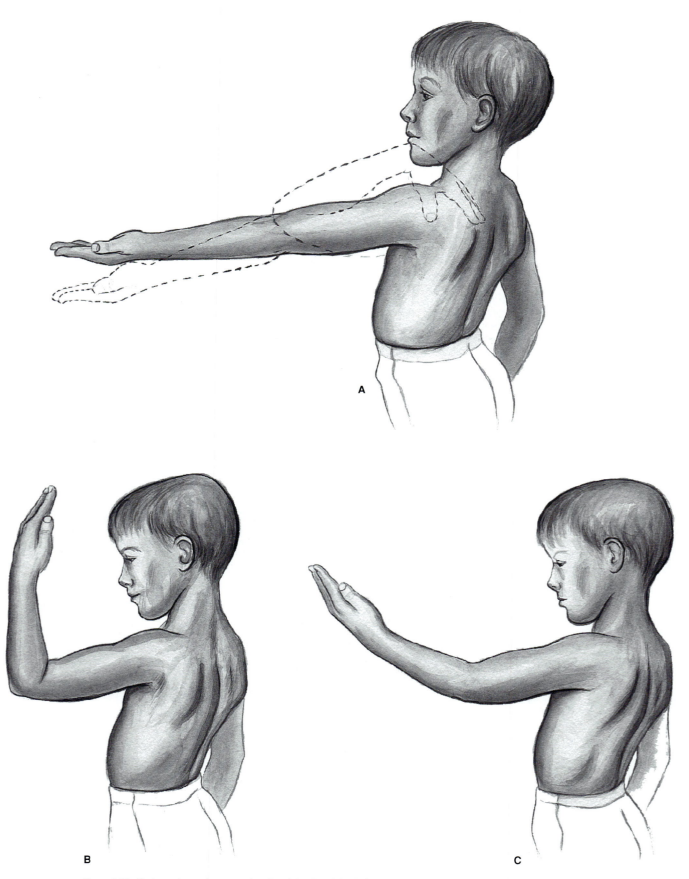

Figure 4–23. Flexion and extension range of motion of the elbow joint. **A–C.** Note that the zero starting position is the extended straight elbow with the forearm in full supination.

elbow. *Extension* is the movement of straightening of the elbow. The normal range of elbow extension is 0 degrees. At this point the olecranon process touches the olecranon fossa. When the ligamentous and capsular tissues are hyperlax, the elbow extends beyond neutral (0 degrees); in such an instance the term *hyperextension* is used to describe the abnormal extensibility of the elbow joint. In the female, 5 degrees of hyperextension is normal. Athletic, muscular adolescents may have a few degrees of lack of elbow extension from neutral position because of increased tension in the biceps brachii muscle. In spastic paralysis and arthritis of the elbow (inflammatory or traumatic), limitation of elbow extension commonly occurs. Osseous causes of flexion deformity of the elbow are epiphyseal dysplasia, a malunited supracondylar fracture of the humerus, or intraarticular loose bodies blocking extension.

As you flex and extend the elbow, palpate and listen for *crepitation* from the elbow joint; it may be due to loose bodies, chondromalacia of the joint due to arthritis, or synovial or bursal bands.

Palpation. Next, gently *palpate* the soft tissues and bones on the medial, lateral, posterior, and anterior aspects of the elbow. Is there any effusion in the joint? Is the synovium thickened? Is there any elevation of local temperature? Feel the elbow with the dorsum of the proximal phalanges of your hands and compare the temperature with the opposite side. Is there any soft tissue mass or enlarged epitrochlear lymph nodes? Gently palpate the lateral epicondyle and lateral supracondylar line of the humerus, the olecranon process and olecranon fossa, and the medial epicondyle and medial supracondylar line of the humerus. Is there any local tenderness?

Then test the *ligamentous stability* of the elbow joint. First, place one hand on the medial side of the distal arm immediately above the elbow joint, and with your other hand, apply varus stress at the elbow joint by pushing the forearm medially. With one hand grasp the lateral aspect of the distal arm just above the elbow joint, and exert valgus stress by pushing the forearm laterally with your other hand. The elbow should be in a few degrees of flexion. Palpate for tenderness over the medial and lateral collateral ligaments of the elbow and for a gap of the joint medially when valgus stress is applied and laterally when varus stress is applied.

In the adolescent or adult in whom tennis elbow is suspected, perform the following test. Ask the patient to make a fist and extend the wrist with the forearm in full pronation. With one hand steady the proximal forearm immediately distal to the elbow joint with your thumb over the lateral epicondyle and the tendon of the common extensors at its origin, and with your other hand push the extended wrist into flexion. The patient experiences acute pain at the origin of the tendons of the common extensor in the presence of tennis elbow.

Next test the *deep tendon reflexes* in the upper limb. First test the *biceps reflex.* Rest the patient's forearm on your forearm and put your thumb on the biceps tendon near its insertion. Tap your thumb nail with a reflex hammer or with the ulnar border of your opposite hand. The elbow should jerk into some flexion with contraction of the biceps brachii muscle. The biceps is innervated by the musculocutaneous nerve, which is a function of the C5 neurologic level. To test the *brachioradialis reflex,* place the patient's upper limb in the same position as for the biceps reflex. With the reflex hammer or ulnar border of your hand, tap the brachioradialis tendon distally over the radius; the wrist deviates radially. The brachioradialis is innervated by the radial nerve, and the brachioradialis reflex is the test for C6 neurologic level function. For the *triceps reflex,* tap the triceps tendon over the olecranon fossa. The elbow jerks into extension. The position of the patient's arm is the same as above. The triceps reflex is a function of the C7 neurologic level (see Figs 4–2 through 4–6, pp. 267–271).

Inspect the general alignment of the forearm. Is it bowed ulnarward or radially? What is the resting posture? Is it in neutral position, supination with the palm up, or pronation with the palm down? Look for the relationship of the distal radius and ulna. In the normal wrist, the radial styloid process is 1 to 1.5 cm distal to the ulnar styloid process. Is the distal end of the ulna prominent dorsally, indicating Madelung's deformity? Is the radial head prominent proximally, indicating radial head subluxation or dislocation? Test range of motion of the forearm. It is important that you hold the lower arm steady with one hand and hold the wrist at the lower end of the radius and ulna and pronate and supinate it. Normal range of motion is 90 degrees of supination and 90 degrees of pronation. Ranges of wrist motion are palmar flexion, dorsiflexion, and ulnar and radial deviation. Ranges of metacarpophalangeal and interphalangeal joints of the fingers are palmar flexion and dorsiflexion. The fingers abduct and adduct (Fig 4–24). The thumb ranges are flexion, extension, abduction-adduction, and opposition (Fig 4–25).

PULLED ELBOW (TRAUMATIC SUBLUXATION OF THE RADIAL HEAD)

This is a common injury in children under 4 years of age; it rarely occurs in a child 5 years of age or older. It is produced by sudden forceful longitudinal traction on the hand with the forearm pronated and the elbow extended. Ordinarily it occurs when the child is lifted by the hand to prevent falling over a curb or is pulled by the hand during play. Often it is referred to as nursemaid's elbow or temper tantrum elbow.

Following injury the child cries with pain and holds the partially flexed elbow and pronated forearm of the affected arm with the opposite hand. He refuses to move or use the involved limb.

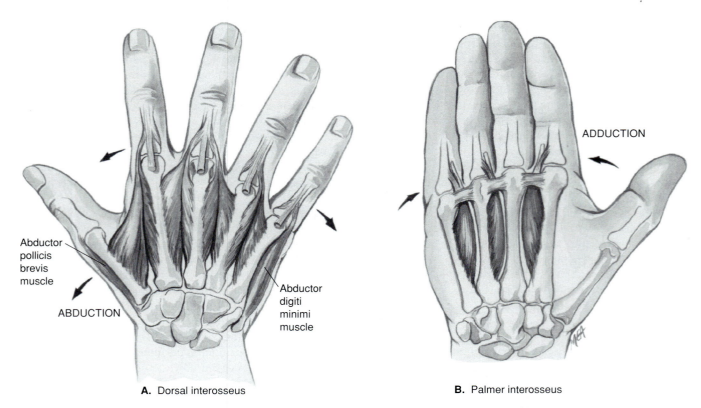

A. Dorsal interosseus

Abductor pollicis brevis muscle

ABDUCTION

Abductor digiti minimi muscle

B. Palmer interosseus

ADDUCTION

Figure 4–24. Range of abduction and adduction of the fingers. **A.** Dorsal view. **B.** Palmar view.

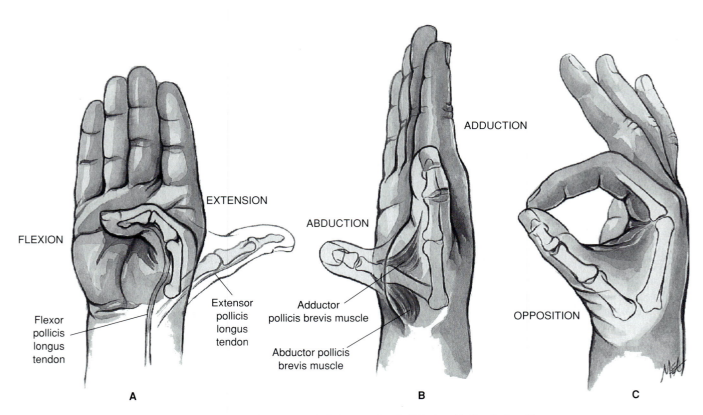

EXTENSION

FLEXION

Flexor pollicis longus tendon

Extensor pollicis longus tendon

ADDUCTION

ABDUCTION

Adductor pollicis brevis muscle

Abductor pollicis brevis muscle

OPPOSITION

A

B

C

Figure 4–25. Range of thumb motion. **A.** Flexion-extension. **B.** Abduction-adduction. **C.** Opposition.

Palpation reveals local tenderness over the anterolateral part of the radial head. Supination of the forearm is markedly restricted and resisted by the child. On gentle examination, flexion and extension of the elbow are painless and full range of motion is possible. The diagnosis of subluxated elbow is made by these characteristic physical findings. Radiograms are normal.

Ultrasonography of the elbow demonstrates that the distance between the radial head and capitellum of the humerus is increased in cases of pulled elbow, probably due to interposition of the annular ligament.[153]

Mechanism of Injury. In the infant and young child the radial head is larger than the radial neck, in a ratio varying from 1.3:1 to 1.6:1. The smallest ratio in the fetus is 1.1:1, whereas in the adult it is 1.25:1. Therefore, the injury is not caused by the radial head pulling through the annular ligament because of the smaller size of the radial head in relation to the radial neck.

The configuration of the radial head is somewhat oval rather than circular. The anterior part of the radial head elevates acutely from the radial neck, whereas the posterior and lateral parts of the radial head rise rather gradually. When longitudinal traction is applied on the wrist with the forearm in *supination,* the annular ligament is held firmly in place by the acute elevation of the radial head. When the forearm is in *pronation,* longitudinal traction on the wrist results in the annular ligament slipping over the radial head.

The experimental anatomic studies of Salter and Zaltz demonstrated that in children under 5 years of age, sudden forceful pull on the head with the elbow extended and the forearm supinated did not cause subluxation of the radial head, whereas when the forearm was in pronation the sudden longitudinal traction force on the forearm resulted in (1) a transverse tear of the thin, weak distal attachment of the annular ligament to the radial neck, (2) the anterior part of the radial head sliding through the anterior part of the annular ligament, and (3) the detached portion of the annular ligament slipping over the radial head and becoming trapped in the radiohumeral joint. In children over 4 years of age a tear in the annular ligament could not be produced by forceful traction with the elbow in extension and the forearm in pronation; this is due to the thick and strong annular ligament.[156]

The subluxated radial head could be easily reduced by passive supination of the forearm when the detached interposed portion of the annular ligament did not extend beyond the equator (transverse diameter) of the radial head; however, when the interposed annular ligament extended beyond the equator, the subluxated radial head could not be reduced by passive supination of the forearm. When greater force is applied, the entire humero-ulnar-radial joint dislocates.

Treatment. Simply hold the elbow with one hand to prevent rotation of the shoulder and with the other hand rotate the child's forearm into full supination. Upon reduction of the subluxation a click may be felt and/or heard. The relief from pain is immediate. The child smiles and begins to use the limb.

Ordinarily immobilization of the elbow is not required when it is the first subluxation and treatment is not delayed; however, immobilization is advisable if reduction is delayed for more than 12 hours or reduction is unstable, as shown when, on pronation of the forearm, pain and clicking occur and the child refuses to use the forearm. It is best to immobilize the upper limb for 10 to 14 days in an above-elbow posterior mold or cast with the forearm in full supination and the elbow in 90 degrees of flexion. Recurrent subluxation of the radial head requires splinting for 2 to 3 weeks, particularly when the child has generalized ligamentous hyperlaxity.

Occasionally the subluxated radial head cannot be reduced by closed supination of the forearm. This occurs in the older child in whom the interposed detached annular ligament extends beyond the equator of the radial head. These very rare cases are treated by open surgery. The entrapped annular ligament is sectioned, and its divided ends are withdrawn from the radiohumeral joint and repaired with several interrupted sutures.

CONGENITAL DISLOCATION OF THE RADIAL HEAD[158–162]

This rare abnormality is usually not detected in the newborn or infant. It is diagnosed later on in childhood when the parents note that the elbow does not straighten or bend fully. The condition is not painful, and no local tenderness is present. Occasionally, the dislocation is noted on radiograms taken following some minor trauma.

The displacement of the radial head may be posterior, anterior, or lateral. Restriction of range of motion of the elbow joint is due to bony contact between the radial head and lower end of the humerus. In posterior dislocation, extension of the elbow is limited. The displaced radial head is prominent and palpable posteriorly, and the ulna is bowed dorsally in its proximal third. By contrast, in anterior dislocation the elbow does not flex fully, the displaced radial head is prominent and palpable anterior in the cubital fossa, and the ulna is bowed volarward in its upper third. Ordinarily pronation or supination of the forearm are not limited, but on rotation of the forearm sometimes a click may be audible and palpable, which is bothersome to the concerned parent although not to the patient.

Involvement may be bilateral or unilateral. In anterior dislocation of the radial head often both elbows are affected. In unilateral anterior dislocation, trauma should be ruled out.

Congenital dislocation of the radial head may occur in congenital radioulnar synostosis or in congenital absence or longitudinal deficiency of the ulna. It may be part of a syndrome such as Larsen's syndrome in which the hips and/or knees are also dislocated, the feet are deformed with talipes equinovarus, and the facial features are characteristic.

Imaging Findings. The ossification center of the radial head does not appear until the age of 5 years in girls and 6 years in boys. Ultrasonograms depict the cartilaginous radial head and demonstrate the dislocation. In the radiograms, a line is drawn through the longitudinal axis of the radial shaft and its relationship to the center of the capitellum of the humerus is determined in true lateral radiograms of the elbow, including the forearm and wrist. In the normal elbow joint, regardless of the degree of flexion or extension of the elbow, the line drawn through the longitudinal axis of the radial shaft bisects the center of the ossific nucleus of the capitellum of the humerus; when it does not, the radial head is subluxated or dislocated (Fig 4–26).

In congenital dislocation of the radial head, the radius is overgrown and it is too long in relation to the ulna. As the child gets older, secondary changes develop. The radial head becomes club-shaped and elliptic and the capitellum of the humerus dysplastic and flattened because of loss of contact and growth stimulation from the dislocated radial head.

Treatment. Closed reduction is often impossible. An attempt may be made in the newborn if the diagnosis is made that early, especially when the dislocation is anterior.

The question arises as to whether open reduction should be performed with shortening of the radius. This issue is controversial. Many surgeons prefer to ignore and accept the dislocation and leave it alone until skeletal growth is complete; then when it becomes symptomatic the radial head is excised. Do not excise the radial head in the young child, as doing so causes proximal migration of the radius, wrist instability and pain, and progressive cubitus valgus.

In the young child (up to 3 years of age) I recommend open reduction of anterior dislocation of the radial head, with Z-lengthening of the biceps brachii and shortening of the radius in its mid-shaft, which is fixed internally with a compression plate. When the annular ligament is fibrosed and irreparable, it is excised and a strip of triceps brachii or triceps fascia is used to reconstruct the annular ligament (Bell Tawse procedure).

DEVELOPMENTAL DISLOCATION OF THE RADIAL HEAD

The radial head subluxates in any bone dysplasia in which the ulna shortens and the radius outgrows the ulna. It is common in multiple hereditary exostosis (Fig 4–27). Other causes of ulnar shortening are fibrous dysplasia of the ulna, osteofibrous dysplasia (Campanacci syndrome) of the ulna, and traumatic or infectious growth arrest of the distal or proximal physis of the ulna.

Another cause of radial head subluxation in multiple exostosis is the pressure of an enlarging exostosis between the upper part of the radius and ulna, pushing the radial head posterolaterally.

Treatment. This consists of elongation of the ulna when the radial head is only subluxated. Ulnar lengthening may have to be combined with radial shortening in its mid-shaft when the radial head is dislocated. The radial head is excised in the skeletally mature patient when it is dislocated and bothersome to the patient, causing limited range of motion or rubbing of the bony protuberance on hard surfaces (Fig 4–27).

TRAUMATIC DISLOCATION OF THE RADIAL HEAD

Radial head dislocation due to trauma is almost always anterior and unilateral. In the infant it may not be detected until later in childhood and may be mistaken for congenital dislocation. In traumatic dislocation of the radial head—either Monteggia fracture-dislocation or the occasional primary traumatic anterior dislocation without associated fractures, the ulna is bowed, the shape of the radial head is not deformed, and the capitellum of the humerus is normal.

An attempt at closed or open reduction is appropriate when diagnosis is made early.

ACQUIRED DISLOCATION OF THE RADIAL HEAD

This dislocation occurs in neuromuscular disorders. In spastic cerebral palsy, the spastic, taut pronator teres causes fixed pronation forearm contracture and displaces the radial head posterolaterally. A simple surgical release of the pronator teres near its insertion prevents dislocation of the radial head and loss of rotation of the forearm.

In brachial plexus paralysis, the radial head may be displaced anteriorly due to paralysis of the triceps brachii and the unopposed pull of the biceps brachii; the subluxation of the radial head may be posterolateral when the forearm is fixed in pronation with loss of active supination.

CONGENITAL SYNOSTOSIS OF THE ELBOW

The presenting complaint is a stiff elbow that is fixed in varying degrees of flexion and pronation, with moderate to

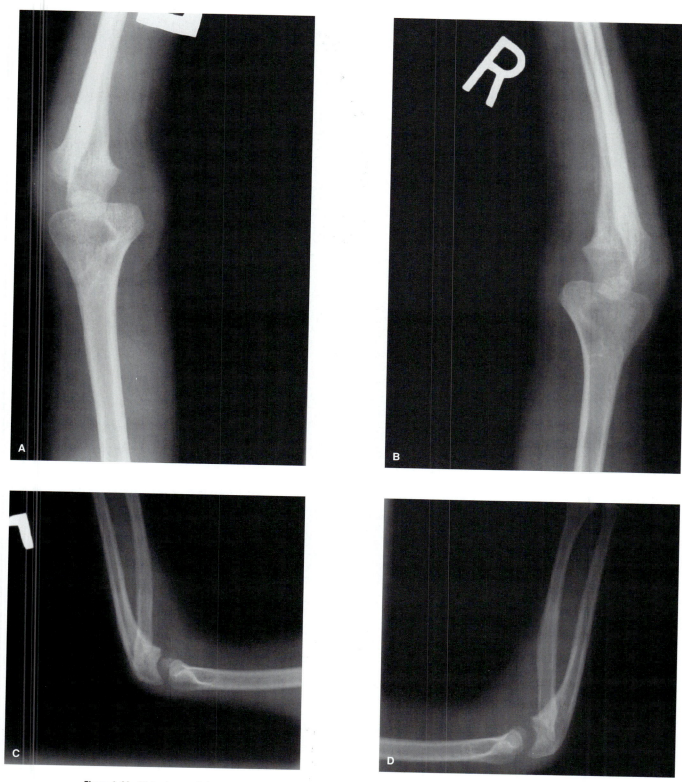

Figure 4–26. Bilateral congenital posterior dislocation of the radial heads. **A–D.** AP and lateral radiographic views of both elbows. Note that a line drawn through the longitudinal axis of the radius traverses posterior to the ossific nucleus of the capitellum of the humerus and does not bisect it.

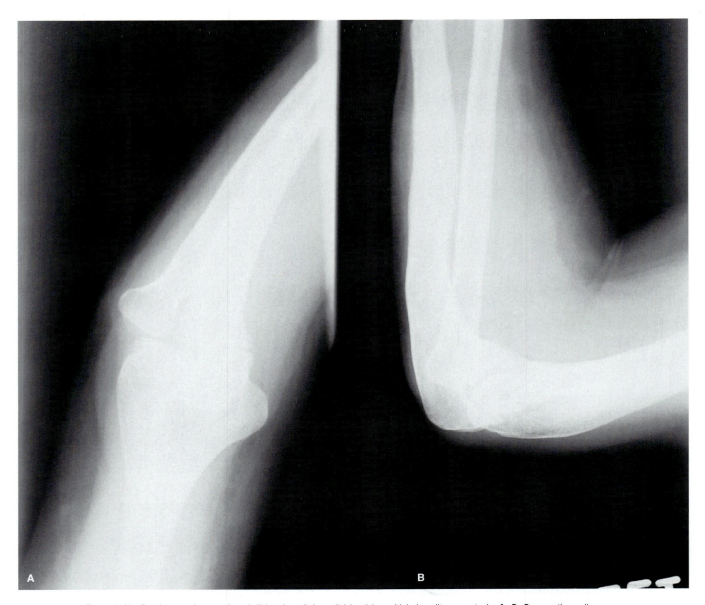

A   B

Figure 4–27. Developmental posterolateral dislocation of the radial head in multiple hereditary exostosis. **A, B.** Preoperative radiograms. *(Continues)*

severe atrophy and shortening of the upper limb. The diagnosis is obvious at birth. It may occur as an isolated anomaly or in association with major congenital malformations of the upper limb. Often the ulna is absent and the synostosis is humeroradial. Involvement may be unilateral or bilateral.

Treatment is individualized. The hyperpronated single-bone forearm is derotated into neutral position to improve functional posture of the hand. Lengthening of the upper limb—humerus and/or radius (in absence of the ulna)—is performed when the upper limb shortening is severe. Arthroplasty of the elbow should not be attempted because it does not succeed.

OSTEOCHONDROSIS OF THE CAPITELLUM OF THE HUMERUS (PANNER'S DISEASE)

This condition occurs in children, presenting with pain and stiffness of the elbow. Examination reveals effusion, minimal to moderate synovial thickening, and local tenderness over the capitellum. Its cause is unknown and is most probably nontraumatic in origin. Radiograms show fragmentation of the capitular epiphysis. Loose fragments do not detach into the elbow joint. The condition is self-limited and benign in its course. The capitellum spontaneously reossifies.[163–165] Treatment is symptomatic; surgical intervention is not indicated.

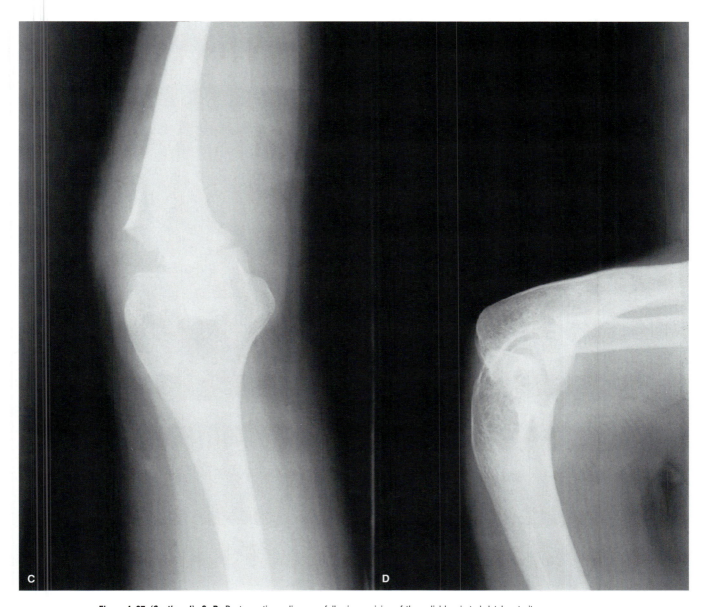

Figure 4–27 *(Continued).* **C, D.** Postoperative radiograms following excision of the radial head at skeletal maturity.

OSTEOCHONDRITIS OF THE CAPITELLUM OF THE HUMERUS (LITTLE LEAGUE ELBOW OR PITCHER'S ELBOW)

This occurs in adolescents between the ages of 11 and 17 years and involves the dominant upper limb. It is more common in boys and in female gymnasts. It is traumatic in its pathogenesis, caused by repetitive valgus stress, and compressive forces of the radial head on the capitellum.

Pain over the lateral condyle of the humerus, stiffness of the elbow in the form of flexion deformity, and limitation of flexion are the findings on physical examination. Radi-ograms show irregular rarefaction of the capitellum of the humerus (Fig 4–28). There may be loose bodies in the elbow joint (Fig 4–29).

Treatment. When there are no loose bodies in the elbow joint, initially the elbow may be supported in an above-elbow cast for a period of 4 to 6 weeks. If there is no response to treatment, the lateral condyle of the humerus is treated with multiple holes drilled through an arthroscope to expedite revascularization. Any loose bodies in the elbow joint are removed either through the arthroscope or more simply through an open arthrotomy.

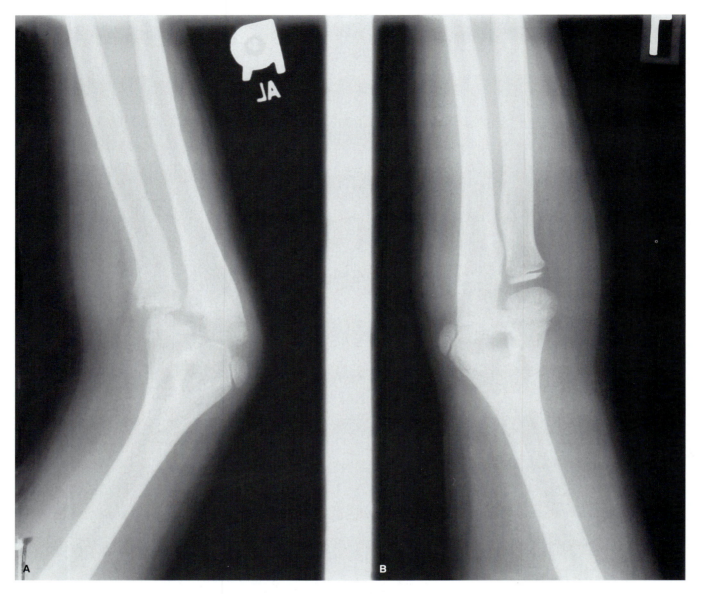

Figure 4–28. Osteochondritis of the capitellum of the humerus of the right elbow. The left elbow is normal. **A–D.** AP and lateral radiograms of both elbows. Note the irregular rarefaction and the radiopacity of the capitellum of the right humerus. *(Continues)*

CONGENITAL RADIOULNAR SYNOSTOSIS[161–171]

The presenting complaint is loss of rotation of the forearm, which is fixed in a position of neutral rotation to hyper-pronation. The deformity is prenatal and present in the new-born; however, it often escapes notice until early childhood.

Etiology. The radius and ulna originate from the same me-sodermal tissue as cartilage. An arrest of development re-sults in failure of longitudinal segmentation and separation of the cartilaginous anlage of the radius and ulna. Bony fusion between the upper ends of both bones of the forearm occurs when the mesodermal tissue between the two bones ossifies.

Classification. There are two types of congenital synos-tosis of the radius and ulna. In *type I* the upper ends of the radius and ulna are completely fused, with no cortical bone between their spongiosa. The radial head may be absent (the "headless type") or completely synostosed to the ulna. The extent of fusion varies; the distal end of the radius and ulna are almost always separate. In *type II* the radial head is dislocated posteriorly and the upper shafts of the radius and ulna are fused (Fig 4–30).

In a third type of radioulnar coalition, the upper parts of the radius and ulna are bound together by a short, thick interosseous ligament that checkreins rotation of the fore-arm. The proximal metaphyseal parts of the radius and ulna are separate.

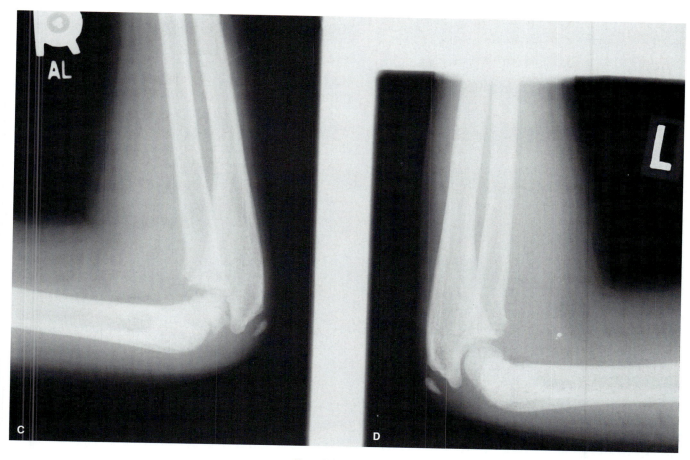

Figure 4–28 *(Continued).*

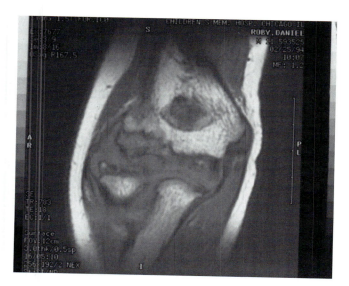

Figure 4–29. Magnetic resonance imaging of the elbow showing osteochondrosis of the capitellum of the humerus with loose bodies in the elbow joint.

Diagnosis. The characteristic finding of radioulnar synostosis is loss of rotation of the forearm. Check it by holding the elbow with one hand and the distal radius and ulna with the other hand and attempt rotation.

When involvement is unilateral, the involved forearm is atrophic with varying degrees of bowing of the radius. In type II radioulnar synostosis, the dislocated radial head may be palpable posteriorly. In type I, in which the radial head is completely fused to the ulna or absent, a dimple (depression) may be present at the site of the normally located radial head. The wrist and shoulder joints have normal range of motion. Lack of supination of the forearm is compensated by excessive rotation at the shoulder joint. Often varying degrees of flexion deformity of the elbows are present.

The degree of functional deficit depends upon the position of the forearm in which it is fixed and whether involvement is unilateral or bilateral. When the forearm is hyperpronated the disability is great; the child can bring only the dorsum of the hand to his mouth and has great difficulty in handling eating utensils. When involvement is bilateral, activities of daily living that require supination-pronation of the forearm, such as turning door knobs or buttoning shirts, are difficult.

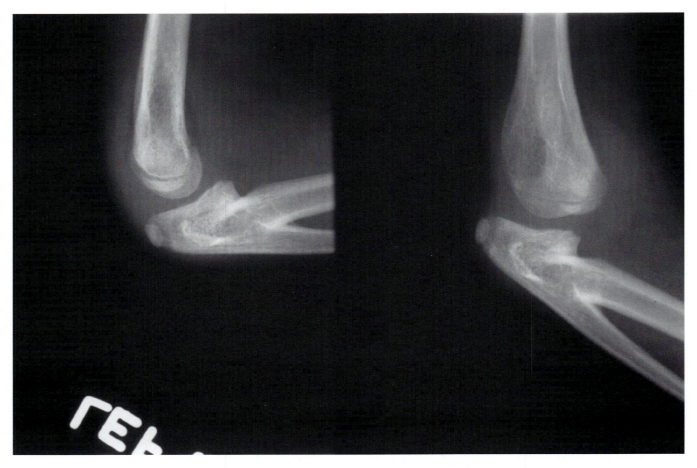

Figure 4–30. Proximal congenital radioulnar synostosis (Type II) with posterior dislocation of the radial head.

Treatment. Surgical separation of the synostosis should not be performed, as the results have been poor and disappointing. Rotation osteotomy is indicated when the functional disability is great because of the hyperpronated fixed position of the forearm. In bilateral cases the dominant side is placed in 30 to 45 degrees of pronation and the contralateral side in 10 to 30 degrees of supination, whereas in unilateral cases the forearm is fixed in neutral rotation. When the degree of rotation required is greater than 45 degrees, osteotomy of both the radius and ulna is performed proximally at the level of the synostosis.

It is simpler to osteotomize the radius only at its middle third. It is best to release the contracted pronator teres near its insertion to prevent recurrence of deformity. The potential risk of compartment syndrome and Volkmann's ischemic contracture should be explained to the patient and family.

CONGENITAL LONGITUDINAL DEFICIENCY OF THE RADIUS[172–178]

The deformity is obvious at birth as the hand is clubbed radially. The severity varies from partial to total absence of the radius. The forearm is short, and the distal radius and radial styloid process cannot be palpated. The ulnar styloid process and distal ulna are prominent, appearing as a knob. The whole forearm is bowed radially. It is often associated with hypoplasia or absence of the thumb and with varying degrees of flexion deformity of the elbow joint. Functional disability varies according to the severity of the deformity and whether involvement is unilateral or bilateral and whether a thumb is absent or present. Ordinarily, the affected child is disabled and has difficulty in self-care such as dressing, feeding, and washing.

The exact cause of congenital absence or hypoplasia of the radius is unknown. It is usually sporadic with no hereditary problem. It is often associated with severe anomalies. Of these, blood dyscrasia (Fanconi pancytopenia and thrombocytopenia with absence of the radius, or TAR syndrome) clinically is the most significant. In the heart, atrial septal defect (Holt-Oram syndrome), ventricular septal defect, coarctation of the aorta, and pulmonary stenosis are common. In the genitourinary tract, hypoplasia or absence of a kidney, horseshoe kidney, and hydronephrosis are not uncommon. In the spine there may be congenital scoliosis due to hemivertebrae, Klippel-Feil syndrome, or sacral agenesis.

It behooves the surgeon to examine the whole child.

Classification. Longitudinal deficiency of the radius may be classified into three types. Type A is simple hypoplasia of the radius in which the distal radial physis is deficient with delay in the ossification center of its epiphysis. Proximally the radial epiphysis and elbow are normal. Type B is partial absence of the radius. The distal and middle portions of the radius are completely absent and are not visible on radiograms at birth (Fig 4–31). The radial deviation of the carpus is moderate. Type C is complete absence of the radius (Fig 4–32).

Treatment. This varies according to the severity of deficiency. In type A the radius is lengthened. In types B and C the carpus is centralized over the distal ulna. An osteotomy is performed to straighten a markedly bowed ulna. The Ilizarov technique is preferred by some surgeons.

CONGENITAL LONGITUDINAL DEFICIENCY OF THE ULNA

This deformity is very rare. The presenting deformity is ulnar clubbing, which is very obvious at birth. It is often associated with congenital ankylosis of the elbow, and the forearm is flexed in hyperpronation, a position of poor function.

Treatment consists of derotation osteotomy of the radius to place the forearm in 30 degrees of supination. When the ulna is very short, it is elongated with the Orthofix callotasis or Ilizarov technique.[179]

■ WRIST AND HAND

MADELUNG'S DEFORMITY[181–189]

The presenting complaint is deformity of the wrist. The distal end of the ulna is prominent, appearing as a knob on

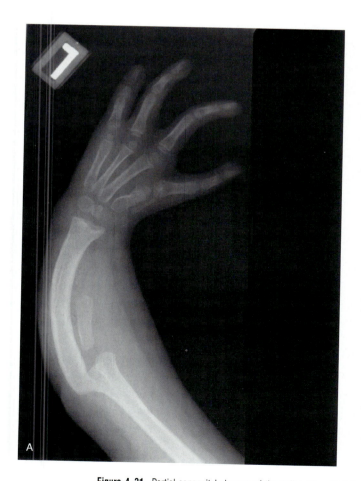
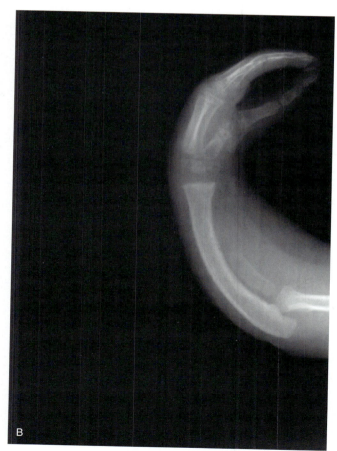

Figure 4–31. Partial congenital absence of the radius (Type B) following centralization of the carpus over the distal end of the ulna. AP **(A)** and lateral **(B)** radiograms.

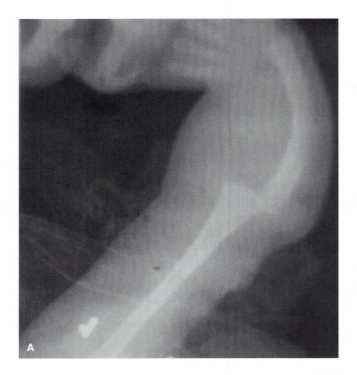

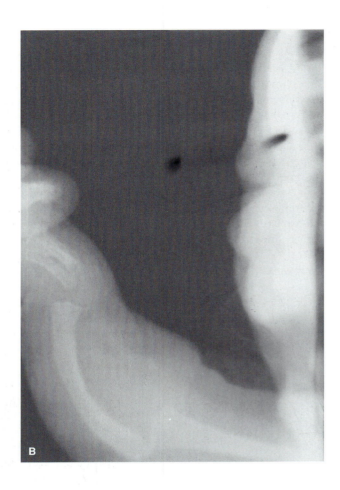

Figure 4–32. Type C congenital longitudinal deficiency of the radius. Note the complete absence of the radius. AP **(A)** and lateral **(B)** radiogram of the left forearm showing longitudinal deficiency of the radius. Note the radial club hand appearance.

the dorsal and ulnar aspects of the wrist (Fig 4–33). The deformity is caused by partial asymmetric growth retardation or arrest of the ulnar and volar aspects of the distal radial physis. The radius is shortened; in the normal wrist the distal radial styloid process is 1 to 1.5 cm distal to the ulnar styloid process; in Madelung's deformity the radial styloid process is at the same level as the ulnar styloid process or proximal to it. The forearms are short. Rotation of the forearm, especially supination, is restricted. The deformity is ordinarily detected between 8 and 12 years of age. The stature of the affected individuals is short, averaging less than 5 feet. The wrists may become painful in late adolescence or early adult life. Both wrists are often involved. Madelung's deformity is an hereditary disorder, transmitted as an autosomal dominant trait.

Imaging. Make radiograms of both wrists to include the forearms and elbows. In the normal wrist the distal articular surface of the radius is tilted 5 degrees volar and 25 degrees toward the ulna; in Madelung's deformity it is tilted volarward as much as 80 degrees and ulnarward as much as 90 degrees. The shortening of the radius is evident. An MRI or CT scan shows the physeal narrowing or closure of the volar and ulnar aspects of the distal radial physis.

Perform a skeletal radiographic survey to rule out gen-

eralized bone dysplasias, which present with Madelung-like deformity of the wrist, such as multiple hereditary exostosis, Ollier's enchondromatosis, Turner XO gonadal dysgenesis syndrome, or Léri-Weill syndrome, in which the tibiae and fibulae are deformed and the phalanges of the hands are short. Partial arrest of the distal radial growth plate may be acquired as a result of trauma or infection.

Treatment. This depends upon the severity of deformity. When the wrist is painful with increasing stiffness, surgery is indicated. Asymmetric growth of the distal radius is controlled by excision of the prematurely fused ulnar and volar parts of the distal radius and interposition of fat. Marked bowing of the distal radius is straightened by osteotomy. Disparity of length between the radius and ulna is treated either by shortening the ulna or by elongating the radius by either the Ilizarov or the Orthofix callotasis technique. Factors to consider in the choice of operation are the age of the patient, the severity of instability of the wrist, and the intensity of pain.

SYNDACTYLY[190–202]

Webbing or fusion of two fingers is the most common congenital anomaly of the hand, occurring once in every 2250

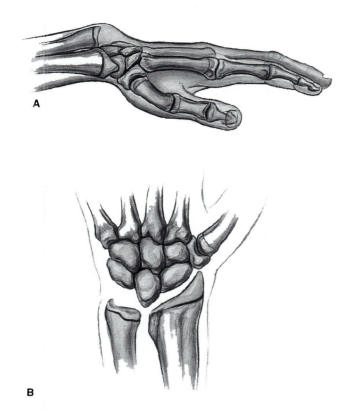

Figure 4–33. Drawing showing Madelung's deformity. **A.** Lateral view. **B.** Posteroanterior view.

births. Syndactyly is caused by failure of differentiation between adjacent fingers. In one of two cases, both hands are involved. Syndactyly between the long and ring fingers is the most common—about 60 percent; next most frequent is syndactyly between the little and ring fingers (27 percent). The thumb develops earlier than the fingers; therefore, syndactyly between the thumb and index finger is rare, occurring in only about 3 percent of cases.

There is a definite sex predilection for the male, boys being affected twice as commonly as girls. Occurrence is sporadic in 80 percent of the cases. A family history is present in 20 percent.

Assessment. Determine the degree of soft tissue webbing and whether it involves only the skin (simple syndactyly) or a bony fusion is present (complex syndactyly). When the webbing between the fingers does not reach the fingertip and stops at a point between the fingertip and the normal commissure, it is classified as incomplete syndactyly (Fig 4–34A). When the fusion of the skin between the fingers extends to the fingertips, the syndactyly is complete (Fig 4–34B).

In complex syndactyly there is osseous connection between the two digits (Fig 4–34C). This is best shown by radiography. Syndactyly may be associated with polydactyly (Fig 4–34D).

It is important to examine the whole child to rule out syndromes. Syndactyly is common in Apert's syndrome (cranial stenosis with syndactyly of hands and feet); in Poland's syndrome, in which the ipsilateral pectoral muscles are absent; and in congenital constriction syndrome (Streeter's dysplasia).

Treatment. The webbed fingers are separated to improve function by restoration of the normal spread between them and to improve appearance. Webbed digits of unequal length, i.e., thumb and index finger and little and ring fingers, develop lateral angulation and flexion deformity. Therefore, they should be separated early in life, between 6 and 12 months of age. There is no urgency to separate syndactylies between long and index fingers and between the ring and long fingers; they can wait until 2 to 3 years of age.

POLYDACTYLY[203–215]

A supernumerary digit is readily diagnosed at birth. It is caused by twinning or duplication of a single embryologic bud.

The extra digit may be lying to the side of the little finger (postaxial), it may be lying on the side of the thumb (preaxial), or occasionally it is central—the ring, middle, and/or index finger is duplicated.

Palpate the extra digit to determine its type: (1) Does it consist of only soft tissue with no bones, joints, or tendons, (2) does part or all of the duplicated digit articulate with a common metacarpal or phalanx, or (3) is the entire digit with its own metacarpal duplicated (Fig 4–35)?[208]

Passively manipulate the interphalangeal and metacarpophalangeal joints to determine their range of motion. Next, by stimulation technique, determine the motor control of the digit. Is there associated simple or complex syndactyly between the duplicated digits, nail dystrophy, and brachydactyly? Examine the whole child to rule out associated anomalies and syndromes. Examine the pectoral region; there may be a duplication of the breast in the female and the nipple in the male.

Incidence and Heredity. Little finger duplication is very common in blacks, occurring in 1 in 300, whereas in whites it occurs in only 1 in 3000. In blacks the extra little finger is not associated with other anomalies or syndromes; it is inherited as an autosomal dominant trait. In whites, associated anomalies and syndromes are commonly present. When the duplication of the little finger in whites appears as a part of a syndrome, it is often inherited as an autosomal recessive trait. Duplication of the thumbs is ordinarily sporadic.

Duplication of the thumb (preaxial polydactyly) occurs in 0.08 per 1000; there is no racial predilection. The inci-

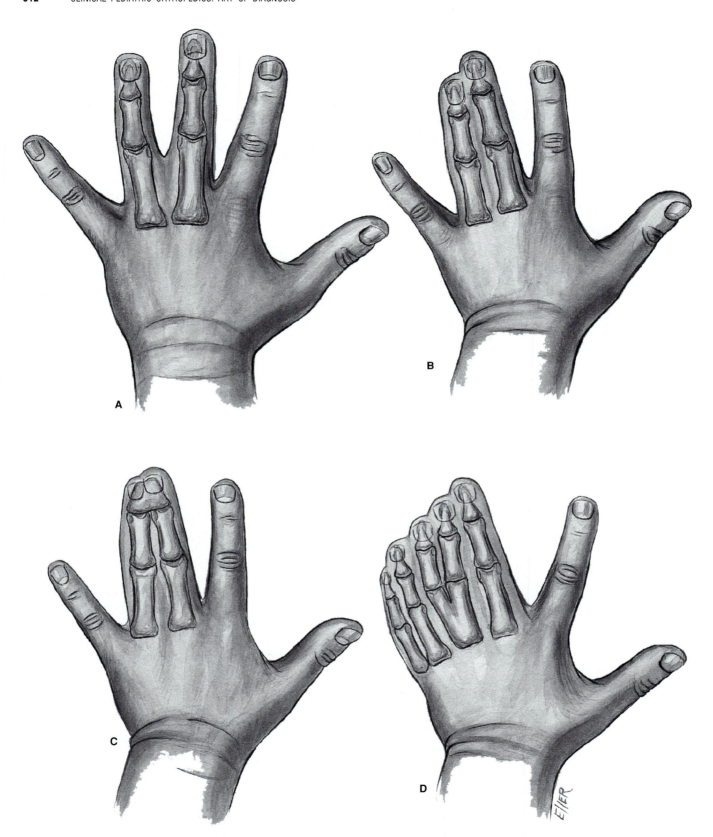

Figure 4–34. Classification of syndactyly. **A.** Incomplete simple syndactyly. Note that the webbing between the two digits stops short of the fingertip. **B.** Complete simple syndactyly. The fusion of the skin between the fingers extends to the fingertips. **C.** Complex syndactyly. Note the bony fusion between the distal phalanges and the complete skin–soft tissue fusion between the long and ring fingers. **D.** Syndactyly associated with polydactyly.

dence is the same in whites and blacks.[209–211,215] Involvement is often unilateral. Seven types of thumb polydactyly have been described by Wassel (Fig 4–36).[212] One of the duplicated thumbs may be underdeveloped, or both thumbs may be of equal size. Assess circulation carefully, as both thumbs may be supplied by one digital vessel.

Treatment. When the little finger is duplicated, the entire extra little finger is simply ablated. When it is a hypoplastic soft tissue mass attached to the little finger by a narrow pedicle, it is removed in the nursery. A fully duplicated little finger is removed in the operating room when the infant is 6 to 12 months of age.

Ablation of the duplicated thumb is more complex. It is important to provide joint alignment and stability and establish adequate motor control and strength.

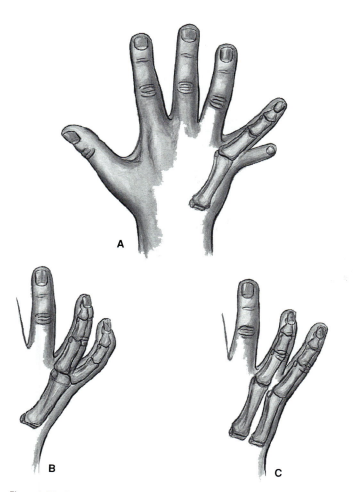

Figure 4–35. Types of postaxial polydactyly. **A.** Type I. The extra digit consists only of soft tissue mass with no bony phalanges. **B.** Type II. Note that the phalanges of the extra finger have normal bony, cartilaginous, and tendinous components; they articulate with an enlarged or bifid single metacarpal. **C.** Type III. The duplicated little finger consists of its own three phalanges, metacarpal, and soft tissue components.

CONGENITAL LONGITUDINAL DEFICIENCY OF THE THUMB[216–220]

This condition manifests in a range of severity from complete absence of the thumb to a floating thumb to simple hypoplasia. The hypoplastic absent thumb is readily detectable at birth, but be cautious. Often longitudinal deficiency of the thumb is associated with shortening of the radius and is a manifestation of a generalized syndrome such as Fanconi or Holt-Oram syndrome. When the first metacarpal of the thumb is short and broad, one should rule out Cornelia de Lange syndrome. Examine the feet. If a short thumb is associated with a short great toe, rule out myositis ossificans progressiva. If the hypoplastic thumb is associated with brachydactyly, it may be a manifestation of Carpenter's or Rubenstein-Taybi syndrome. The importance of examining the whole child in congenital longitudinal deficiency of the thumb cannot be overemphasized. The patient with an absent or hypoplastic thumb has difficulty in grasping, prehension, and opposition.

Treatment. In the floating thumb (pouce flottant) the metacarpal is partially or completely absent. The hypoplastic thumb with a nail and two phalanges has no tendons or motor function; it is useless. It is treated by simple ablation of the vestigial thumb.

The hypoplastic thumb may be elongated by deepening the web proximally between the thumb and index finger; when the interphalangeal and metacarpophalangeal joints are stable, motor function of the thumb is good. The absent thumb is managed by pollicization of the index finger (Fig 4–37). Tendon transfers are performed to provide opposition and abduction of the pollicized index finger. Toe transfers by microsurgical technique are no longer recommended.

WEB CONTRACTURE BETWEEN THUMB AND INDEX FINGER

This is usually associated with other congenital abnormalities such as hypoplasia of the thumb and syndactyly. The restriction of the spread between the thumb and index metacarpal interferes with function. A Z-plasty is performed to deepen the thumb web and improve function (Fig 4–38).

TRIGGER THUMB[221–224]

In this relatively rare deformity the interphalangeal joint of the thumb is locked in flexion, appearing like a trigger (Fig 4–39). Palpation reveals a nontender nodule of varying size on the tendon of the flexor pollicis longus in the vicinity of the metacarpophalangeal joint. The fibrous sheath of the flexor pollicis longus tendon is thickened and constricted. Pathologic examination of the fibrous sheath shows non-

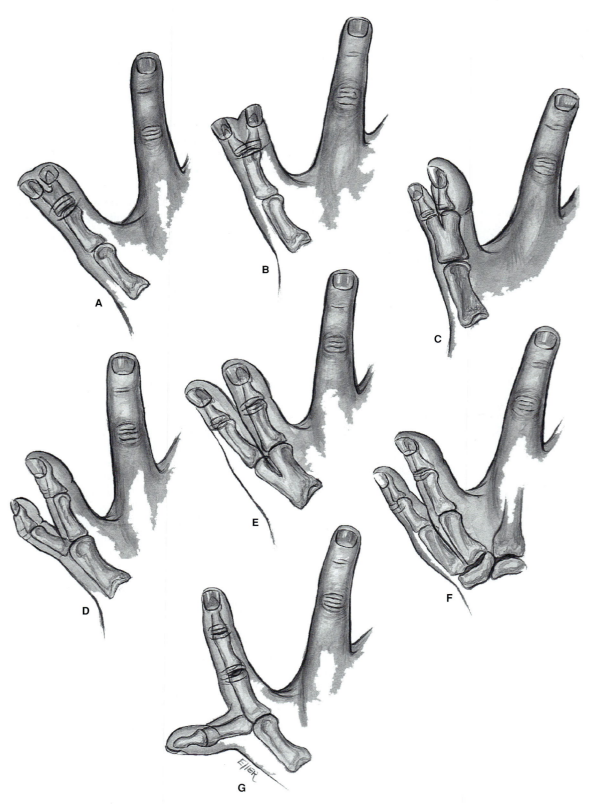

Figure 4–36. Classification of duplication of the thumb according to Wassel. **A.** Type I. The distal phalanx is bifid—very rare—2 percent. **B.** Type II. The distal phalanx is duplicated—15 percent. **C.** Type III. The distal phalanx is duplicated, articulating with a bifid proximal phalanx—6 percent. **D.** Type IV. Both the proximal and distal phalanges of the thumb are duplicated—43 percent. **E.** Type V. Both proximal and distal phalanges are duplicated and the metacarpal is bifid—10 percent. **F.** Type VI. Both phalanges and the metacarpals are duplicated—4 percent. **G.** Type VII. The entire thumb is duplicated and the thumb is triphalangeal—20 percent.

specific chronic inflammatory cells. The constriction is due to stenosing tendovaginitis of the flexor pollicis longus; however, the exact cause is unknown. Sometimes it is familial in incidence; there is no genetic pattern.

Clinical Features. The deformity is present at birth (in 25 percent of the cases) or develops later on in childhood, ordinarily by 2 years of age. In the congenital form, involvement is bilateral in about 50 percent of the cases, whereas in the childhood form both thumbs are involved in about 25 percent of the cases.

Ordinarily the thumb is locked in flexion at the interphalangeal joint (not at the metacarpophalangeal joint). Occasionally the thumb is locked in extension and does not flex at the interphalangeal joint. The nodule on the volar surface of the thumb at the level of the metacarpophalangeal joint is readily palpable. Do not mistake the nodule for a tumor.

Radiograms in the AP, lateral, and oblique projections are made to rule out an osseous lesion such as an osteochondroma. MRI is not indicated.

Treatment. Initially management should be nonsurgical because of the possibility of spontaneous recovery within 12 months, which occurs in 30 percent of cases in the congenital form and 12 percent in the childhood form. During this period of observation parents are instructed to perform gentle passive stretching exercises several times a day;

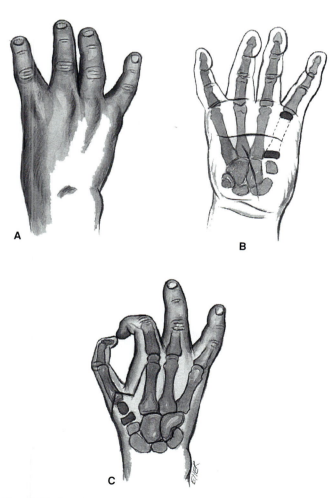

Figure 4–37. Congenital absence of the thumb managed by pollicization of the index finger. **A, B.** Drawings showing the anomaly and skeletal pathology. **C.** Drawing showing the result after pollicization of the index finger. Note that the first metacarpal is shortened, with its distal epiphysis left behind to articulate with the carpus. Tendon transfers are performed to provide opposition and abduction of the pollicized index finger.

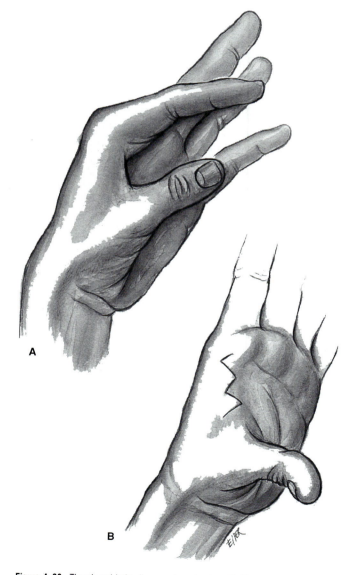

Figure 4–38. Thumb and index finger web contracture. **A.** Note limitation of spread between the two digits. **B.** Appearance after Z-plasty.

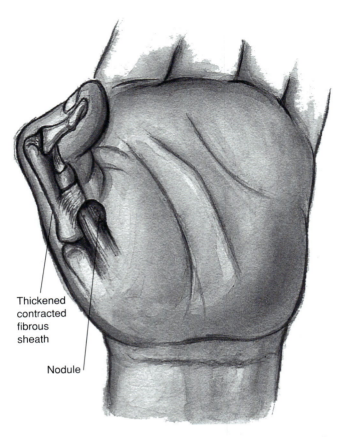

Thickened
contracted
fibrous
sheath

Nodule

Figure 4–39. Trigger thumb in the infant. The interphalangeal joint is locked in flexion. Note the nodule on the volar surface of the flexor pollicis longus tendon and the thickened, contracted fibrous sheath at the level of the metacarpophalangeal joint.

exercises should not be painful. Part-time splinting of the thumb in extension can be attempted, but ordinarily the splints are not tolerated by the infant and young child; they are difficult to fit and the thumb slides out of the splint.

In the 2- to 3-year-old child in whom the deformity persists, surgical correction is indicated; it consists of simple release by partial excision of the contracted fibrous sheath of the flexor pollicis longus tendon through a transverse incision at the flexor crease of the metacarpophalangeal joint of the thumb. The procedure is done as an outpatient surgical procedure under general anesthesia. The result of surgery is excellent. Complications are inadvertent sectioning of the digital nerves or flexor tendon and infection. Adherence of the tendon can be prevented by partial excision of the fibrous sheath instead of simple release by dividing the sheath.

CONGENITAL CLASPED THUMB[225–227]

In this deformity the metacarpophalangeal joint of the thumb is acutely flexed, lying across the palm of the hand (Fig 4–40). It is caused by anomalies of the extensor-flexor mechanism of the thumb. Congenital clasped thumb should

be distinguished from trigger thumb, in which the flexion deformity is at the interphalangeal joint.

Treatment depends upon the type of anomaly. When the deformity is due to simple hypoflexion or aplasia of the extensor pollicis brevis, initially the thumb is splinted into extension-abduction. At about 2 to 3 years of age, the extensor indicis proprius tendon is transferred for restoration of thumb extension-abduction. In the more severe type of clasped thumb, soft tissue release of the contracted thumb and webbed skin is performed by Z-plasty or a full dorsal rotation flap and a full-thickness skin graft.

KIRNER DEFORMITY[232,238]

In this deformity the terminal phalanx of the little finger is deviated radially and into volar flexion (Fig 4–41). It is hereditary, transmitted as an autosomal dominant trait. In-

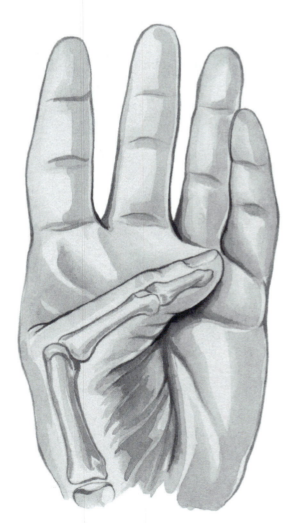

Figure 4–40. Congenital clasped thumb. Note that the thumb is markedly flexed at the metacarpophalangeal joint and adducted across the palm.

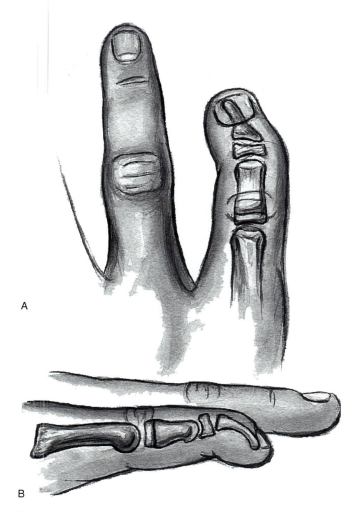

A

B

Figure 4–41. Kirner deformity. **A.** Dorsal view. **B.** Lateral view. Note that the terminal phalanx of the little finger is deviated palmoradially.

volvement is almost always bilateral. Treatment is rarely indicated.

MISCELLANEOUS FINGER DEFORMITIES

Clinodactyly[230,231,239]

In this rather common hereditary autosomal dominant deformity, the finger is curved and deviated in the radioulnar plane at either the proximal or the distal interphalangeal joint (Fig 4–42). The little finger is most commonly affected. Ordinarily there is no functional impairment. Clinodactyly is a common finding in Down syndrome and other chromosomal abnormalities.

Surgical treatment is indicated in the rare case in which the deformity is so severe that it interferes with grasp and cosmetic appearance is objectionable. The deformity is corrected by a closing wedge osteotomy.

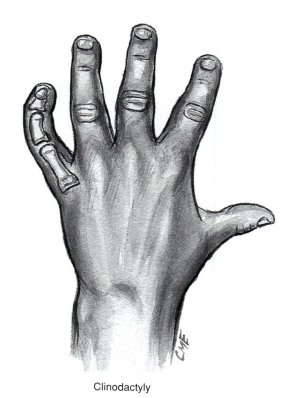

Clinodactyly

Figure 4–42. Clinodactyly of the little finger. Note that it is curved radially at the distal interphalangeal joint.

Camptodactyly[233,240]

The Greek word for bent finger is camptodactyly. This condition is characterized by flexion deformity of a digit, occurring commonly at the proximal interphalangeal joint and occasionally at the distal interphalangeal joint (Fig 4–43). The little finger is commonly involved; the ring finger is next in frequency of affection.

Examination reveals no increased local temperature, redness, or local tenderness. The degree of flexion deformity varies.

Mild to moderate flexion deformity does not require surgery. Some deformities are treated by extension–dorsal wedge osteotomy. The arc of motion does not improve.

Constriction Ring Syndrome[228,234,235,237]

Ringlike constriction bands may involve any of the digits, most commonly in the distal part of the thumb and least commonly in the short little finger (Fig 4–44). Premature rupture of the amniotic sac and sudden reduction of amniotic fluid volume may be the cause of the amniotic bands. The syndrome is sporadic and nonhereditary in occurrence.

The ring constriction may involve only the skin and subcutaneous tissue or extend deep to involve muscle, tendons, and even bone.

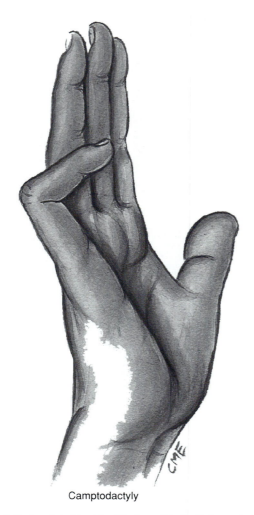

Camptodactyly

Figure 4–43. Camptodactyly of the little finger. Note the flexion contracture at the proximal interphalangeal joint.

Rings that do not interfere with lymphatic drainage and circulation do not require treatment. The deeper bands are surgically released.

Macrodactyly[229]

Macrodactyly presents as a localized symmetric enlargement of one or more digits (Fig 4–45). It is more common on the radial side of the hand and in about 9 of 10 cases, only one hand is involved. It is classified into four types: type I—gigantism with lipofibromatosis; type II—gigantism and neurofibromatosis; type III—gigantism and digital hyperostosis; and type IV—gigantism and hemihypertrophy. In the differential diagnosis one should consider other causes of a swollen finger such as fibrous dysplasia, osteoid osteoma, hemangioma, and arteriovenous fistula.

Treatment depends upon the type. In those associated with lipofibromatosis and neurofibromatosis, bulk reduction is performed early and growth arrest is performed to retard the longitudinal growth of the finger. For very grotesque enlarged digits, amputation is carried out.

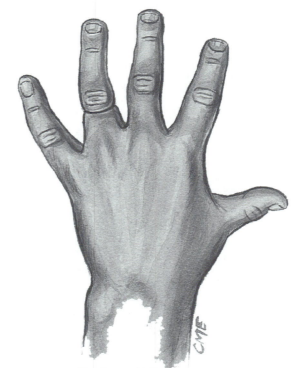

Simple constriction ring

Figure 4–44. Congenital constriction ring of the left ring finger. It is simple, involving only skin and subcutaneous tissue. In severe cases, it may extend deep to muscles and tendons and may involve bone.

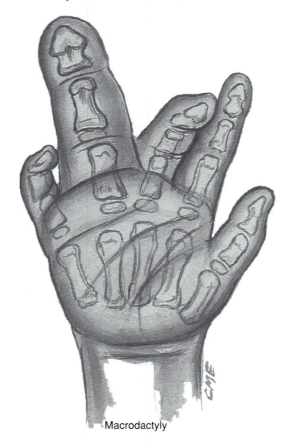

Macrodactyly

Figure 4–45. Simple macrodactyly of the ring finger.

REFERENCES

Congenital Muscular Torticollis

1. Brackbill Y, Douthit TC, West H: Psychophysiologic effects in the neonate of prone versus supine placement. *J Pediatr* 82:84, 1973
2. Brooks B: Pathologic changes in muscle as a result of disturbances of circulation. *Arch Surg* 5:188, 1922
3. Brougham DI, Cole WG, Dickens DRV, Menelaus MB: Torticollis due to a combination of sternomastoid contracture and congenital vertebral anomalies. *J Bone Joint Surg* 71B: 404, 1989
4. Canale ST, Griffin DW, Hubbard CN: Congenital muscular torticollis. *J Bone Joint Surg* 64A:810, 1982
5. Chandler FA: Muscular torticollis. *J Bone Joint Surg* 30A: 566, 1948
6. Chandler FA, Altenberg A: "Congenital" muscular torticollis. *JAMA* 125:476, 1944
7. Cheng JCY, Au AWY: Infantile torticollis: A review of 624 cases. *J Pediatr Orthop* 14:802, 1994
8. Coventry MB, Harris L: Congenital muscular torticollis in infancy. Some observations regarding treatment. *J Bone Joint Surg* 41A:815, 1959
9. Davids JR, Wenger D, Mubarak SJ: Congenital muscular torticollis: Sequelae of intrauterine or perinatal compartment syndrome. *J Pediatr Orthop* 13:141, 1993.
10. Dubousset J: Torticollis in children caused by congenital anomalies of the atlas. *J Bone Joint Surg* 68A:178, 1986
11. Ferkel RD, Westin GW, Dawson EG, Oppenheim WL: Muscular torticollis. A modified surgical approach. *J Bone Joint Surg* 65A:894, 1983
12. Hummer CD Jr, MacEwen GD: The coexistence of torticollis and congenital dysplasia of the hip. *J Bone Joint Surg* 54A: 1255, 1972
13. Ippolito E, Tudisco C, Massobrio M: Long-term results of open sternocleidomastoid tenotomy for idiopathic muscular torticollis. *J Bone Joint Surg* 67:30, 1985
14. Itoi E, Funayama K, Suzuki T, Kamio K, Sakurai M: Tenotomy and postoperative brace treatment for muscular torticollis. *Contemp Orthop* 20:515, 1990
15. Jepson PN: Ischemic contracture. Experimental study. *Ann Surg* 84:785, 1926
16. Jones PG: *Torticollis in Infancy and Childhood. Sternomastoid Fibrosis and the Sternomastoid "Tumor."* Springfield, IL, Charles C Thomas, 1968
17. Lidge RT, Bechtol RC, Lambert CN: Congenital muscular torticollis. Etiology and pathology. *J Bone Joint Surg* 39A: 1165, 1957
18. Ling CM, Low YS: Sternomastoid tumor and muscular torticollis. *Clin Orthop* 86:144, 1972
19. MacDonald D: Sternomastoid tumor and muscular torticollis. *J Bone Joint Surg* 51B:432, 1969
20. Middleton DS: The pathology of congenital torticollis. *Br J Surg* 18:188, 1930
21. Morrison DL, MacEwen GD: Congenital muscular torticollis: Observations regarding clinical findings, associated conditions and results of treatment. *J Pediatr Orthop* 2:500, 1982

22. Pirsing W: Kongenitaler Schiefhals mit kemlkopf-trachea-verlagerung durch. Kontraktur des Musculus omohyoideus. *Arch Otorhinolaryngol* 215:335, 1977
23. Ramenofsky ML, Buyse M, Goldberg MJ: Gastroesophageal reflux and torticollis. *J Bone Joint Surg* 60A:1140, 1975
24. Weiner DS: Congenital dislocation of the hip associated with congenital muscular torticollis. *Clin Orthop* 121:163, 1976

Hemiatlas

25. Dubousett J: Torticollis in children caused by congenital anomalies of the atlas. *J Bone Joint Surg* 68A:178, 1986

Inflammatory Torticollis

26. Fried JA, Athreya B, Gregg JR, Das M, Doughty R: The C-spine in juvenile rheumatoid arthritis. *Clin Orthop* 179: 102, 1983
27. Halla JT, Fallahi S, Hardin JG: Nonreducible rotational head tilt and atlantoaxial lateral mass collapse. Clinical and roentgenographic factors in patients with juvenile rheumatoid arthritis. *Arch Intern Med* 143:471, 1983
28. Hensinger RN, DeVito PD, Ragsdale CG: Changes in the cervical spine in juvenile rheumatoid arthritis. *J Bone Joint Surg* 68A:189, 1986

Traumatic Acquired Torticollis

29. Birney TJ, Hanley EN Jr: Traumatic cervical spine injuries in childhood and adolescence. *Spine* 14:1277, 1989
30. deBeer J de V, Hoffman EB, Kieck CF: Traumatic atlantoaxial subluxation in children. *J Pediatr Orthop* 10:397, 1990
31. Floman Y, Kaplan L, Elidan J, Umansky F: Transverse ligament rupture and atlanto-axial subluxation in children. *J Bone Joint Surg* 73B:640, 1991
32. Pennecot GF, Leonard P, Peyrot Des Gachons S, Hardy JR, Pouliquen JC: Traumatic ligamentous instability of the cervical spine in children. *J Pediatr Orthop* 4:339, 1984
33. Sherk HH, Nicholson JT, Chung SMK: Fractures of the odontoid process in young children. *J Bone Joint Surg* 60A: 921, 1978
34. Steel HH: Anatomical and mechanical considerations of the atlantoaxial articulation. *J Bone Joint Surg* 50A:1481, 1968

Neuromuscular Torticollis

35. Reimer R, Onofrio BM: Astrocytomas of the spinal cord in children and adolescents. *J Neurosurg* 63:669, 1985
36. Tachdjian MO, Matson DD: Orthopaedic aspects of intraspinal tumors in infants and children. *J Bone Joint Surg* 47A:230, 1965

Atlantoaxial Instability

37. Bhatnagar M, Sponseller PD, Carroll C, Tolo VT: Pediatric atlantoaxial instability presenting as cerebral and cerebellar infarcts. *J Pediatr Orthop* 11:103, 1991
38. Brook DC, Burkus RJK, Benson DR: Asymptomatic occipital atlantal instability in Down's syndrome. *J Bone Joint Surg* 69A:293, 1987

39. Dawson EG, Smith A: Atlantoaxial subluxation in children due to vertebral anomalies. *J Bone Joint Surg* 61A:582, 1979

40. Dzentis AJ: Spontaneous atlanto-axial dislocation in a mongoloid child with spinal cord compression. Case report. *J Neurosurg* 25:458, 1966

41. El-Khoury GY, Clark CR, Dietz FR, Harre RG, Tozzie JE, Kathol MH: Posterior atlanto-occipital subluxation in Down's syndrome. *Radiology* 159:507, 1986

42. Fielding JW, Hensinger RN, Hawkins RJ: Os odontoideum. *J Bone Joint Surg* 62A:376, 1980

43. Fielding JW, Hawkins RJ, Ratzan S: Spinal fusion for atlanto-axial instability. *J Bone Joint Surg* 58A:400, 1976

44. Fraser RA, Zimbler SM: Hindbrain stroke in children caused by extracranial vertebral artery trauma. *Stroke* 6:153, 1975

45. Gelch MM, Senft KE, Goldberg MJ: Symptomatic atlanto-axial subluxation in persons with Down's syndrome. *J Pediatr Orthop* 4:682, 1984

46. Locke GR, Gardner JI, Van Epps EF: Normal values of atlas odontoid distribution in children. *Am J Radiol* 97:135, 1966

47. Miyakawa G: Congenital absence of the odontoid process resulting in dislocation of atlas and axis. *J Bone Joint Surg* 15:988, 1952

48. Pueschel SM, Scola FH, Perry CD, Pezzullo JC: Atlanto-axial instability in children with Down's syndrome. *Pediatr Radiol* 10:129, 1981

49. Pueschel SM, Scola FH, Tupper TB, Pezzullo JC: Skeletal anomalies of the upper cervical spine in children with Down syndrome. *J Pediatr Orthop* 10:607, 1990

50. Semine AA, Ertel AN, Goldberg MJ, Bull MJ: Cervical spine instability in children with Down syndrome (trisomy 21). *J Bone Joint Surg* 60A:649, 1978

51. Shikata J, Yamamuro T, Mikawa Y, Iida H, and Kobori M: Atlanto-axial subluxation in Down's syndrome. *Int Orthop* 13:187, 1989

52. Steel HH: Anatomical and mechanical considerations of the atlantoaxial articulation. *J Bone Joint Surg* 50A:1481, 1968

53. Tredwell SJ, Newman DE, Lockitch G: Instability of the upper cervical spine in Down syndrome. *J Pediatr Orthop* 10:602, 1990

Klippel-Feil Syndrome

54. Bailey RW: *Congenital Deformities of the Cervical Spine.* Philadelphia, Lea & Febiger, 1974, pp 6–9

55. Bonola A: Surgical treatment of the Klippel-Feil syndrome. *J Bone Joint Surg* 38B:400, 1956

56. Duncan PA: Embryologic pathogenesis of renal agenesis associated with cervical vertebral anomalies (Klippel-Feil phenotype). *Birth Defects* 13:91, 1977

57. Feil A: L'absence et la diminution des vertébrés cervicales (étude clinique et pathogénique); le syndrome de réduction numérique cervicale. Thèse de Paris, 1919

58. Feil A, Roland J, Vanbockstael: Les hommes sans cou. Considérations sur la réduction numérique et le tassement des vertébrés cervicales. *Rev Orthop* 11:281, 1924

59. Hall JE, Simmons ED, Danylchuk K, Barnes PD: Instability of the cervical spine and neurological involvement in Klippel-Feil syndrome. A case report. *J Bone Joint Surg* 72:460, 1990

60. Hensinger RN, Lange JE, MacEwen GD: Klippel-Feil syndrome: A constellation of associated anomalies. *J Bone Joint Surg* 56A:1246, 1974

61. Herring JA, Bunnell WP: Klippel-Feil syndrome with neck pain. *J Pediatr Orthop* 9:343, 1989

62. Klippel M, Feil A: Anomalies de la colonne vertébrale par absence des vertébrés cervicales cage thoracique remontant jusqu'a la base du craine. *Bull Soc Anat Paris* 87:185, 1912

63. Klippel M, Feil A: The classic: A case of absence of cervical vertebrae with the thoracic cage rising to the base of the cranium (cervical thoracic cage). *Clin Orthop* 109:3, 1975

64. Lowry RB: The Klippel-Feil anomalad as part of the fetal alcohol syndrome. *Teratology* 16:53, 1977

65. Nagib MG, Maxwell RE, Chou SN: Identification and management of high risk patients with Klippel-Feil syndrome. *J Neurosurg* 61:523, 1984

66. Ritterbusch JF, McGinty LD, Spar J, Orrison WW: Magnetic resonance imaging for stenosis and subluxation in Klippel-Feil syndrome. *Spine* 16:39, 1991

67. Shoul ML, Ritvo M: Clinical and roentgenological manifestations of the Klippel-Feil syndrome (congenital fusion of the cervical vertebrae, brevicollis). *AJR* 68:369, 1972

Intervertebral Disc Calcification

68. Eyring EJ, Peterson CA, Bjornson DR: Intervertebral disc calcification in childhood. *J Bone Joint Surg* 46A:1432, 1964

69. Newton TH: Cervical intervertebral-disc calcification in children. *J Bone Joint Surg* 40A:107, 1958

70. Peck FC Jr: A calcified thoracic intervertebral disc with herniation and spinal cord compression in a child; case report. *J Neurosurg* 14:105, 1957

71. Schechter LS, Smith A, Pearl M: Intervertebral disk calcification in childhood. *Am J Dis Child* 123:608, 1972

72. Silverman FN: Calcification of the intervertebral discs in childhood. *Radiology* 62:801, 1954

73. Sonnabend DH, Taylor TK, Chapman GK: Intervertebral disc calcification syndromes in children. *J Bone Joint Surg* 64B:25, 1982

74. Weens HS: Calcification of the intervertebral discs in childhood. *J Pediatr* 26:178, 1945

Sprengel's Deformity

75. Bagg HJ: Hereditary abnormalities of the limbs, their origin and transmission. II. A morphological study with special reference to the etiology of club feet, syndactylism, hypodactylism, and congenital amputation in the descendants of x-rayed mice. *Am J Anat* 43:167, 1929

76. Bagg HJ, Halter CR: Further studies on the inheritance of structural defects in mice exposed to roentgen ray irradiation. *Am J Anat* 33:119, 1924

77. Bagg HJ, Little CC: Hereditary structural defects in the descendants of mice exposed to roentgen ray irradiation. *Am J Anat* 33:119, 1924

78. Bazan UB von: The association between congenital elevation of the scapula and diastematomyelia. *J Bone Joint Surg* 61B:49, 1979

79. Bazan UB von, Redlich H, Puhl W, Best S: The omovertebral bone—new possibility of pre-operative examination by computed axial tomography. *Z Orthop* 116:795, 1978

80. Blair JD, Wells PO: Bilateral undescended scapula associated with omovertebral bone. *J Bone Joint Surg* 39A:201, 1957

81. Bonnevie K: Embryological analysis of gene manifestation in Little and Bagg's abnormal mouse tribe. *J Exp Zool* 67:443, 1934

82. Carson WG, Lovell WW, Whitesides TE Jr: Congenital elevation of the scapula. *J Bone Joint Surg* 54B:395, 1972

83. Cavendish ME: Congenital elevation of the scapula. *J Bone Joint Surg* 54B:395, 1972

84. Chung SMK, Farahvar H: Surgery of the clavicle in Sprengel's deformity. *Clin Orthop* 116:138, 1976

85. Engel D: The etiology of the undescended scapula and related syndromes. *J Bone Joint Surg* 25:613, 1943

86. Eulenberg M: Beitrag zur Dislocation der Scapula. *Amtliche Berichte uber die Versammlungen deutscher Naturforscher und Aerzte fur die Jahre* 37:291, 1863

87. Eulenberg M: Casuistische Mittheilungen aus dem Begiete der Orthopadie. *Arch Klin Chir* 4:301, 1863

88. Green WT: The surgical correction of congenital elevation of the scapula (Sprengel's deformity). Proceedings of the American Orthopedic Association. *J Bone Joint Surg* 39A:1439, 1957

89. Greitemann B, Rondhuis JJ, Karbowski A: Treatment of congenital elevation of the scapula. 10 (2–18) year follow-up of 37 cases of Sprengel's deformity. *Acta Orthop Scand* 64:365, 1993

90. Jeannopoulos CL: Congenital elevation of the scapula. *J Bone Joint Surg* 34A:883, 1952

91. Klisiç P, Filipovic M, Uzelac O, Milinkovic Z: Relocation of congenitally elevated scapula. *J Pediatr Orthop* 1:43, 1981

92. Ogden JA, Conlogue GJ, Phillips MS, Bronson ML: Sprengel's deformity. Radiology of the pathologic deformation. *Skeletal Radiol* 4:204, 1979

93. Otter G den: Bilateral Sprengel's syndrome with situs inversus totalis. *Acta Orthop Scand* 41:402, 1970

94. Rigault P, Pouliquen JC, Guyonvarch G, Zujovic J: Congenital elevation of the scapula in children. Anatomopathological and therapeutic study apropos of 27 cases. *Rev Chir Orthop* 62:5, 1976

95. Ross DM, Cruess RL: The surgical correction of congenital elevation of the scapula. *Clin Orthop* 125:17, 1977

96. Sprengel O: Die angeborene Verschiebung des Schulterblattes nach oben. *Arch Klin Chir* 42:545, 1891

97. Woodward JW: Congenital elevation of the scapula. Correction by release and transplantation of muscle origins. *J Bone Joint Surg* 43A:219, 1961

Congenital Pseudarthrosis of the Clavicle

98. Ahmadi B, Steel HH: Congenital pseudarthrosis of the clavicle. *Clin Orthop* 126:129, 1977

99. Gardner E: The embryology of the clavicle. *Clin Orthop* 58:9, 1968

100. Gibson DA, Carroll N: Congenital pseudarthrosis of the clavicle. *J Bone Joint Surg* 52B:629, 1970

101. Grogan DP, Love SM, Guidera KJ, Ogden JA: Operative treatment of congenital pseudarthrosis of the clavicle. *J Pediatr Orthop* 11:176, 1991

102. Lloyd-Roberts GC, Apley AG, Owen R: Reflections upon the aetiology of congenital pseudarthrosis of the clavicle. *J Bone Joint Surg* 57B:24, 1975

103. O'Rahilly R: *In* Frantz CH (ed): *Normal and Abnormal Embryological Development*. National Research Publication 1497, Washington, DC, US Government Printing Office, 1967, p 10

104. Russo MT, Maffulli N: Bilateral congenital pseudarthrosis of the clavicle. *Arch Orthop Trauma Surg* 109:177, 1990

105. Schnall SB, King JD, Marrero G: Congenital pseudarthrosis of the clavicle: A review of the literature and surgical results of six cases. *J Pediatr Orthop* 8:316, 1988

106. Støren H: Old clavicular pseudarthrosis with late appearing neuralgias and vasomotoric disturbances cured by operation. *Acta Chir Scand* 94:187, 1946

107. Young MC, Richards RR, Hudson AR: Thoracic outlet syndrome with congenital pseudarthrosis of the clavicle: Treatment by brachial plexus decompression, plate fixation and bone grafting. *Can J Surg* 31:131, 1988

Cleidocranial Dyplasia

108. Anspach WE, Heupel RG: Familial cleidocranial dysostosis (cleidal dysostosis). *Am J Dis Child* 58:786, 1939

109. Cole WR, Levin S: Cleidocranial dysostosis. *Br J Radiol* 24:549, 1951

110. Fairbanks HAT: Cranio-cleido dysostosis. *J Bone Joint Surg* 31B:608, 1949

Congenital Absence of Pectoral Muscles

111. Beals RK, Crawford S: Congenital absence of the pectoral muscles. A review of twenty-five patients. *Clin Orthop* 119:166, 1976

112. Brown JB, McDowell I: Syndactylism with absence of the pectoralis major. *Surgery* 7:599, 1940

113. Clarkson P: Poland's syndactyly. *Guy's Hosp Rep* 111:335, 1962

114. David TJ: Nature and etiology of the Poland anomaly. *N Engl J Med* 287:487, 1972

115. Ireland DCR, Takayama N, Flatt A: Poland's syndrome. *J Bone Joint Surg* 58A:52, 1976

116. Poland A: Deficiency of the pectoral muscles. *Guy's Hosp Rep* 6:191, 1841

117. Resnick E: Congenital unilateral absence of the pectoral muscles often associated with syndactylism. *J Bone Joint Surg* 24:925, 1942

118. Soderberg BN: Congenital absence of the pectoral muscle and syndactylism: A deformity association sometimes overlooked. *Plast Reconstr Surg* 4:434, 1949

119. Sugiura Y: Poland's syndrome. Clinicoroentgenographic study on 45 cases. *Cong Anom* 16:17, 1976

Obstetrical Brachial Plexus Paralysis

120. Aitken J: Deformity of the elbow joint as a sequel to Erb's obstetrical paralysis. *J Bone Joint Surg* 34B:352, 1952

121. Babbitt DP, Cassidy RH: Obstetrical paralysis and dislocation of the shoulder in infancy. *J Bone Joint Surg* 50A:144, 1967

122. Blount WP: Osteoclasis for supination deformities in children. *J Bone Joint Surg* 22:300, 1940

123. Carlioz H, Brahimi L: La place de la désinsertion interne du sous-scapulaire dans le traitement de la paralysie obstetricale du mêmbre superieur chez l'enfant. *Ann Chir Infant* 12:159, 1971

124. Chung SMK, Nissenbaum MM: Obstetrical paralysis. *Orthop Clin North Am* 6:393, 1975.

125. Erb WH: Ueber eine eigenthumliche Localisation von Lahmungen im Plexus brachialis. *Verhandl Naturhist Med Heidelberg N.F* 2:130, 1874

126. Erb W: On a characteristic site of injury in the brachial plexus (reprinted). *Arch Neurol* 21:433, 1969

127. Fairbank HAT: Birth palsy: Subluxation of shoulder joints in infants and young children. *Lancet* 1:1217, 1913

128. Gilbert A: Obstetrical brachial plexus palsy, in Tubiana R (ed): *The Hand.* Philadelphia, WB Saunders Co, 1991, pp 575–601

129. Gilbert A, Khouri N, Carlioz H: Exploration chirurgicale du plexus brachial dans la paralysie obstetricale. Constatations anatomiques chez 21 maladies opères. *Rev Chir Orthop* 66: 33, 1980

130. Gilbert A, Razaboni R, Amar-Khodja S: Indications and results of brachial plexus surgery in obstetrical palsy. *Orthop Clin North Am* 19:91, 1988

131. Green WT, Tachdjian MO: Correction of residual deformities of the shoulder in obstetrical palsy. *J Bone Joint Surg* 45A: 1544, 1963

132. Greenwald AG, Schute PC, Shiveley JL: Brachial plexus birth palsy: A 10-year report on the incidence and prognosis. *J Pediatr Orthop* 4:689, 1984

133. Hardy AE: Birth injuries of the brachial plexus. *J Bone Joint Surg* 63B:98, 1981

134. Hoffer MM, Wickenden R, Roper B: Brachial plexus birth palsies. Results of tendon transfers to the rotator cuff. *J Bone Joint Surg* 60A:691, 1978

135. Kennedy R: Suture of the brachial plexus in birth paralysis of the upper extremity. *B M J* 1:298, 1903

136. L'Episcopo JB: Tendon transplantation in obstetrical paralysis. *Am J Surg* 25:122, 1934

137. Mallet J: Paralysie obstetricale. *Rev Chir Orthop* 58(Suppl 1):115, 1972

138. Millesi H: Indications et résultats des interventions directes dans la paralysie traumatique du plexus brachial chez l'adulte. *Rev Chir Orthop* 63:82, 1977

139. Putti V: Due sindromi paralitiche del'arto superiore. Note di fisiopatologia della rotazione antibrachiale. *Chir Organi Mov* 26:215, 1940

140. Rossi LN, Vassella F, Mumenthaler M: Obstetrical lesions of the brachial plexus: Natural history in 34 personal cases. *Eur Neurol* 21:1, 1982

141. Seddon HJ: *Surgical Disorders of the Peripheral Nerves.* London, Churchill-Livingstone, 1972

142. Sever JW: Obstetric paralysis: Its etiology, pathology, clinical aspects and treatment with a report of 470 cases. *Am J Dis Child* 12:541, 1916

143. Sever JW: The results of a new operation for obstetrical paralysis. *Am J Orthop Surg* 16:248, 1918

144. Zancolli EA: Classification and management of the shoulder in birth palsy. *Orthop Clin North Am* 12:433, 1981

145. Zancolli EA: Paralytic supination contracture of the forearm. *J Bone Joint Surg* 49A:1275, 1967

146. Zancolli EA, Aponte F, Zancolli ER: Paralisis obstetrica. Clasificacion de las secuelas. *Bol Trab Sociedad Arg Ortop Traumatol* Ano XLIV, No 3, 1979

147. Zancolli EA, Aponte F, Zancolli ER: Paralisis obstetrica de tip braquial superior. Clasificacion de sus secuelas y su correcion quirurgica. *Bol Trab Sociedad Arg Ortop Traumatol* Ano XLIV, No 5, 1979

148. Zancolli EA, Mitra H: Latissimus dorsi transfer to restore elbow flexion. *J Bone Joint Surg* 55A:1265, 1973

149. Zancolli EA, Zancolli ER Jr: Palliative surgical procedures in sequelae of obstetrical palsy, in Tubiana R (ed): *The Hand.* Philadelphia, WB Saunders Co, 1991, pp 602–623

150. Zaoussis AL: Osteotomy of the proximal end of the radius for paralytic supination deformity in children. *J Bone Joint Surg* 45B:523, 1963

Pulled Elbow

151. Green JT, Gay FH: Traumatic subluxation of the radial head in young children. *J Bone Joint Surg* 36A:655, 1954

152. Griffin ME: Subluxation of the head of the radius in young children. *Pediatrics* 15:103, 1955

153. Kosuwon W, Mahaisavariya B, Saengnipanthkul S, Laupattarakasem W, Jirawipoolwon P: Ultrasonography of pulled elbow. *J Bone Joint Surg* 75B:421, 1993

154. McRae R, Freeman P: The lesion in pulled elbow. *J Bone Joint Surg* 47B:808, 1965

155. Ryan JR: The relationship of the radial head to the radial neck diameters in fetuses and adults with reference to radial head subluxation in children. *J Bone Joint Surg* 51A:781, 1969

156. Salter RB, Zaltz C: Anatomic investigation of the mechanism of injury and pathologic anatomy of "pulled elbow" in children. *Clin Orthop* 77:134, 1971

157. Stone CA: Subluxation of the head of the radius—report of a case and anatomical experiments. *JAMA* 1:28, 1916

Congenital Dislocation of the Radial Head

158. Almquist EE, Gordon LH, Blue AI: Congenital dislocation of the head of the radius. *J Bone Joint Surg* 51A:1118, 1969

159. Brennan JJ, Krause MEH, Harvey DM: Annular ligament construction for congenital anterior dislocation of both radial heads. *Clin Orthop* 29:205, 1963

160. Exarhou EI, Antoniou NK: Congenital dislocation of the head of the radius. *Acta Orthop Scand* 41:551, 1970

161. Good CJ, Wicks MH: Developmental posterior dislocation of the radial head. *J Bone Joint Surg* 65B:64, 1983

162. Lloyd-Roberts GC, Bucknill TM: Anterior dislocation of the radial head in children: Aetiology, natural history and management. *J Bone Joint Surg* 59B:402, 1977

Osteochondrosis of the Capitellum of the Humerus

163. Laurent LE, Lindstrom BL: Osteochondrosis of the capitellum of the humeri (Panner's disease). *Acta Orthop Scand* 26:111, 1956

164. Panner HJ: A peculiar affection of the capitulum humeri, resembling Calvé-Perthes of the hip. *Acta Radiol* 10:234, 1929

165. Smith MGH: Osteochondritis of the humeral capitulum. *J Bone Joint Surg* 46B:50, 1964

Osteochondritis of the Capitellum of the Humerus

166. Brogdon BG, Crow NE: Little Leaguer's elbow. *AJR* 83: 671, 1960

Congenital Radioulnar Synostosis

167. Green WT, Mital MA: Congenital radioulnar synostosis: Surgical treatment. *J Bone Joint Surg* 61A:738, 1979

168. Hansen OH, Andersen NO: Congenital radioulnar synostosis: Report of 37 cases. *Acta Orthop Scand* 41:225, 1970

169. Jancu J: Radioulnar synostosis. A common occurrence in sex chromosomal abnormalities. *Am J Dis Child* 122:10, 1971

170. Kelikian H: *Congenital Deformities of the Hand and Forearm*. Philadelphia, WB Saunders Co, 1974, pp 310–407, 714–752, 939–975

171. Mital MA: Congenital radioulnar synostosis and congenital dislocation of the radial head. *Orthop Clin North Am* 76: 375, 1976

Congenital Longitudinal Deficiency of the Radius

172. Bora FW Jr, Nicholson JT, Cheema HM: Radial meromelia: The deformity and its treatment. *J Bone Joint Surg* 52A:966, 1970

173. Carroll RE, Louis DS: Anomalies associated with radial dysplasia. *J Pediatr* 84:409, 1974

174. Flatt A: *The Care of Congenital Hand Anomalies*, 2nd ed. St. Louis, Mosby-Year Book, 1993, pp 366–410

175. Lamb DW: Radial club hand, a continuing study of sixty-eight patients with one hundred and seventeen club hands. *J Bone Joint Surg* 59A:1, 1977

176. Lamb DW: The treatment of radial club hand. Absent radius, aplasia of the radius, hypoplasia of the radius, radial paraxial hemimelia. *Hand* 4:22, 1972

177. Lidge R: Congenital radial deficient club hand. *J Bone Joint Surg* 51A:1041, 1969

178. Zaricznyj B: Centralization of the ulna for congenital radial hemimelia. *J Bone Joint Surg* 59A:694, 1977

Congenital Longitudinal Deficiency of the Ulna

179. Carroll RE, Bowers WH: Congenital deficiency of the ulna. *J Hand Surg* 2:169, 1977

180. Ogden JA: Ulnar dysmelia. *J Bone Joint Surg* 58A:467, 1976

Madelung's Deformity

181. Beals RK, Lovrien EW: Dyschondrosteosis and Madelung's deformity. Report of three kindreds and review of the literature. *Clin Orthop* 116:24, 1976

182. Berdon WE, Grossman H, Baker DH: Dyschondrosteosis (Léri-Weill syndrome). Congenital short forearms, Madelung-type of wrist deformities and moderate dwarfism. *Radiology* 85:678, 1965

183. Gelberman RH, Bauman T: Madelung's deformity and dyschondrosteosis. *J Hand Surg* 5:338, 1980

184. Golding JSR, Blackburne JS: Madelung's disease of the wrist and dyschondrosteosis. *J Bone Joint Surg* 58B:350, 1976

185. Madelung V: Die spontane Subluxation der Hand nach vorne. *Verh Dtsch Ges Chir* 7:259, 1878; Reprinted in *Arch Klin Chir* 23:395, 1979

186. Matev I, Karagancheva S: The Madelung deformity. *Hand* 7:152, 1975

187. Nielsen JB: Madelung's deformity: A follow-up study of 26 cases and a review of the literature. *Acta Orthop Scand* 48: 379, 1977

188. Ranawat CS, DeFiore J, Straub LR: Madelung's deformity: An end-result study of surgical treatment. *J Bone Joint Surg* 57A:772, 1975

189. Vickers DW: Madelung's technique of surgery, in Tachdjian MO (ed): *Pediatric Orthopedics*, 2nd ed. Philadelphia, WB Saunders Co, 1990, pp 214–215

Syndactyly

190. Apert E: De l'acrocephalosyndactylie. *Bull Mem Soc Med Hop Paris* 23:1310, 1906

191. Brooksaler FS: Poland's syndrome. *Am J Dis Child* 121:263, 1971

192. Brown JB, McDowell F: Syndactylism with absence of the pectoralis major. *Surgery* 7:599, 1940

193. Flatt AE: Practical factors in the treatment of syndactyly, in Littler JW, Cramer LM, Smith JW (eds): *Symposium on Reconstructive Hand Surgery*. St. Louis, CV Mosby Co, 1974, pp 144–156

194. Flatt AE: *The Care of Congenital Hand Anomalies*. St. Louis, Mosby-Year Book 1993, pp 228–275

195. Hoover GH, Flatt AE, Weiss MW: The hand and Apert's syndrome. *J Bone Joint Surg* 52A:878, 1970

196. Ireland DCR, Takayama N, Flatt AE: Poland's syndrome: A review of forty-three cases. *J Bone Joint Surg* 58A:52, 1976

197. Kelikian H: *Congenital Deformities of the Hand and Forearm*. Philadelphia, WB Saunders Co, 1974, pp 331–407

198. Poland A: Deficiency of the pectoralis muscle. *Guys Hosp Rep* 6:191, 1841

199. Poznanski AK: *The Hand in Radiologic Diagnosis*. Philadelphia, WB Saunders Co, 1974, pp 278–283

200. Temtamy SA: Carpenter's syndrome: Acrocephalopolysyndactyly, an autosomal recessive syndrome. *J Pediatr* 69:111, 1966

201. Temtamy SA: *Genetic Factors in Hand Malformations*. Thesis. Baltimore, Johns Hopkins University, 1966

202. Walsh RJ: Acrosyndactyly: A study of 27 patients. *Clin Orthop* 71:99, 1970

Polydactyly

203. Barsky AJ: *Congenital Anomalies of the Hand and Their Surgical Treatment*. Springfield, IL, Charles C Thomas, 1958, pp 48–64

204. Barsky AJ: Congenital anomalies of the thumb. *Clin Orthop* 15:96, 1959

205. DeMarinis F, Sobbota A: On inheritance and development of preaxial and postaxial types of polydactyly. *Acta Genet* 7:215, 1957

206. Flatt AE: *The Care of Congenital Hand Anomalies.* St. Louis, Mosby-Year Book 1993, pp 120–145

207. Kelikian H: *Congenital Deformities of the Hand and Forearm.* Philadelphia, WB Saunders Co, 1974, pp 408–456

208. Stelling F: The upper extremity, in Ferguson AB (ed): *Orthopedic Surgery in Infancy and Childhood,* 3rd ed. Baltimore, Williams & Wilkins, 1967, pp 292–334

209. Temtamy SA: *Genetic Factors in Hand Malformations.* Thesis. Baltimore, Johns Hopkins University, 1966

210. Temtamy SA, McKusick VA: Polydactyly. *Birth Defects* 14: 364, 1978

211. Temtamy S, McKusick VA: Synopsis of hand malformations with particular emphasis on genetic factors. *Birth Defects* 5: 125, 1969

212. Wassel HD: The results of surgery for polydactyly of the thumb. A review. *Clin Orthop* 64:175, 1969

213. Wood VE: Polydactyly and the triphalangeal thumb. *J Hand Surg* 3:436, 1978

214. Wood VE: Treatment of central polydactyly. *Clin Orthop* 74: 196, 1971

215. Woolf CM, Myrianthopoulos NC: Polydactyly in American Negroes and whites. *Am J Hum Genet* 25:397, 1973

Congenital Longitudinal Deficiency of the Thumb

216. Buck-Gramcko D: Pollicization of the index finger: Method and results in aplasia and hypoplasia of the thumb. *J Bone Joint Surg* 53A:1605, 1971

217. Gilbert A: Toe transfer for congenital hand defects. *J Hand Surg* 7:118, 1982

218. Littler JW: On making a thumb: One hundred years of surgical effort. *J Hand Surg* 1:35, 1976

219. Manske PK, McCarroll HR: Index finger pollicization for congenitally absent or non-functioning thumb. *J Hand Surg* 10A:606, 1985

220. Percival NJ, Sykes PJ, Chandraprakasam T: A method of assessment of pollicization. *J Hand Surg* 16B:141, 1991

Trigger Thumb

221. Bollinger J, Fahey J: Snapping thumb in infants and children. *J Pediatr* 41:445, 1952

222. Compere EL: Bilateral snapping thumbs. *Ann Surg* 97:773, 1933

223. Dinham JM, Meggitt BF: Trigger thumbs in children. A review of the natural history and indications for treatment in 105 patients. *J Bone Joint Surg* 56B:153, 1974

224. Fahey JJ, Bollinger JA: Trigger-finger in adults and children. *J Bone Joint Surg* 36A:1200, 1954

Congenital Clasped Thumb

225. Weckesser EC, Reed JR, Heiple KG: Congenital clasped thumb (congenital flexion-adduction deformity of the thumb). *J Bone Joint Surg* 50A:1417, 1968

226. White JW, Jensen WE: The infant's persistent thumb clutched hand. *J Bone Joint Surg* 34A:680, 1952

227. Zadek I: Congenital absence of the extensor pollicis longus of both thumbs. Operation and cure. *J Bone Joint Surg* 16: 432, 1934

Miscellaneous Finger Deformities

228. Askins G, Ger E: Congenital constriction band syndrome. *J Pediatr Orthop* 8:461, 1988

229. Barsky A: Macrodactyly. *J Bone Joint Surg* 49A:1255, 1967

230. Burke F, Flatt AE: Clinodactyly. A review of a series of cases. *Hand* 3:269, 1979

231. Carstam N, Theander G: Surgical treatment of clinodactyly caused by longitudinally bracketed diaphysis. *Scand J Plast Reconstr Surg* 9:199, 1975

232. Dykes RG: Kirner's deformity of the little finger. *J Bone Joint Surg* 60B:58, 1978

233. Engber WM, Flatt AE: Camptodactyly: An analysis of sixty-six patients and twenty-four operations. *J Hand Surg* 2:216, 1977

234. Field JH, Krag DO: Congenital constricting bands and congenital amputation of the fingers: Placental studies. *J Bone Joint Surg* 55A:1035, 1973

235. Higginbottom MC, Jones KL, Hall BD, Smith DW: The amniotic band disruption complex: Timing of amniotic rupture and variable spectra of consequent defects. *J Pediatr* 95:544, 1979

236. Katz G: A pedigree with anomalies of the little finger in five generations and seventeen individuals. *J Bone Joint Surg* 52A:7171, 1970

237. Kino Y: Clinical and experimental studies of the congenital constriction band syndrome, with an emphasis on its etiology. *J Bone Joint Surg* 57A:636, 1975

238. Kirner J: Doppelseitige Verkrummungen des Kleinfingerendgliedes als selbstandiges. *Fortschr Gen Rontgen* 36:804, 1927

239. Poznanski AK, Pratt GB, Manson G, Weiss L: Clinodactyly, camptodactyly, Kirner's deformity, and other crooked fingers. *Radiology* 93:573, 1969

240. Smith RJ, Kaplan EB: Camptodactyly and similar atraumatic flexion deformities of the proximal interphalangeal joints of the fingers. *J Bone Joint Surg* 50A:1187, 1968

THE SPINE

The presenting complaints are back pain and/or deformity of the spine, which may be scoliosis, lordosis, kyphosis, poor posture with exaggerated dorsal roundback, rounding of the shoulders, and swayback.

Scoliosis is lateral angulation and rotation of the vertebral column. It is subdivided into structural and nonstructural. A curve is structural when it does not have normal flexibility as demonstrated in supine, side-bending radiograms. *Structural scoliosis* is subdivided into idiopathic, neuromuscular, and congenital.

Structural scoliosis may also be post-traumatic due to fracture or dislocation or secondary to irradiation or surgical laminectomy of the vertebral column. Paraspinal soft tissue contractures can produce scoliosis.

Scoliosis and other spinal deformities are frequently present in connective tissue disorders such as Ehlers-Danlos and Marfan's syndromes and various bone dysplasias such as spondyloepiphyseal dysplasia, Morquio's disease, diastrophic dwarfism, and osteogenesis imperfecta.

In spondylolisthesis and spondylolysis there is a definite increased incidence of scoliosis. Intraspinal tumors such as astrocytomas may present with scoliosis, hyperlordosis, or hyperkyphosis. In tumors of the vertebral column such as osteoid osteoma, osteoblastoma, and eosinophilic granuloma, scoliosis may be the presenting complaint.

Nonstructural scoliosis corrects or overcorrects in supine side-bending radiograms. It may be due to poor posture, secondary to lower limb length disparity, or due to pelvic obliquity resulting from adduction or abduction contracture of the hips. A herniated lumbar disc in the adolescent may be caused by scoliosis, discitis, or other inflammatory diseases of the spine.

Kyphosis is posterior convexity of a segment of the spine in the sagittal plane. In hyperkyphosis the degree of posterior convexity is more than the normal. It may be postural, due to Scheuermann's disease, or due to congenital anomalies such as defects of formation or segmentation.

In bone dysplasia, osteogenesis imperfecta, and juvenile osteoporosis, kyphosis is often present. In myelomeningocele, kyphosis may be present at birth due to congenital deformities of the vertebral column or may develop later due to paralysis. Following trauma to the vertebral column, either with or without spinal cord injury, kyphosis may develop. In skeletal dysplasias such as mucopolysaccharidosis and neurofibromatosis, kyphosis is a common deformity.

Lordosis is anterior convexity of a segment of the spine. It may be (1) postural, (2) congenital, due to vertebral anomalies, (3) neuromuscular, (4) postlaminectomy, or (5) due to hip flexion contracture.[1,2]

■ POSTURAL ROUNDBACK AND SWAYBACK

Postural roundback and swayback in the orthopedic practice are very common complaints of parents. The child presents with exaggerated roundback with drooping of the shoulders and forward tilting of the neck and exaggerated swayback. Frequently the grandparents who accompany them have severe kyphosis with backache. The parents' concern is that they don't want their child to appear like the grandparents. The adolescent girl or boy has no backache, is not concerned about posture, and is rebellious that the parents are constantly correcting his or her poor posture—"Stand up straight!"

Somatotypes are familial, and there is a strong hereditary pattern of exaggerated postural roundback. The parents demand that something be done, but can exercises or orthotic devices alter or improve the roundback determined by the genetic code? The body image of an adolescent is an important consideration. A maturing female with rapid development of large breasts may be shy and may try to hide her breasts by hunching her shoulders, which accentuates the roundback appearance. The male who is having a tremendous growth spurt and is much taller than his peers may also hunch his shoulders to appear shorter.

What is posture? Posture is the relationship of the parts of the body to the line of the center of gravity. Posture varies greatly between individuals and varies with age as well. In a normal perfect posture, the line of the center of gravity as viewed from the lateral side passes through the mastoid process to the cervical thoracic junction, crosses the bodies of the vertebrae at the thoracolumbar junction, and falls just anterior to the sacroiliac joint and slightly posterior to the hip joint; then it passes through the anterior knee joint and ends at the front of the talus in the ankle. The lower limbs are straight, with the hips and knees in neutral extension, and the pelvic inclination is 60 degrees to the vertical. The chin is tucked in, the shoulders are level, the abdomen is flat, and the posterior convexity of the thoracic spine and anterior convexity of the lumbar spine are within normal limits (Fig 5–1A). In the frontal plane there is no scoliosis. A plumb line dropped from the spinous process of C7 falls in the intergluteal cleft.

In poor posture, the center of the line of gravity from the mastoid process falls behind the sacrum, and the vertebral column is decompensated in the sagittal plane. The head is held markedly forward, the roundback in the thoracic spine is exaggerated, and hyperlordosis is present. The shoulders droop, the chest is depressed, and the abdomen protrudes (Fig 5–1B).

The normal posture of an infant prior to walking age is a total convex curve. When the child begins to stand and walk, exaggerated lumbar lordosis with a protuberant abdomen is normal. With further growth and development and improvement of motor strength of antigravity muscles (the gluteus maximus, erector spinae, abdominal, quadriceps, and triceps surae), the child assumes normal posture.

History. When a child presents with poor posture, first ask whether he or she has back pain. Poor posture alone in a child or adolescent is not painful. When the child complains

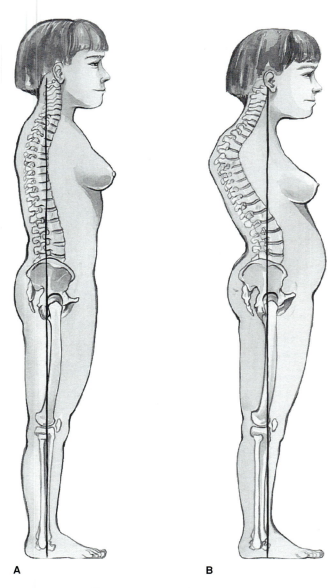

A   **B**

Figure 5–1. Posture. **A.** Normal. **B.** Poor.

Inquire about milestones of motor development. When there is a delay in walking, one should be suspicious of neuromuscular affections such as hypotonia, myopathies (muscular dystrophy), central nervous system damage, and peripheral nerve disease. Has the child had any chronic, debilitating diseases or congenital heart disease? Any trauma? Is there "loose-jointedness" in the family? Do other family members have postural defects?

Examination. First inspect the patient from the front, back, and side, and determine the severity of the postural defect. Drop a plumb line from C7 or the base of the occiput and determine if there is any decompensation of the spine to the right or the left. Inspect the trapezius neckline and level of the shoulders. Is the head tilted forward? Are the shoulders rounded? Is there any asymmetry of the flank creases? Look at the child from the side and determine whether there is pelvic inclination and whether the shoulders are carried behind the pelvis with the neck hyperflexed and the head tilted forward. Are the knees hyperextended? Does the abdomen protrude? How severe is the lordosis? From the front, assess the pectoral muscles. Are they taut, pulling the shoulders forward? In an adolescent female, large breasts may be a factor in poor posture.

Next ask the patient to pinch the glutei together and to retract the abdominal muscles to see if he can actively correct the pelvic inclination and exaggerated lumbar lordosis. Inspect the lower limbs for valgus, varus, and medial or lateral torsional deformity. Do the feet provide normal weight-bearing, or are they deformed into valgus or varus? Assess the gait of the patient for any abnormality. Determine if there is any laxity or contracture of the ligamentous tissues. On adduction does the thumb protrude beyond the ulnar border of the hand, or does the thumb touch the volar surface of the forearm on hyperflexion of the wrist? Do the fingers become parallel to the dorsal surface of the forearm on hyperextension of the wrist? Do the elbows or knees hyperextend into recurvatum? All of these findings indicate extreme laxity of ligamentous tissues and are important causes of poor posture. Pinch and pull the skin to rule out Ehlers-Danlos syndrome. Inspect the child's hands and feet. Is there any arachnodactyly to suggest Marfan's syndrome? Measure the standing and sitting heights of the patient. Rule out contracture of the fascial and musculotendinous structures, especially the hip flexors (Thomas test), rectus femoris (Ely test), fascia lata (Ober test), and pectoral muscles (ask the patient to bring his or her shoulder blades together). Is there any bony deformity such as pectus carinatum or excavatum? Ask the patient to bend forward, and inspect the contour of the thoracic kyphosis. Is it flexible or rigid? Is it sharp and angular, indicating Scheuermann's disease, or is it smooth and arcuate, indicating physiologic roundback (Fig 5–2A, B)? Next, perform the *thoracic hyperextension test;* with the patient prone, ask him or her to raise the head, neck, and shoulders off the table to see if

of pain, inquire about the location. Is it in the neck, thoracic spine, or lumbar region? Does it radiate to the posterior part of the thigh and legs? Lumbosacral pain with or without sciatica suggests spondylolisthesis or herniated disc. Thoracic or thoracolumbar pain suggests Scheuermann's disease. Pain in the neck with the held tilted forward and severe cervical lordosis suggests an intraspinal, space-occupying lesion such as astrocytoma of the spinal cord. Bone lesions such as osteoid osteoma, osteoblastoma, eosinophilic granuloma, or infectious inflammatory lesions such as discitis, vertebral osteomyelitis, tuberculosis, or rheumatoid arthritis cause back pain.

Next inquire about the flexibility or rigidity of the exaggerated dorsal roundback and swayback. A stiff, painful back demands diligent investigation to rule out serious pathology.

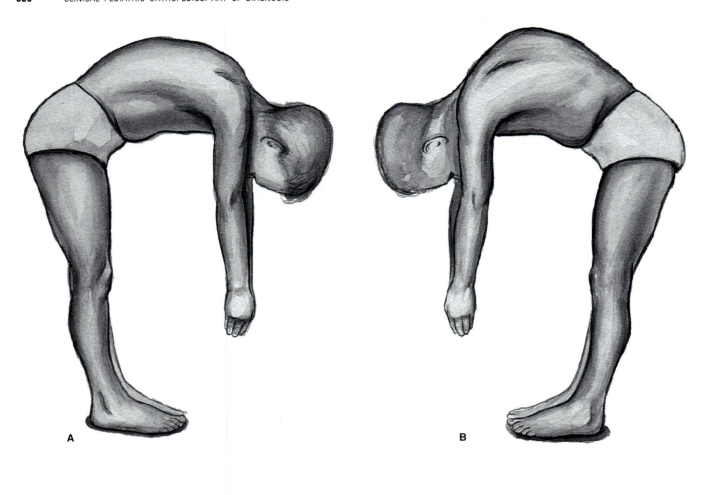

A

B

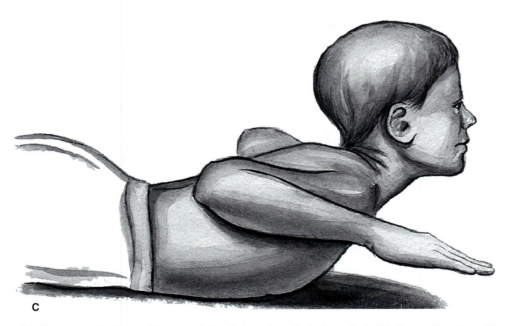

C

Figure 5–2. Postural roundback versus Scheuermann's juvenile kyphosis. **A.** Postural roundback. Note the smooth contour of the thoracic kyphosis. **B.** Scheuermann's juvenile kyphosis. Note the sharp angular contour of the thoracic kyphosis. **C.** Thoracic hyperextension test. In postural roundback the dorsal angulation corrects, whereas in Scheuermann's juvenile kyphosis the deformity is fixed due to wedging of the vertebrae. The kyphosis does not straighten.

the thoracic kyphosis is flexible (dorsal roundback) or rigid (Scheuermann's disease) (Fig 5–2C). Is there hypokyphosis of the thoracic spine with exaggerated posterior angulation of the thoracolumbar junction? With the patient supine, perform a knee-chest test to determine whether the lumbar lordosis disappears (Fig 5–3). Rule out hamstring tautness by performing a straight-leg raising test and determining popliteal thigh-leg angle by extending the flexed knees with the hips in 90 degrees of flexion. Hamstring tightness is frequently associated with Scheuermann's disease, spondylolisthesis, and spinal cord lesions. Determine the motor strength of the abdominals (flexed knee sit-up), gluteus maximus (ask the patient to extend the hip with the knees flexed in prone position), and erector spinae (ask him to raise his shoulders, head, and neck off the table). In the child, always perform Gower's test (getting up off the floor from the supine position—does he or she turn over to prone and climb up the knees with his or her hands, indicating myopathy?).

Gently palpate the spine for painful areas. There is no local tenderness in roundback poor posture, whereas in Scheuermann's disease local tenderness is elicited by palpation of the involved vertebrae. Perform the *Goldthwaite test.* (With the patient prone, elevate his or her knees off the examining table) (Fig 5–4). Are the paraspinal muscles in the lumbar area rigid, indicating an irritating lesion in the intraspinal canal or spondylolisthesis? Is there local tenderness over the L5–S1 or L4–L5 disc interspace? Is there local tenderness over the sacroiliac joint? Are there any external stigmata of spinal dysrhaphism?

Always examine the skin reflexes, the superficial abdominal by stimulating the skin around the umbilicus and

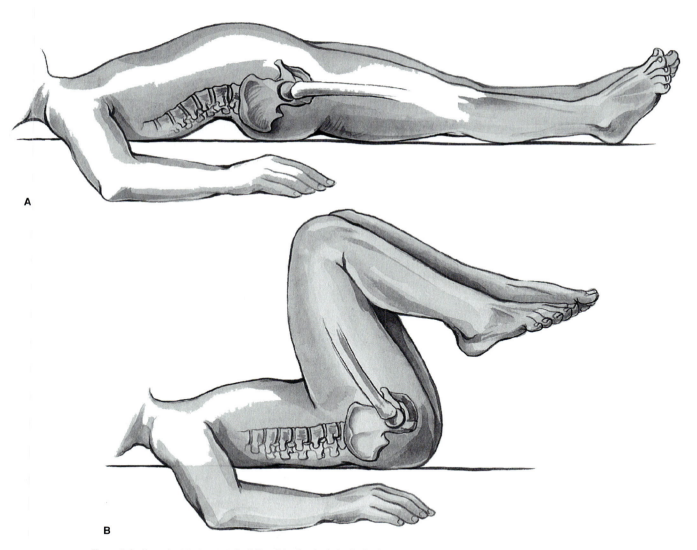

Figure 5–3. Knee-chest test to test flexibility of lumbar lordosis. **A.** Supine with the hips fully extended. Note the severe lumbar hyperlordosis. **B.** On acute flexion of the hips, bringing the knees toward the chest, the lumbar spine straightens, demonstrating the flexibility of the lumbar spine.

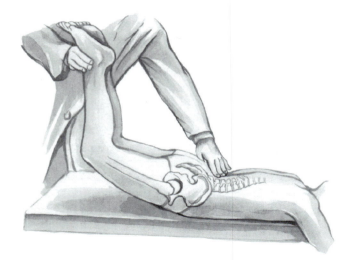

Figure 5–4. Goldthwaite test. With the patient prone, elevate the flexed knees off the examining table. When the lumbar spine is rigid due to spasm of the paraspinal muscles, the pelvis and lumbar spine rise in one piece.

the cremasteric reflex in boys by stroking the upper, inner thigh. Is there any sensory loss in the trunk or limbs? Determine the deep tendon reflexes (DTR) to rule out hypotonia (the DTR are absent or depressed) or an upper motor neuron lesion (the DTR are exaggerated).

Imaging. Routine radiograms should not be made in simple physiologic roundback or swayback. Radiograms are made when there is a suspicion of structural deformation of the vertebrae or an intraspinal lesion. Bone imaging with technetium-99m is performed when a bone lesion such as osteoid osteoma, spondylolisthesis, or Scheuermann's disease is suspected. Magnetic resonance imaging (MRI) is performed only occasionally when an intraspinal tumor is suspected.

Treatment. Treatment consists of postural exercises in the form of pelvic tilt, abdominal and gluteus maximus exercises, and passive stretching of contracted muscles and fascia (hip flexors, rectus femoris, and fascia lata). An orthosis to improve roundback deformity is ordinarily not indicated except in very severe cases, when a Milwaukee brace is worn for a period of 6 to 12 months.

■ BACK PAIN

Back pain in children and adolescents is a rare complaint. It is usually poorly localized and nonspecific. Often it is caused by serious pathology, requiring diligent investigation. The cause of back pain varies in different age groups.

History. Ask the following questions: (1) What is the *location* of the pain: Is it in the lower back—the thoracolumbar region or thoracic area? (2) Does it *radiate* to the buttocks and the posterolateral aspect of the thigh and leg, indicating a lumbosacral level lesion? Does it radiate to the front of the abdomen, indicating a thoracolumbar level lesion, or the front of the chest, indicating a thoracic level lesion? (3) What is the nature of the pain—is it sharp or dull? (4) Is the pain severe, moderate, or mild? Is the pain severe enough to force the patient to stay in bed? Have any days been missed from school? (5) Is it aggravated by coughing, sneezing, or straining at stool? (6) Is there pain at night? Does the pain respond to salicylates, acetaminophen (Tylenol), or other medications such as nonsteroidal anti-inflammatory drugs? (7) Was the *onset of pain* sudden or gradual? Did the pain follow an acute episode of lifting weights, trauma, or a fall? (8) Is the *duration of pain* weeks, months, or years? Is it constant or intermittent? What is the *frequency*—once a day or once a week? (9) What is the relation to physical activity? Is it aggravated by prolonged standing or walking? (10) Is there any sensory disturbance of the lower limbs such as numbness or tingling? (11) Is there any bowel or bladder or sphincter dysfunction? (12) Is there any motor weakness of the feet, legs, or hips? Any stumbling or falling? (13) Is there any fever or skin rash? Herpes zoster? (14) Is there any family history of herniated disc, spondylolisthesis, or kyphosis?

Examination. Follow the same steps as for examination of a patient with scoliosis. *Inspect* the patient from the back, front, and side with the patient standing and then bending forward. Rule out scoliosis. Are the shoulders and pelvis level (iliac crests and anterosuperior iliac spine)? Is there any rotation of the vertebrae—a rib or lumbar paravertebral muscle hump? Is the spine compensated in the frontal projection? Does a plumb line dropped from C7 fall in the intergluteal cleft? Is there hyperkyphosis and hyperlordosis? Are there any external stigmata of spinal dysraphism such as hairy patches or hemangioma? Any café-au-lait spots, axillary or inguinal freckling, or neurofibroma to suggest neurofibromatosis?

Look at the feet for claw toes and pes cavus or equinus deformities. Is there any obvious atrophy of the calves or thighs? Document this by measuring their circumferences.

Observe the gait of the patient. Are there any abnormalities such as drop foot? Ask the patient to walk on his toes, heels, and inner and outer borders of the feet. How does he get out of a chair? Is he in pain?

Next, *palpate* the entire spine. Begin with the soft tissues. Rule out spasm of the *paraspinal muscles,* which seem prominent and feel rather rigid. Examine the paraspinal muscles with the patient standing on both legs and then on one leg at a time. Marked paravertebral muscle spasm obliterates the normal lumbar lordosis. Then gently palpate the supraspinous and intraspinous ligaments; when stretched out and strained, they are tender. Palpate and percuss the kidney region posteriorly. Renal pathology causes low back pain. Next palpate the bones. First feel the spinous processes: Local tenderness or tumorous enlargement suggests aneurysmal bone cyst or osteoblastoma. Any *step-off* between L5–S1 or L4–L5 spinous processes suggests spondylolisthesis. Any defect between the lamina indicates spina bifida. Laterally, gently press over the facet joints and the transverse processes. Palpate the posterior aspect of the sacrum, sacrococcygeal region, posterior iliac spines, sacroiliac joints, and iliac crests. Inferiorly palpate the greater sciatic notch and the sciatic nerve. Perform the pelvic compression test by pushing the iliac bones toward each other with the palms of your hands. Do not forget to palpate the abdomen, inguinal area, and symphysis pubis anteriorly.

Next, test *range of motion* of the spine—flexion and extension, lateral bending, and rotation. Determine the mobility of the hips, knees, and ankles and feet. Rule out hamstring tightness. Extend the flexed knee with the hip in 90 degrees of flexion and determine the popliteal angle. Then perform the *straight-leg raising test*—it may be limited because of hamstring tautness or sciatic nerve irritation.

Is the pain in the posterior thigh or does it radiate distally to the leg and foot? In severe sciatica and particularly in midline disc protrusion, the patient complains of pain in the opposite thigh and occasionally in the leg.

Then perform the Lasègue test—straight leg raise 20 to 30 degrees and dorsiflex the foot and ankle; when the test is positive, it reproduces sciatic pain.

Ask the patient to lie prone and carefully palpate the entire spine for areas of tenderness. Perform the Goldthwaite test by raising the flexed knees off the examination table (see Fig 5–4).

With the patient supine, perform a *Faber-Patrick test* to determine sacroiliac pathology; place the foot of the test side on the opposite knee with the hip flexed, abducted, and laterally rotated. With one hand on the opposite ilium, hyperextend the hip by pushing the knee toward the floor (Fig 5–5); when painful the test is positive, indicating sacroiliac pathology, which is rare in children and adolescents. It is usually seen in osteomyelitis of the iliac bone or in rheumatoid arthritis.

Another way to test sacroiliac pathology is by the *Gaenslen test* (Fig 5–6). With the patient supine with the knees flexed on the abdomen, move the buttocks of the test side off the edge of the table and let the thigh and leg fall off the table into hyperextension while keeping the opposite hip flexed. The test is positive when the patient complains of pain in the sacroiliac joint.

Test for *Beevor's sign*. With the patient's upper limb across the chest and the hips and knees flexed 45 degrees, ask the patient to sit up part way and hold that position. Observe the umbilicus! When the innervation of rectus abdominus muscle (anterior primary division of T5 to T12) is intact, the umbilicus does not move. When there is asymmetric weakness of the rectus abdominus, the umbilicus moves to the stronger side of the muscle—up or down or to one side or the other (Fig 5–7).

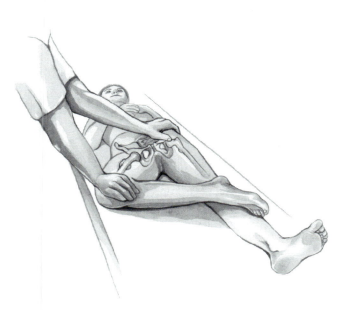

Figure 5–5. Faber-Patrick test to demonstrate sacroiliac pathology. With the patient supine, place the foot of the test side on the opposite knee with the hip flexed, abducted, and laterally rotated. With one hand on the opposite ilium, stabilize the pelvis. With the other hand, hyperextend the hip, pushing the knee toward the floor.

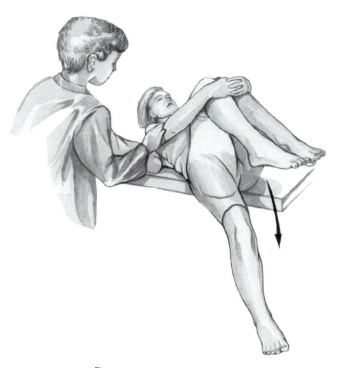

Figure 5–6. Gaenslen test. See text.

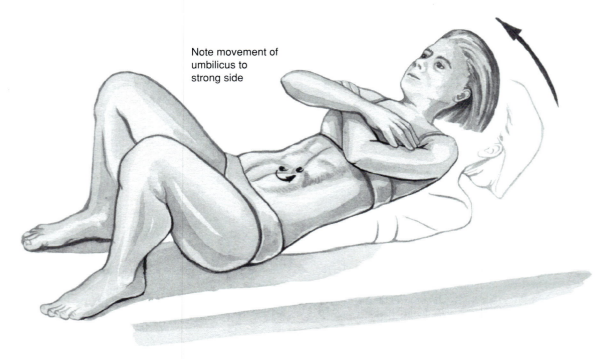

Note movement of
umbilicus to
strong side

Figure 5–7. Beevor's sign. See text.

Next, perform a thorough neurologic examination. First, determine *motor strength* of the following muscles according to *neurologic level.*

S1 to S4 Levels.   (1) Peroneus longus and brevis (S1 level innervated by the superficial peroneal nerve); (2) gastrocnemius-soleus (S1–S2 levels supplied by the tibial nerve); (3) gluteus maximus (S1 level supplied by the inferior gluteal nerve). (4) S2, S3, and S4 neurologic levels innervate the bladder and intrinsic muscles of the foot.

L5 Level.   (1) Extensor hallucis longus and extensor digitorum longus and brevis (supplied by the deep peroneal nerve); (2) gluteus medius (innervated by the superior gluteal nerve).

L4 Level.   (1) Tibialis anterior (supplied by the deep peroneal nerve).

T12, L1, L2, and L3 Levels.   (1) The iliopsoas is a difficult muscle to test. With the hip at right angles as the patient sits at the edge of the examining table and the hip in neutral or slight medial rotation, ask the patient to raise his or her thigh toward the ceiling.

Next, test *sensation* to touch and pinprick according to the *neurologic level* (Fig 5–8).

S2 to S4 Level.   This supplies sensation around the anus. A simple way to test the superficial anal reflex is to touch and stimulate the skin around the anus and see if the anal

sphincter muscle contracts (it is best to postpone this step of examination until the end and to have a female nurse carry this out in the female patient).

S1 Level.   Determine sensation on the plantar and lateral sides of the foot and over the lateral malleolus.

L5 Level.   Test sensation on the dorsum of the foot and lateral aspect of the leg.

L4 Level.   Test sensation on the medial aspect of the leg.

L1 to L3 Level.   Anterior aspect of the thigh. L3—above the knee, L4—middle two thirds of the thigh, and L2—immediately below the inguinal ligament.

Next, determine the superficial skin reflexes: (1) In boys the *cremasteric reflex* is innervated by T12; (2) the *abdominal reflex*—the lower abdomen is innervated by T10 to L4 and the upper abdomen by T7 to T10. The superficial abdominal reflex is tested by stimulating each quadrant of the abdomen with a sharp object. The umbilicus moves toward the side being stimulated (Fig 5–9). The cremasteric reflex is tested by stimulating the inner aspect of the upper thigh with a sharp object (such as your fingernail). The testicle pulls upward (Fig 5–10).

Next, test the *deep tendon reflexes.* The Achilles tendon reflex or ankle jerk determines the neurologic status of S1, whereas the patellar tendon reflex or knee jerk is a function of L4.

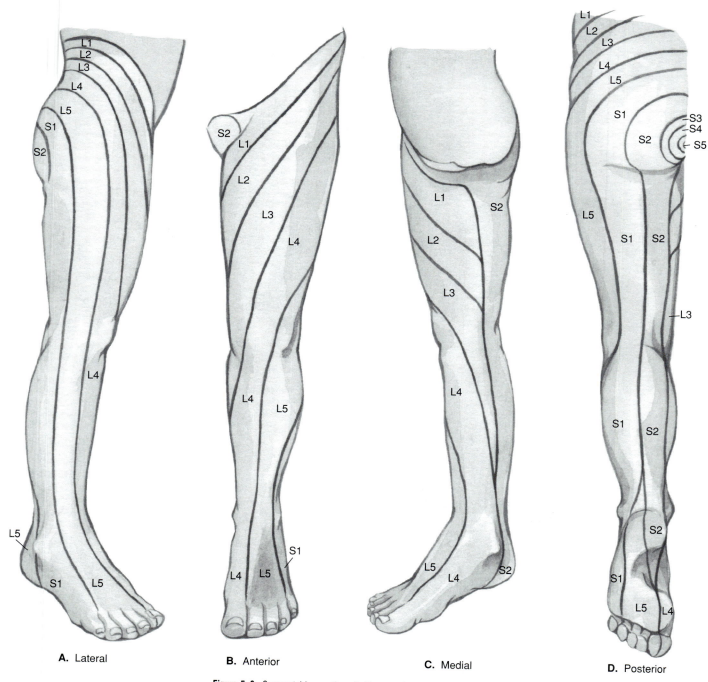

Figure 5–8. Segmental innervation of skin sensation of the lower limbs.

A. Lateral

B. Anterior

C. Medial

D. Posterior

Imaging Studies. Initially, simple radiograms in the AP and lateral projections are made. When spondylolysis or spondylolisthesis is suspected, oblique projections and dynamic flexion-extension views of the lumbosacral spine are made along with a spot lateral film. Sacroiliac joints are best depicted in oblique projections. Bone scan with technetium-99m is an important investigative tool. Computed tomography (CT) and MRI are performed as necessary.

Various causes of back pain in children and adolescents are given in Table 5–1. Only the most common causes of back pain and deformities of the spine are discussed in this section.

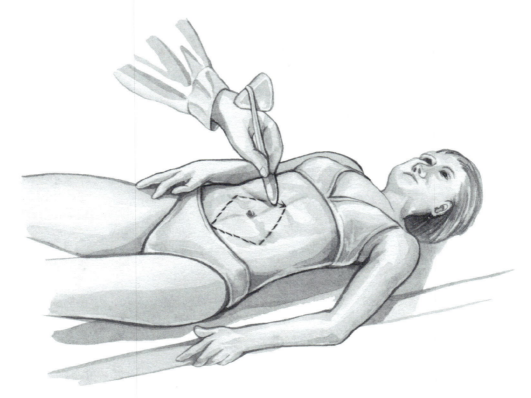

Figure 5–9. Superficial abdominal skin reflex. See text.

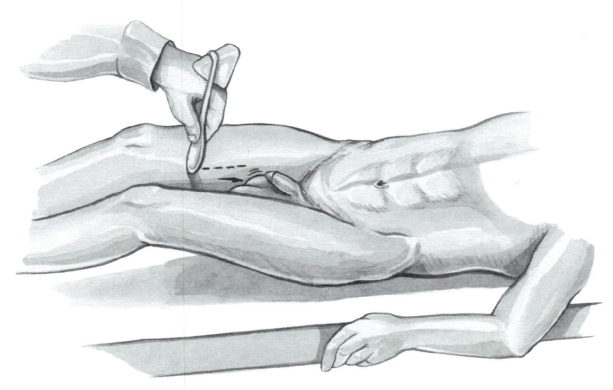

Figure 5–10. Cremasteric reflex. See text.

■ KYPHOSIS

SCHEUERMANN'S JUVENILE KYPHOSIS

The presenting complaints are poor posture with exaggerated roundback and back pain. The kyphosis is angular (not round) and is fixed due to structural changes of the involved vertebrae; that is, it is not flexible and does not correct on extension of the thoracic spine.

Scheuermann, a Danish radiologist, is credited with being the first to describe juvenile kyphosis in 1920, an era of high prevalence of tuberculosis of the spine. He insisted that a definitive diagnosis could be made only by radiograms. The characteristic radiographic findings in advanced stages of the disease are (1) wedging of 5 degrees or more of the three apical vertebrae (commonly T7, T8, and T9), (2) vertebral end-plate irregularity, (3) disc space narrowing, and (4) Schmorl node formation, which may or may not be present (Fig 5–11).

The age of presentation is usually around puberty. The age of onset is difficult to determine because radiographic changes such as wedging and kyphosis are visualized at 11 to 12 years of age and not in the younger child.

The prevalence of Scheuermann's juvenile kyphosis is estimated to be 1 percent, according to Ascani, with a higher preponderance in the female, with a female:male ratio of 1.4:1.[3]

In about 85 to 90 percent of the cases of Scheuermann's disease, the thoracic spine is involved, and in the remaining cases the kyphosis is in the thoracolumbar or lumbar area.

Etiology. The cause of Scheuermann's disease is not known. It is not due to aseptic necrosis of bone. The ring

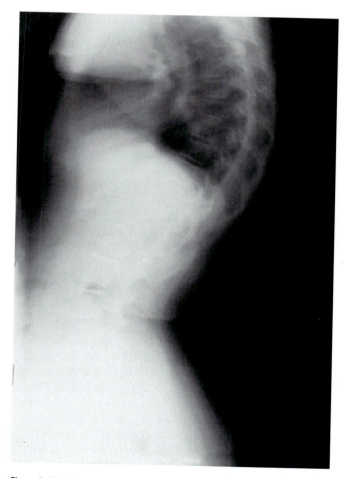

Figure 5–11. Scheuermann's juvenile kyphosis. Radiographic findings of the spine as seen in a lateral radiogram of the spine. Note the severe kyphosis and wedging of the apical thoracic vertebrae.

apophysis does not contribute to the longitudinal growth of the vertebral body.[4,5] It is not caused by rupture of bulging discs into the spongiosa through traumatic tears of the vertebral end-plates.[31] It is not due to inflammatory apophysitis. Taut hamstrings, contracture of the iliopsoas, and mechanical static forces have been implicated in the pathogenesis of Scheuermann's disease.[15]

Scheuermann's disease may be familial with a dominant inheritance, and it may also be sporadic in its occurrence.[16,20,25]

In thoracic Scheuermann's disease, the kyphotic deformity is readily apparent; however, one should remember that the range of normal thoracic kyphosis varies widely and increases with increasing age. In a growing child, 20 to 45 degrees of thoracic kyphosis are normal. A posterior curvature of the thoracic spine greater than 50 degrees is excessive. In the lumbar spine and at the thoracolumbar junction any posterior angulation is abnormal.

History. Determine the age of the patient when the roundback deformity was first noted, whether it has been progressive or static, and whether it is associated with back pain. Is there any history of weight-lifting or gymnastics? Mechanical forces may be pathogenic factors in Scheuermann's disease. Does the patient complain of fatigue? Has the patient had previous multiple fractures, indicating juvenile osteoporosis or metabolic bone disease as a cause of wedging of the vertebrae? Has the patient had any spinal surgery such as laminectomy or irradiation for Wilms' tumor or neuroblastoma? Radiation to the growth areas causes kyphosis. Is there any history of exposure to tuberculosis or bacille Calmette-Guérin (BCG) vaccination? Inquire about a family history of kyphosis and café-au-lait spots or other stigmata to suggest neurofibromatosis.

When the thoracic level is involved, the pain is an intermittent dull ache and not severe, incapacitating, or constant. In thoracolumbar or lumbar Scheuermann's disease, the pain is the principal complaint.

Examination. The physical findings vary according to the anatomic level of involvement. The severity of the deformity varies from mild to severe.

Scheuermann's juvenile kyphosis is angular. Examine the patient from the side and also in the prone position. The kyphosis is fixed and does not correct on dorsal hyperextension (see Fig 5–2). The shoulders droop and the thoracic spine is held backward, with the center of gravity falling behind the sacrum. The neck and lumbar spine are hyperlordotic compensating the thoracic kyphosis. The pectoral muscles are contracted. In thoracolumbar Scheuermann's kyphosis, the posterior angulation of the spine is rather long, with a short lower lumbar lordosis. In the occasional lumbar Scheuermann's kyphosis, the lower spine is straight and has a slight prominence of the spinous processes of the involved vertebrae, and the thoracic spine is hypokyphotic. Ask the patient to bend forward and check for associated scoliosis, which is present in 20 to 30 percent of the cases.[9]

Palpate the spinous processes for any local tenderness that may be present. Ask the patient to bend to the right and left and forward and backward to test for spasm of the paravertebral muscles. Ask the patient to touch his or her toes with the knees straight and to perform straight-leg raising to assess tightness of the hamstrings, which is a very common finding in Scheuermann's disease. Next, perform a thorough neurologic examination to rule out spinal cord compression, which is rare. Is there any spasticity or hyperreflexia? Test the umbilical skin reflex and cremasteric reflex and perform a thorough sensory examination to rule out sensory deficit. Determine the motor strength of muscles in the lower limbs to rule out paresis.

Imaging. The following radiographic views are made: (1) a lateral standing view of the spine with the arms in 90 degrees of flexion holding a support, the head erect, and the knees and hips in neutral extension; (2) an AP standing view of the spine, iliac crests as high as possible, to rule out associated scoliosis; (3) lateral view of the thoracolumbar spine in hyperextension to determine flexibility of the kyphosis; (4) spot lateral films of L5–S1 if clinical findings suggest spondylolysis or spondylolisthesis.

The radiographic findings depend upon the age of the patient. Wedging of the vertebrae is usually not present in the patient less than 12 years of age. The wedging is most marked in the vertebrae at the apex of the kyphosis. According to Sørenson, 5 degrees is the limit between normal and abnormal wedging.[34] By definition, the kyphosis should include the last three adjacent vertebrae with wedging of each vertebra of 5 degrees or more. Wedging is a late radiographic finding. In the early stages of Scheuermann's kyphosis, radiograms disclose irregular lumbothoracic vertebral end-plates, narrowing of the disc interspace, and Schmorl's nodes, which represent disc protrusion into the spongiosa of the vertebrae. Schmorl's nodes may be present in the vertebrae without Scheuermann's juvenile kyphosis, and juvenile kyphosis may be present without Schmorl's nodes.

Bone imaging with technetium-99m shows increased localized uptake of the anterior part of the wedged vertebrae. An MRI demonstrates the irregularity of the vertebral end-plates, Schmorl's nodes, the disc pathology, and wedging of the vertebrae.

In the *differential diagnosis* one should consider *postural roundback,* in which the degree of the posterior angulation of the thoracic spine is less than 45 degrees. The wedging of the involved vertebrae is less than 5 degrees, and there is no irregularity of the vertebral end-plates or narrowing of the disc interspaces. The kyphosis in postural roundback is smooth and flexible. Postural roundback is not painful. *Congenital kyphosis* should be distinguished from

Scheuermann's disease. It may be due to defective formation or the failure of segmentation of the vertebral bodies. Because congenital kyphosis may cause paraplegia, early diagnosis is crucial. Localized kyphosis may be present in neurofibromatosis and following laminectomy or radiation. Careful history-taking and examination of the patient settle the diagnosis.

Congenital absence of the posterior elements in myelodysplasia, bone dysplasias such as spondyloepiphyseal or Morquio's disease, metabolic bone diseases such as osteoporosis, osteogenesis imperfecta, and post-traumatic kyphosis should be ruled out. Tuberculous kyphosis is rare in developed countries but still occurs. It is important to consider the possibility of Pott's disease in the differential diagnosis.

Treatment. This varies according to the severity of the deformity, age of the patient, and stage in the course of the disease. Mild cases (40 to 60 degrees) are treated with physical therapy consisting of hyperextension exercises, pelvic tilt, and motor strengthening of the gluteus maximus, abdominal, and erector spinae muscles. Flexion stresses on the spine, such as weight-lifting, should be avoided.

Orthotic treatment in the form of a Milwaukee brace with posterior pads is indicated in thoracic juvenile hyperkyphosis when the deformity is moderate (60 to 75 degrees) or severe (over 75 degrees) and progressive and clinically symptomatic (Fig 5–12). Orthoses are effective in the growing spine (vertebral end-plates not fused to vertebral bodies). Orthoses are less effective when the curve is greater than 75 degrees and are ineffective after completion of vertebral growth. An important factor in achieving successful correction of the kyphosis is the duration of the brace wear. Ordinarily, 2 years of full-time wear and 1 year of part-time wear are required for successful management.

Surgical treatment is indicated in the skeletally mature patient with severe pain, progressive deformity, and neurologic compromise. It is important that surgery be both anterior and posterior. Preoperatively perform an MRI scan to rule out thoracic disc herniation. Short fusions are doomed to failure. Serious complications of surgery include superior mesenteric artery syndrome, sublaminar hooks causing cord compression, hooks pulling out, and functional kyphosis caudal and cephalad to the site of fusion.

In *thoracolumbar Scheuermann's kyphosis,* treatment is more conservative. Surgery is seldom necessary. Orthotic support, rest, and stretching of the hamstrings relieve symptoms in most cases. Occasionally the deformity is very severe and requires surgical intervention.

In the adult patient, especially females with osteoporosis after menopause, untreated severe Scheuermann's disease can be catastrophic. It should not be considered a benign, cosmetic problem. Disabling pain, reduced pulmonary function, and thoracic cord compression are major problems.

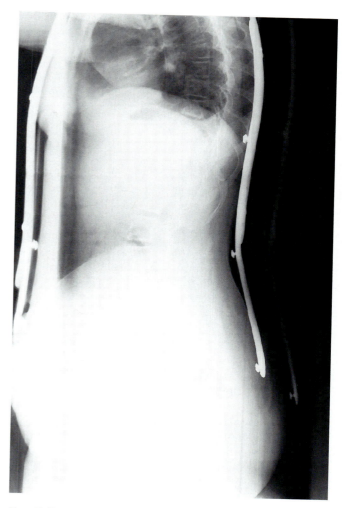

Figure 5–12. Lateral of the spine of a patient with Scheuermann's juvenile kyphosis being treated by a Milwaukee brace.

CONGENITAL KYPHOSIS

Acute posterior angulation is the presenting manifestation of congenital kyphosis. It is classified into two types: (1) failure of formation—absence or hypoplasia of part or all of a vertebral body with preservation of the posterior elements (Fig 5–13E, F) and (2) failure of segmentation of the anterior part of two or more adjacent vertebrae (Fig 5–14B). With posterior growth of the vertebral bodies and failure of growth anteriorly, the degree of kyphosis progressively increases.

The most common site of kyphosis is between T10 and L2. A compensatory hyperlordosis develops in the lumbar spine which may cause backache. Acute posterior angulation of the spine is usually detected in infancy. The kyphosis gradually increases in severity and may result in paraplegia if not treated. The deformity is evident in a radiogram. Prior to surgery, MRI is performed to delineate

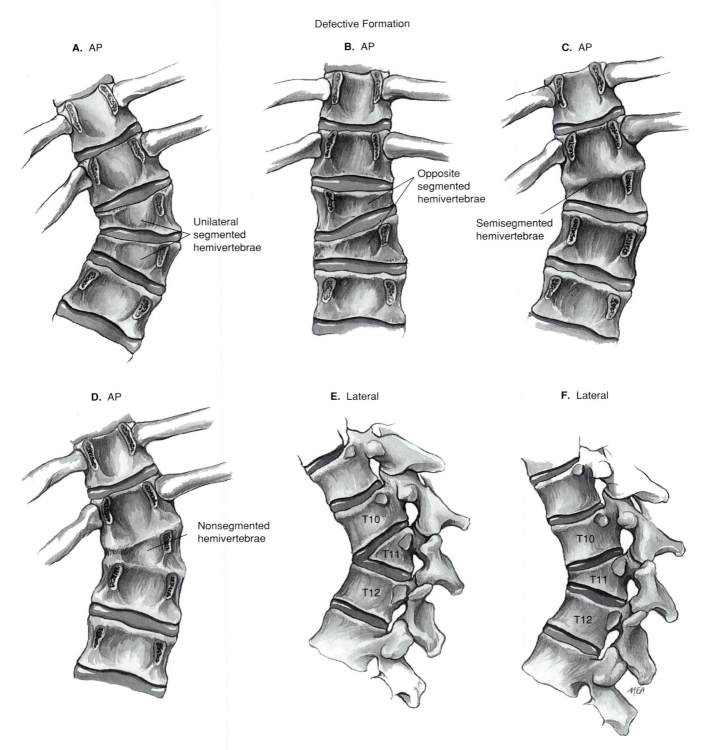

Figure 5–13. Congenital deformities of the spine due to defective formation. **A.** Unilateral hemivertebrae with intact vertebral growth plate and disc. **B.** Segmented hemivertebrae on opposite sides. Note that the vertebral growth and discs are intact. **C.** Unilateral segmented hemivertebra fused to the adjacent vertebra superiorly. Note that the vertebral growth plate and disc are intact inferiorly. **D.** Nonsegmented hemivertebra fused to the adjacent vertebra. Note that the vertebral growth plates and discs are absent. **E** and **F.** Lateral view of the spine showing defective anterior formation of the 11th thoracic vertebra. Note the posterior angulation at the site of the vertebral anomaly.

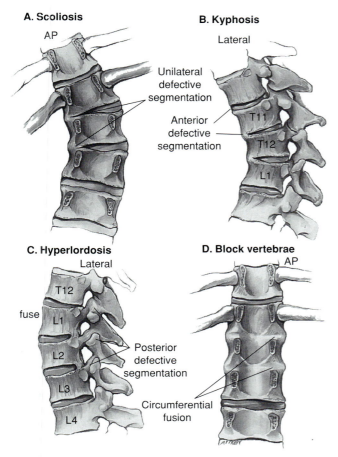

A. Scoliosis
AP

Unilateral
defective
segmentation

Anterior
defective
segmentation

B. Kyphosis
Lateral

T11

T12

L1

C. Hyperlordosis
Lateral

T12

fuse   L1

L2

Posterior
defective
segmentation

L3

L4

D. Block vertebrae
AP

Circumferential
fusion

Figure 5–14. Congenital deformities of the spine due to defective segmentation. **A.** AP view of the spine showing unilateral bar between T12–L1 and L1–L2. Note the scoliosis, which will relentlessly increase with asymmetric growth. **B.** Lateral view of the spine showing failure of segmentation anteriorly between T11 and T12 and L1. Note the kyphosis, which will progressively increase because of failure of growth anteriorly and continued growth posteriorly. **C.** Lateral view of the spine showing failure of segmentation of the posterior part of the vertebra and posterior elements of L1–L2 and L2–L3. **D.** Block vertebrae due to circumferential fusion of the vertebral bodies between L1–T12 and L1–L2.

associated spinal cord pathology, especially in the presence of neurologic deficit.

Orthotic devices are of no value and should not be prescribed. Treatment consists of early posterior fusion, which should be performed before the age of 3 years. When the degree of kyphosis exceeds 60 degrees in older children, both anterior and posterior fusions are performed. In the adolescent patient, when there is enough bone stock, the compression type of instrumentation is carried out posteriorly.

KYPHOSIS IN NEUROFIBROMATOSIS

This condition is caused by deformity of the vertebral bodies. Clinically it presents as acute posterior angula-

tion of the spine. The presence of other clinical features of neurofibromatosis makes the diagnosis. Severe deformity leads to paraplegia. Once the degree of kyphosis exceeds 50 degrees, braces are ineffective. Treatment consists of both anterior and posterior fusion. Posterior instrumentation should be used. Halo casts are utilized for cervical and high thoracic kyphosis. When associated dural ectasia and neurofibromatosis are present in the spinal canal, laminectomy is performed, followed by spinal fusion.

KYPHOSIS IN BONE DYSPLASIA

This is a common finding in achondroplasia. It is often associated with compensatory hyperlordosis and a hip flexion deformity. It is also seen in mucopolysaccharidoses such as Morquio's disease, osteoporosis such as osteogenesis imperfecta, juvenile osteoporosis, and Turner's syndrome. In the young child, three-point hyperextension thoracolumbosacral orthosis (TLSO) is used to prevent anterior wedge compression of the vertebral bodies and contracture of the anterior longitudinal ligament. If bracing does not stop the progression of kyphosis, posterior spinal fusion is indicated with or without instrumentation.

POSTRADIATION KYPHOSIS

This is seen in young children who, during the first few years of life, were treated for malignant tumors such as Wilms' tumor or neuroblastoma. Treatment consists of posterior fusion and instrumentation if the kyphosis is detected early and is not severe. Once the degree of kyphosis exceeds 60 degrees, both anterior and posterior fusions are required.

POSTLAMINECTOMY KYPHOSIS

This is seen in children who had laminectomy performed for excision of a spinal cord tumor. The neurosurgeon is so concerned about the tumor that he ignores the mechanical integrity of the posterior elements of the spine. It is important that a unilateral laminotomy be performed and that the lamina be replaced. Once the patient presents with severe kyphosis, usually in the juvenile or adolescent age group, both anterior and posterior fusions must be performed. Anteriorly the contracted ligaments are sectioned, and fusion is carried out along the entire length of the deformity. Halo gravity traction is employed for 2 to 3 weeks; then a diligent posterior fusion is performed. Posterior instrumentation is carried out if the bone stock is sturdy. Postoperatively the spine is supported in a halo cast until solid fusion has taken place.

TUBERCULOUS KYPHOSIS

This is very rare in developed countries but can still occur, and it should always be considered in the differential diagnosis. It is caused by collapse of vertebral bodies. Treatment consists of excision of the tuberculous bone, replacement with bone grafts through an anterior approach and posterior fusion, and antituberculous drug therapy.

CONGENITAL HYPERLORDOSIS

This is caused by unsegmented bars of the posterior part of the vertebral bodies or congenital synostosis of the posterior lamina and articular parts with arrest of growth posteriorly and continued growth anteriorly (Fig 5–14C). It is usually not detected early on simple radiograms because of the cartilage stage of congenital fusion. The deformity progressively increases. CT or MRI is often required to delineate the specific pathology.

Braces are of no value. Treatment consists of anterior fusion. If the deformity is severe and lordosis is very marked, correction is achieved by shortening the anterior column by removal of wedges at the disc interspaces and posterior osteotomies of the synostosis at the same levels.

■ SPONDYLOLISTHESIS AND SPONDYLOLYSIS

SPONDYLOLISTHESIS

Spondylolisthesis is the slipping forward of one vertebra onto another, usually affecting the fifth lumbar vertebra over the sacrum. The term is derived from two Greek words, *spondylos*, meaning spine, and *olisthanein*, meaning to slip. The term spondylolysis is used when a defect is present in the pars interarticularis but no forward slipping has occurred.

Spondylolisthesis is classified into five different types: *Type I—dysplastic* is a congenital dysplasia of the lumbosacral junction with a deficiency of the superior facet of S1 or the arch of L5, allowing forward slipping of L5 onto S1. The pars interarticularis is intact but may be attenuated and elongated. Ordinarily the degree of slip is progressive and severe (Fig 5–15A). Neurologic deficit is common because of the pressure on the dural sac with an anteriorly pulled lamina of L5. In *type II—isthmic*, there is a break—"stress fracture"—of the pars interarticularis (Fig 5–15B). With repeated stress fractures, the pars interarticularis may become elongated and attenuated. An acute fracture of the pars interarticularis is also classified as isthmic spondylolisthesis. In *type III—traumatic*, there is an acute fracture of the pedicle lamina or facet with consequent instability and forward slip of the vertebrae. In this type, the pars interarticularis is intact. *Type IV—degenerative*, also known as

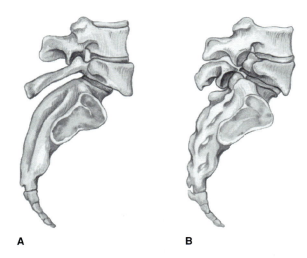

Figure 5–15. Common types of spondylolisthesis seen in children and adolescents. **A.** Type I—dysplastic. **B.** Type II—isthmic. See text.

pseudospondylolisthesis, is not seen in children. Longstanding degenerative arthritis causes facet deficiency. The disc interspace is narrowed. It commonly involves the fourth lumbar level and is seen in patients over 40 years of age. In *type V—pathologic*, the bone structure is insufficient and weak from a developmental dysplasia such as osteogenesis imperfecta, neurofibromatosis, or a neoplastic lesion. This section does not cover traumatic or pathologic spondylolisthesis because of its rarity or degenerative spondylolisthesis because it does not occur in children.

Etiology. The pars interarticularis defect is caused by two factors: (1) inherited dysplasia in the cartilage model of the affected vertebrae, and (2) increased loading and strain on the weakened pars interarticularis due to the upright posture and lumbar lordosis of the human. With repetitive stress and microfractures, the pars interarticularis elongates and develops lysis and the vertebra slips forward under body weight. The trauma is usually hyperextension, occurring commonly in gymnasts, weight-lifters, and football linemen. There is a positive family history in 35 percent of the dysplastic cases and 15 percent of the isthmic cases. Whites are more commonly affected than blacks, and it is twice as common in males as in females. It is not seen in nonambulatory patients. It is more common in early walkers and is present in 35 percent of patients with thoracolumbar Scheuermann's disease.

Isthmic Spondylolisthesis

This is the most common type of spondylolisthesis. The presenting complaint depends upon the age of the patient and the severity of the slipping. The child under 10 years of age often has no pain. Poor posture and increased swayback are the presenting complaints. With an adolescent growth spurt, the patient develops low back pain that is aggravated by prolonged standing or walking and relieved by rest. The pain is in the region of the low back and buttocks and is due to instability of the fifth lumbar segment. When there is pressure on the nerve root, the patient develops sciatica, with pain radiating to the posterolateral aspect of the thigh and leg. Sensory and motor deficits may develop due to irritation of the fifth lumbar and first sacral nerve roots by the fibrocartilaginous mass at the defect in the pars interarticularis.

On examination, excessive lumbar lordosis is evident. The hamstrings are taut and in spasm. Straight-leg raising is restricted. The paravertebral muscles are in spasm, as demonstrated by limitation of lateral bending and a positive Goldthwaite test. On palpation there is local tenderness at the L5–S1 junction. On forward bending, the trunk may deviate to the side. In symptomatic spondylolisthesis, the gait is awkward, with a pelvic waddle and a shortened stride length. This bizarre gait abnormality is referred to as the Phalen-Dickson sign.[90] Depending upon the degree of nerve root irritation, there will be evidence of neurologic deficit such as decreased ankle deep tendon reflexes, sensory motor deficit, and bladder control problems (which, when present, require urgent relief of nerve root compression). In severe spondylolisthesis there is a marked increase in lumbosacral kyphosis, with increase of the forward tilt of the pelvis. There is increased incidence of scoliosis in spondylolisthesis.[51,60,70,71,78]

Imaging Findings. Radiograms should include AP, lateral, right and left 45-degree oblique views of the lumbosacral spine, and a spot lateral view of the L5–S1 interspace. Make the lateral radiograms standing to determine the slip angle.

Spondylolysis is unilateral in 20 to 25 percent of the cases. The pars interarticularis defect is best seen in the oblique view with the lamina flattened. The appearance of a Scottish terrier outline can be seen, with the neck of the dog corresponding to the pars interarticularis (Fig 5–16).

In spondylolisthesis, the defect in the pars interarticularis can be visualized in the lateral projection (Fig 5–17). The degree of slip of spondylolisthesis can be graded as follows: Grade I—Anterior displacement is 25 percent or less; grade II—between 25 and 50 percent; grade III—between 50 and 75 percent; and grade IV—greater than 75 percent (Fig 5–18). The *slip angle* is the most important determination in the radiogram (Fig 5–19). In the lateral projection of a standing film, determine the angle between the line drawn on the superior surface of the L5 and the inferior surface of the S1 vertebral bodies. It is vital that it be a true spot lateral radiogram.

Treatment. The modality of treatment depends upon the following factors: (1) whether it is spondylolysis or spondylolisthesis; (2) the type and degree of slip; (3) whether

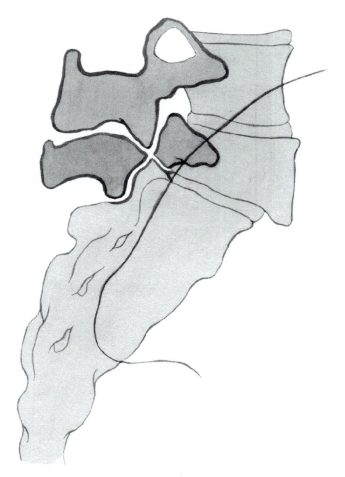

Figure 5–16. Pars interarticularis defect as depicted in the oblique radiogram. Note the Scottish terrier outline. The neck of the dog corresponds to the pars interarticularis.

the slip is static and stable or progressive and unstable; (4) whether it is asymptomatic or symptomatic: An asymptomatic spondylolysis has a better prognosis than a symptomatic one. The severity of back pain, the degree of disability, and the limitation of normal physical activity are other important factors to consider.

Risk factors for progression of slippage are (1) the *type* of slip; dysplastic spondylolisthesis is more prone to progressive slip and persistence of symptoms than the isthmic type. (2) Anatomic configuration of L5 and S1; when the superior surface of the sacrum is dome-shaped and perpendicular and the fifth lumbar vertebra is trapezoid, the probability of progressive slip is great. (3) The slip angle; when the sagittal rotation of the L5 vertebral body on S1 is greater than 50 degrees, the probability of progression and anterior displacement is great. (4) The degree of slip. Grades III and IV spondylolisthesis (i.e., slips 50 percent or greater) are at great risk for progression, whereas spondylolysis or minimal spondylolisthesis in the adolescent is unlikely to slip further. (5) Mobility of the defect—dynamic

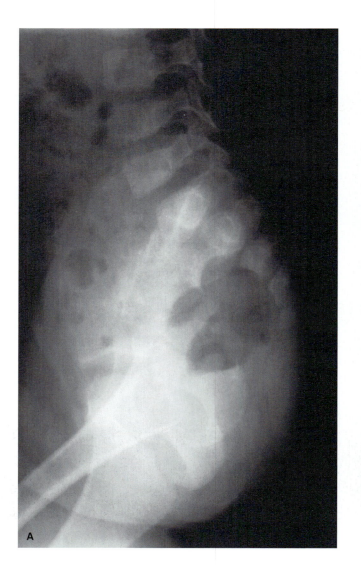

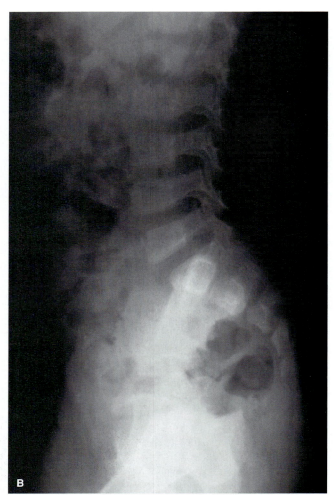

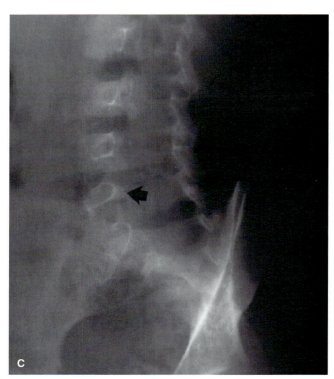

Figure 5–17. Spondylolisthesis of L5–S1. **A** & **B.** Lateral flexion-extension views. Note the defect in the pars interarticularis and the slip. **C.** Oblique view showing the defect in the pars interarticularis.

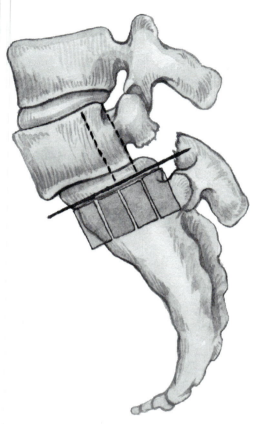

Figure 5–18. Four classifications of spondylolisthesis according to degree of anterior displacement. See text.

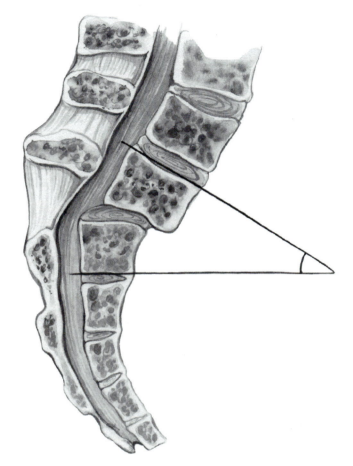

Figure 5–19. Slip angle in spondylolisthesis. See text.

radiograms; lateral views of the lumbosacral spine in flexion and extension or standing versus supine demonstrate mobility of the defect. An unstable and mobile spondylolisthesis is likely to displace further. (6) Marked ligamentous hyperlaxity such as seen in Down's or Marfan's syndrome or osteogenesis imperfecta carries a poor outlook; the probability of progressive slip is great. (7) Age; the younger the patient at onset, the greater the risk for progression. (8) Sex; the female is at greater risk for further slip than is the male.

SPONDYLOLYSIS

Most cases of spondylolysis are asymptomatic and do not require treatment or restriction from participating in normal physical activities and sports. It is best to forewarn the parents that weight-lifting, gymnastics, and football (particularly linemen) increase mechanical loading of the lumbar spine, with the highest concentration of forces at the pars interarticularis, and that an asymptomatic spondylolysis may become symptomatic. When these adolescents present with lower back and/or sciatica pain, radiograms (AP, lateral and obliques of L5 spine, and spot laterals of L5–S1)

are repeated. CT scan or MRI demonstrates the spondylolytic lesion. Bone scan and SPECT imaging with technetium-99m is performed; the pars interarticularis shows increased uptake, indicating stress fracture. Involvement may be unilateral or bilateral.

Symptomatic spondylolysis is treated with a TLSO, usually a reverse Boston brace with anterior opening. The excessive lordosis should be corrected and diminished to zero degrees if possible. The orthosis is worn during the waking hours but not at night. When the patient is in very acute pain, bed rest for a few days is appropriate and usually ameliorates the severe symptoms. Pelvic tilt and abdominal and gluteus maximus exercises are performed several times a day. Avoid acute flexion of the trunk. Curtail contact sports and gymnastics. The back pain and hamstring spasm gradually subside and the bone scan becomes normal within 4 to 6 months. Return to sports is resumed gradually.

Surgical treatment of spondylolysis is rarely indicated. Very occasionally conservative measures fail to relieve symptoms. When severe back pain and disability persist after a 6- to 12-month period of conservative treatment, posterolateral fusion between L5 and the midsacrum is performed. When the lesion is between L4 and L5 and symptomatic, direct repair of the defect with autogenous bone grafting and internal fixation with screws is carried out. The natural history of symptomatic L4–L5 spondylolysis is poor; the back pain almost always persists and increases in severity.[97]

Spondylolisthesis. In decision-making as to modality of treatment, consider the age of the patient, the degree of slip, the mobility and instability of the defect, the presence or absence of symptoms, the severity of disability when symptomatic, and its response to conservative treatment.

Asymptomatic spondylolisthesis, less than 25 percent slip, does not require treatment. When posture is poor with excessive lumbar lordosis and tight hamstrings, physical therapy is in order: Abdominal pelvic tilt, gluteus maximus, and hamstring stretching exercises are performed several times a day. These adolescents are allowed to participate in normal physical activities. Patients with asymptomatic spondylolisthesis with greater than 50 percent slip are advised not to lift weights, participate in contact sports, or perform gymnastics because such mechanical stresses cause pain.

Symptomatic grade I and grade II spondylolisthesis is treated similarly to symptomatic spondylolysis—TLSO support to the lumbar spine, restriction of physical activity and strain to the spine, and physical therapy. Nonsteroidal anti-inflammatory medications are given as necessary.

Operative Treatment. This is indicated when (1) moderate or severe back pain and disability and neurologic deficit persist and interfere with normal activities of daily life despite conservative treatment; (2) when the slip progresses beyond 50 percent—that is, grade II slip becomes grade III or IV; (3) when grade III or grade IV spondylolisthesis with severe hamstring spasm, abnormal gait, and marked postural deformity does not respond to conservative therapy; and (4) when cauda equina and bladder symptoms develop; these cases require urgent care. MRI or CT scanning with metrizamide myelography is performed to delineate the pathology. Often the displaced vertebral body tilts anteriorly and the upper segment of the pars interarticularis of L5 compresses the fifth lumbar nerve root. Sacral nerve root compression causes urinary retention or bladder-sphincter loss. Cauda equina syndrome is more common in the dysplastic type with an intact ring of L5 and 50 percent or greater slip.

Operative treatment of L5–S1 spondylolisthesis consists of bilateral posterolateral fusion from L5 to the midsacrum. The fusion extends to L4 when the transverse process of L5 is small or when the L4–L5 disc space angle is high.

Decompression is performed when there is neurologic deficit. Do not mistake hamstring tautness for neurologic deficit! Following in situ fusion without decompression, hamstring tautness subsides in 6 to 12 months. Never perform decompression without arthrodesis. Postoperative immobilization in a bilateral hip spica cast is mandatory when decompression and fusion are performed.

Reduction of Spondylolisthesis. When the slip angle is high, restoration of sagittal alignment of the lumbar spine may be attempted. In children and adolescents, reduction by cast is safest. In the Edwards technique, gradual reduction is carried out by modular contact. Transpedicular devices are best. It is wise to avoid distraction implants. Following reduction, serious complications are loss of sphincter control, sensory loss of genital areas, loss of fixation, and pseudarthrosis.

■ DISCITIS[118–136]

The presenting complaints are back pain, refusal to sit or stand, or walking with a limp in an older infant or a young child between 2 and 7 years of age. The pain is often vague. Depending upon the level of the lesion, it may radiate to the buttock and posterior thigh or it may be in the anterolateral aspect of the thigh and knee or the abdomen.

Discitis is a nonspecific inflammatory lesion of the disc; it is benign and self-limiting. It should be distinguished from pyogenic infection of the disc space and adjacent vertebral osteomyelitis. In the infant and young child the discs do receive their blood supply from the adjacent vertebral bodies.[120]

History. Ask the parents about the occurrence of an upper respiratory infection, otitis media, a urinary tract infection, or diarrhea prior to the onset of pain. Inquire about the location of pain, whether it radiates, and if any antibiotics were given which may mask pyogenic infection. Is there any history of trauma?

Examination. The child is irritable but not acutely ill. Systemic signs such as temperature elevation are slight or nil. The paraspinal muscles at the level of discitis are in marked spasm. When the lumbar spine is involved (75 percent of the cases) the *Goldthwaite test* is positive (in prone extension of the hips with the knee flexed 90 degrees); the lumbar spine is rigid and moves in one piece with the pelvis (see Fig 5–4). Lateral tilting and rotation of the spine are limited. When the thoracic or cervical spine is involved, the *anvil test* is positive; that is, on percussion of the top of the head, the patient complains of pain at the site of the discitis; also, when the neck is acutely flexed, the patient complains of pain in the back.

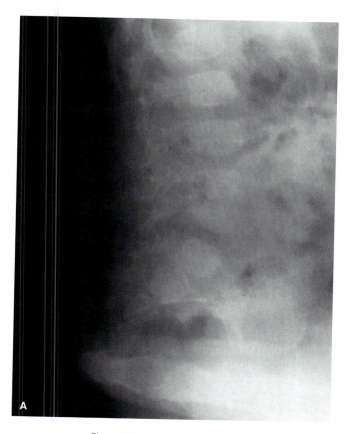

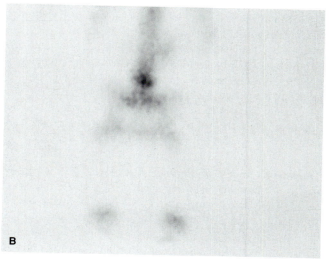

Figure 5–20. Discitis between L4 and L5 in a 2-year-old infant. **A.** Initial lateral radiogram showing narrowing of the disc interspace between L4 and L5 and irregularity of the vertebral end-plates. **B.** Bone scan with technetium-99m showing increased uptake between L4 and L5.

On palpation, the site of discitis is acutely tender, as shown by change in the pitch of the cry of the infant or child.

Imaging. Initially the plain radiograms are normal; when the level of discitis is lumbar the only finding is loss of the normal lordosis.[122] Within 10 to 14 days the disc interspace narrows, with haziness and irregularity of the vertebral end-plates (Fig 5–20). Later the vertebral end-plates develop sclerosis and irregular erosion.

Bone scan with technetium-99m should be performed. It shows increased local uptake.[118] CT or preferably MRI is indicated when pyogenic osteomyelitis cannot be ruled out.[123,125] Discitis should be differentiated from vertebral osteomyelitis.[130]

Laboratory Studies. The white blood count and differential are usually within normal limits; the sedimentation rate may be slightly elevated. Blood cultures are rarely positive.

Needle aspiration is performed only when infection is suggested because of the presence of paraspinal soft tissue mass and erosion and destruction of the vertebrae. Biopsy, preferably open, is indicated when neoplasm is suspected.

Treatment. This consists of simple rest and immobilization of the spine in a TLSO. Antibiotic therapy is not indicated. Prognosis is good.

■ HERNIATED INTERVERTEBRAL DISC[137–147]

A herniated disc is very rare in a child and rather uncommon in the adolescent. When it occurs, the clinical findings and treatment are similar to those in an adult. The presenting complaints are low back pain with or without sciatica and stiffness of the back.

On examination, motions of the lumbar spine are markedly restricted with paravertebral muscle spasm. Sciatic scoliosis may be present. It is more common in boys than girls. In about one half to two thirds of the cases, a definite episode of trauma or mechanical stress can be identified, such as lifting a heavy object from the floor with the lumbar spine acutely flexed.

Imaging.   Plain radiograms are ordinarily normal; they do not show narrowing of the intervertebral disc spaces. They are made to rule out other causes of back pain. A definitive diagnosis is usually made by MRI. The level of disc herniation is equally distributed between the L4–L5 and L5–S1 interspaces. Myelography is not indicated except preoperatively in nonconclusive cases when multiple-level lesions are suspected.

When MRI is normal, bone scan with technetium-99m radionuclide is performed to rule out other causes of back pain such as spondylolysis or osteoid osteoma.

Treatment.   In the absence of neurologic defect, conservative nonsurgical measures such as bed rest and support to the spine in the form of a TLSO are employed first. If they fail to relieve symptoms, surgery in the form of discectomy is performed. Simultaneous fusion is not indicated. Short-term results of surgery are excellent, but in time with long-term follow-up, the results deteriorate and back pain and sciatica recur. About 10 percent of the cases require further surgery in the form of re-exploration at the same level or exploration at different levels. Some adult patients require fusion for stabilization of the spine.

■ SCOLIOSIS

When a series of vertebrae deviate from their anatomic midline position and rotate, the spinal deformity is called scoliosis. The following definition of terms, endorsed by the Scoliosis Research Society, is provided for clarity of language and communication.

TERMINOLOGY

When the curve corrects or overcorrects on side-bending or lying down, it is referred to as a *nonstructural* curve. With progression of the scoliosis, contracture of soft tissues and structural changes in the bony vertebrae develop and the curve loses its flexibility—it does not correct on side-bending in supine posture; the curve becomes *structural.* The vertebra in the curve that is most deviated and rotated from the midline is referred to as the *apical vertebra.* The *end vertebrae* are the most cephalad and caudal vertebrae that are maximally rotated to the concavity of the curve (the superior surface of the most upper vertebra and the inferior surface of the most inferior vertebra). The curve that is more structural, greater in degree, and more deforming is referred to as the *major curve,* whereas the curve that is less structural and smaller in degree is referred to as the *minor curve.* The use of the term *primary* is discouraged because it is difficult to identify. When scoliosis has two structural curves, it is called a *double major curve.*[194,246]

Postural Scoliosis.   This is characterized by a long thoracolumbar curve with no compensatory curves and rotation of the vertebrae to the concavity of the curve and not to the convexity as in structural scoliosis. The curve is flexible; it disappears when the patient is prone. It does not progress and does not become structural. Treatment consists of postural exercises for the poor posture. No specific treatment is indicated for the scoliosis.

Functional Scoliosis.   This is caused by disparity of the lower limb lengths. The curve is a single, long thoracolumbar curve with the convexity to the side of the short lower limb. There are no compensatory curves. Again, the rotation of the vertebrae is to the concavity of the curve, and the curvature disappears upon leveling the pelvis by placing an appropriate lift under the shorter lower limb. Treatment consists of equalizing the limb lengths when there is significant decompensation of the spine with a tilt to the short side.

Scoliosis Due to Infrapelvic Obliquity.   This is due to either adduction or abduction contracture of the hips. It is seen in infants due to intrauterine malposture or in the older child due to paralytic pelvic obliquity, as in cerebral palsy, myelomeningocele, or poliomyelitis. The curve is single—either lumbar or thoracolumbar—with a convexity on the low side of the pelvis. Treatment consists of passive stretching exercises to correct the contractural deformity around the hips and the pelvic obliquity. Occasionally in paralytic pelvic obliquity, soft tissue release of the hip abductors or adductors is performed.

IDIOPATHIC SCOLIOSIS

Scoliosis of unknown cause is called idiopathic. It is identified by exclusion; that is, clinically there is no neuromuscular disorder, and in the radiograms the vertebrae do not show any congenital or developmental abnormality. Idiopathic scoliosis is the most common type, with a prevalence of 2 to 3 percent for curves of 10 degrees or less and a prevalence of 0.2 to 0.3 percent for curves of 20 degrees or more.

The presenting complaint is the deformity of the spine which is detected by the parents, pediatrician, or a nurse during school screening. The deformities are asymmetry of the shoulders (one higher than the other), asymmetry of the flank creases with a high prominent hip, list of the trunk, and prominence of a shoulder blade or breast.

Idiopathic scoliosis is subdivided according to the age of onset into three types: (1) *infantile,* developing in the first 3 years of life; (2) *juvenile,* developing between the ages of 4 and 10 to 12 years (prior to beginning of adolescence); and (3) *adolescent,* onset during the adolescent pubertal growth spurt. Some degree of overlap between these three types is often present, as an adolescent detected with scoliosis may have developed it in childhood and scoliosis in a 5-year-old child may have its onset before 3 years of age.

Etiology. The cause of idiopathic scoliosis remains unknown. Its pathogenesis is most probably multifactorial.[182,191,225] Research has shown changes in the axial skeleton, collagen, and neuromuscular tissues; however, this may be secondary and not primary. Vestibular dysfunction has been implicated. Heredity may play a role.[177,260]

History. An adequate history assists in determining the cause of scoliosis. When was the deformity first noted? Who detected it—the pediatrician during routine examination, the nurse at a school screening, or the parents, or was it discovered incidentally in a radiogram of the chest or an intravenous pyelogram?

Inquire as to the nature of imaging or other diagnostic studies performed after detection of the scoliosis. What was the degree of the curvature? How was it treated—simple observation, exercises, or orthosis? Has the degree of scoliosis increased while under observation or treatment? Have any operative procedures been done?

Pain is not a clinical feature of idiopathic scoliosis in children and adolescents. When pain is present it is usually due to some other cause such as spondylolisthesis; Scheuermann's juvenile kyphosis; lesions in bone such as osteoid osteoma, osteoblastoma, or aneurysmal bone cyst; inflammatory conditions such as rheumatoid arthritis or discitis; or tumors of the spinal cord. A child with back pain and spinal deformity should have thorough clinical, neurologic, and imaging studies consisting of routine radiograms, bone scan with technetium-99m, CT, and/or MRI.

Inquire as to muscle weakness in the lower limbs and spasm or stiffness in the back. Does the patient have any disturbance of the sphincters, rectal or urinary?

In severe scoliosis, cardiopulmonary function may be compromised. Is there any shortness of breath or difficulty in breathing?

Ask about past growth. Did the patient have a rapid growth spurt? Inquire about the onset of the menarche in girls and the development of secondary sex characteristics in both girls and boys.[244,245] Try to estimate the future growth potential. Does the child come from a tall family? What are the heights of the parents, uncles and aunts, and siblings?

Take a careful orthopedic and medical history. Has the child had any fracture of bone, joint infection, or arthritis in the lower limbs which may cause lower limb length inequality?

Physical Examination. Inspect the patient standing without clothing but properly draped with an examination gown open in the back, no bra, and preferably brief panties or shorts that expose the iliac crests and posterior and anterior superior iliac spines. Thoroughly inspect the skin for findings such as café-au-lait spots (suggesting neurofibomatosis), a tuft of hair or hemangioma in the midline of the spine (suggesting spinal dysrhaphism), or dimples and sinus tract in the sacrum (suggesting intraspinal teratoma).

Measure the standing height (with bare feet) and the sitting height. Then note the alignment of the spine in the posterior, anterior, and lateral projections (Fig 5–21A to D). The patient's knees should be straight, the feet together, and the upper limbs dependent at the sides of the body. Are the head, neck, and shoulders balanced over the pelvis? Is the spine compensated or decompensated? Drop a plumb line from the occipital protuberance at the base of the skull; in the normal compensated spine it should fall in the intergluteal cleft. When the spine is decompensated with a list of the trunk, the plumb line falls to the right or left of the intergluteal cleft (Fig 5–21E). The distance between the plumb line and the intergluteal cleft denotes the amount of the list. Note the symmetry or asymmetry of the waistline (is one flank deeper than the other?), the position of the scapulae, and the level of the shoulders (Fig 5–22). On the side with the high shoulder, the trapezius neckline is shortened. Project a horizontal line from the top of the acromioclavicular joint of the lower shoulder and another horizontal line from that of the higher shoulder. Measure the vertical distance between the two lines in centimeters. Determine the level and extent of lateral deviation of the spinous processes from the median level. Identify the pattern of the curve or curves on inspection—left thoracolumbar, right thoracic and left lumbar, and the like.

Next perform Adam's forward bending test (Fig 5–23).[148] For thoracolumbar and lumbar scoliosis, inspect the spine from the back as the child bends forward at the waist with the upper limbs dependent and his or her palms in opposition. Be sure the knees are fully extended

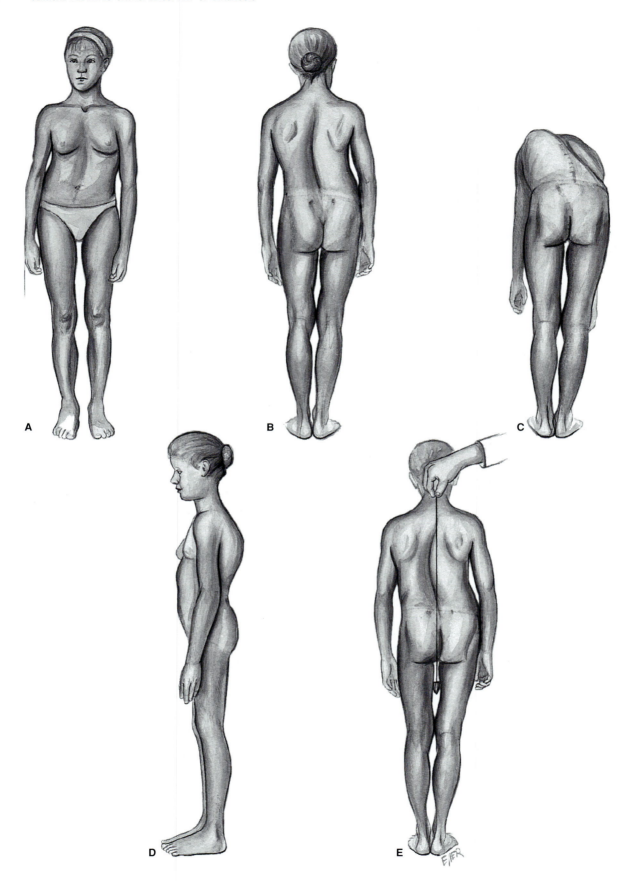

Figure 5–21. Clinical appearance of a girl with scoliosis. **A, B.** Note the asymmetry of the shoulders, the flank creases, and the rotation of the vertebrae to the convexity. This is a left thoracolumbar curve, which is an unusual pattern. One should be suspicious of underlying pathology such as syringomyelia. **C.** Note that on forward bending the rotation of the vertebrae is to the convexity from the posterior view, indicating that the scoliosis is structural and not postural. **D.** Lateral view showing the exaggerated lumbar lordosis and thoracic kyphosis. **E.** Plumb line test. The line is dropped from C7 to the intergluteal cleft. Note that the trunk is decompensated to the left.

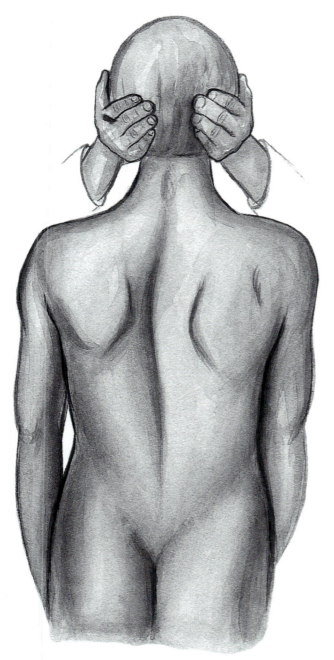

Figure 5–22. Left thoracolumbar scoliosis. Note the asymmetry of the level of the shoulders and scapulae. The left side is higher and the trapezius neckline is shorter on the left.

and the feet are together. For cervical and thoracic scoliosis, inspect the patient anteriorly. Note the degree and direction of rotation of the vertebrae. In structural scoliosis the curve persists and the spinous processes rotate to the concavity of the curve, as shown by the prominence of the ribs of the thoracic cage and paravertebral muscles and transverse processes in the lumbar spine on the convex side of the curve. In postural scoliosis the spinous processes rotate to the convexity of the curve, with the ribs and paravertebral muscles prominent on the concave side of the curve when the patient is viewed posteriorly. The degree of rotation is measured in centimeters by determining the height of the thoracic and paraspinal lumbar prominence. A scoliometer is often used because it is an accurate method of measuring vertebral rotation (Fig 5–24).[168]

Determine the flexibility of the curve by right and left lateral bends while observing the patient from the back (Fig 5–25). In the smaller child, longitudinal traction by pulling the head vertically upward is another way to test flexibility of the curve.

Next examine the patient from the front. Note the level of the shoulders and the alignment and symmetry of the trunk. Determine the level of the anterior superior iliac spines. Is there any pelvic obliquity? Is there asymmetry of the breasts, rib cage, or pectoral region? Is there any pectus excavatum or carinatum?

Then examine the patient from the side for assessment of the sagittal contour of the spine (see Fig 5–21D). What is the general posture? Most patients with scoliosis have poor posture and carry their shoulders behind their sacrum. Note the degree of lordosis; is there hyperlordosis? Note the degree of pelvic inclination. Is the thoracic roundback normal, hyperkyphotic, or hypokyphotic? Assess the anteroposterior diameter of the thoracic cage and the amount of chest expansion by measuring its circumference with normal deep breathing and exhalations. At this point of the examination, it is important to ask the patient to touch his toes with his knees fully extended to rule out hamstring tautness.

Next the patient is asked to lie prone on the examination table. Inspect the spine. Do the curves decrease in severity? Test flexibility of the curves by bending the spine to the right and left. Ask the patient to lift his head and shoulders into hyperextension to test flexibility of the

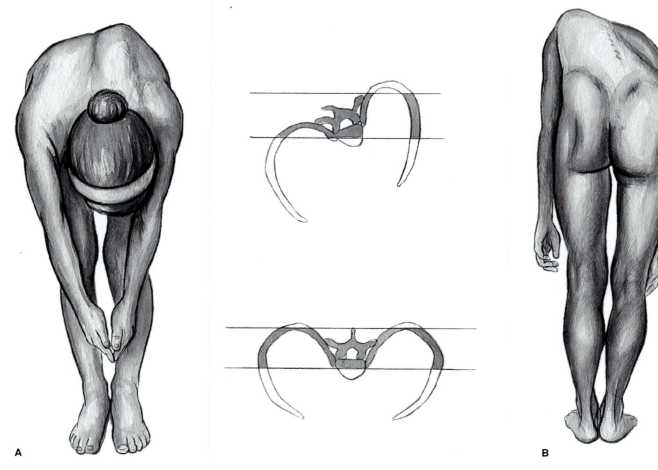

Figure 5–23. Adam's forward bending test. See text.

thoracic kyphosis. Rule out paravertebral muscle spasm. Methodically palpate the spine for any area of local tenderness.

In prone and supine positions, assess the level of the anterior and posterior, superior iliac spines and iliac crests and rule out pelvic obliquity. If obliquity is present, is it infrapelvic or suprapelvic or both in its origins? Is the pelvic obliquity fixed or flexible?

Test range of motion of the hips. Is there any contractural deformity about the hips? Perform Ober's test to rule out hip abduction contracture and the Thomas test for hip flexion contracture, and maximally abduct the hips for adduction contracture. Test range of motion of the elbows, knees, and ankles. Is there hyperlaxity of ligaments with genu recurvatum or hyperextension of the elbows? Do the feet dorsiflex excessively at the ankles? Measure apparent and actual lower limb lengths and thigh and calf circumferences. Does the child have any foot deformity? Friedreich's ataxia or intraspinal pathology should be ruled out when pes cavus is present.

The next step is to assess the neuromuscular system to rule out paralytic scoliosis. Perform a thorough neurologic examination. Test deep tendon reflexes, superficial abdominal skin reflexes, the cremasteric reflex in boys, and the motor strength of muscles. Observe gait for any abnormality or ataxia.

A general physical examination, particularly of the pulmonary, cardiovascular, and genitourinary systems, is carried out next. Is there any deformity of the teeth or mandible, overbite or underbite? Steps in the examination of a patient with scoliosis are outlined in Table 5–2.

Imaging. *Radiographic Assessment.* At the initial presentation of the patient with scoliosis, radiograms of the entire spine are made to determine the cause and type of scoliosis, the site of deformity, the curve pattern, the magnitude of the curvature, and skeletal maturity. Initially only upright AP and lateral radiographs of the entire spine are made. In the lateral projection, the presence or absence of associated

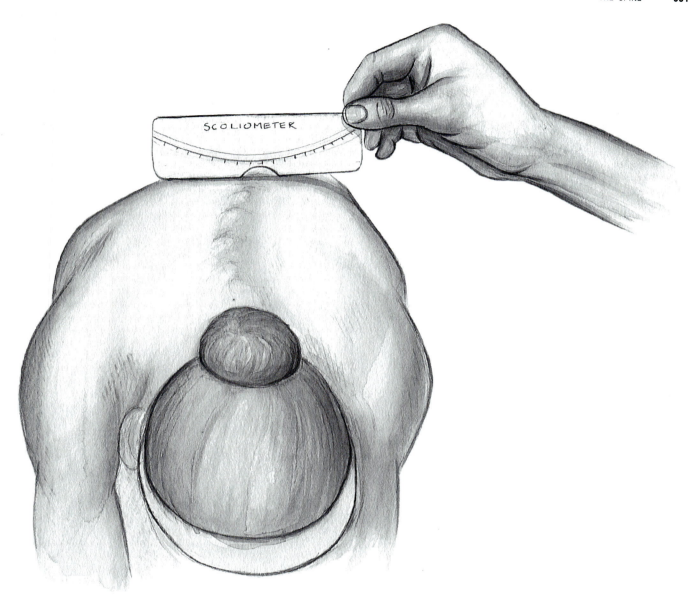

Figure 5–24. Measurement of degree of rotation of the vertebrae by the scoliometer.

kyphosis, hyperkyphosis, or hypokyphosis; lordosis or hypolordosis; and spondylolisthesis is determined. Bending views to test flexibility are made only when treatment by surgery or orthosis is being considered.

Measurement of the Degree of the Curve. Two methods are available. In the *Cobb method,* draw a line perpendicular to the superior surface of the cephalad end vertebra and another line perpendicular to the inferior surface of the caudal end vertebra; the angle formed between the two perpendicular lines is the degree of the curve (Fig 5–26). This is the most common method used.[174] The Oxford Cobb meter is a quick way to measure the degree of the curve.

In congenital spine deformity with multiple anomalies, the subchondral bony plates of the vertebrae are difficult to determine. In such curves, the Ferguson method is used to measure the degree of the curve.[189] Identify the superior and inferior end vertebrae and the apical vertebrae. Mark a dot in the center of these vertebral bodies. Draw lines from the dot of the apex vertebra to the dots of the end vertebrae. The angle of divergence between these two lines from 180 degrees is the degree of the curve (Fig 5–27).

The degree and direction of rotation of the vertebral bodies are determined by noting the relationship of the spinous processes and the pedicles to the center of the vertebral body in the AP radiogram. Also note if there is any

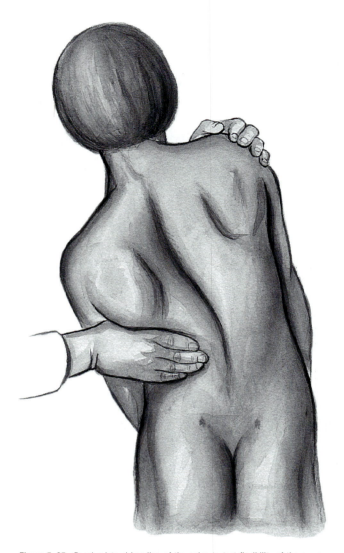

Figure 5–25. Passive lateral bending of the spine to test flexibility of the curve.

TABLE 5–2. STEPS IN EXAMINATION OF PATIENT WITH SCOLIOSIS

Inspection of skin
   Café-au-lait spots—neurofibromatosis?
   Tuft of hair, hemangioma—spinal dysrhaphism?
   Dimple, sinus tract—intraspinal teratoma?

Height—standing and sitting

Alignment of spine—PA, AP, and lateral

Determine level and extent of curves and curve pattern by clinical inspection.

Plumb line test—measure degree of decompensation of spine.

Level of shoulders and scapulae.

Perform Adam's forward bending test.

Use scoliometer to determine degree of rotation of vertebrae.

Perform lateral bending test to determine flexibility of curves.

Assess the degree of thoracic kyphosis, lumbar lordosis, and pelvic tilt.

Assess AP diameter of thoracic cage, circumference of chest, and amount of chest expansion.

Perform toe-touch test with knees completely extended to rule out hamstring tautness.

Test flexibility of curves and degree of thoracic kyphosis in prone position by lateral bends and hyperextension of thoracic spine.

Palpate for paravertebral spasm and areas of tenderness.

Rule out pelvic obliquity in supine and prone positions.

Rule out contractural deformities of hips (adduction, abduction, flexion), knees, and ankles. Any foot deformity—Pes cavus?

Measure circumference of thighs and calves. Any atrophy?

Perform thorough neuromuscular examination including deep tendon reflexes and superficial abdominal reflex.

Examine the entire child!

---

wedging of the vertebral bodies by comparing their height on the right and left sides.

In the lateral radiogram of the entire spine the degree of kyphosis of the thoracic spine and lordosis of the lumbar spine is determined. Rule out spondylolisthesis at the L5 and S1 level.

Occasionally special imaging studies are indicated. MRI is performed when there is a neurologic deficit; the absence of an abdominal umbilical reflex; a positive Beevor sign; failure to diminish or obliterate lumbar lordosis on knee-chest test or on forward flexion; rigidity of paraspinal extensor muscles on the Goldthwaite test; presence of skin lesions such as a hair patch, pigmentation, hemangioma, or a dimple in the midline of the spine, particularly in congenital scoliosis; a history of back pain; early age of onset with progression; a left thoracic curve, especially if long, or other unusual curve patterns; rapid curve progression; interpediculate space widening; and/or pedicle erosion (this suggests spinal cord tumor, syringomyelia, diastematomyelia, or spinal dysrhaphism) (Table 5–3).

CT scanning is indicated when the presence of a benign bone tumor such as osteoid osteoma or metastatic bone disease is suspected clinically and in plain radiograms; it accurately localizes the lesion and shows the extent of bone destruction and assists in planning the surgical approach. CT is also performed when spinal cord compression is suspected; in such an instance, it is often combined with myelography.

Ultrasonography of the kidneys and abdomen and intravenous pyelogram are performed to rule out associated anomalies of the urinary tract, particularly in congenital scoliosis.

Skeletal Maturity. Assess the skeletal maturity of the patient from the AP film of the spine by the Risser sign—the ossification of the iliac apophysis, which begins anteriorly at the anterior superior iliac spine and extends posteriorly toward the posterior superior iliac spine. The iliac crest is

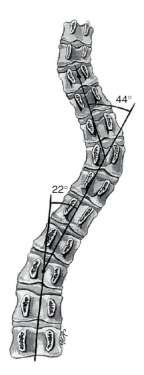

Figure 5–27. Ferguson method of measuring scoliosis. See text.

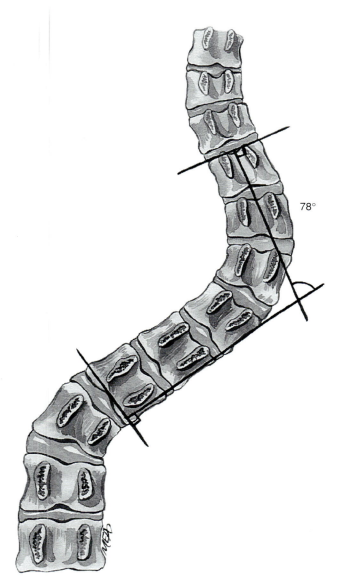

Figure 5–26. Cobb method of measuring scoliosis. See text.

subdivided into four quadrants. Risser 0 is no ossification of the iliac apophysis, Risser 1 is ossification at the anterior one fourth, Risser 2 is at the anterior half, Risser 3 is at the anterior three fourths, Risser 4 is complete excursion, and Risser 5 is fusion of the ossific center of the apophysis to the body of the ilium (Fig 5–28).[236,262]

In the lateral radiogram the stage of ossification of the ring apophysis is determined. It appears as a separate ossification area. Skeletal maturation of the vertebrae is completed, and the spine stops growing when the ring apophysis fuses with the vertebral body.

The skeletal age is determined by comparison of the radiograms of the left hand and wrist with the standards of the Greulich and Pyle bone age atlas.[196]

Hazards of Radiation Exposure. The areas of concern are the gonads and the organs, with the breast, thyroid, and bone marrow the most sensitive. Irradiation to the organs is cumulative, whereas radiation to the gonads increases the mutation rate but its effect is noncumulative.

In initial assessment and follow-up examinations of patients with scoliosis and other spinal deformities, radiation should be minimized. Take as few radiograms as possible; do not repeat radiograms because of poor quality films. Be selective—do not order "routine radiographic series." Always examine the patient prior to ordering radiograms. Techniques to minimize radiation are listed in Table 5–4.[184,203,233]

Screening. All large curves were small initially. The goal of screening is to detect spinal deformity when small and by effective treatment to prevent its progression to a large curve. School screening programs of children 10 to 16 years old, an age group in which children are most at risk for progression, is an effective way to detect scoliosis early. The education of parents through Parent-Teacher Association presentations, primary care physicians, and nurses increases awareness of spinal deformity in children. The screening techniques recommended are Adam's forward bending test of the naked back and Bunnell's scoliometer

TABLE 5–3. INDICATIONS FOR MRI ASSESSMENT OF SPINE IN SCOLIOSIS

1. Presence of neurologic deficit
2. Absence of abdominal umbilical reflex
3. Positive Beevor's sign
4. Failure to diminish or obliterate lumbar lordosis on knee-chest test or on forward flexion
5. Rigidity of paraspinal extensor muscles on the Goldthwaite test (prone hip extension with knee flexed 90 degrees)
6. Presence of skin lesions such as hair patch, pigmentation, hemangioma or dimple in midline of the spine, particularly in congenital scoliosis
7. History of back pain
8. Early age of onset of curvature with progression
9. Left thoracic curve, especially if long, or other unusual curve pattern
10. Rapid curve progression
11. Interpediculate space widening and/or pedicle erosion. In the plain radiograms this finding suggests spinal cord or intraspinal tumors, syringomyelia, diastematomyelia, or spinal dysrhaphism

TABLE 5–4. TECHNIQUES TO MINIMIZE RADIATION

Use high-speed films.
Use quanta rare earth intensifying screens.
Collimate the x-ray beam to include only the body.
Use antiscatter grids.
Use aluminum beam filtration.
Appropriately shield the gonads and breasts.
Use anteroposterior instead of posteroanterior projection.

for measuring trunk rotation. These are the most effective; they are accurate and inexpensive.

Orthotic treatment is effective in altering the natural history and preventing progression of adolescent idiopathic scoliosis. School screening programs have decreased the number of patients requiring surgery.

The problems with school screening are (1) over-referral, (2) the risk and danger of unnecessary diagnostic radiation, and (3) noncompliance by the parents. These problems are being resolved by the education of primary care physicians and parents. Screening of children between 10 and 14 years of age is justified.[152,167,239,255]

Curve Pattern. First determine the *curve site* by location of the apical vertebra: (1) cervical, (2) cervicothoracic (apex at either C7 or T1), (3) thoracic, (4) thoracolumbar (apex at either T12 or L1), (5) lumbar, and (6) lumbosacral (apex between L5 and S1). Lumbosacral curves are compensatory to the thoracic curve above them. A curve pattern may be single or double major or multiple. Ordinarily multiple curve patterns are short and nondeforming and do not progress.

Cephalocaudally curve patterns may be classified as (1) single, major high thoracic curve, (2) single, major thoracic curve, (3) single, major thoracolumbar curve, (4) single, major lumbar curve, (5) major thoracic and minor lumbar curve, (6) double major thoracic and lumbar curves, (7) double major thoracic and thoracolumbar curves, and (8) double major thoracic curve.

King's classification of curve patterns of thoracic curves is of great value in the selection of the fusion area: Type I—Double major thoracic and lumbar curves. Clinically both the thoracic and lumbar curves are predominant (Fig 5–29). Type II—Major thoracic and compensatory flexible lumbar curve. Clinically the thoracic prominence is marked, whereas the lumbar prominence is minimal. Radiographically both curves cross the midline. In this type selective fusion of the thoracic curve is possible as the unfused lumbar curves spontaneously balance the fused thoracic curve. Type III—Thoracic curve with minimal or no decompensation. The lumbar curve does not cross the midline. Type IV—Long thoracic curve with marked decompensation with the curve reaching the midline at L4, which tilts into the curve. Type V—Double thoracic curve with both curves structural, with high left and right thoracic

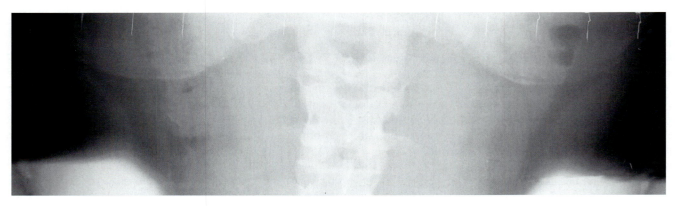

Figure 5–28. Risser sign (3). Note that the ossification center of the iliac apophysis is three fourths of the way across the iliac crest anteroposteriorly.

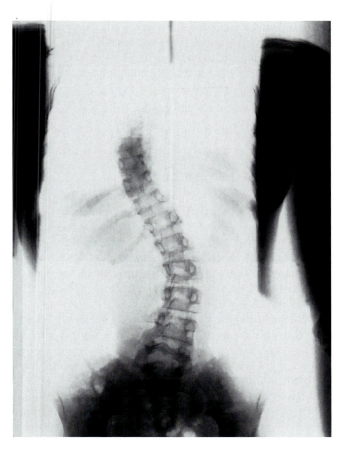

Figure 5–29. Double major thoracic and lumbar curve.

prominence. The left neckline is prominent with a positive tilt of T1. In this double thoracic pattern, fusion of both curves is necessary.

Infantile Idiopathic Scoliosis

It is very rare in North America but not infrequent in Europe. The scoliosis is structural, develops before 3 years of age, and is of unknown cause. There are no congenital or developmental anomalies of the vertebrae and no evidence of hypotonia or other neuromuscular diseases.

Infantile scoliosis is more common in boys, and the curve pattern is frequently left thoracic. There are two types of infantile scoliosis—resolving and progressive. The *resolving type* comprises about 85 percent of the cases; it spontaneously decreases with growth and disappears in 2 to 3 years. The progressive type (15 percent of the cases) increases in severity without treatment. One can distinguish the resolving type from the progressive type by the rib-vertebra angle difference (RVAD) and the relationship between the head of the rib and the vertebral body (Mehta). On the posteroanterior radiograph of the spine the rib-vertebra angle (RVA) is formed between the line drawn perpendicular to the end-plate of the apical vertebra and the

lines drawn along the center of the rib. RVA is measured on the convex and concave sides of the curve (Fig 5–30). The RVAD is the difference of the angles between the two sides of the apical vertebra; if it is less than 20 degrees, the curve is of the resolving type; an angle greater than 20 degrees indicates the progressive form of infantile scoliosis.

When there is no overlap between the head of the rib and the vertebral body (phase 1 of Mehta) the curve is the resolving type, whereas when the head of the rib overlaps the vertebral body (phase 2 of Mehta) the curve is the progressive type (Fig 5–31).[226] Other prognostic factors in the natural history of infantile scoliosis are (1) the age of onset—when the curve develops during the first year of life the probability (90 percent) is that it is the resolving type; (2) the absence of secondary curves indicates a resolving type; and (3) the degree of the curve—a curve greater than 35 degrees has a poor prognosis.

Assessment. Diagnosis of infantile idiopathic scoliosis is made by exclusion. Thoroughly examine the neuromuscular system to rule out hypotonia and neurologic disorders. Rule out congenital and developmental anomalies of the vertebral column. During the first 4 months of life, ultrasonography of the spine can detect a cartilaginous bar and intraspinal pathology. Examine the hips to rule out dislocation.

Juvenile Idiopathic Scoliosis

This type of curve develops between 3 and 10 years of age. The natural history is variable: Mild juvenile curves may resolve or follow a nonprogressive, mildly progressive, or markedly progressive course. Curves detected before 6 years of age and greater than 30 degrees tend to be pro-

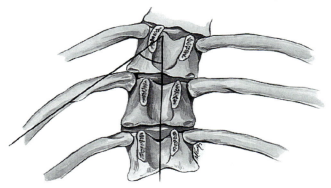

Rib-vertebra angle difference (RVAD) of Mehta

Figure 5–30. Diagram of the rib-vertebra angle difference (RVAD) in posterolateral radiogram of the spine. (1) Draw a line perpendicular to the end-plate of the apical vertebra. (2) Draw a line along the center of the rib. (3) Measure the angle formed by the intersection of the two lines on the concave and convex sides. This is the rib-vertebra angle (RVA). (4) Calculate the RVAD by subtracting the convex value from the concave value. (The RVA is more acute on the convex side than on the concave side of the curve.)

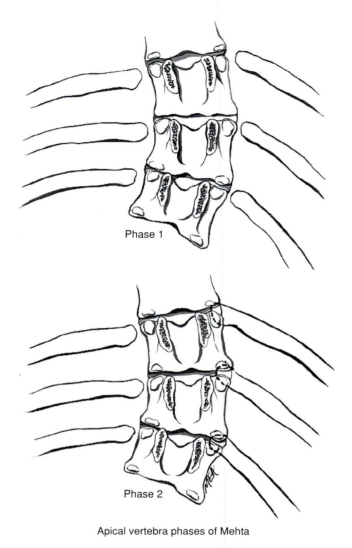

Phase 1

Phase 2

Apical vertebra phases of Mehta

Figure 5–31. Apical vertebra phases of Mehta determined by the relationship between the head of the rib and vertebral body. **A.** Phase 1—No overlap between the head of the rib and vertebral body. This indicates a resolving type. **B.** Phase 2—The rib head overlaps the vertebral body. This indicates progressive type of infantile scoliosis.

gressive. Mehta RVAD is not useful in juvenile idiopathic scoliosis.

Treatment. Three categories of management are available: (1) observation, (2) orthosis, and (3) surgery. Surface electric stimulation is no longer used.[230] Physical therapy exercises per se do not improve or prevent progression of scoliosis. However, they do improve posture, correct contractural deformity of pelvifemoral muscles, provide flexibility of the spine, and increase motor strength of abdominal, erector spinae, and gluteal muscles.

Observation. The objective of nonsurgical treatment is to prevent progression of the scoliosis. Curves that are less

than 20 degrees and have not shown any progression do not require any treatment. They are assessed every 3 to 4 months. Do not make radiograms of the spine at each office visit; examine the patient first. Be conscious of the hazards of radiation.

Orthotic Treatment.[151, 157, 159, 160, 162, 172, 183, 188, 198, 212, 235, 257] A brace is indicated in a skeletally immature patient with a 30- to 45-degree curve or a curve between 20 and 29 degrees which has a documented definite progression on follow-up examinations. An important requisite of orthotic treatment is a minimum of 12 months of remaining skeletal growth, a Risser sign of $3\pm$, or vertebral ring apophyses that are not fused, and a girl who is premenarchal or has had recent menarche (within the past 6 months).

Curves between 30 and 45 degrees should be treated immediately. Curves between 25 and 29 degrees are also treated immediately if the Risser sign is 0 or 1.

Contraindications to orthotic treatment are (1) skeletally mature patient (Risser 4 to 5 and ring apophyses fused), (2) presence of thoracic lordosis, (3) curves greater than 45 degrees, and (4) patients with unstable and psychologically disturbed personalities.

Two basic types of orthoses are available: (1) the cervicothoracolumbosacral orthosis (CTLSO) or the Milwaukee brace, and (2) the TLSO, which may be *high,* extending to one or both axillae for thoracic curves, or *low,* used in thoracolumbar and lumbar curves; many designs of TLSO are available named after the city of origin such as Boston, Wilmington, and Charleston. These orthotics are either prefabricated or custom made.

The corrective forces exerted by the orthosis are (1) *transverse*—applied at the apex of the lateral and/or posterior angulation with three-point fixation and (2) *longitudinal* traction. It is questionable as to whether compression by muscle contraction is an effective force exerted by spinal orthosis. Asymmetric growth by uneven loading of the cartilaginous vertebral growth plates is not provided by orthotic treatment.

The brace-wearing schedule may be *full time* (22 hours per day; out for bathing or sports such as swimming, physical education, and physical therapy) or *part time,* either 16 hours per day or only at night. Curves greater than 30 degrees and curves that are progressive require full-time wear; when the Risser becomes 4+ or vertebral growth is complete and a girl is 18 months past menarche, the patient is weaned from the brace, initially wearing it 18 hours per day and then only at night. Discontinue brace wear in 3 to 6 months.

In juvenile scoliosis, indications for orthotic treatment are the same as in adolescent idiopathic scoliosis. Initially brace wear is full time; once curve progression is controlled, brace wear is part time. When the curve increases with part-time brace wear, full-time brace wear is resumed.

GENERALIZED AFFECTIONS OF THE MUSCULAR SKELETAL SYSTEM

In this chapter, common generalized disorders affecting the neuromusculoskeletal system are presented.

■ DELAY IN MOTOR DEVELOPMENT

Common complaints are delay in holding the head up, sitting, crawling, or walking. Some infants stand and take steps at 10 months of age and others at 12 months, whereas some are delayed in walking until 15 months of age. Such variation in motor development is normal. Delay in walking until 18 months of age is not abnormal, provided that the child can stand with support and take reciprocal steps while holding a parent's hand or furniture.

Normally motor skills develop at the following average ages: At 3 months of age the infant lifts the head up when prone. At 6 months he or she holds the head steady when lifted to sitting posture from supine and turns the head side to side and begins to roll over from prone to supine and then supine to prone. At 9 months he sits without support and begins to pull himself to standing posture and stand with two-handed support. At 12 months of age, he stands without support and begins walking forward without assistance. At 18 months of age, he ascends stairs with two-handed support. At 2 years of age, he begins to ascend stairs with no support, one foot at a time. At 3 years, he begins to ascend stairs without support foot over foot. At 4 years of age, he begins to descend stairs without support foot over foot and begins to balance on one foot.

HISTORY

Take a detailed prenatal and birth history. What was the length of the pregnancy? When an infant is the product of a premature birth, delay of motor development is more or less commensurate with the early birth; for example, 2 months premature equals 2 months late in development of motor skills. Was there any bleeding during pregnancy or threatened abortion? Any history of prenatal infection, radiation, or trauma? Ask about fetal movements—during which week of pregnancy did the mother feel movement?

What was the condition of the newborn? Any history of seizures or cyanosis? Were resuscitation and oxygen required? Was the umbilical cord wrapped around the neck? Any jaundice? Were bili lights used? What was the length of the hospital stay?

Depending upon the stage of motor development, inquire as to when the child held the head up, rolled over from front to back and back to front, sat, crawled, or stood.

Ask about functional development of the upper limbs. Does the child hold a bottle, reach for and grasp toys, and transfer objects from hand to hand? Has he or she shown any hand preference? What about language development? Has he or she begun to talk? What about toilet training? Ask about general health and previous illnesses, and review the systems. Finally, take a detailed family history.

The cause of delayed motor development may be a lesion in the central or peripheral nervous system, a myopathy, or generalized skeletal disorders.

It is vital to determine whether the neuromuscular condition and motor weakness are static or progressive. Obtain a pediatric neurology consultation as required.

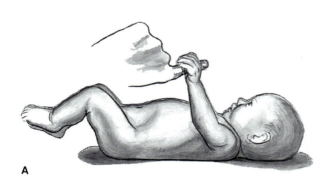

A

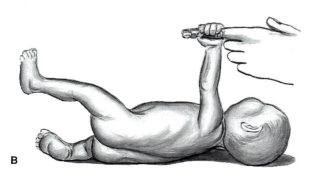

B

Figure 6-1. Hand grasp reflex. See text.

EXAMINATION

Perform a thorough neurologic and musculoskeletal examination. Any child with delayed motor development should have routine evaluation of the following reflexes to determine the level of neurophysiologic maturation.

Hand Grasp Reflex. Present in all normal newborns and young infants, it disappears between 2 and 4 months of age. Place your index or little finger on the ulnar aspect of the infant's hand; the fingers of the infant automatically flex and grasp the examiner's finger (Fig 6–1A). Pulling on the infant and lifting the baby increases the flexor tone, and the infant may be suspended by his hold on your finger (Fig 6–1B). Persistence of the hand grasp reflex after 4 to 6 months indicates spastic cerebral palsy.

Moro Reflex. Place the patient supine with both upper and lower limbs in full extended position. Elicit the reflex either by supporting the back of the head on the palm of your hand and then suddenly dropping the head or by gently raising the trunk of the baby off the table by holding his or her hands and rapidly releasing them (Fig 6–2A, B). Both methods suddenly extend the cervical spine. When the Moro reflex is positive, the child hyperextends the spine and abducts and extends all four limbs and digits (Fig 6–2C, D). The child then flexes and adducts all of the limbs as if hugging himself or herself (Fig 6–2E). In the normal infant, the Moro reflex begins to fade at 3 months of age and gradually disappears at 4 to 6 months of age. When the Moro reflex persists after the age of 6 months, central nervous system (CNS) maturation is delayed such as is seen in cerebral palsy. Do not mistake the startle reflex for the Moro reflex. The startle reflex is elicited by a sudden loud noise or by tapping the sternum. The response is flexion of the elbows and clenched fists. This is different than the Moro reflex, in which the elbows and digits are extended.

Crossed Extension Reflex. This reflex is tested by holding one lower limb extended at the knee and applying firm pressure on the sole of the extended limb. The opposite free limb flexes, adducts, and extends as if kicking the examiner. This is sometimes referred to as Philippson's reflex. It should not be obtained after the first month of life. Persistence indicates partial or complete spinal cord lesion.

Asymmetric Tonic Neck Reflex. With the patient supine and all four limbs in neutral extension, rotate the head to one side and maintain the rotation to the count of five; then rotate the head to the opposite side and keep it in rotation to the count of five. The reflex is positive when the limbs on the side toward which the chin is rotated go into extension, whereas the limbs on the opposite side go into flexion (Fig 6–3A, B). In the normal child the asymmetric tonic

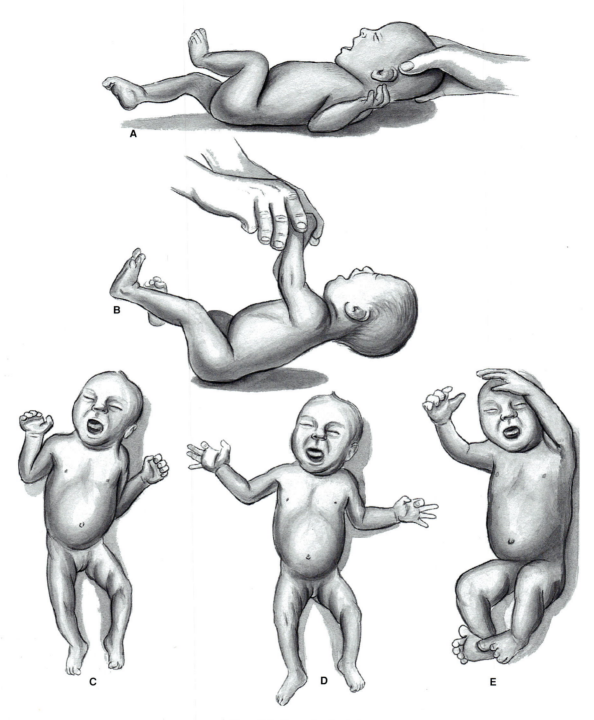

Figure 6–2. Moro reflex. See text.

neck reflex disappears by the age of 4 to 6 months. In spastic cerebral palsy it persists.

Placing Reaction. This is tested by holding the infant horizontal from the waist. Bring the dorsum of the ulnar aspect of the forearms against the edge of the table. The normal child places the hands on the table (Fig 6–4A, B). In the lower limbs, the placing reaction is tested by holding the infant upright supported from the waist, and the anterior aspect of the tibiae or dorsa of the feet are brought against the edge of the table. The normal infant flexes the hips and knees and places the feet on the table (Fig 6–5A–C). The

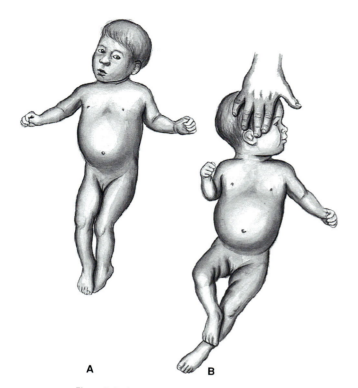

Figure 6–3. Asymmetric tonic neck reflex. See text.

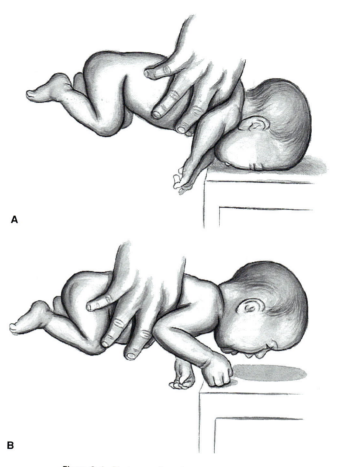

Figure 6–4. Placing reaction of upper limbs. See text.

placing reaction is present in all full-term newborn infants. When absent, there is damage to the CNS.

Walking Reflex or Stepping Reflex. This is tested by holding the infant upright with the soles of the feet pressing on the table; push the infant gently forward. When the reflex is present, the infant begins reciprocal flexion and extension of the lower limbs as if he or she is walking (Fig 6–6A–C). This walking reflex is present in the normal newborn but disappears by the age of 1 to 2 months. If present at 3 months or older, it indicates CNS damage.

Plantar Grasp Reflex. Exert light digital pressure on the plantar aspect of the foot near the metatarsal heads. The toes flex similar to palmar grasp reflex in all normal newborn infants; the reflex disappears by 12 months of age (Fig 6–7). Its persistence beyond 1 year indicates brain damage.

Symmetric Tonic Neck Reflex. The child is placed prone on your lap or on the mother's lap with the hips and neck flexed. Extend the head and neck. In the normal infant, the elbows extend and the knees flex (Fig 6–8A). When the neck is flexed, the elbows flex and the knees go into extension (Fig 6–8B). Symmetric tonic neck reflex develops by 6 months of age, and there is no time limit for its disappearance. Its absence indicates CNS damage.

Protective Extension of Arms Reflex. Support the infant in the air by the waist in prone posture and suddenly lower

his head toward the floor (Fig 6–9A,B). When the reflex is positive, the elbows immediately extend to protect the head from hitting the floor. This reflex appears at 6 months of age and persists throughout life. Absence of a positive response suggests severe brain damage.

Neck Righting Reflex. Hold the infant in the air by his waist and tilt him 45 to 60 degrees to either side. When neck righting reflex is present, the child lifts his or her head up to align it with the trunk (Fig 6–10). This reflex develops normally between 6 and 8 months of age. Its absence indicates CNS damage.

Tilting Reaction. Support the child by holding him under the arm pits and bearing weight on his feet as much as possible and suddenly move him forward, backward, and sideways. He hops to maintain balance (Fig 6–11A–D). This hopping reaction develops between 12 and 18 months of age, and its absence indicates brain damage.

Galant Reflex or Trunk Incurvation. This is tested by placing the patient prone. With your index finger, stroke the

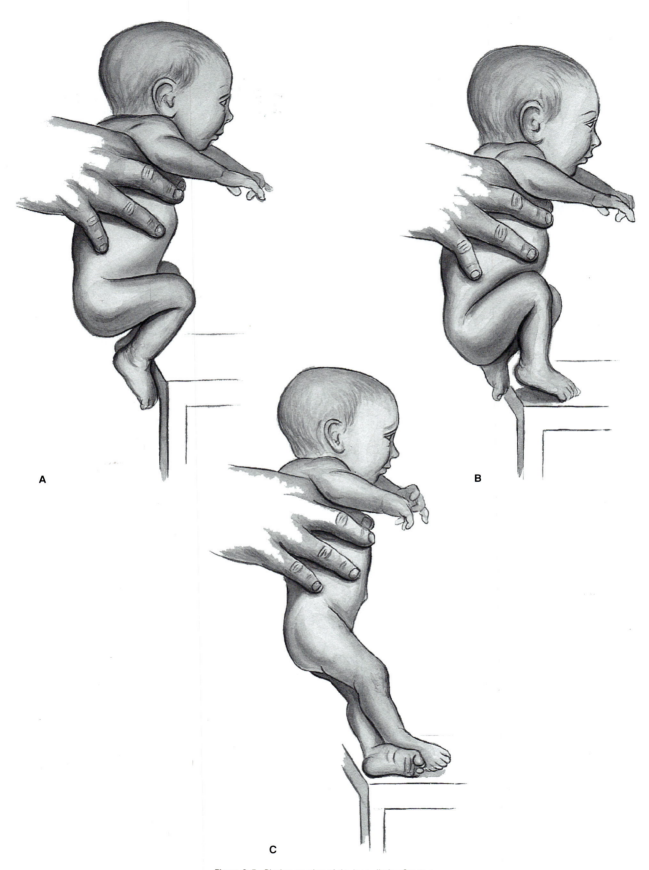

Figure 6–5. Placing reaction of the lower limbs. See text.

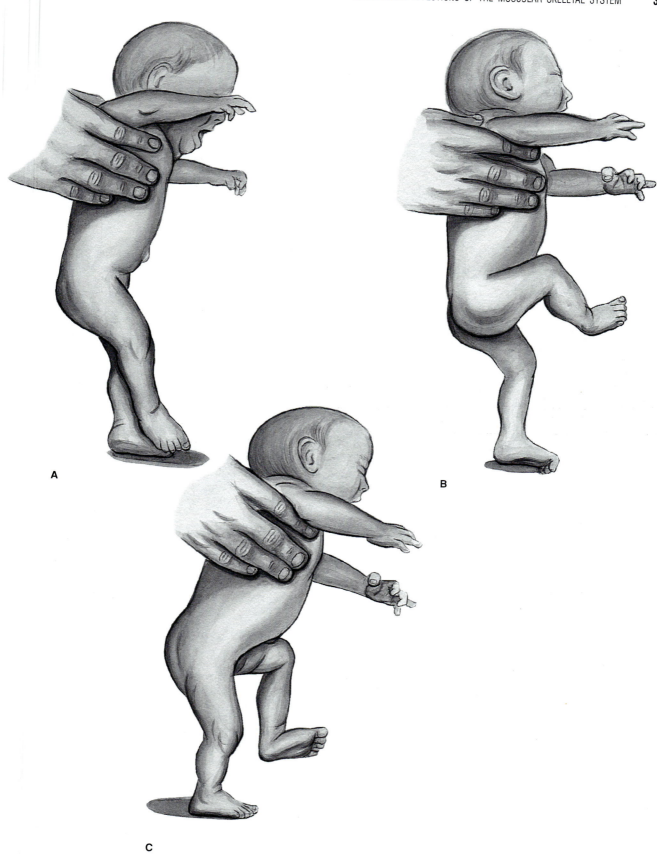

A

B

C

Figure 6–6. Walking reflex. See text.

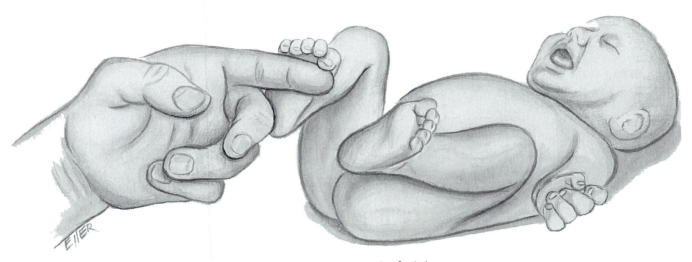

Figure 6–7. Plantar grasp reflex. See text.

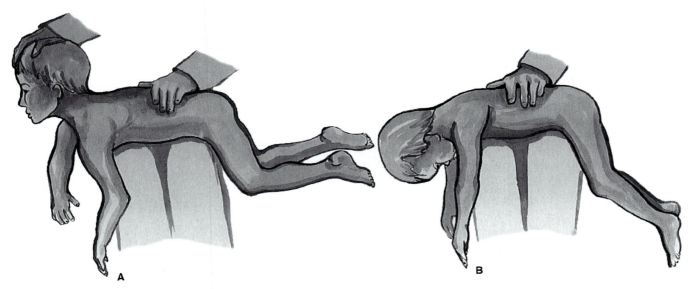

Figure 6–8 A,B. Symmetric tonic neck reflex. See text.

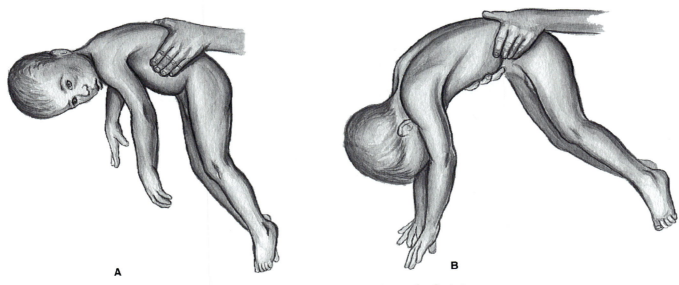

Figure 6–9 A,B. Progressive extension of arms reflex. See text.

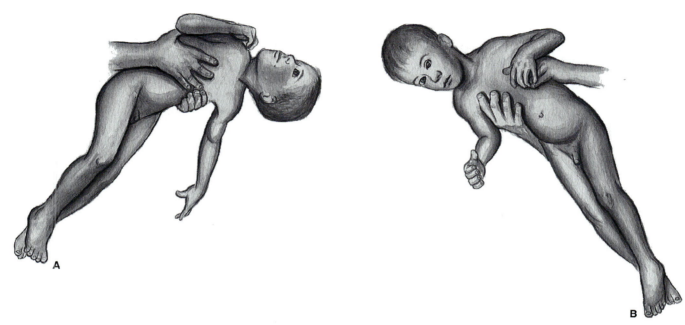

Figure 6–10 A,B. Neck righting reflex. See text.

paraspinal muscles. The trunk flexes toward the side of the stimulus (Fig 6–12). A strong persisting Galant reflex after 2 to 3 months of age suggests CNS damage.

Muscle Strength and Motor Function.   A common cause of delay in motor development is hypotonia with joint laxity. The presenting complaint is that when the child is put in stance, the knees collapse and the ankles and feet go into severe valgus. It is important to perform muscle strength testing and to palpate the muscles to be sure the muscle tone is normal. Feel the skin and make sure it is not hyperextensible. Test for hyperlaxity of ligaments (see pp. 452 and 453).

■ BENIGN CONGENITAL HYPOTONIA

This is the most common cause of delayed motor development. The presenting complaint is delayed walking in a 15- to 18-month-old child. There is generalized hypotonia of the skeletal muscles involving the lower and upper limbs and the trunk. The muscle weakness is mild and symmetric. The deep tendon reflexes are present. Muscle atrophy is minimal to moderate. There is no pseudohypertrophy and no sensory deficit.

The serum creatine phosphokinase (CPK) and aldolase levels are normal. Electromyography (EMG) shows no denervation atrophy; the amplitude potentials are normal or low. Pathologic examination of the muscles does not show neuronal atrophy; the muscle fibers are simply small.

The prognosis is good. The natural course is one of gradual improvement. The child affected with benign congenital hypotonia ordinarily walks by 24 to 30 months of age. In severe cases, developmental therapy is appropriate.

■ SPINAL MUSCULAR ATROPHY (SMA)

This progressive degenerative disease of the anterior horn cells of the spinal cord and motor nuclei of the cranial nerves (5th to 12th inclusive) manifests clinically by hypotonia due to motor weakness of the voluntary muscles. The hypotonia is greater in the lower than in the upper limbs because the degenerative process begins and is more marked in the distal part of the spinal cord, and then it progresses and extends proximally. Involvement is sequential, with more severe affection of the proximal than the distal muscle groups. The paralysis is flaccid with absence of deep tendon reflexes. Pyramidal long tract signs and spasticity are absent. Sensation is normal. SMA is a hereditary condition, transmitted as an autosomal dominant trait. The prevalence is 1 in 15,000 live births. Its exact cause is unknown.

There is marked variation in the degree of muscle atrophy, severity of muscle weakness, and length of survival. In general, the younger the age of onset, the more extensive and severe the hypotonia and the shorter the life span. Byers and Banker subdivided SMA into three types: (1) acute infantile, (2) chronic infantile, and (3) juvenile. Clinical features vary according to the type of SMA.[5]

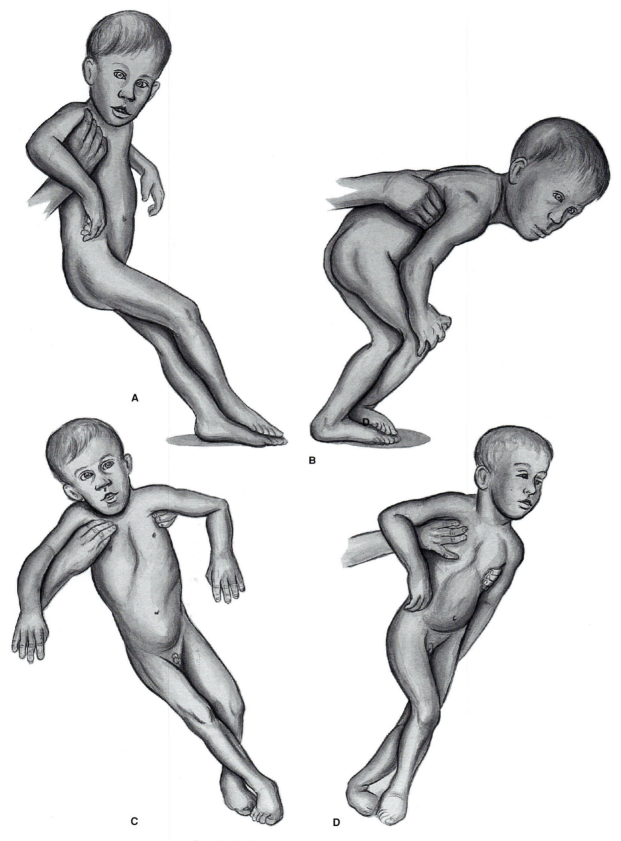

Figure 6–11. Tilting reactions in standing position. See text.

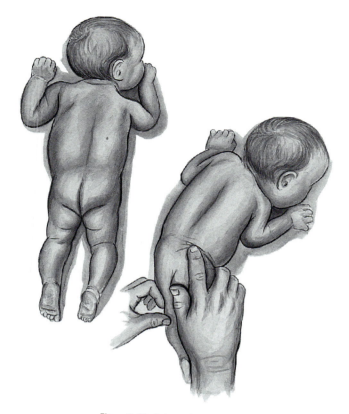

Figure 6–12. Galant reflex. See text.

In the *acute infantile type,* the involvement is very severe and extensive. The degenerative process of the anterior horn cells begins in utero. During the last trimester of pregnancy, the movements of the fetus are diminished or absent. At birth the baby is limp and "floppy" due to generalized severe weakness of the voluntary muscles.[8] The limbs are motionless. The resting posture of the infant is typical; the hips are flexed, abducted, and laterally rotated, and the elbows are flexed. Head and neck control is very poor or absent. Sitting balance does not develop. With progression of the disease, bulbar paralysis and respiratory failure develop and death occurs between 10 and 12 months of age.

In the *chronic infantile type* (Werdnig-Hoffman) the onset of paralysis occurs between 2 and 12 months of age.[10,16] Involvement is more severe in the lower than in the upper limbs. Initially the patellar tendon reflex is absent, but the triceps and biceps reflexes are present. Soon, fine tremors of the hands and fasciculations of the tongue develop. The disease progresses slowly but steadily. Most of the children with this type of SMA sit and stand holding onto furniture; death occurs around 4 to 5 years of age.

In the *chronic juvenile type,* the hypotonia develops after 12 months of age. It manifests as weakness of the gluteus maximus and thigh muscles. Tremors and muscle fasciculations develop soon thereafter. Motor development is delayed; the patients sit by 12 months of age and stand and walk by 2 years of age. These patients live to the age of 30 years.

Kugelberg-Welander disease is the most benign form of SMA. The hypotonia manifests between 2 and 15 years of age in the form of muscle weakness of the hip extensors and abductors.[11] The gait is waddling, and Gowers' test is positive. The patient has difficulty in climbing stairs. Progression of muscle weakness is very slow. These patients can ambulate until 40 to 45 years of age, when they become wheelchair bound. Their life span is normal.

Diagnosis. Definite diagnosis of SMA is made by muscle biopsy and the demonstration of denervation atrophy of skeletal muscles; the muscle fibers are small and narrow, the sarcolemmal nuclei are increased, the longitudinal and transverse striations are preserved, and the internal architecture of muscles is normal. EMG shows denervation atrophy. Nerve conduction velocities are normal. Determine CPK and serum aldolase levels; they are normal in the chronic and acute infantile types of SMA, but elevated in the juvenile SMA and Kugelberg-Welander disease. The dystrophin test for muscular dystrophy is negative.

In the differential diagnosis, rule out benign congenital hypotonia, which is distinguished clinically from Werdnig-Hoffman disease by the presence of deep tendon reflexes, lack of progression of paralysis, and absence of denervation atrophy on EMG. Infantile muscular dystrophy, cerebral palsy, and traumatic or infectious transverse myelitis are other entities to consider in the differential diagnosis.

Treatment. In infancy, passive stretching exercises are performed several times a day to prevent development of contractural deformation of the joints. Splinting of the limbs in functional position is appropriate in the older child. Symmetric posturing prevents development of pelvic obliquity.

Spinal deformity is the most serious problem. Scoliosis appears early and progresses rapidly. Initially the spine is supported in orthotics, but progression of the curvature cannot be prevented by bracing. Ordinarily, spinal fusion and internal fixation with segmented instrumentation are required to stabilize the trunk over a level pelvis.[6,13]

■ CEREBRAL PALSY

The term *cerebral palsy* (CP) comprises a spectrum of affections of the CNS due to a fixed, nonprogressive lesion or lesions that occurred prenatally, at birth, or in the immediate postnatal period. Interference with the developing CNS results in varying degrees of disorders of movement and posture, deformation of the musculoskeletal system, sensory disturbances, and mental retardation. Hearing, eyesight, and speech may be affected. Some patients may have seizures. The presenting complaint varies according to the type of CP and the age of the patient.

CLASSIFICATION

When classifying CP, one should consider the state of muscle tone, presence or absence of involuntary movements, and distribution of paralysis.[66] Abnormal muscle tone is a sign of neuromuscular affection and not a disease entity. Muscle tone alters with maturation of the CNS; it also varies according to the position, posture, state of physical fatigue, and emotional condition of the child.

Are the muscles *spastic* or *rigid?* Rapidly move a part of the limb—dorsiflex the ankle with the knee in extension and flexion or flex the hip 90 degrees and abduct it. When the muscle is *spastic,* the tension of the muscle increases following an initial free interval and "blocks" further movement; then the muscle relaxes and the part of the limb can be moved further. A spastic muscle has a "clasp knife" type of waxing and waning resistance to abrupt and sudden movement.

A *rigid* muscle resists constantly throughout the range of motion. Rigidity is not velocity sensitive. It is present in either slow or rapid movement of the limb. In rigidity, resistance to passive movement is not intermittent; it is present throughout the entire range of motion. The increased muscular tension is present in equal degrees in agonist and antagonist muscles such as flexors and extensors of the knees or elbows. When the resistance to passive movement is continuous, it is referred to as waxy; when it is discontinuous, it is cogwheel rigidity.

Spasticity occurs as a result of lesions of the cerebrum and pyramidal pathways; the alpha and gamma neuron balance is disturbed. Rigidity results from diffuse damage of the brain.

In spasticity the deep tendon reflexes are exaggerated, and the *Babinski* and *Hoffman* signs are positive. The Babinski sign is tested by stroking the plantar aspect of the foot; when the sign is positive, the toes extend and fan out. The Hoffman sign is elicited by sudden passive extension of the distal phalanx of the ring finger with the fingers and thumb in flexed posture; when the test is positive, the adjacent fingers automatically extend.

Clonus, a state of rapid alternate spasm and relaxation of the agonist and antagonist muscles, may be present in spasticity. It is tested by sudden dorsiflexion of the ankle or rapid distal movement of the patella.

In classifying CP, one should carefully observe the patient for the presence or absence of *abnormal movements* (hyperkinesia), which are involuntary contractions of voluntary muscles. These disordered movements of the limbs are frequently present with lesions of the extrapyramidal system of the brain. *Athetosis* is the term ordinarily used to denote these abnormal movements. The site of the lesion and the type of pathologic changes determine the part and extent of the body involved and the type and pattern of abnormal movement, which may be flexion-extension, rotatory, tension, or dystonic. Ask the patient to extend the hand-wrist-elbow or the foot-ankle-knee and maintain it in extended posture and observe for abnormal movements.

Spasticity and athetosis may coexist when both the pyramidal and extrapyramidal systems are involved. The term *mixed CP* is used to describe this type of involvement. Look for *tremor* of the hands; it may be constant or intention.

Ataxia results from lesions of the cerebellum. This type of cerebral palsy is rare and demands thorough neurologic assessment by a competent pediatric neurologist. In ataxia, the kinesthetic sense, equilibrium, and muscle-coordinated function are lost. Movements are disorderly. The gait is wide-based, staggering, and unsteady. Ask the patient to walk in tandem (one foot in front of the other) and follow a straight line on the floor; he or she is unable to do so. Ask the patient to successively pronate and supinate the forearms—such alternate movements are performed clumsily and with difficulty. With eyes closed, ask the patient to touch the tip of his or her index finger to the tip of the nose; he or she past points. Ask the patient to stand still with his or her eyes closed—he or she sways and tends to fall toward the side of the lesion—a positive *Romberg* sign. Inspect the eyes for *nystagmus.*

Next, determine the distribution of the paresis. The term *hemiplegia* is used when the upper and lower limbs are involved on the same side, *monoplegia* when one limb is involved, and *quadriplegia* or *tetraplegia* when all four limbs are involved. The term *double hemiplegia* is used when all four limbs are involved, but one side is more severely affected than the other. The term *diplegia* is employed when paresis of the lower limbs is more severe than that of the upper limbs and the paresis is symmetric between the right and left sides. The term *total body involved* is used when the head, neck, trunk, and all four limbs are involved.[23]

Spastic Hemiplegia

The presenting complaint depends upon the age of the patient and the severity of involvement. When involvement is *minimal,* diagnosis is not made until the child begins to walk and is noted to walk on his or her toes.

Ordinarily independent walking is slightly delayed; the child begins to walk between 18 and 24 months of age. Another observation by the parents is that the baby is right or left hand dominant. Hand dominance does not develop normally until 2 to 3 years of age. Be suspicious of contralateral hemiplegia or other abnormalities of the upper limb when strong hand dominance is present in an infant under 1 year of age.

Observe the child's gait—it is either toe-toe, toe-heel, or plantigrade. When the heel touches the floor, the knee may hyperextend because of the spasticity of the soleus. Determine the degree of genu recurvatum at heel strike in gait. When the hamstrings are spastic and contracted, the knees are flexed in gait. In severe spasticity, the hip is adducted and medially rotated to a varying degree.

The posture of the upper limb in moderate or severe spastic hemiplegia is typical: The shoulder is adducted and medially rotated, the elbow is flexed, the forearm is pronated, the wrist and fingers are flexed, and the thumb is adducted across the palm (Fig 6–13). In minimally involved cases, the posture of the upper limb may be almost normal. Ask the child to run; under stress the spasticity increases and the upper limb assumes the posture of elbow flexion, forearm pronation, and wrist and finger flexion.

Perform the *Crothers' slap* test. Ask the patient to slap your hand; he has difficulty in doing so because of incoordination.

Inspect the child for *atrophy* of the upper and lower limbs. In spastic hemiplegia there is underdevelopment of the involved upper and lower limbs. Measure the maximal circumference of the calves, thighs, forearms, and arms. The spastic limbs are atrophic. Determine the disparity of lower limb lengths by measuring the actual and apparent lengths. The spastic limb is short. The more severe the involvement, the greater the amount of shortening and atrophy. Ask the patient to stand with his or her hips and knees straight and the feet flat on the floor (an assistant or mother may have to assist you in proper posturing of the limbs). Are the iliac crests level? When the lower limb is short on the hemiplegic side, the ipsilateral iliac crest is low. Is there scoliosis? If present, is the scoliosis postural (rotation to the concavity) or structural (rotation to the convexity)?

Put blocks of various heights under the short leg and determine the raise required to level the pelvis. Ordinarily it is no greater than 1/4 to 3/8 inch. Does the scoliosis disappear when the pelvis is level? A greater degree of shortening of the lower limb exaggerates the toe-heel gait pattern.

Assess the *foot progression angle* (FPA). A spastic posterior tibial muscle and varus foot and/or abnormal medial tibial torsion and/or excessive femoral antetorsion or spastic hip adductors make the child toe in. Pes valgus due to spastic peroneal and/or fixed contracture of the triceps surae and excessive lateral tibiofibular torsion make the child toe out.

Determine the *range of motion of the joints:* (1) dorsiflexion and plantar flexion of the foot and ankle with the knee in 90 degrees of flexion and full extension; (2) eversion and inversion of the subtalar joint, and forefoot ab-

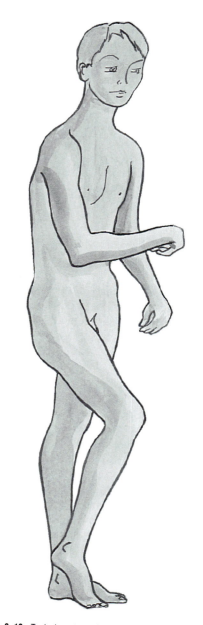

Figure 6–13. Typical posture of a child with spastic hemiplegia.

duction-adduction; (3) knee flexion-extension; (4) straight-leg raising and popliteal-thigh-foot angle; (5) range of hip motion; (6) perform the Thomas test for hip flexion contracture; (7) determine the degree of anterior pelvic tilt. Is there pelvic obliquity? In the upper limb, test range of motion of all joints. Rule out dislocation of the radial head.

Assess *motor function* of muscles. Test the deep tendon reflexes and determine the reflex maturation level. Are the Hoffman and Babinski signs positive?

Assess *sensory function in the hand* in the older child. Forty to 50 percent of spastic hemiplegic children have asterognosis, impaired two-point discrimination, and loss of position sense.[111] Hemianopsia and visual peripheral defects may be present. Suggest to the parents that they obtain ophthalmologic consultation.

Prognosis. Ninety percent of the children with spastic hemiplegia walk independently by the age of 3 years; the remaining 10 percent do so by 4 to 6 years of age. They attend regular school, are able to self-care, perform activities of daily living, and become employed in some type of occupation. They cannot perform skilled work using both upper limbs. The main problems of the hemiplegic patient are epilepsy, mental retardation, and behavioral dysfunction.

Spastic Diplegia

This type of CP is characterized by moderate or marked spasticity of the lower limbs and minimal spasticity of the upper limbs. Most cases of spastic diplegia are due to prematurity; others are caused by hypoxia, cerebral vascular accident, head trauma, encephalitis, or rubella. In history taking, an attempt should be made to determine the cause of the spastic diplegia.

Examine the upper limbs carefully to detect spasticity of the pronators of the forearm, elbow flexors and wrist-finger flexors, and thumb adductor. The radial periosteal, biceps, and triceps tendon reflexes are exaggerated. On Crothers' slap test the incoordination of the hands and upper limbs is evident. Gross hand function is normal; but the fine motor activities of the fingers and thumb are impaired.

The trunk is grossly normal. Ordinarily there is some motor weakness of the rectus abdominis and lateral abdominal muscles.

The spasticity of the lower limb muscles is marked or severe. The hips develop adduction-flexion-medial rotation contracture. The feet and ankles have an equinus deformity with oblique or vertical tali. When the peroneal muscles are spastic, the feet are in valgus, whereas when the posterior tibial muscle is spastic, the hindfoot and midfoot are in varus. The patient has no cerebral control over the anterior tibial muscle. The hamstrings are spastic and contracted, as shown by the restricted straight-leg raising and decrease in the popliteal thigh-leg angle, which is performed by extending the knee with the hip in 90 degrees of flexion. Ankle and patellar deep tendon reflexes are exaggerated, and the Babinski sign is positive.

Intellect and speech are usually normal or slightly impaired. Spastic diplegic children ordinarily attend regular school. The prognosis for independent ambulation is fairly good. Most children with spastic diplegia are community ambulators; however, about 20 percent require a walker or crutches for ambulation. It is very rare that they are non-walkers.

Spastic Quadriplegia with Total Body Involvement

The newborn with total body involved CP is hypotonic at birth, and the severe CNS damage is not suspected. Diagnosis in the neonatal period and in early infancy is not made unless seizures or some other acute life-threatening episodes such as apnea requiring resuscitation occur.

The presenting complaint is delayed motor development, such as inability to hold the head up at 3 to 4 months of age or sitting supported or turning over prone to supine or supine to prone at 5 to 6 months of age.

In time, usually between 3 and 6 months of age, these infants gradually develop spasticity or rigidity of the muscles in their limbs and trunk. The lower limbs are more severely affected than the upper limbs. Head and neck control are poor. Spastic posture of the limbs is typical. When supine, the shoulders abduct and laterally rotate, elbows flex, and the forearms are pronated. The hips are adducted, flexed, and medially rotated; the knees are flexed due to hamstring contracture or extended due to contracture of the rectus femoris; the foot and ankle are in equinus. These patients have a strong extensor thrust.

Drooling, defects in speech, mental retardation, seizures, and strabismus are common.

Prognosis for independent ambulation is poor. Standing balance and assisted ambulation with external support are achieved in about 30 to 40 percent of the cases, enabling them to be household ambulators. Most patients are sitters.

History. Make an attempt to determine the cause of the nonprogressive brain lesion. Is it due to birth injury, developmental abnormality, or an insult to the CNS sustained in the immediate postnatal period? In general, asymmetric paralysis is produced by vascular, infectious, or destructive lesions, and diffuse symmetric paralysis with total body involvement is caused by developmental malformation of the CNS.

Definite neurologic sequelae result from certain etiologic factors; for example, prematurity causes spastic diplegia, birth trauma causes spastic hemiplegia or quadriplegia, anoxia causes athetosis, and maternal rubella causes spasticity, deafness, and congenital heart disease.

Determine whether there was fetal distress due to hypoxia or anoxia. Was there any antepartum hemorrhage due to placenta previa? Was there any pre-eclamptic toxemia? In pregnancies complicated by pre-eclampsia, the oxygen saturation of the umbilical vessels is markedly decreased. How was the health of the mother during pregnancy? Hypoxia of the fetus may occur in a pregnant mother with severe cardiopulmonary disease.

Examination. The feet, ankles, knees, hips, and trunk are interdependent, and in the assessment and management of the child with cerebral palsy it is vital to consider them as a functional unit. The posture of each level depends on that of the other. Deformity at one level causes compensatory accommodations at a level proximal or distal to it. For example, fixed equinus of the ankle is compensated by hyperextension of the knee and flexion posture of the hip. In calcaneus deformity of the ankle due to a weak triceps surae, the center of body weight falls behind the ankle axis; to compensate the mechanical axis deviation, the knees are flexed and the body weight is brought forward. Hip flexion deformity is compensated by excessive lumbar lordosis of the trunk, flexion of the knee, and equinus of the ankles and feet.

Deformities of the hips, knees, ankles, feet, and trunk are presented individually; the importance of examination of the entire musculoskeletal system cannot be overemphasized.

The sequence of examination steps is modified and varies according to the type of CP, severity of involvement, age of the patient, and level of motor development. Begin the examination with the child on the mother's lap, a comfortable and secure environment for the frightened child in a strange atmosphere. Be gentle! Touch the child's foot and leg to develop some physical contact. Talk to and smile at the patient. Examine the child supine and prone on the examining table and then assess his or her stance and gait.

Finally, evaluate the appliances—splints, braces, walking casts, and seating devices. If possible, communicate with the therapists (physical and occupational) and find out why the child has been brought to your office. What are the concerns of the parents and the therapist, and what has been the previous management by the therapist? Historically, try to determine the level of motor development of the patient and tailor your examination steps accordingly.

First observe the general appearance of the child. Does he or she drool? Is there strabismus or nystagmus? How is the eyesight? Does he or she follow objects? What is the communication and speech development level? Any vocalization, words, or sentences?

Does the child have head-neck control? Can he or she hold the head in midline? Does he or she lift up the head against gravity from supine and prone positions? On inspection, is there microcephaly or hydrocephaly? Measure the circumference of the head. Are the fontanelles open (the posterior fontanelle closes at 2 months of age and the anterior fontanelle at 18 months). Are the fontanelles bulging, normal, or sunken?

Does the infant have sucking reflex? What about the teeth and palate? How many teeth? Is the palate normal, high-arched, or cleft?

Next have the mother place the child on the examination table in supine position and ask her to stay with the patient. Initially it may be comforting to the child to have his or her head on the mother's lap prior to resting flat on the examining table.

What is the resting posture of the upper limbs? Are the elbows flexed, forearms pronated, wrist and fingers flexed, and the thumb adducted and flexed across the palm? This is a common feature in moderate or severe spastic CP. Note the posture of the shoulders; are they adducted and medially rotated or abducted and laterally rotated?

Next, observe the posture of the pelvis and the lower limbs. In spasticity the hips are adducted, flexed, and medially rotated, the knees are in flexion, and the feet and ankles are in equinus. Is there pelvic obliquity and apparent shortening of the lower limbs due to abduction contracture of the contralateral hip and/or adduction contracture of the ipsilateral hip? Is there exaggerated anterior pelvic tilt?

Then have the child lie prone and inspect the spine for trunk incurvation and suprapelvic obliquity.

In assessing deformities in CP, try to determine their pathogenesis. Spasticity is the major deforming force; it causes limitation of movement of the part. The muscles do not elongate and develop permanent shortening and myostatic contracture. The muscles antagonist to the spastic muscle are hypotonic with poor cerebral control. The long bones develop torsional and angular deformity in response to muscle imbalance; a common example is excessive femoral antetorsion. The joints become misshapen and eventually dislocate. Habitual malposture and persisting strong primitive and pathologic reflexes aggravate the deformity.

In testing *range of motion of joints,* distinguish between *functional* and *fixed* deformity. Exaggerated stretch reflex due to spasticity of the muscle causes functional deformity, whereas permanent shortening and myostatic contracture produces a fixed deformity.

Begin with the *hips.* The common deformities of the hips are adduction, flexion, and medial rotation.

First determine the range of *hip abduction* and record the degree of *hip adduction deformity.* The hip adductors are (1) adductor longus, (2) adductor brevis, (3) adductor magnus, and (4) gracilis and medial hamstrings (semitendinosus and semimembranosus). With the patient supine, level the anterosuperior iliac spines and iliac crests. A common pitfall is failure of correction of pelvic obliquity prior to testing range of hip abduction. Determine range of hip abduction first with the hips and knees in 90 degrees of flexion, next with the hips and knees maximally extended, and then with the hips extended and the knees flexed 90 degrees at the edge of the examining table (Fig 6–14).

In addition to their primary function as hip adductors, the adductor longus and anterior part of the adductor brevis are secondary hip flexors, and medial rotators. The adductor magnus is both a hip adductor and hip extensor. When the hips are flexed, the adductor longus is somewhat relaxed and the adductor magnus is stretched. Testing hip abduction with the hips flexed and then extended differentiates the degree of hip adduction deformity caused by adductor longus and adductor brevis from adductor magnus. Palpate the hip adductor muscles for tautness. Testing the range of hip abduction with the hips and knees in extension and then the hips extended and the knees flexed differentiates the

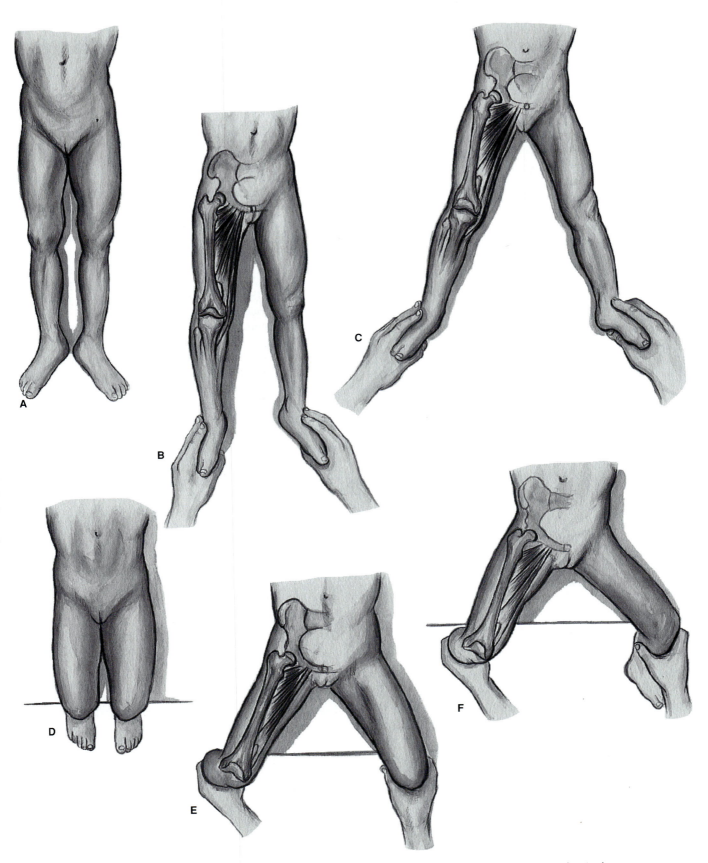

Figure 6–14. Testing spasticity and contracture of the hip adductors in cerebral palsy. **A–C.** With the hips and knees in extension, abduct the hips suddenly to elicit the stretch reflex of the hip adductors and then gently and firmly abduct them maximally to determine the degree of hip adduction contracture. With the knees in extension, both the hip adductors and gracilis are tested. **D.** With the hips extended, flex the knees at the edge of the examining table to relax the medial hamstrings. **E, F.** Suddenly abduct the hips to elicit stretch reflex of the hip adductors and then maximally abduct the hips to determine the degree of contracture of the hip adductors.

adduction contracture caused by the adductors (longus, brevis, and magnus) from that of the gracilis and medial hamstrings; the flexed posture of the knees relaxes the gracilis and medial hamstrings (Fig 6–14D–F). Carefully note any asymmetry of passive hip abduction between the right and left sides.

Next perform the *Phelps gracilis test*. Turn the patient to prone position with the hips in maximal abduction and the knees in 90 degrees of flexion; extend one knee at a time. If the gracilis and medial hamstrings are spastic and contracted, the hip automatically adducts on passive full extension of the knee.

Determine the range of hip adduction while the patient is prone with the hips extended and the knee flexed on the tested side; not infrequently in unilateral hip subluxation there is pelvic obliquity and an abduction contracture of the contralateral hip.

Determine the range of hip extension and flexion deformity, which is caused primarily by spasticity and contracture of the iliopsoas and secondarily by the rectus femoris. The two deforming forces are distinguished by performing the Thomas test with the knees in extension and then in flexion. When rectus femoris and iliopsoas are both contracted, hip flexion deformity is increased with the knee in flexion and decreased with the knee in extension. When the position of the knee has no effect on the degree of hip flexion deformity, iliopsoas is the major deforming force. Palpate the muscle fibers of the rectus femoris at their pelvic origin; are they taut?

Next turn the child to prone position and perform the *prone rectus or Ely test*. With the hip and knee in complete extension, passively flex the knee. When the rectus femoris is spastic and contracted, the pelvis rises from the table. Record the degree of knee flexion when the pelvis begins to elevate and the maximum elevation of the pelvis on complete knee flexion (Fig 6–15).

Steel elicits stretch reflex of the rectus femoris as follows: With the patient in prone position, sharply slap the patient's buttocks; the rectus femoris contracts, the hip flexes, and the pelvis elevates from the table.[102] This method of testing may not be tolerated by some parents and patients. To elicit stretch reflex of the rectus femoris, this author prefers the sudden rapid flexion of the knee while performing the Ely test.

Determine the degree of anterior tilt of the pelvis with the patient supine. Is there exaggerated lumbar lordosis? Is it fixed or flexible? When flexible, lumbar lordosis disappear on acute flexion of the hips.

Assess range of *medial and lateral rotation of the hips*. Medial rotation deformity of the hips is caused by spasticity, myostatic contracture of the medial rotators of the hip (gluteus minimus, anterior part of gluteus medius, tensor fascia femoris, medial hamstrings, adductor longus, and the anterior part of adductor brevis), and/or excessive femoral antetorsion. First, determine range of medial and lateral rotation of the hip with the patient supine and the hip flexed

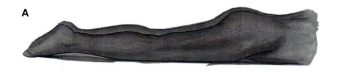

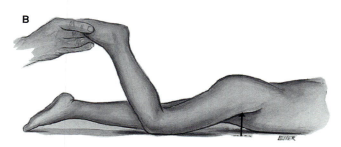

Figure 6–15. Prone rectus or Ely test. **A.** Position of patient. **B.** Passive flexion of the knee raises the pelvis off the table when the rectus femoris is spastic and contracted.

90 degrees (Fig 6–16A). Place the patient in prone position with the hip in extension and the knee in 90 degrees flexion. Test range of motion of one hip at a time. With one hand, steady the pelvis on the table and rotate the hip laterally by pushing the bent leg toward the opposite limb—first suddenly to determine the degree of lateral rotation at which the spastic medial rotators of the hip grab, and then gradually and steadily. Then rotate the hip medially by pushing the bent leg away from the opposite leg. The angle at which the greater trochanter rotates to midlateral position is the degree of femoral antetorsion. Medially rotate the hip and record its maximal range. Finally, maximally rotate the hip medially to determine range of medial rotation of the hip (Fig 6–16B).

While the patient is in prone position, determine the thigh-foot angle and the degree of tibial torsion and alignment of the foot and ankle. In spastic diplegia the most common pattern of rotational abnormality is excessive femoral antetorsion and lateral tibial torsion and pes valgus.

At this point, if the patient is able to ambulate, ask him or her to stand and walk. When there is medial rotation deformity of the hip and excessive femoral antetorsion, the lower limbs are adducted and rotated medially and the patellae face inward in stance.[28,109] In gait, the patient toes in, that is, with a negative FPA. Often there is a gluteus medius limp and a Trendelenburg lurch due to hip abductor muscle weakness and lever arm dysfunction caused by malposition of the greater trochanter due to excessive femoral antetorsion. In addition, excessive femoral antetorsion and in-toeing gait (1) interfere with stance phase stability because the patient rolls off toward the anterolateral border of the foot, (2) cause inadequate clearance of the foot in

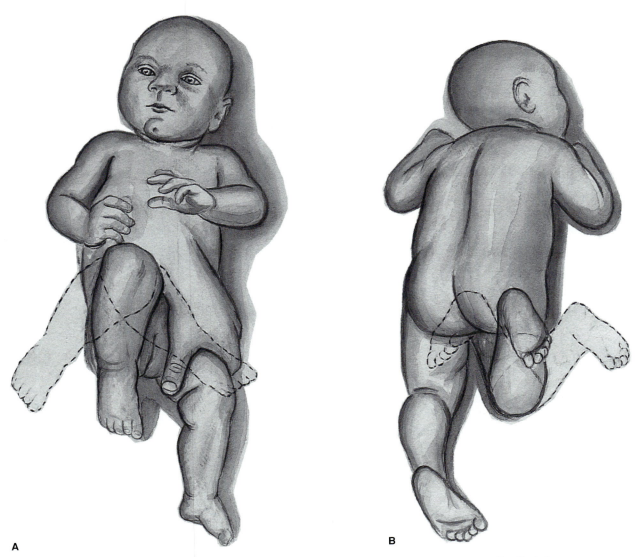

Figure 6–16. Testing range of medial and lateral rotation of the hips. **A.** In flexion. **B.** In extension in prone position. See text.

swing phase, and (3) make it difficult to appropriately pre-position the foot for the next gait cycle at the end of the terminal swing.

Next, with the patient supine, flex the hips and knees 90 degrees and with the hips in neutral adduction-abduction and rotation, determine whether the knees are level (Gal-leazi sign). A subluxated or dislocated hip causes apparent shortening of the femur. Are the greater trochanters abnor-mally prominent? Inspect the gluteal, inguinal, thigh, and popliteal creases. Are they symmetric? In dislocation of the hip the inguinal crease extends posterior to the anal aper-ture. Perform the Ortolani and Barlow tests to determine stability of the hip.

Deformities of the *knee* are flexion, extension, recur-vatum, and patellar tendon lag (loss of complete active ex-tension of the knee due to elongation of the patellar ten-don).[38,106]

Deformities of the hip and ankle affect the knee; the problem is compounded by the presence of "two-joint" muscles that cross the knee. The hamstrings flex the knee and extend the hip; the gastrocnemius plantar flexes the ankle and flexes the knee; and the quadriceps (direct head of rectus femoris) extends the knee and flexes the hip.

Flexion deformity of the knee may be *primary,* caused by spasticity and contracture of the hamstrings; *secondary,* to compensate for flexion deformity of the hip and/or equinus deformity of the ankle; or *functional,* because when the triceps surae is weak, the knee assumes flexion posture to lower the center of gravity of the body.

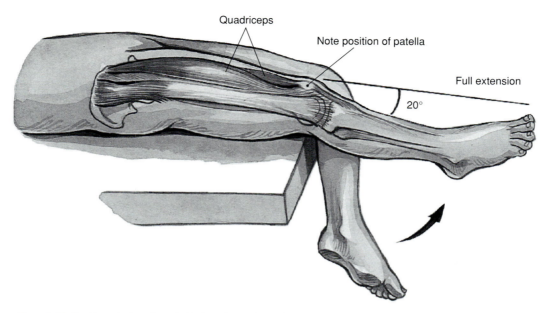

Figure 6–17. Quadriceps lag is performed with the patient supine and/or sitting. Ask the patient to actively extend the knee fully against gravity. When he or she cannot do this through the complete range of passive knee extension, quadriceps lag is present due to elongation of the patellar tendon.

First, passively extend the knee with the hip in extension (not flexion) and determine the degree of fixed flexion deformity of the knee. Palpate the patellar retinaculi; are they contracted? What is the position of the patella; is it riding high because of elongation of the patellar tendon? Ask the patient (while supine and/or sitting) to actively extend the knee as completely as possible against gravity. Is there *quadriceps lag*—that is, the knee does not actively extend fully, but passively the examiner can fully extend it (Fig 6–17)? Determine the degree of lack of complete *active* knee extension.

Palpate the proximal tibial tubercle; is it prominent and tender? Are there callosities and thickened bursa in the prepatellar region of the knees? They are present in patients who ambulate on their knees.

Next, test spasticity and contracture of the hamstrings by the *straight-leg raising test.* Perform it with the patient supine and the hips and knees in full extension. With one hand, steady the pelvis flat on the examination table, and with your other hand, lock the knee in full extension. With your forearm, raise the leg off the floor by flexing the hip (Fig 6–18). The degree of straight-leg raising is the angle between the lower limb and the examination table when the pelvis begins to tilt.

Determine the degree of spasticity and contracture of the hamstrings by the Holt method. Flex the hip of the tested limb to 90 degrees, and passively extend the knee as completely as possible. The degree of hamstring contracture is the angle subtended between the anterior surface of the leg and thigh (Fig 6–19A). An alternate method, recommended by Bleck, is to measure the popliteal angle between

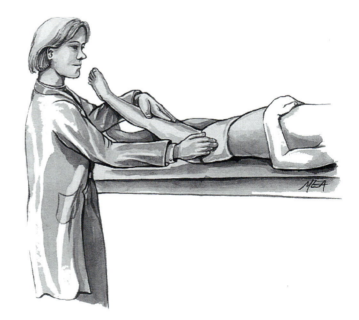

Figure 6–18. Straight leg raising test to determine hamstring tautness. The patient lies supine with the contralateral hip resting in extension. Note that the examiner stabilizes the pelvis with one hand and with his other hand holds the knee in complete extension, with the patient's ankle and foot resting on his forearm. Passively flex the hip; when the pelvis begins to tilt, determine the angle between the lower limb and the examination table.

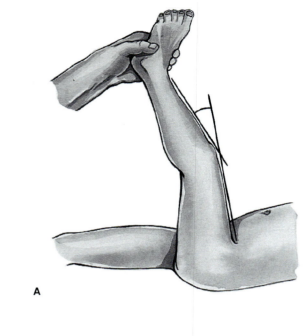

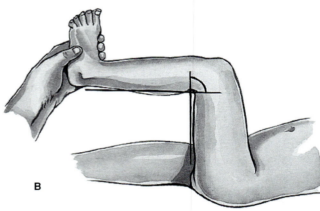

Figure 6–19. Holt and Bleck methods of determining hamstring contracture. With the patient supine and the contralateral hip in complete extension, flex the hip to be tested to 90 degrees and extend the knee passively. **A.** In the Holt method, measure the angle between the anterior aspects of the leg and thigh. **B.** In the Bleck method, measure the popliteal angle between the posterior aspects of the thigh and hip.

the posterior aspects of the leg and thigh (Fig 6–19B). Caution! Be sure that the hip is always in 90 degrees of flexion at each determination![23]

Ask the patient to sit and note the sitting posture. The hamstrings are two-joint muscles; they flex the knee and extend the hip. Contracture of the hamstrings limits the range of hip flexion because of the pull of the short hamstrings on the ischium and pelvis. In moderate hamstring contracture the patient has difficulty sitting with the knees in extension; he or she has to flex the knees, and the lumbar spine flattens and assumes a kyphotic posture (Fig 6–20A). In severe contracture of the hamstrings the patient cannot

sit; he or she slides down the chair even with the knees in flexion (Fig 6–20B).[84]

In *jump knee gait,* knee flexion is increased in early stance phase through initial double support; in the mid and late stance phase of gait, the knee extends to normal or near normal range. In late swing phase, the knee extension is decreased. The ankles and feet are in equinus. The patient has decreased stability while standing and sustains frequent falls. The swing limb advancement is poor.[53,106]

Jump knee gait is caused by overactivity of the hamstring muscles. The quadriceps femoris has good motor strength. Knee extension in mid and late single stance phase is facilitated by strong plantar flexors of the ankle. The iliopsoas is overactive. EMG studies show overactivity of the hamstrings, the iliopsoas, the triceps surae, and sometimes the rectus femoris.

Kinetic studies show increased hip-knee flexion early in stance, with extension of the knee in late stance and equinus of the ankles. Force plate studies show an equinus pattern of the center of pressure during progression.

In *crouch gait,* knee flexion is increased throughout the stance phase, with variable alignment in the swing phase. It is caused by contracture-spasticity of the hamstrings, as shown by limitation of straight-leg raising and decrease in the popliteal-thigh angle.[105] Often hip flexion deformity due to spasticity of the iliopsoas is present. The anterior pelvic tilt is exaggerated. Not infrequently, associated increased lateral tibiofibular torsion and pes valgus deformity increase the degree of knee flexion posture. The foot may be in neutral position, calcaneus, or equinus. Crouch gait is often seen after injudicious overlengthening of the triceps surae.

EMG studies show quadriceps and hamstring overactivity with stance phase prolongation.

Extension deformity of the knee is caused by spasticity and contracture of the quadriceps, specifically the rectus femoris. EMG studies show prolonged hyperactivity during the swing phase. With the patient prone and the hips and knee fully extended, passively flex the knee (the Ely test). Determine the degree of knee flexion at which the quadriceps grabs; measure the amount of elevation of the pelvis off the table on maximal passive knee flexion.

Next, with the patient supine, hips in extension, and the knees dangling at the edge of the examining table, determine the range of knee flexion; when the quadriceps is contracted (particularly the direct head of rectus femoris, which takes origin from the pelvis), the knee does not flex fully (Fig 6–21A). Ask the patient to sit; the range of knee flexion increases because the direct head of the rectus femoris relaxes with the hip in flexion (Fig 6–21B).

The child with extension contracture of the knee walks with a *stiff knee gait,* which is characterized by excessive knee extension throughout swing phase with variable alignment in stance phase. The normal reciprocal hip and knee

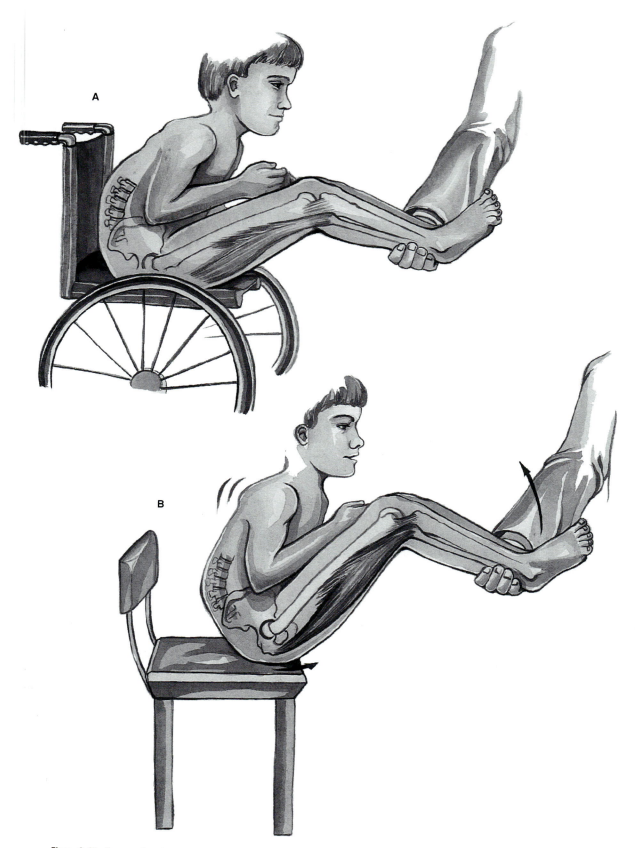

Figure 6–20. Compromise of sitting posture in contracture of the hamstrings. **A.** Note that he or she cannot sit with his or her knees in extension; he or she has to flex the knees to decrease the pull of the hamstrings on the ischium and pelvis. The lumbar spine assumes a kyphotic posture. **B.** In severe contracture of the hamstrings, the knees are flexed, the lumbar spine is in marked hyper-kyphosis, and the patient slides off the chair.

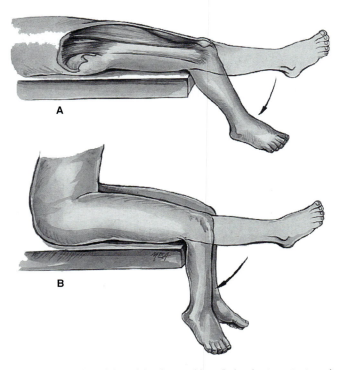

Figure 6–21. Method of determining decreased knee flexion due to contracture of the rectus femoris. **A.** Determine range of knee flexion with the patient supine, the hip in extension, and the knee dangling at the edge of the table. **B.** Ask the patient to sit with the hip in 90 degrees of flexion; the reflected head of the rectus femoris (which takes origin from the pelvis) relaxes. Determine the range of knee flexion; it is increased when extension deformity of the knee is due to contracture of the rectus femoris.

flexion is lost. The patient has difficulty in clearing the swing limb, compensating by circumduction-abduction of the hip, vaulting, increased lateral rotation of the pelvis during swing phase, and pelvic obliquity. The stride length is short.[31,42,69,70,74,108,116]

Genu recurvatum is caused by spasticity and contracture of the quadriceps or equinus deformity of the ankle due to contracture of the triceps surae (particularly the soleus) in the presence of weak hamstrings. Test the range of hyperextension of the knee with the patient lying supine. Observe the posture of the knee in gait; in mid and terminal stance phase, the knee hyperextends. In prone, perform the Ely test to assess the degree of spasticity and contraction of the quadriceps; also, test motor strength of hamstrings by asking the patient to flex the knee against gravity. Are there operative scars of a previously performed hamstring release or Eggers' procedure (transfer of hamstrings to the femoral condyles)? Test for AP and lateral (varus-valgus) instability of the knee—it is often absent except in severe longstanding cases.

Determine the degree of equinus deformity by testing the range of dorsiflexion of the ankle with the knees in extension and flexion and the patient in prone and supine positions. Distinguish between dynamic equinus elicited by

stretch reflex and fixed equinus due to myostatic contracture of the triceps surae. Is there ankle clonus?

Gait analysis in mid and late stance phase shows that the knee hyperextends, and the range of knee flexion in the swing phase is diminished to a varying degree. The stride length is shortened and the velocity is diminished, interfering with forward momentum. EMG discloses overactivity of the triceps surae in stance phase.

Next examine the foot and ankle. *Equinus* is the most common deformity; it is caused by spasticity and contracture of the triceps surae due to involvement of both the soleus and gastrocnemius muscles or the gastrocnemius alone.[22] Equinus deformity may be *functional*—due to spasticity and exaggerated reflex of the triceps surae without myostatic contracture; or it may be *fixed*—caused by permanent shortening of the triceps surae muscle.

Determine range of passive dorsiflexion of the ankle with the patient supine and prone, first with the knee extended and then with the knee flexed. Be sure the patient does not actively dorsiflex the ankle. Active dorsiflexion of the ankle relaxes the triceps surae because of reciprocal innervation of agonist-antagonist muscle, and greater range of dorsiflexion of the ankle is obtained. The gastrocnemius portion of the triceps surae (because it takes origin from the femoral condyles) is relaxed when the knee is flexed, and the range of ankle dorsiflexion is greater when equinus deformity is due primarily to contracture of the gastrocnemius. When dorsiflexing the ankle, do not apply dorsiflexion force on the forefoot; that stimulates and stretches the peroneals, posterior tibial, and long toe flexor muscles. Grab the heel and pull the hindfoot distally and gently dorsiflex the ankle. Dynamic EMG studies have shown that on sudden passive ankle dorsiflexion with the knee in flexion, both gastrocnemius and soleus are stimulated and fire. Testing passive ankle dorsiflexion with the knee in flexion and then extension differentiates fixed contractural deformity caused by gastrocnemius and soleus and not spasticity and dynamic functional equinus deformity (Fig 6–22).

A common pitfall is mistaking *extensor thrust* for dynamic or fixed equinus deformity of the ankles. When the patient is held vertically upright, both ankles and feet are in severe plantar flexion and the knees are extended. When the child is postured supine, plantar flexion position of the ankles persists, but to a lesser degree than when upright. Turn the patient to prone position and test range of passive ankle dorsiflexion with the knee extended; it is much greater. Flex the knees to 90 degrees; with the hips extended and the patient prone, the ankles automatically dorsiflex 15 to 25 degrees (Fig 6–23). The importance of distinguishing extensor thrust from true equinus deformity cannot be overemphasized. Not infrequently, the heel cord is lengthened for extensor thrust in the absence of true equinus deformity, causing calcaneus deformity.

In stance (supported or independent), ask the patient to place the foot on the floor; do the heels touch the floor?

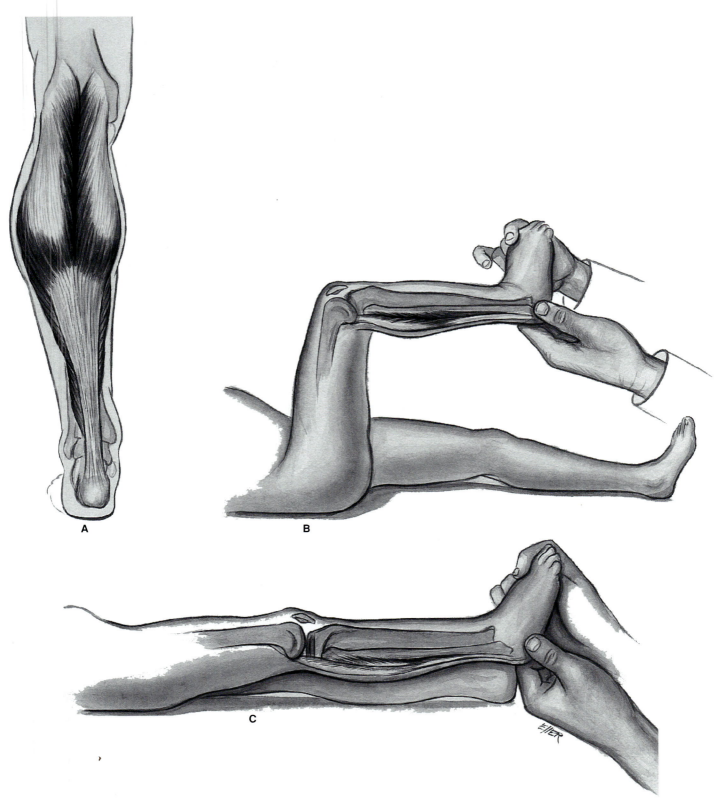

Figure 6–22. Testing contracture of the triceps surae by passive dorsiflexion of the ankle. **A.** Triceps surae muscle. Note that the gastrocnemius takes its origin from the femoral condyle. **B.** Determine the range of dorsiflexion of the ankle with the knee flexed. In this position, the gastrocnemius portion of the triceps surae is relaxed. **C.** Determine the range of dorsiflexion of the ankle with the knee in complete extension. In this position, the contractural deformities of both the gastrocnemius and soleus are tested.

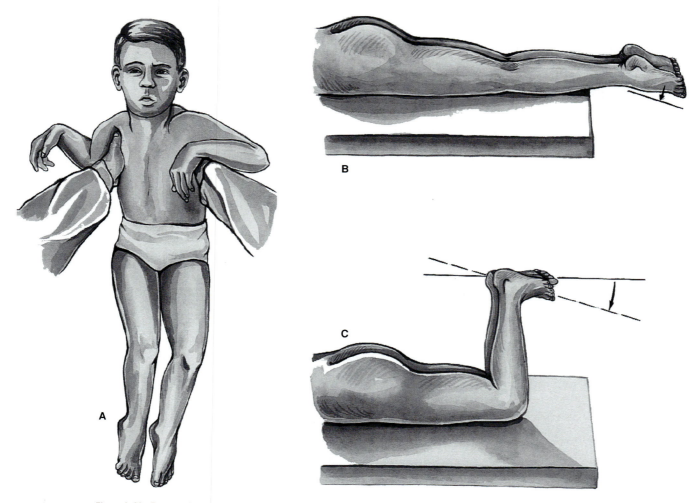

Figure 6–23. Extensor thrust—clinical detection. **A.** In upright vertical posture, the feet and ankles are in marked plantar flexion and the knees are extended. **B.** In prone position with the hips and knees extended, the range of passive dorsiflexion of the ankle is limited, but to a lesser degree than in supine or upright. **C.** Flex the knees with the child prone and the hips extended. In extensor thrust, the ankles dorsiflex through normal range. Do not mistake extensor thrust for true equinus deformity.

Ask the patient to walk (assisted or alone, depending upon the degree of involvement); the gait pattern may be toe-toe, toe-heel, or plantigrade.

Observe the position of the knee when the heel strikes the floor. Is the knee flexed, neutral, or hyperextended? A contracted soleus muscle prevents dorsiflexion of the ankle, and the tibia, acting as a lever, thrusts the knee into recurvatum.

Assess the *alignment of the foot* in prone, supine, and upright posture. Is there *pes valgus* deformity? Determine the range of passive inversion of the foot with the ankle in neutral dorsiflexion and maximal plantar flexion. Are the peroneal muscles spastic, pulling the foot into eversion and valgus, or is the valgus position of the hindfoot due to the bowstringing effect of the triceps surae on the ankle and subtalar joint, displacing the calcaneus posterolaterally under the talus? Note the position of the talus: Is it normal,

oblique in equinus, or vertical? Is there rocker-bottom deformity of the foot? What is the calcaneal pitch—neutral, plantar flexion, or dorsiflexion?

Spasticity of the posterior tibial muscle causes *varus deformity of the hindfoot and midfoot*. Passively dorsiflex the ankle and evert the hindfoot; the tendon of the spastic-contracted posterior tibial muscle is prominent in the lower leg behind the groove posterior to the medial malleolus and restricts range of eversion of the hindfoot. When there is marked contracture, the posterior tibial tendon tends to slip anteriorly over the medial malleolus.

Spastic long toe flexors curl the toes and force the forefoot into *metatarsus varus*. Passive dorsiflexion of the ankle aggravates these deformities. Push the forefoot into valgus and rule out spasticity and contracture of the abductor hallucis muscle. Spasticity and contracture of adductor hallucis cause *hallux valgus* deformity.

Assessment of Motor Strength of Muscles by Muscle Testing This is difficult because of inadequate coordinated cerebral control of the muscles. Often the patient does not have selective cerebral control over individual muscle or muscle groups; he cannot voluntarily activate an individual muscle on command. In the spastic lower limb, frequently cerebral control of the anterior tibial muscle is cerebral zero. Ask the patient to dorsiflex the ankle with the knee in extension; the anterior tibial muscle does not contract voluntarily. Extensor hallucis longus contracts and the big toe hyperextends (Fig 6–24). Ask the patient to dorsiflex the ankle with the knee flexed; with the gastrocnemius portion of the triceps surae relaxed, the patient may have some cerebral control over the anterior tibial muscle. Then perform the *Strumpell* test (which is also referred to as the "confusion" or automatic reflex); ask the patient to flex the hip against resistance with the knee bent 90 degrees. This maneuver makes the anterior tibial contract, bringing the ankle and foot into dorsiflexion (Fig 6–24B). Diligently perform a motor strength grading of all of the spastic muscles and their antagonists. It is also best for muscle testing to be performed by a competent pediatric physical therapist who is an expert in CP.

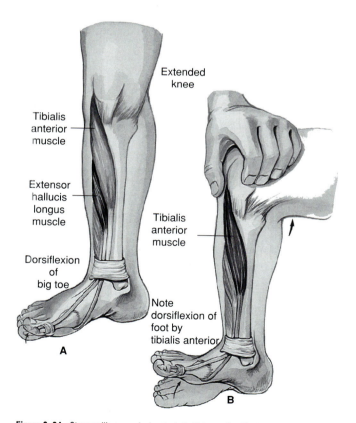

Tibialis anterior muscle

Extensor hallucis longus muscle

Dorsiflexion of big toe

Extended knee

Tibialis anterior muscle

Note dorsiflexion of foot by tibialis anterior

A

B

Figure 6–24. Strumpell's or confusion test. **A.** Note on dorsiflexion of the ankle, with the knee in extension, that the anterior tibial muscle does not contract; instead the extensor hallucis longus contracts and the big toe hyperextends. **B.** Ask the sitting patient to flex the hip against resistance with the knee flexed 90 degrees. Note that the anterior tibial contracts, bringing the foot and ankle into dorsiflexion.

Examination of the Upper Limbs. In infancy and childhood, the orthopedic surgeon, parents, and therapist are concerned primarily with their patient's inability to stand and walk and, unfortunately, the upper limb is often ignored. In spastic diplegia, the upper limbs are minimally involved; whereas in spastic quadriplegia, with total body involvement, the upper limbs are moderately or severely affected. In spastic hemiplegia, the upper limb involvement may be minimal, moderate, or severe.

In assessment and management of the upper limbs in cerebral palsy, the level of intelligence and communication of the patient are important considerations. The process of cognition involves perception and abstract reasoning. In the infant and young child, testing of intelligence quotient is difficult; however, an approximate general impression can be made. In the older child, IQ is determined. Children with normal IQ or an IQ of 50 to 70 are educable. Surgery and therapy of the upper limbs in these children achieve functional improvement, whereas in CP children with an IQ below 50, functional results from upper limb surgery are of dubious value. Therefore, the first step in assessing the upper limb in the CP child is determining the *level of intelligence and cognition.*

The second step is to perform the *hand placement test.* Ask the patient to place his dominant and then the involved hand on top of his head and then the opposite knee (Fig 6–25A, B). This simple activity requires range of motion, coordinated movements of the shoulder, elbow, wrist, and hand, and selective cerebral muscle control. Spasticity and contracture of the muscles limit range of motion of the joints, and motor disorders such as athetosis hinder precision. Determine the precision of placement of the hand and the time required to do so. When a CP child cannot place his or her hand on the head and the opposite knee within 5 seconds, functional results of upper limb surgery are not satisfactory.

Third, perform the *"cookie test."* Ask the parents whether, when a cookie is given to their child, he or she grasps and takes it to his or her mouth. Then have the parents give a cookie to their child and observe what he or she does. When a CP child fails the "cookie" test, functional improvement from therapy and surgery of the upper limb should not be expected.

Does the child transfer objects from one hand to the other? Can the child grasp and release objects (Fig 6–26A, B)? Palmar grasp reflex is a primitive one and is normal in infants up to 3 months of age. Do not mistake it for grasp and release, which require coordinated selective cerebral muscle control. Is the thumb flexed across the palm, interfering with grasp?

Can the child oppose the thumb to the index finger (Fig 6–27A)? This refined opposition pinch is present in a normal child by 1 year of age. In the spastic child attempting to oppose, the adductor pollicis adducts the thumb toward the index finger and he is unable. Instead he pinches

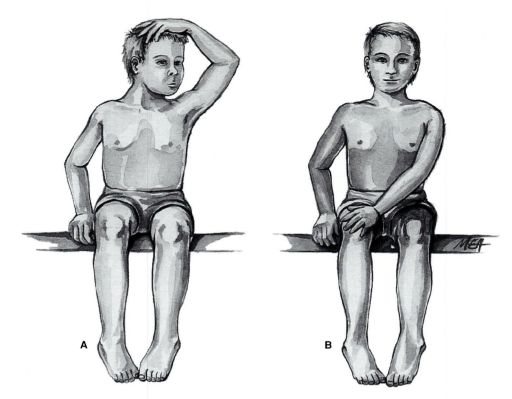

Figure 6–25. Hand placement test. **A.** Ask the patient to place his hand on top of his head. **B.** Then ask the patient to place his hand on the opposite knee. Observe the precision of placement and the time required to perform the test.

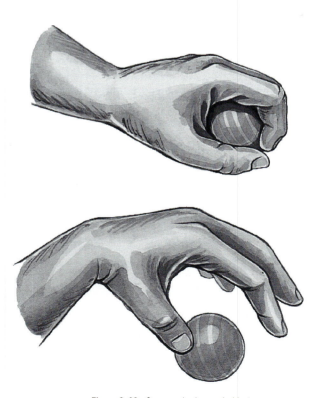

Figure 6–26. Grasp and release of objects.

the sides of the thumb and index finger together (key pinch) (Fig 6–27B). In severe involvement, there is no selective cerebral control over the thumb.

Next, ask the patient to dorsiflex the wrist, extend the fingers, abduct or extend the thumb, supinate the forearm, extend the elbow, and abduct, elevate, and laterally rotate the shoulder. Does the child have selective cerebral muscle control to carry out these motions (or the motions are in pattern)?

An attempt is made to assess *motor strength of key muscles* controlling motion of the fingers, thumbs, wrists, forearms, and elbows. Ask for an official muscle strength grading and functional assessment by an occupational therapist. Can the patient feed himself or herself, dress, attend to toilet functions, and perform two-handed assisted work?

Is there any *sensory disturbance?* About 40 to 50 percent of the patients with hemiplegia have sensory deficits. Lesions of the somatosensory cortices affect perceptual sensory function—namely stereognosis (object identification), texture discrimination, two-point discrimination, number perception in the palm, and position sense. Homonymous hemianopsia is present in one of four hemiplegic CP children. Thalamic sensation, that is, pain, sharp, dull, and touch are normal. In the pathogenesis of sensory deficits, inexperience in using the hand may be a factor in sensory

luxation or dislocation of the radial head; (7) pronation contracture of the forearm; (8) subluxation or dislocation of the radial head; (9) flexion deformity of the elbow; (10) medial rotation and adduction contracture of the shoulder; and (11) in acquired CP, abduction contracture of the shoulder due to spasticity of the deltoid.

Begin your examination with the thumb. *Adduction contracture of the thumb* is caused by spasticity and contracture of the adductor pollicis and first dorsal interosseous muscles. On inspection, the thumb metacarpal is adducted next to the index metacarpal, and the MCP joint of the thumb may be neutral or in varying degrees of flexion (Fig 6–28A). The skin web between the thumb and index metacarpals is contracted. Ask the patient to extend, flex, and abduct the thumb and determine degree of selective cerebral control over these muscles. The MCP joint of the thumb does not subluxate on active and passive extension-abduction of the thumb.[54]

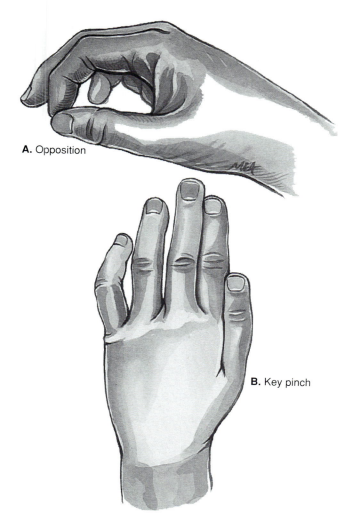

A. Opposition

B. Key pinch

Figure 6–27. Opposition. **A.** Opposition between thumb and index finger. **B.** Key pinch. Note that the sides of the thumb and index finger oppose instead of normal pulp-to-pulp opposition.

deficit. The results of upper limb surgery in CP are adversely affected by sensory deficit. It is a relative, but not absolute, contraindication to surgery.[111]

In examination and assessment of the deformities of the hand and upper limb in CP, make an effort to determine their cause. Is the deformity due to hypertonicity of muscle (spastic or tension athetoid), muscle imbalance, myostatic contracture, joint contracture, or hyperextensibility of joints due to ligamentous stretching? Is there any bony deformity?

Inspect the resting posture of the entire upper limb and determine the passive range of motion of each joint. In spastic CP, the deformities of the upper limb are (1) adducted thumb; a thumb-in-palm; (2) dorsal subluxation of the metacarpophalangeal (MCP) joint of the thumb; (3) flexion of the fingers; (4) swan-neck deformity of the fingers; (5) flexion and ulnar deviation of the wrist; (6) sub-

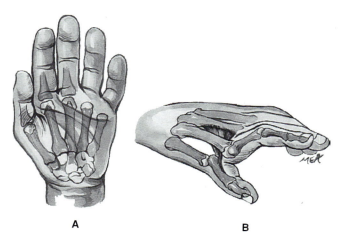

A   **B**

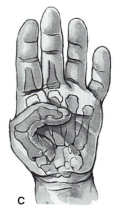

C

Figure 6–28. Deformities of the thumb in spastic cerebral palsy. **A.** Adduction contracture of the thumb. The thumb is in poor functional position. Pulp-to-pulp opposition between the thumb and index finger is not possible. Side-to-side pinch is lost. **B.** Thumb metacarpal adduction contracture associated with instability and dorsal subluxation of the MP joint. **C.** Thumb metacarpal contracture combined with flexion deformity of the MP and IP joints of the thumb.

Flexion deformity of the MCP joint of the thumb may be associated with adduction contracture of the thumb. This is due to spasticity and contracture of the flexor pollicis brevis. The interphalangeal joint of the thumb has normal range of motion.

Contracture of the thumb adductor may be associated with instability, hyperextension, and *dorsal subluxation of the MP joint* (Fig 6–28B). This is caused by ligamentous and capsular hyperlaxity of the MCP joint and hypertonicity of the extensor pollicis longus and brevis. The patient is unable to oppose and pinch with the pulp of the thumb and index fingers.

Thumb metacarpal adduction contracture may be combined with *flexion deformity of the MCP and interphalangeal (IP) joints of the thumb* (Fig 6–28C). This is caused by spasticity and contracture of the flexor pollicis longus and the intrinsic muscles of the thumb. The clasped thumb in the palm stimulates the gripping reflex, and the fingers clench over the thumb in the palm. Placement of objects in the palm is interfered with, and the patient is unable to grasp, causing marked functional disability.

Differentiate between muscle-tendon contracture and joint contracture by asking the patient to hyperflex the wrist; when the deformity is due to muscle contracture, the fingers and thumb extend out of the palm on hyperflexion of the wrist whereas in joint contracture they do not extend (Fig 6–29A, B). The position and stability of the wrist affect function of the thumb.

In the spastic hand, *finger deformities* are flexion and swan-neck. Flexion deformities of the MCP and IP joints of the fingers are caused by spasticity and myostatic contracture of the flexor digitorum profundus and sublimus muscles. This is usually associated with flexion deformity of the wrist. Passively flex the fingers and test the range of wrist extension; this maneuver differentiates spasticity and contracture of the finger flexors from that of wrist flexors.

Next, with the wrist in extension, passively extend first the proximal interphalangeal (PIP) and then the distal interphalangeal (DIP) joints of each finger and determine the tension elicited at each joint; the test distinguishes spasticity and contracture of the flexor digitorum superficialis from that of the flexor digitorum profundus. Flexion deformity of the fingers and weak finger extensor muscles cause inadequate or poor release.

Perform *Bunnell's intrinsic test* to assess the degree of spasticity and contracture of the intrinsic muscles of the hand. Ask the patient to flex the PIP and DIP joints, first with the MCP joints fully extended and then fully flexed. In the normal hand, when the MCP joints are flexed the IP and DIP joints have greater range of motion than with the MCP joints extended. When the intrinsic muscles are contracted and fibrosed, the range of motion of the IP joints does not increase with the MCP joints flexed.

Swan-neck deformity of the fingers is caused by contracture of the middle extensor band, which is shorter in relation to the lateral extensor bands.[110] The deformity is

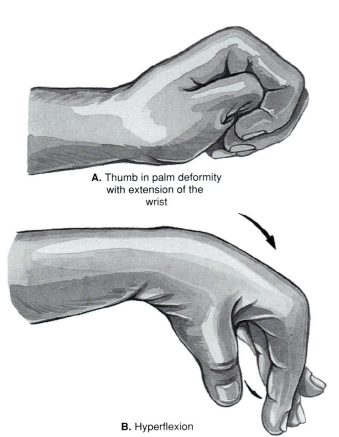

A. Thumb in palm deformity with extension of the wrist

B. Hyperflexion

Figure 6–29. Thumb-in-palm deformity with fingers clenched over the thumb. **A.** The gripping reflex and exaggeration of the deformity on extension of the wrist. **B.** On hyperflexion of the wrist, the fingers and thumb extend out of the palm because of the relaxation of the thumb and finger flexors.

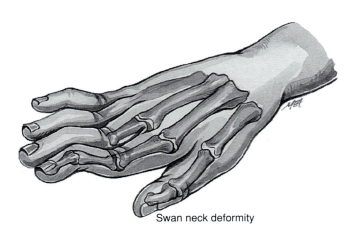

Swan neck deformity

Figure 6–30. Swan neck deformity of the digits. Note the hyperextension of the PIP joints and flexion of the DIP joint.

characterized by hyperextension of the PIP joint and flexion of the DIP joints (Fig 6–30). The volar capsule and retinacular ligaments of the PIP joint are stretched and lax. Moderate and severe swan-neck deformity of the fingers interferes with grasp.

Flexion and ulnar deviation deformity of the wrist weakens the grasp (Fig 6–31). It is caused primarily by spasticity and contracture of the flexor carpi ulnaris and weak dorsiflexors of the wrist (extensor carpi radialis, longus, and brevis and extensor carpi ulnaris).

The strength of long finger extensors may be good or weak; test by asking the patient to extend the fingers with the wrist in acute flexion and with the wrist in dorsiflexion.

Flexion deformity of the wrist is often associated with *pronation contracture of the forearm.* Ability to dorsiflex the wrist and rotate the forearm into supination and pronation are essential movements for functional use of the hands. Pronation contracture of the forearm is caused by spasticity and contracture of the pronator teres. In severe cases the pronator quadratus may also be contracted. Test the degree of rotation of the forearm. Hold the distal radius and ulna with one hand; with your other hand hold the elbow steady in 90 degrees of flexion and rotate the forearm from full pronation to maximal supination (Fig 6–32). Record the degree at which the pronator teres grabs and the maximal degree of supination. Palpate the radial head. Is it dislocated or does it subluxate?

Flexion deformity of the elbow is caused by spasticity and contracture of biceps brachii and brachialis muscles.

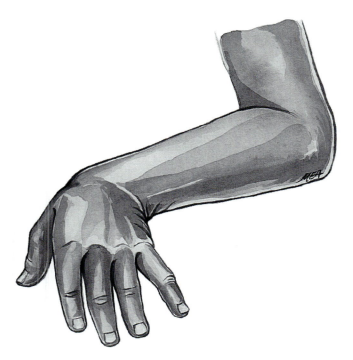

Figure 6–31. Flexion and ulnar deviation deformity of the wrist. This posture weakens the strength of the grasp. Note the associated pronation contracture of the forearm.

Minimal to moderate deformity of the elbow is not a functional handicap. Severe flexion deformity of the elbow, however, causes hygiene and cosmetic problems and may limit crutch or walker use and restrict reach and activities that require two hands.

Shoulder deformity in spastic CP is usually medial rotation and adduction. In acquired CP the deltoid muscle may be spastic and cause abduction deformity of the shoulder.

Deformities of the Spine. Examine the trunk and spine in prone, supine, sitting, and standing posture at the initial examination and at each subsequent office visit. Weakness of the trunk extensors and abdominal muscles causes exaggerated thoracic or thoracolumbar kyphosis. Scoliosis is common, occurring in 15 to 25 percent of the total body involved CP patients. Most curve patterns are long thoracolumbar or lumbar. Idiopathic scoliosis does occur in CP patients. Other causes of scoliosis are pelvic obliquity, asymmetric paresis, and/or spasticity of the trunk muscles and congenital deformities such as hemivertebrae and unsegmented vertebral bars.

Management. The orthopedic surgeon's concerns are the deformities of the musculoskeletal system, poor posture, and disorders of movement. In the management of CP, however, other disciplines are involved, including neurology, neurosurgery, pediatrics, ophthalmology, audiology, speech therapy, physical and occupational therapy, sociology, vocational counseling, and habilitation. Always bear in mind the importance of provision of total care to the CP child. Concerned parents and an adequate home situation are vital.

The orthopedic surgeon is principally involved in the management of patients with spastic diplegia, spastic hemiplegia, and spastic quadriplegia with total body involvement.

CP is an incurable and life-long disorder. The care of the child with CP extends over a period of many years. Management is a more appropriate term than treatment. The problem is very complex and dynamic; it changes with growth and maturation of the CNS. Management should be goal oriented. The child should be assessed thoroughly at intervals, realistic goals set, and a program of management provided accordingly. The objectives of management of the musculoskeletal system are to prevent and correct deformity and improve function.

A team effort is provided by the orthopedic surgeon and the physical and occupational therapist. The immediate goals of therapy are provision of mobility and ambulation. A total body involved child is a sitter and can stand with support. He is a nonwalker and wheelchair dependent for all activities of daily living. Nonwalkers may be able to transfer independently, that is, to get in and out of a wheelchair, be able to transfer with assistance, or be totally dependent. Walking is subclassified into community walkers, household walkers, and physiologic walkers; that is, they

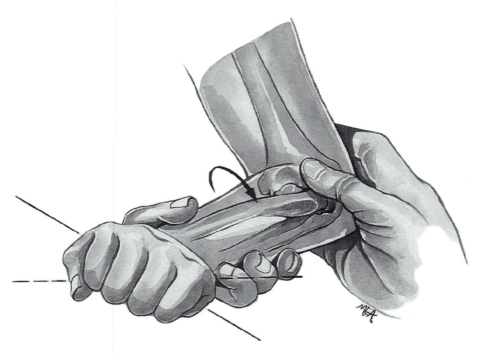

Figure 6–32. Method of testing the degree of pronation contracture of the forearm. Note that the examiner steadies the elbow in 90 degrees of flexion with one hand and with the other hand holds the distal ends of the radius and ulna and rotates the forearm into supination. Palpate the radial head to rule out subluxation.

can walk with the assistance of therapists or parents. As the child gets older and heavier, the total body involved CP child requires more assistance for mobility. It is beyond the scope of this textbook to discuss modalities of physical therapy management. The various deformities and their management are discussed briefly.

Spine deformity, scoliosis, and kyphosis can be prevented by having these children sleep prone in a total body splint or bivalved cast. It is important to provide a level pelvis and prevent pelvic obliquity by soft tissue release around the hips. When the scoliosis and kyphosis cannot be controlled in a sitting patient, a thoracolumbosacral orthosis (TLSO) is prescribed for support of the trunk. If scoliosis progresses beyond 40 degrees, a spinal fusion with internal instrumentation is indicated.[27]

Multilevel surgery is in vogue, but it has its advantages and definite disadvantages. Patients who have hip flexion-adduction deformity, knee flexion deformity, and equinus deformity are managed in many medical centers by hip flexor-adductor myotomies, hamstring lengthening, and heel cord lengthening. The older child who also has rotational malalignment undergoes derotation osteotomies of the femur and/or tibia. This author strongly recommends a more conservative approach, as often unnecessary hamstring lengthening is performed for knee flexion deformity, ignoring the fact that hamstrings are also hip extensors. A child who has a weak gluteus maximus and undergoes hamstring lengthening is unable to extend the hips, increasing his or her disability. Often a simultaneous heel cord length-

ening is performed with release of the hip adductors and flexors. When the triceps surae motor strength is weak, the result is calcaneus deformity and a crouch posture and gait. One cannot overemphasize that each case must be individualized and that adequacy of postoperative care must be carefully determined. Often success or failure of a surgical procedure depends upon how the patient is cared for after surgery.[21-23]

Hip flexion and adduction deformity of the hip often co-exist. They are corrected by myotomy of the adductor longus and brevis and the gracilis muscles and by fractional lengthening of the iliopsoas, which is performed at the pelvic brim in ambulators. Preservation of hip flexion is important.

Hip subluxation and dislocation in cerebral palsy are preventable by appropriate soft tissue release in the young child. When hip dislocation or subluxation develops in the older patient, derotation varization osteotomy of the femur to correct femoral antetorsion and coxa valga, and a shelf acetabuloplasty or Chiari's medial displacement innominate osteotomy are performed (Fig 6–33).*

Equinus deformity of the foot and ankle in the young child and infant is managed by splinting the foot and leg in neutral position and by physical therapy to maintain normal range of motion of the ankle.[22] Exercises are performed to develop cerebral control over the anterior tibial muscle.

*19–21, 24, 26, 29, 46, 49, 50, 52, 57, 61, 67, 71, 78, 79, 90, 91, 96, 115

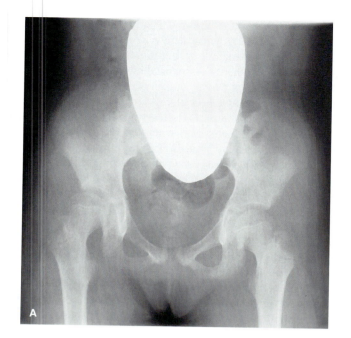

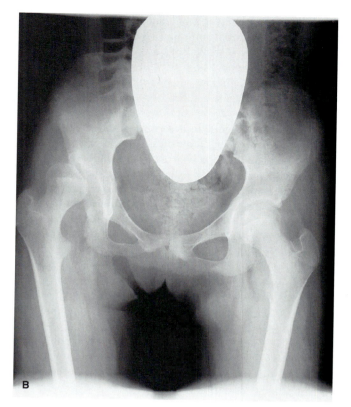

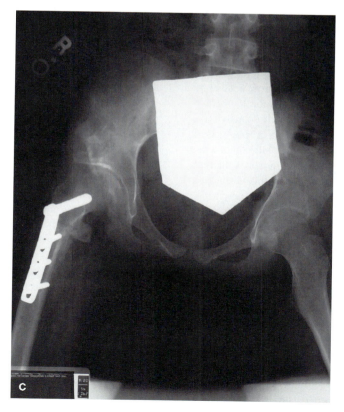

Figure 6–33. Hip subluxation in cerebral palsy. **A.** AP view of the pelvis. Note the minimal subluxation of the right hip at 3 years of age. **B.** At 10 years of age, note the marked dislocation of the hip. This is a preventable deformity. **C.** Six months postoperative showing concentric reduction of the right hip following derotation varization intertrochanteric osteotomy and shelf acetabuloplasty.

When the child begins to stand and walk, a solid and then articulating ankle-foot orthosis (AFO) is given. Fixed equinus deformity is treated by serial casting or botulinum toxin (Botox) injection, both of which are temporary measures providing a window of opportunity for the patient to develop control over a cerebral zero anterior tibial muscle and to develop power of ankle dorsiflexion. If the above measures fail, fixed equinus deformity is corrected by a heel cord lengthening. The requisites are the following: (1) Good sitting and standing balance and potential for walking with or without assistance and (2) Good motor strength of the triceps surae. Do not perform heel cord lengthening when the triceps surae muscle has poor motor strength because calcaneus deformity results, which is more disabling than the equinus deformity. (3) Absence of hip flexion deformity, which should be corrected prior to correction of equinus deformity. (4) A patient who is motivated and cooperative postoperatively. (5) A patient who is at least 3 years of age.

Many techniques of heel cord lengthening are described in the literature; sliding lengthening of the heel cord is carried out when both the gastrocnemius and soleus are contracted and the Vulpius technique of gastrocnemius lengthening when only the gastrocnemius is contracted.

When the posterior tibial muscle is spastic, causing varus deformity of the foot, and dynamic EMG shows continuous activity in both phases of gait, it is lengthened at its musculotendinous juncture. When the posterior tibial is active only during the swing phase of gait and causes varus deformity of the hindfoot, it is split and one half of the tendon is transferred laterally to the peroneus brevis.[45]

An oblique and vertical talus causing hindfoot valgus is treated by the Crawford procedure of subtalar arthroereisis when the deformity can be corrected by passive manipulation.[30] A subtalar stabilization with a bone graft (Grice procedure) or a triple arthrodesis is indicated when the foot is painful and unstable due to muscle weakness. The growth of the foot is not disturbed by the Grice procedure; it is extra-articular. Triple arthrodesis is performed in the skeletally mature foot (10–12 years in girls and 12–14 years in boys).[56]

Flexion deformity of the knee is treated by a fractional lengthening of the hamstrings distally.[34,35,53,55] The requisites are (1) normal or good motor strength of hamstrings and gluteus maximus, (2) ability to flex the knees against gravity and resistance in prone, and to extend the hips against gravity with knees flexed, (3) absence of genu recurvatum, and (4) absence of equinus deformity.

Extension contracture of the knee is managed by passive exercises to elongate the contracted rectus femoris and by active exercises to develop simultaneous knee and hip flexion in gait with dorsiflexion of the ankles. Surgical release of the rectus femoris is indicated when the deformity is severe. An operative prerequisite is that quadriceps femoris muscle strength is at least good. It is contraindicated when there is quadriceps lag and the patient cannot extend the knees fully against gravity. The rectus femoris release is performed distally when there is no associated rotational malalignment (in-toeing or out-toeing); it is performed proximally when there is associated hip flexion contracture. When stiff knee gait is accompanied by in-toeing or out-toeing, the distal insertion of the rectus femoris is transferred to the biceps femoris tendon when the FPA is medial and to the medial hamstrings when the FPA is lateral.[42]

Genu recurvatum is a difficult problem to treat. Initially, always try nonsurgical measures in the form of a solid or articulating AFO in neutral alignment with heel elevation.[93] In mild recurvatum, a simple measure is a rocker sole.

When equinus deformity is present and is a pathogenic factor in genu recurvatum, it is corrected by serial casting and/or Botox injection into the triceps surae; if these nonsurgical measures fail, the triceps surae is lengthened by Vulpius musculotendinous technique. Postoperatively, an aggressive physical therapy regimen is carried out to develop simultaneous knee flexion and ankle dorsiflexion in gait.

In the *upper limbs* surgical measures are delayed until maturation of the CNS is adequate for functional training postoperatively. The objectives of surgery are to improve function, reach, grasp, and release with the hand. Coordination and cerebral control over individual muscles and muscle groups are not provided by surgery.

The adduction and flexion deformities of the thumb are managed by passive stretching exercises in the infant and young child. Several times a day the thumb metacarpal is pulled into abduction and the whole thumb into extension. Do not subluxate the MCP joint of the thumb.

An opponens hand splint for night use and part-time day use is fitted as soon as the child is 2 years of age. The splint holds the thumb metacarpal in maximal abduction and the thumb in neutral extension. The MCP joint should be stabilized, and the thumb should not slip proximally through the splint and cause dorsal subluxation. Such nonsurgical measures may prevent development of myostatic contracture of the thumb adductors and flexors.

Surgery is indicated when the thumb-in-palm posture hinders grasp by the fingers and/or when the thumb cannot be opposed or side-pinched to the index finger.

Botox injection in the thumb adductors may be tried preoperatively; it causes temporary paralysis for a period of about 3 to 6 months.[59] Aggressive postinjection therapy and splinting are carried out to determine whether the patient will develop active thumb abduction and extension.

Adduction contracture of the thumb is released in the palm at its origin from the metacarpal; releasing the adductor pollicis at its origin preserves some function of thumb abduction, which is important for pinch.[63,64] In severe thumb web contracture, in addition to the release of the thumb adductor, the first dorsal interosseous is released by stripping it from the first metacarpal. Occasionally Z-plasty of the contracted thumb web is performed.

Flexion contracture of the thumb is treated by fractional lengthening of the flexor pollicis longus at its musculotendinous juncture. Do not overlengthen the long thumb flexor!

Hyperextension and dorsal subluxation of the MCP joint of the thumb is treated by capsulodesis of the MCP joint.[36] Detach the volar capsule proximally from the metacarpal, advance it proximally, and fix it to the metacarpal neck with a pull-out suture. Use a smooth pin for internal fixation with the MCP joint in 30 degrees of flexion for a period of 3 weeks. The procedure is effective in providing stability to the MCP joint.

Tendon transfer to develop thumb abduction and extension is indicated when the thumb abductors and extensors continue to remain cerebral zero following adductor and flexor release and the patient is unable to actively abduct and extend the thumb. Prerequisites for tendon transfers to the thumb abductor and extensor pollicis are a stable MCP joint of the thumb and full passive range of abduction of the first metacarpal and extension of the thumb. The procedure should not be performed when pinch is weak. The muscles that may be transferred are the brachioradialis, flexor digitorum sublimus of the ring finger, and palmaris longus.[65]

Swan-neck deformity of long fingers is treated by the Swanson procedure, in which the PIP joint is tenodesed. A single slip of the flexor digitorum superficialis is divided proximally, leaving its distal attachment and the other slip intact. The sectioned stub of the superficialis slip is tautly sutured with pull-out technique to the distal end of the proximal phalanx with the PIP joint in 30 degrees of flexion. A small, smooth pin is used for internal fixation, which is removed in 3 weeks and the pull-out suture in 6 weeks.[110]

Flexion deformity of the fingers is corrected by fractional lengthening of the flexor digitorum superficialis and profundus at its musculotendinous juncture.

Pronation contracture of the forearm is treated by musculotendinous lengthening of the pronator teres near its insertion.

Flexion and ulnar deviation deformity of the wrist and pronation deformity of the forearm are treated by transfer of the flexor carpi ulnaris to the extensor carpi radialis longus and brevis when the patient can actively extend the fingers with the wrist in functional extended position.[47,48] When the patient cannot extend the fingers with the wrist in neutral dorsiflexion, the flexor carpi ulnaris is transferred to the finger extensors.[51]

■ PROGRESSIVE MUSCULAR DYSTROPHY

The term *progressive muscular dystrophy* encompasses a spectrum of primary degenerative noninflammatory diseases of voluntary muscles which are genetically determined. The pathologic changes in the dystrophic muscles are primary and not secondary to abnormality of the CNS or peripheral nerves.

The heredity, age of onset, group of muscles involved by the dystrophic process, clinical picture, and rate of progression of muscular weakness vary in the different types of muscular dystrophy. Molecular and genetic studies are making great strides in our understanding of muscular dystrophies.

Muscular dystrophies can be classified into two general categories: (1) pure muscular dystrophy and (2) dystrophies with myotonia.

From the *genetic standpoint,* they can be subclassified into (A) *X-linked recessive:* (1) Duchenne muscular dystrophy, (2) Becker muscular dystrophy, and (3) Emery-Dreifuss muscular dystrophy; (B) *autosomal dominant:* (1) facioscapulohumeral muscular dystrophy (Landouzy-Déjérine), (2) distal muscular dystrophy (Gowers), and (3) myotonic dystrophy; and (C) *autosomal recessive:* (1) limb girdle, (2) infantile facioscapulohumeral, and (3) congenital muscular dystrophy.

DUCHENNE MUSCULAR DYSTROPHY

This is the most common type of muscular dystrophy, occurring at a rate of 1 of every 3500 live male births. It is inherited as an X-linked recessive trait. Only males are affected, and only females are carriers. When the mother is a carrier, 50 percent of the daughters are carriers. In about one third of the patients, the disorder occurs as a new mutation. The defective gene is located on the Xp 21 region of the X chromosome, spanning 2 million pairs and including 65 exons. It encodes the 400-kilodalton protein dystrophin.[144,145]

History and Examination. The presenting complaint is walking on toes or a waddling gait. The patient runs clumsily; he has difficulty in rising from the floor, climbing stairs, hopping, or jumping. These symptoms develop insidiously and are noted by the parents between 2 and 4 years of age. Ask about details of motor development—holding the head up, unsupported sitting, standing, and independent walking are delayed. Obtain a family history. Duchenne muscular dystrophy is hereditary; a positive family history is present in about two thirds of the cases. It is important to rule out CNS disorders such as CP and peripheral neuropathy.

On examination the calf muscles are enlarged due to pseudohypertrophy caused by accumulation of fat. In stance, the posture is poor, with excessive lumbar lordosis, a protuberant abdomen, and the shoulders carried behind the pelvis. Ask the child to stand on one leg; it is difficult. The Trendelenburg test is positive. The gait is toe-heel or toe-toe with a gluteus maximus, gluteus medius, and quadriceps limp. He walks on a wide base, placing his feet wide apart to increase his base of support. Perform Gowers' test.[140] Ask him to lie supine on the floor and get up from the floor without the use of his upper limbs for support.

He cannot; he rolls over from supine to prone, puts his hands on his knees, and pushes his trunk upward by "climbing" his hands up his thighs (see Fig 1–29C). There is an extension lag of the quadriceps. Muscle weakness is symmetric.

Initially the muscles of the pelvic girdle are involved, followed by those of the shoulder girdle. Lift the patient under his axillae; he slides through the examiner's hands. This is referred to as Meryon's sign or "slip-through" sign.[156]

Natural Course. The course of Duchenne muscular dystrophy is one of steady, rapid, relentless progression of muscle degeneration and weakness. The average age when walking ceases is about 10 years, with a range of 8 to 14 years. The weak gluteus maximus and medius and quadriceps are unable to stabilize the hips and knees. Periods of bed rest due to acute illness or operations cause rapid deterioration. Aggressive rehabilitation and orthopedic measures (release of contractures and KAFO) prolong ability to walk by 1 to 3.5 years. Ordinarily by age 12 years the patient is unable to walk even with orthotic support and is wheelchair bound. Motorized electric wheelchairs provide some independence in ambulatory performance.

Equinus deformity of the ankles develops first, followed by progressive flexion contracture of the hips, knees, and elbows. Weakness of the trunk and abdominal muscles leads to gravitational collapse of the spine and progressive scoliosis. The onset of scoliosis always follows losing the ability to walk; prolongation of walking ability delays the onset of scoliosis.[166] The apex of the long C curve is at the lower thoracic level, and the curve extends into the pelvis, causing pelvic obliquity and making sitting difficult and painful. The collapsing spine also results in thoracolumbar kyphosis.

By age 16 years the patient loses the ability to sit and is bedridden. Instability of the spine and severe kyphoscoliosis are the causes of loss of sitting ability. The patient is unable to go to school. With progression of dystrophy, the patient loses the ability to move his limbs. There may be some flexion-extension of the fingers and toes. By age 19 years the patient dies because of respiratory failure and pulmonary infection and collapse. Life may be prolonged by tracheostomy and a portable respirator; but the indications for such heroic measures are controversial. Eventually the cardiac muscles degenerate, infiltrate with fat, and undergo fibrosis. Intellectual development is impaired in patients with Duchenne muscular dystrophy. When a patient lives past the age of 22 years, he most probably has Becker's muscular dystrophy and not the Duchenne type.

Diagnosis. Tentative diagnosis of muscular dystrophy is made by the clinical findings. The following laboratory tests are performed to confirm the diagnosis of muscular dystrophy and to specify its type: (1) *Serum enzymes—CPK and aldolase* are markedly elevated—10 to 50 times the normal. The high level of CPK is due to release of the enzymes with degeneration of the muscle cells. The severity of muscle dystrophy is not reflected by the level of CPK. With progression of the dystrophy and loss of muscle tissue, the elevated CPK levels gradually decline. The level of serum aldolase correlates rather well with that of CPK. In neuromuscular disorders due to abnormality of the CNS or peripheral nerves, the levels of CPK and aldolase are normal or only slightly elevated. CPK differentiates a myopathic process from a neurogenic affection. (2) *Electrophysiologic tests.* Nerve conduction is normal. EMG shows a pattern of low amplitude, short duration, and polyphasic motor unit potentials; these EMG changes are nonspecific. EMG and nerve conduction studies are performed to distinguish neuropathy from myopathy. (3) *Muscle biopsy.* Histologic confirmation of muscular dystrophy is an integral part of the diagnostic work-up. In Duchenne's muscular dystrophy a biopsy of the vastus lateralis is performed. Open biopsy is performed in most patients. Needle biopsy is indicated when small pieces of tissue are required for specific tests. Specimens for light microscopy are frozen in liquid nitrogen immediately, whereas those for electromicroscopic studies are fixed immediately in 4 percent glutaraldehyde in the operating room. The stage of dystrophy determines the histologic findings. In the *early phase* there is variation in fiber size intermixed with focal areas of degenerating or regenerating fibers. With progression of the dystrophy, variation in fiber size becomes more severe, with round dark-staining fibers and areas of endomysial connective and fatty tissue. Later on the muscle fibers are lost and replaced by fibrous and fatty tissue. It is important to obtain muscle tissue that grossly appears normal and is not fibrofatty. (4) *Dystrophin testing and DNA mutation analysis.* The dystrophin test (dystrophin blotting) makes a definitive biochemical diagnosis of Duchenne muscular dystrophy and differentiates it from the less severe Becker muscular dystrophy. In Duchenne muscular dystrophy the intracellular protein dystrophin is completely absent, whereas in Becker muscular dystrophy it is present but is either decreased in amount or altered in size. It also predicts the severity of these two types of muscular dystrophy. Only a small amount of frozen muscle tissue is required, and the test is readily available in most medical centers.

In the early stages, the clinical picture of limb-girdle muscular dystrophy, Emery-Dreifuss muscular dystrophy, congenital myopathy, and dermatomyositis is similar to the Duchenne and Becker types of muscular dystrophy. In these muscle disorders, the dystrophin test is normal.

DNA mutation analysis (polymerase chain reaction or DNA [Southern] blot analysis) is performed on a small sample of blood. It makes a definitive diagnosis and identifies carriers. It also provides prenatal diagnosis in 75 percent of the cases by amniocentesis and amniotic fluid analysis.

Treatment. Prevention by detection of carriers of Duchenne muscular dystrophy is possible in about 65 percent of the cases. If the mother is known to be a carrier and the fetus is determined to be male, termination of pregnancy may be considered as a preventive measure. Prenatal diagnosis of Duchenne muscular dystrophy with complete certainty is not possible at present.

Myoblast transfer therapy and DNA gene transfer therapy appear to hold a definite promise in reversing the biochemical defect in Duchenne muscular dystrophy. At present these modalities of therapy are exploratory.

Prednisone provides some short-term benefit in ameliorating progressive weakness, but long-term use of steroids is contraindicated because of its side effects—weight gain, osteoporosis, and myopathy.

Orthopedic Management. The objectives are to align and support the musculoskeletal system and initially prolong ambulation and then sitting as long as possible. It is vital to be honest and realistic in management of the child with Duchenne muscular dystrophy; care is best provided in a muscle disease multidisciplinary treatment clinic.

Factors to assess are (1) the degree of motor weakness, (2) contractural deformity of joints (equinus, flexion deformity of the knees and hips, lateral rotation-abduction contracture of the hips), (3) obesity, and (4) emotional and intellectual development of the child. The outlook is poor for fat, poorly motivated, noncommunicative, and nonintelligent boys. Inactivity causes disuse atrophy of muscles.

Sequentially the following stages of surgical care are provided: (1) *ambulatory* (the patient is still able to walk), (2) *rehabilitative*—when the patient has lost the ability to walk, but with appropriate release of contractural deformities and external support, within 3 to 6 months walking can be resumed and prolonged for an additional 2 to 3 years; (3) *palliative*—to provide comfort in sitting in a wheelchair or in lying posture.

In the walking patient, beware of premature lengthening of the heel cord, as it shifts weight-bearing posteriorly and destabilizes the knee. The use of night splints to prevent equinus and knee flexion deformity is questionable; they aggravate atrophy.

Walking ability is prolonged by a Vulpius heel cord lengthening when moderate equinus of the ankle has developed but the quadriceps femoris function is still good, with minimal or no flexion contracture of the hips and knees. Anterior transfer of the posterior tibial tendon through the interosseous route removes a deforming force and prevents recurrence of equinovarus deformity. Although it does not adequately function as a dorsiflexor, it does provide a tenodesing effect. Passive stretching exercises are performed to attempt delay of development of flexion deformity of the hips and knees.

Iliotibial band release and lengthening of hamstrings are performed when flexion deformities of the hips and

knees develop. KAFOs are used to lock the knees in extension and stabilize them. The usefulness of KAFOs is limited; walking with KAFOs is difficult. The patient stands with support. It is best to perform surgical correction of contractural deformities prior to loss of ability to walk; it is easier for the patient to maintain than to regain walking.

Collapsing spine and progressive scoliosis cannot be controlled by orthotic support because the patient cannot shift his trunk from pressure areas; the muscles are weak. TLSOs do not work; the curve progresses relentlessly.

Spinal fusion is indicated when the scoliosis is 30 degrees or more or the vital capacity is 40 percent or less—whichever occurs first. A double L-shaped unit rod segmental instrumentation inserted into the pelvis by the Galveston technique provides adequate correction of the degree of the curvature and control of the pelvic obliquity. Sitting in a wheelchair is improved. The vital capacity of the lungs increases.[130,136,180,187] When respiratory failure occurs, tracheostomy and a portable respirator prolong life.

BECKER MUSCULAR DYSTROPHY[126–128,144,145,148,177]

This benign form of muscular dystrophy occurs in 1 in 30,000 live male births. Clinically it is characterized by later onset in childhood than the Duchenne type and a course of slower progression of muscle weakness. Inheritance is X-linked. Muscle weakness is less severe, and the affected patients are able to walk until late in adolescence or into their 20s and occasionally into adulthood. Respiratory problems are much less, and they live longer than those with the Duchenne type. Becker's muscular dystrophy can be distinguished from Duchenne muscular dystrophy by molecular and genetic studies.[127,145]

Treatment. Equinus deformity is corrected by heel cord lengthening. The posterior tibial tendon is transferred anteriorly if functioning. In general, AFOs or KAFOs are better tolerated in patients with Becker's muscular dystrophy than in the Duchenne type. In late stages of the disease when the patient becomes wheelchair bound, scoliosis may develop. It is managed by stabilization of the spine with fusion and instrumentation when severe and progressive.

EMERY-DREIFUSS MUSCULAR DYSTROPHY[132,134,170]

The presenting complaints are an awkward gait, toe-walking, and muscle weakness. These symptoms gradually develop during childhood. In the adolescent the distinctive clinical features become fully established: (1) fixed equinus deformity of the foot and ankle; (2) flexion deformity of the elbows; (3) contracture of the extension of the neck and paravertebral muscles of the lumbar and thoracic spine; and (4) cardiac abnormalities consisting of bradycardia and atrioventricular heart block. Muscle weakness progresses slowly; most affected patients maintain the ability to walk until the fifth or sixth decade of life. Obesity and equinus deformity impede ambulation, causing loss of ability to walk when the patient is 30 to 40 years of age. Scoliosis of a minimal to moderate degree develops in most patients; however, it does not progress relentlessly. It seems that soft tissue rigidity of the spine stabilizes the spinal curvature.

Genetics. Emery-Dreifuss muscular dystrophy is transmitted as an X-linked recessive disorder. The fully developed phenotype is seen only in the male. Linkage studies have shown that the site of the gene locus is in the long arm of the X chromosome at xq28.[132]

Treatment. Equinus deformity is treated by heel cord lengthening. Anterior transfer of the posterior tibial muscle and appropriate night and day orthotics prevent recurrence of deformity. Flexion deformity of the elbow and extension contracture of the neck and thoracolumbar spine are managed by active and passive stretching range-of-motion exercises.[170] The most serious problem is the bradycardia and the atrioventricular heart block; they are treated by implantation of a cardiac pacemaker.

CONGENITAL MUSCULAR DYSTROPHY[125,192]

This form of muscular dystrophy manifests at birth. It is autosomal recessive in inheritance and is present in both genders. The presenting complaint is motor weakness of the limbs, trunk, and facial muscles. The infant has difficulty in sucking and swallowing. Most patients have marked contracture of their joints, a common deformity is talipes equinovarus. The stiffness of the joints tends to increase with growth and immobilization in splints or casts.

Diagnosis is made by muscle biopsy, which shows variation in the diameter of the fibers within each fascicle and increased perimysial and endomysial fibrosis—dystrophic changes similar to those of Duchenne muscular dystrophy. The CPK level is markedly elevated. There are no abnormalities of the dystrophin protein or genes.

The course and prognosis are variable. In type I, the weakness stabilizes or improves with time. The affected child is able to walk by 2 years of age and lives well into adulthood. A few patients deteriorate rapidly with marked progressive degeneration of the muscles and do not survive after the first year of life.[192] In type II (referred to as Fukuyama congenital muscular dystrophy), there is marked retardation of motor and mental development and severe contracture of the joints; these patients do not survive the first decade of life.

Treatment in type I congenital muscular dystrophy should be aggressive in the form of passive range-of-mo-

tion exercises, splints, and soft tissue release. Developmental therapy is beneficial in these affected infants and children. Orthotic support is well tolerated.

LIMB GIRDLE MUSCULAR DYSTROPHY

This type comprises a heterogeneous group in which the proximal muscles of the limbs—scapulohumeral and/or pelvicofemoral—are involved. Inheritance is autosomal recessive; however, autosomal dominant forms and sporadic cases do occur. Onset is usually in the adolescent age group, and the course of the disease is one of slow progression.

The presenting complaints are forward drooping of the shoulders, winging of the scapulae, difficulty in elevating the arms in the scapulohumeral type, and difficulty in getting up from the floor and climbing stairs in the pelvicofemoral type. Ordinarily the shoulder girdle is affected first. When it begins in the pelvic girdle, it is referred to as the Leyden form.[155]

Diagnosis. CPK levels are elevated 10 times normal. EMG and histology findings of muscle tissue are those of myopathy. A dystrophin test establishes the diagnosis.

Treatment is similar to that of Becker's muscular dystrophy.

FACIOSCAPULOHUMERAL MUSCULAR DYSTROPHY (LANDOUZY-DÉJÉRINE)[153]

The presenting complaints are (1) weakness of the facial muscles, which manifests by absence of wrinkles on the forehead and eyes, difficulty in closing the eyes, a transverse smile, and progressive muscle weakness causing indistinct speech, and (2) shoulder girdle muscle weakness, limitation of shoulder abduction, and winging of the scapulae.

The pattern of muscle weakness in the shoulder is unique; the weak muscles are those that fix the scapula to the thoracic wall (the trapezius, levator scapulae, and rhomboids) and the muscles that elevate and control the glenohumeral joint (deltoid, supraspinatus, infraspinatus, and subscapularis) are strong.

The defective gene is located on chromosome 4q.[189] Inheritance is autosomal dominant. The prevalence is 1 in 20,000.[161]

Onset of the dystrophy is usually late childhood or early adolescence. Progression of muscle weakness is insidious and gradual with periods of arrest. Eventually the disease spreads to the lower limbs with weakness of the dorsiflexors of the foot and ankle, resulting in drop foot. This type is referred to as scapuloperoneal dystrophy. Longevity is normal.

Treatment. Stabilization of the scapulae to the rib cage by soft tissue (fascia lata or Mersilene tape) eliminates winging of the scapulae and improves motor strength and range of shoulder elevation and abduction.[151] Arthrodesis of the shoulder to the ribs with internal fixation with a wire plate is another alternative but is not recommended by this author because of complications.[154] Later on when drop foot develops, it is managed by an AFO and tendon transfer.

INFANTILE FACIOSCAPULOHUMERAL MUSCULAR DYSTROPHY

This rare form of muscular dystrophy presents in infancy with weakness of facial muscles, sensorineural loss of hearing, scapular winging, severe lumbar lordosis due to weak gluteus maximus muscle, with normal strength of antagonist hip flexors and foot drop due to weakness of peroneal muscles.

Inheritance appears to be autosomal recessive; the gene responsible has not yet been identified.

Natural History. The children begin to ambulate at a normal age, but the muscle weakness increases rapidly. They use their hands to stabilize the hips posteriorly. Most patients lose their ability to walk in adolescence and become wheelchair bound. Progressive weakness of the thoracic muscles results in respiratory problems.

Treatment. Severe lordosis and fixed flexion contractures of the hips are very disabling and difficult to manage. Orthotic devices are ineffective. Lordotic posture is required to maintain sitting or standing balance. Scapuloplexy is indicated to stabilize scapulocostal articulation and increase range of shoulder abduction.[172]

DISTAL MUSCULAR DYSTROPHY (GOWERS')

In this rare type initial involvement is that of the distal limb musculature; the small muscles of the hands and feet are affected. The presenting complaint is clumsiness and loss of fine coordination in the hands and drop foot gait due to weakness of the dorsiflexors of the foot and ankle. It affects primarily adults. Inheritance is autosomal dominant, affecting both genders equally. The course of the disease is benign; the affected patients can expect normal longevity.[139]

MYOTONIC DYSTROPHY (DYSTROPHIA MYOTONICA)

The onset of this type of muscular dystrophy is usually in late adolescence or early adult life. In women, not infrequently the diagnosis is made following the birth of a child who is affected by the more severe congenital form. Myotonic dystrophy is autosomal dominant in inheritance. The defective gene is linked to chromosome 19q.[167]

The pattern of muscle involvement is that of the face, jaw, eyes, neck, and hands and feet (distal limb musculature). The presenting complaints are generalized clumsiness (particularly of the hands), difficulty in walking and running, and tripping and falling. The characteristic feature in myotonic dystrophy is delayed muscle relaxation. Shake the hand of the patient and let it go. There is delayed release (slowness in relaxation) of the hand grip. The muscle indentation sign is positive—it is elicited by a sharp percussion with the tip of your long finger on the muscle belly of the thenar eminence or tongue. Dimpling persists for a while due to delayed muscle relaxation.

The cervical spine is in exaggerated lordosis due to weakness of the sternocleidomastoid muscles. The facial appearance is expressionless and haggard due to atrophy of the masseters, narrowing of the lower half of the face and mandible, and bilateral drooping of the upper lids. The patient has difficulty in whistling and pursing the lips. Dysarthria is common. Weakness of the laryngeal muscles causes a monotonous and nasal tone to the voice. The course of the disease may be slowly progressive or static. In the adult, frontal baldness develops in men and cataracts and glaucoma in both genders. Mental development may be normal or slightly retarded.

Diagnosis. Diagnosis is made by the EMG findings of dive bomber pattern. The serum CPK and aldolase levels are normal. The muscle biopsy shows some internal nuclei and type I atrophy; these are nonspecific. Genetic studies disclose the abnormality of the chromosome 19q.

Treatment. Musculoskeletal deformities such as varus of the heel are minimal, and no special orthopedic management is required.

CONGENITAL MYOTONIC DYSTROPHY

In this condition, there is a strong family history of myotonic dystrophy, the phenotype becoming increasingly severe with each succeeding generation. The mother has mild or previously undetected myotonic dystrophy, and the baby is born with severe congenital myotonic dystrophy. Prenatal diagnosis can be made when the defective gene is localized to chromosome 19.[178] The severity of the phenotype appears to correlate with the length of the trinucleotide (GTG at the 3' end of a protein-kinin gene on chromosome 19).

The newborn patient presents with severe hypotonia, facial diplegia, a long narrow face, and respiratory stridor. He has difficulty in sucking and swallowing and breastfeeding. Severe clubfoot is present in most patients. Walking is delayed up to 4 to 5 years of age. Some patients never walk independently. Mental retardation from a moderate to severe degree is present in most patients.

Congenital muscular dystrophy should be differentiated from various congenital myopathies such as nemaline (rod-body), central core, centronuclear (myotubular), and congenital fiber-type disproportion. The reader is referred to the excellent reviews by Goebel and Shapiro.[138,169]

Treatment.   Clubfoot is treated by soft-tissue release and support in an AFO. Developmental therapy and walkers are indicated for ambulation. Special sitting devices and TLSO are required for support of the collapsing spine.

MYOTONIA CONGENITA (THOMSEN'S DISEASE)

In this extremely rare condition the presenting complaints are stiffness in walking or running, frequent falling, and clumsiness. After the child has been lying down or sitting for a while, he has difficulty in initiating active movements. Repetitive movements, such as walking, make the patient more supple. Often these children are delayed in motor development. There is no muscle weakness and no associated musculoskeletal deformities. Life expectancy is normal.

Julius Thomsen, who first described myotonia congenita, suffered himself from the disease.[182] The condition is hereditary, and most cases are inherited by autosomal dominant transmission. Some cases are inherited by recessive pattern.

Diagnosis.   Myotonia, the salient feature of the disease, is characterized by a state of delayed relaxation of voluntary muscles following voluntary contraction or mechanical or electrical stimulation. Tap the surface of a voluntary muscle sharply with your fingertip, pencil, or reflex hammer. The muscle at the site of stimulation contracts and remains contracted.

The EMG shows a rapid volley of action potentials. The serum levels of CPK and aldolase are normal. In the differential diagnosis consider myotonic dystrophy and paramyotonia congenita.

Treatment.   Myotonia is ameliorated by oral intake of quinine sulfate or procaineamide.

PARAMYOTONIA CONGENITA OF EULENBERG

In this form of myotonia, onset is in infancy or early childhood, and the proximal muscles of the limbs, eyelids, and tongue are involved. Inheritance is autosomal dominant with equal affection of males and females.

Myotonia is the salient physical finding. The intermittent attacks of muscle weakness may last a few minutes to several hours. Exposure to cold precipitates the myotonia. Activity aggravates it. This is in contrast to myotonia congenita, in which activity improves the myotonia.

EMG shows rapid volley of action potentials. Serum CPK and aldolase levels are normal. Histologic findings are similar to those in myotonic dystrophy.

The natural course is nonprogressive. Paramyotonia congenita improves with age; there is no specific treatment. Musculoskeletal deformities do not develop.

■ HEREDITARY MOTOR AND SENSORY NEUROPATHIES (HMSN)

This heterogeneous group of degenerative disorders of peripheral nerves, nerve roots, and often the spinal cord is characterized by distal muscular atrophy and weakness associated with varying degrees of sensory deficit. According to Dyck and Lambert, HMSN can be subclassified into the following types: (1) HMSN type I—the typical form of Charcot-Marie-Tooth disease, including the Roussy-Levy syndrome. HMSN type I is divided into two subgroups: HMSN type IA—not linked to the Duffy blood group focus and chromosome 1; and HMSN type 1B, which is linked to the Duffy blood group or chromosome 1. The onset of symptoms in type 1 HMSN is between 5 and 15 years of age, whereas type 2 HMSN manifests in the third decade of life. (2) HMSN type II—the neuronal form of Charcot-Marie-Tooth disease. (3) HMSN type III—Déjérine-Sottas disease, the familial hypertrophic interstitial neuritis of infancy and childhood. (4) Type IV—Refsum's disease. (5) HMSN type V—familial spastic paraplegia. (6) HMSN type VI—similar to HMSN type I, but in addition, the patient has optic atrophy. (7) HMSN type VII—which is similar to type I but the patient has retinitis pigmentosa.[203]

CHARCOT-MARIE-TOOTH DISEASE OR PERONEAL MUSCULAR ATROPHY (HMSN TYPE I)*

HMSN type I is inherited as an autosomal dominant trait. The presenting complaint is a high arch of the foot (pes cavus) and/or clawing of the toes. The child has difficulty in running on uneven ground, discomfort under the metatarsal heads, and muscle cramps in the feet and legs.

The muscle weakness is symmetric and distal in distribution; it begins in the intrinsic muscles of the foot and soon involves the peroneals. Imbalance of muscles acting on the foot and ankle results in cavovarus deformity of the foot. Recurrent instability of the ankle is not uncommon.

Later on the muscle weakness slowly extends to the muscles of the anterior compartment, involving the anterior tibial and toe extensors. The weak ankle dorsiflexors opposed by a strong triceps surae cause equinus deformity of the ankle and a toe-heel gait. Muscle atrophy does not in-

---

*195–198, 208–214, 219–220, 229–231

volve the proximal thigh or pelvic girdle. The slender legs with clawed toes and plump thighs give the appearance of "ostrich or stork legs," resembling an inverted champagne bottle.

Much later the muscles of the hands and forearms are involved, resulting in mild to moderate clawing of the fingers and weakness or loss of opposition of the thumb. The arm and shoulder girdle muscles are usually not affected. Mild scoliosis develops in 10 percent of the patients.

On neurologic examination, vibration and position sense are decreased. The ankle jerk is decreased initially and later absent. Loss of radial periosteal reflex develops much later. The patellar, biceps, and triceps reflexes are preserved. In type IA, HMSN motor nerve conduction velocity of peripheral nerves is decreased to 50 percent of normal. Ataxia is not present. Intelligence is normal.

The course of HMSN type IA is one of very slow progression. The final disability is not marked. Life expectancy is normal.

Roussy-Levy syndrome is a forme fruste of Charcot-Marie-Tooth disease. The clinical presence of bilateral pes cavus, atrophy of the intrinsic muscles of the foot and peroneals, and decreased or absent ankle reflex is very similar to HMSN type I. Static tremor of the hands is present in Roussy-Levy syndrome and absent in Charcot-Marie-Tooth disease. Motor nerve conduction is slow in Roussy-Levy syndrome, similar to that of Charcot-Marie-Tooth disease. Ataxia and cerebellar signs are absent in both conditions.[223,224]

Treatment. In the initial stages, passive exercises are performed to maintain flexibility of the toes and forefeet. At periodic intervals the degree of muscle atrophy and progression of the disease are monitored by muscle testing.

When drop foot develops, the posterior tibial tendon is transferred anteriorly through the interosseous route to provide dorsiflexion to the ankle. Triple arthrodesis corrects deformity of the hindfoot and provides stability to the foot; it is performed in the skeletally mature patient.[139]

HYPERTROPHIC INTERSTITIAL NEURITIS OF DÉJÉRINE AND SOTTAS (HMSN TYPE II)[199,215]

This is inherited as an autosomal recessive trait. The presenting complaints are muscle weakness in the lower limbs which causes delay in walking, and an unsteady gait with frequent falls and difficulty in going up and down stairs and running. The child may complain of paresthesia and shooting pains in the limbs. Soon progressive cavus deformity of the feet develops, followed by paralysis of the intrinsic muscles of the hand and flexion deformity of the fingers.

On neurologic examination, sensory loss involves all modalities: anesthesia to light touch, pin prick, vibration,

and position sense. The Romberg sign is positive. The superficial abdominal umbilical skin reflex and cremasteric reflex are lost. The ankle jerk is decreased or absent. On palpation, enlargement of the nerves is noted. Sensory loss and motor weakness cause progressive incoordination.

Diagnostic Studies. Nerve conduction is delayed. EMG shows the finding of muscle atrophy of neural origin. Evoked sensory potentials are decreased or absent. MRI demonstrates spinal nerve root enlargement.

Serum CPK and aldolase are elevated. The total protein of CSF is high. Muscle biopsy shows neural atrophy. Nerve biopsy (usually of the lateral sural nerve) shows enlargement of the nerves due to proliferation of perineural and endoneural connective tissue. The axon cylinders decrease and eventually disappear. Proliferation of the Schwann cells gives the so-called onion bulb formation, which is characteristic of hypertrophic interstitial neuritis.

Treatment. Orthopedic management consists of passive range-of-motion exercises and splinting of the parts to keep them out of deformity. Prednisone ameliorates the symptoms; it is indicated in severe cases.

The disease progresses slowly, with remissions and exacerbations. Life expectancy is normal.

REFSUM'S DISEASE (HMSN TYPE IV)

This is inherited as an autosomal recessive trait. The presenting complaints are similar to other HMSN types— weakness and atrophy of the distal muscles of the limbs, unsteady gait, pes cavus deformity, absence of deep tendon reflexes, and decrease or absence of vibration and position sense.

The distinguishing clinical feature of Refsum's disease is retinitis pigmentosa. The phytic acid level of the serum is elevated, a finding pathognomonic of Refsum's disease.[206,207,222]

Treatment. Dietary deletion of foods containing phytol, phytic acid, or their precursors decreases the level of phytic acid in the blood and provides some relief of symptoms.

CONGENITAL INSENSITIVITY TO PAIN

This rare disorder is characterized by complete sensory loss to pain—protective, subjective, and objective response to noxious stimuli are absent. The central and peripheral nerves and autonomic system are intact and intelligence is normal.[200,218]

The child presents with multiple bruises, burns, sores of the fingertips, lips, and tongue induced by biting. Corneal opacities due to injury are commonly present. The patient does not feel pain and does not cry when hurt.

Deformity of the limbs due to malunion of unrecognized fracture, traumatic dislocations, osteomyelitis, and later on swollen joints due to Charcot-like changes are common.

A thorough evaluation of the CNS and peripheral nervous system is essential, preferably by a pediatric neurologist. In the differential diagnosis of congenital insensitivity to pain, one should consider familial dysautonomia (Riley-Day syndrome), congenital sensory neuropathy, hereditary sensory radicular neuropathy, familial sensory neuropathy with anhidrosis, and acquired sensory neuropathy, toxic or infectious. Riley-Day syndrome is inherited as an autosomal recessive trait and is characterized by absence of fungiform papillae on the tongue, the lack of lacrimation, excessive perspiration, and poor temperature control.

Treatment.   There is no specific treatment. Once the diagnosis is made, the parents and primary care health personnel should have a high index of suspicion for fractures and infections. When treated early they heal. As the child matures he learns how to take care of himself and prevent recurrent trauma.

FRIEDREICH'S ATAXIA (HEREDITARY SPINOCEREBELLAR ATAXIA)[234–254]

A child between 7 and 10 years of age is presented with the complaint of unsteady gait, a tendency to stagger and fall, and difficulty making sudden turns. The parents complain that the child is clumsy. The symptoms have an insidious onset and progress steadily. In time ataxia of the upper limbs develops; the child cannot eat without spilling food because of ineptness in handling a fork or spoon.

Genetic studies have shown the defect on chromosome 9 with two loci (D955 and D9515) that are linked to Friedreich's ataxia. Take a detailed family history. The ataxia is hereditary. Often Friedreich's ataxia can be traced through generations of a family tree. The prevalence is 1 in 50,000 live births. In North America, it is common in people of French Canadian origin. It is transmitted as an autosomal recessive trait; however, autosomal dominant forms do occur.

The disease is caused by degenerative changes in the dorsal and ventral spinocerebellar tracts, the corticospinal tracts, and the posterior column in the spinal cord. The Purkinje cells and the dentate nuclei in the cerebellum undergo progressive atrophy. The anterior horn cells in the spinal cord are usually unaffected. The exact cause of Friedreich's ataxia remains obscure.

Examination.   The gait is ataxic and unsteady. The child cannot walk in tandem—heel to toe to heel. The feet are placed irregularly, and the patient sways and reels.

Ask the patient to stand still on both feet. He is unsteady. Romberg's sign is positive: When standing with his eyes closed, he or she sways and falls. Ataxia is always greater in the lower than the upper limbs. On performing the finger-to-nose test with the eyes closed, the finger past points. Alternating movements of the hands into pronation and supination in opposite directions are slow and difficult. Subsequently nystagmus and head tremors develop. Speech becomes slurred and explosive.

Inspect the feet. The longitudinal arches are markedly elevated. The pes cavus deformity is symmetric and develops early; it may be the initial physical finding. Initially the equinus deformity of the forefoot is flexible, but soon, with progressive contraction of the plantar soft tissues, the cavus deformity becomes fixed and hindfoot varus develops. Muscle imbalance and paralysis of the peroneals and anterior tibial muscles with a strong posterior tibial muscle aggravate the deformity.

Scoliosis is present in almost 90 percent of these patients; it is thoracic and steadily progressive.

The patellar tendon and ankle deep tendon reflexes are absent. The biceps and triceps tendon reflexes are decreased and are eventually absent. The Babinski sign is positive on plantar stimulation. On sensory examination, position, vibration, and two-point discrimination are lost. The course of Friedreich's ataxia is steadily progressive. The patient loses the ability to walk and becomes wheelchair bound.

Myocarditis eventually develops and the patient dies of cardiac failure before the age of 40 years.[236]

Treatment.   Surgical correction of the pes cavus deformity by plantar release and provision of ankle dorsiflexion by anterior transfer of the posterior tibial tendon prolongs the period of walking. AFOs provide stability to the foot.[242]

Progressive scoliosis is treated by arthrodesis with internal instrumentation. Bracing does not control progression of the scoliosis.[239,241]

JUVENILE DERMATOMYOSITIS AND POLYMYOSITIS[255–270]

Juvenile dermatomyositis (JDMS) and polymyositis (PM) are nonhereditary myopathies that are characterized by nonsuppurative inflammation of voluntary muscles associated with degenerative changes and muscle weakness. In dermatomyositis the nonsuppurative inflammatory process involves the skin and manifests in the form of an erythematous skin rash.

JDMS and PM occur in two distinct age groups: (1) juvenile—7 to 15 years of age, and (2) adult—in the fifth and sixth decades of life. Their prevalence is 3 in 1 million per year. In childhood, JDMS is 20 times more common than PM. In North America, JDMS and PM are twice as common in females as in males. The exact cause is unknown; they are considered to be autoimmune disorders.

In JDMS there is a definite association with vasculopathy. Capillary thrombosis involves the skin and nail folds. JDMS with vasculitis involving the gastrointestinal tract is a distinct entity. There is decreased absorption of D-xylose.

Clinical Features. The clinical presentation of JDMS varies greatly. It may have a sudden onset with an acute course or an insidious onset with a chronic course. *Muscle weakness* is the salient feature. Proximal muscle groups are involved first. The child has difficulty in rising from the floor or in climbing stairs. Active elevation of the shoulders is limited—he or she cannot raise the arms to 90 degrees to comb the hair. Soon the disease process involves the sternocleidomastoids: The child is unable to flex his or her neck and lift the head against gravity. Dysphagia and difficulty in swallowing are caused by involvement of the pharyngeal muscles. With progressive involvement of all the muscles of the body, the patient loses the ability to walk and becomes wheelchair bound or confined to bed. In the past, one third of the patients with severe untreated JDMS and PM died, one third were disabled in a wheelchair, and one third resolved. At present, with adequate therapy, the mortality rate has decreased to 2 to 7 percent.

The *skin lesions* in JDMS are quite typical. They consist of (1) an erythematous rash of the cheek, sparing the nasal bridge in a butterfly distribution, (2) heliotype eyelids—a dark lilac discoloration of the upper eyelids, (3) erythematous and atrophic skin on the extensor surface of the elbows, MCP joints, knees, and over the medial malleoli, (4) inflammatory infiltrate of the scalp that may cause partial alopecia, (5) hyperemia of the base of the fingernails, (6) shiny, red, and atrophic fingertips, and (7) vitiligo. In the later stages of dermatomyositis, calcium deposits develop in the subcutaneous tissues.

Nonspecific synovitis of the knees, elbows, wrists, or MCP joints may develop. Vasculitis may cause Reynaud's phenomenon: The fingers become cyanotic or white following exposure to cold or after emotional stress.

Diagnosis. In order to make the diagnosis of polymyositis, the following findings must be present: (1) symmetric proximal (limb-girdle) and sternocleidomastoid muscle weakness, (2) elevation of all or one of the serum enzymes derived from muscle CPK, aldolase, lactate dehydrogenase (LDH), and serum glutamic-oxaloacetic transaminase (SGOT), (3) EMG findings of small, polyphasic motor units, fibrillation, and repetitive discharges—changes indicating inflammation, (4) histopathologic evidence on muscle biopsy of type I and type II fibronecrosis, phagocytosis, regeneration, atrophy in a perifascicular distribution with perivascular inflammatory exudate and occlusion. Criteria for diagnosis of dermatomyositis are a rash characteristic

of dermatomyositis plus three findings listed for differential diagnosis of polymyositis (Table 6–1). In both conditions, rheumatoid diseases should be excluded.

In polymyositis it is vital to perform a muscle biopsy for definitive diagnosis, whereas in dermatomyositis only skin biopsy of the affected sites is carried out. It shows a noninflammatory type of poikiloderma and deposits of mucin, findings distinctive of dermatomyositis.

MRI shows inflammatory changes in muscle and calcification in subcutaneous tissue and muscles. In JDMS and PM the calcium balance is negative due to increased calcium excretion and decreased calcium absorption. The osteocalcin is decreased.

In summary, in a diagnostic work-up of JDMS and PM, the following studies and tests are performed: (1) determination of motor strength by muscle testing performed by a physical therapist, (2) serum CPK, aldolase, LDH, and SGOT, (3) skin biopsy in JDMS and muscle biopsy in PM, (4) EMG of affected muscle, (5) radiography and MRI of the shoulders and pelvic girdle, (6) subungual capillarscopy, and (7) ancillary laboratory tests: (a) erythrocyte sedimentation rate (ESR) normal or slightly elevated in some, (b) complete blood count (CBC) and hemoglobin—white blood count normal or elevated in some; hemoglobin normal or decreased, (d) D-xylose absorption, (e) tests for immunologic and connective tissue disease evaluation—Rh factor, lupus erythematosus cell, and complement activation.

In the differential diagnosis, consider the following: (1) muscular dystrophy, (2) acute myositis, (3) pyomyositis, (4) inclusion body myositis, (5) hereditary myopathies such as McArdle disease.

Treatment. In the acute stages of JDMS and PM, symptomatic relief of the painful muscles is provided by moist applications and rest to the parts. Joint motion is maintained by gentle active and passive exercises. Sun screen greater than SPF16 is applied to the face and exposed areas of the skin, as symptoms often manifest after exposure to sunlight. Corticosteroids (prednisone is preferred) are given to ame-

TABLE 6–1. CRITERIA FOR DIAGNOSIS OF JUVENILE DERMATOMYOSITIS (JDMS) AND POLYMYOSITIS (PM)

	PM	JDMS
1. Symmetric progressive limb girdle and sternocleidomastoid muscle weakness	+	+
2. Elevation of creatine phosphokinase, aldolase, and other muscle-derived enzymes	+	+
3. Electromyography—inflammatory change	+	+
4. Muscle biopsy—histopathology, type I and type II fibronecrosis, perifascicular atrophy, perivascular inflammatory exudate, and vascular occlusion	+	+
5. Skin rash. Erythema typical of dermatomyositis of face, eyelid, and extensor surface of limbs	−	+

liorate the acute inflammatory reaction. In severe cases, immunosuppressants (such as methotrexate, cyclophosphamide, or cyclosporine) are given; this is especially indicated when there is no response to steroid therapy and when vasculitis is present.

Soft tissue calcifications are managed in the early stages by gamma carboxyglutane administration. In the late stages of the disease, the calcified deep fascia and intermuscular septa are excised surgically.

MYELOMENINGOCELE

In this developmental defect of the neural axis, the vertebral arches are not fused and the spinal cord and its membranes are dysplastic. The dura and arachnoid protrude through the defect in the vertebral arches. In myelomeningocele (MM), the dysplastic spinal cord and nerve roots are extruded into the sac. In meningocele, a rare form of spina bifida, spinal cord and nerve roots are not carried out into the sac of the dura and arachnoid.

The exact cause of MM is not known. It most possibly is caused by primary failure of the neural tube secondary to rupture of the once closed neural tube.

The prevalence of MM is 1 to 1.5 per 1000 births. The incidence of MM in the siblings of affected patients is definitely greater than that of the general population. The inheritance pattern of MM is multifactorial.

Antenatal diagnosis can be made by ultrasonography and determination of alpha-fetoprotein (AFP), first in the serum and then in the amniotic fluid obtained by amniocentesis. Longitudinal and transverse scanning by ultrasonography often demonstrates the defect of the vertebral arches and the meningocele sac. AFP level is high. In about 90 percent of cases of open neural tube defects, antenatal diagnosis can be made by combined ultrasonography and determination of AFP levels, first in the serum and then in the amniotic fluid. Amniocentesis is an invasive procedure with 0.5 percent risk of miscarriage.

Following antenatal diagnosis, should the pregnancy be terminated by abortion? This is an individual decision to be made by the parents; it is not acceptable to every parent or physician. During the past decade the incidence of MM has significantly decreased with genetic counseling and prenatal diagnosis.

The external appearance of the meningeal sac filled with cerebrospinal fluid is typical (Fig 6–34). The diagnosis is readily made at birth.

The child with MM has multiple defects in addition to paralysis and musculoskeletal deformities. In the CNS, the Arnold-Chiari malformation, hydrocephalus, hydromyelia, syringomyelia, tethered cord, or diastematomyelia may be present. Paralysis of the bladder and bowel incontinence occur in almost all patients. Sensory loss causes decubitus trophic ulceration of the skin. One half

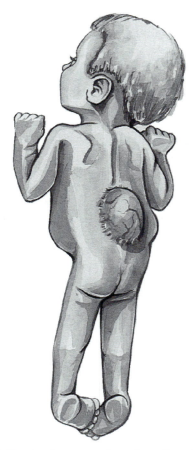

Figure 6–34. The external appearance of a newborn with myelomeningocele.

to one third of the involved patients have intelligence below the normal range.

Assessment. At birth, prior to closure of the meningocele, the orthopedic surgeon determines the neurosegmental level of the lesion and the presence or absence of the deformities of the limbs and spine. In lumbosacral lesions, paralysis of muscles below the neurosegmental level is flaccid; paralysis may be partial or complete. Motor function above the level of involvement is usually normal. Upper limb involvement and disability due to associated lesions at a higher level do occur. Cervicothoracic and higher lesions cause spasticity of muscles.

Determine the presence or absence of deep tendon reflexes. In spastic paralysis they are hyperactive, whereas in flaccid paralysis the deep tendon reflexes are absent. The segmental innervation of the patellar tendon reflex is L3–L4, whereas that of the ankle reflex is S1–S2. Is there clonus? What is the Babinski sign? Is it extensor or plantar stimulation?

Next determine the superficial skin reflexes. The segmental innervation of the abdominal-umbilicus reflex is lower thoracic, whereas that of the cremasteric reflex is

L1–L2. Sensory examination of a newborn or infant is difficult and inadequate; an attempt is made by observing response to pin prick.

Assess motor strength of the muscles of the lower limbs. Accurate grading of muscle strength is difficult. Determine whether muscle activity is absent, present but weak, or present and strong. Often one assesses the power of *muscle groups,* such as the plantar flexors or dorsiflexors of the ankle, knee extensors and flexors, hip abductors and adductors, and hip flexors and extensors. Muscle activity is determined by the active motions of the limb by placing the infant in different positions, use of reflex stimulation techniques, and resting posture of the limb.

Next determine the deformities of the foot, ankle, leg, knee, hip, and trunk. The causes of deformity in MM are (1) intrauterine malposture, (2) static forces of malposture assumed after birth, (3) fibrosis of muscles, (4) dynamic muscle imbalance, and (5) coexisting congenital malformations.

Paralysis of muscles in MM may be *flaccid* due to total loss of spinal cord function distal to a certain neurosegmental level or *reflex spastic* in isolated segments distal to the cord lesion.[343] Muscle imbalance may be between (1) spastic muscle versus flaccid antagonist, (2) spastic muscle versus normal antagonist, or (3) normal muscle versus flaccid antagonist. Deformities and abnormal posture of the limbs are produced by muscle imbalance. Some of the deformities are present at birth, whereas others develop postnatally, either in infancy or later on in childhood or adolescence. Whenever there is asymmetry in paralysis between the right and left sides, the presence of an additional CNS lesion such as diastematomyelia should be ruled out.

Tethering of the spinal cord causes progressive muscle weakness, spasticity, and deformity, such as scoliosis or pes cavus.

When *T12 is the lowest neurosegmental level* functioning, there is complete paralysis of the lower limb muscles. The limb posture is dictated by gravity; the hips posture in flexion, abduction, and lateral rotation, the knees in flexion, and the feet and ankles in equinus. The hips, knees, and ankles develop contractural deformity in the malposture in which they lie. Coxa valga with subsequent hip subluxation may develop later on in childhood. Ordinarily complete hip dislocation does not occur.

When *L1 is the lowest neurosegmental level* functioning, the sartorius muscle is good in motor strength and the iliopsoas muscle is weak (poor). Muscle imbalance with gravity forces of malposture cause flexion and lateral rotation deformity of the hip.

When *L2 is the lowest neurosegmental level* functioning, the sartorius, iliopsoas, hip adductors, and gracilis are strong in motor function. At the L1–L2 neurosegmental level of paralysis, the infant lies supine with the hips in abduction, flexion, and lateral rotation and the knees in flexion. On reflex testing, the cremasteric skin reflex is present,

but the anal skin reflex is absent, and the patellar tendon and ankle deep tendon reflexes are absent.

In the newborn, all hips have flexion deformity; in infancy and childhood, progressive hyperflexion-adduction contracture and coxa valga develop at the L2 neurosegmental level of paralysis. All other muscles are paralyzed and/or fibrotic. In multiple level lesions, there may be reflex spasticity in some muscle groups. Moderate hip subluxation occurs in about four of five patients, and, if untreated, the hips become completely dislocated in about 10 percent of the cases. Contracture of the iliotibial band, paralyzed and fibrosed hamstrings, and posterior capsule of the knee develop in time; these deforming forces cause progressive knee flexion deformity. The feet and ankles develop equinus deformity due to faulty posture.

When *L3 is the lowest neurosegmental level* functioning, the hip flexors, adductors, and quadriceps femoris are strong (good or normal), but the hip abductors and extensors are completely paralyzed. The posture of the infant is flexed, hips are abducted, and knees are extended or hyperextended (because of dynamic imbalance between the strong quadriceps and paralyzed hamstrings). The feet and ankles may be in equinus or equinovarus. On deep tendon reflex testing, the patellar tendon reflex is present, but the ankle reflex is absent. On skin reflex testing, umbilicus, abdominal, and cremasteric reflexes are present, but the anal skin reflex is absent. The deformities are those of hip adduction-flexion and knee extension. Coxa valga is uniformly present, and in about 80 percent of untreated patients, complete dislocation of the hips develops.

When *L4 is the lowest neurosegmental level* functioning, in addition to the strong muscles at the L3 neurosegmental level, the tibialis anterior is strong and the medial hamstrings are weak. Some weak function of the tibialis posterior muscle may be present. The biceps femoris is paralyzed. The hip and knee deformities are as at the L3 neurosegmental level. The feet and ankles develop progressive calcaneovarus deformity because of the dynamic imbalance between the anterior tibial (dorsiflexor of the ankle, invertor of the foot) and the paralyzed plantar flexors and evertors of the feet and ankles.

When *L5 is the lowest neurosegmental level* functioning, muscles acting in addition to L4 neurosegmental level are gluteus medius and minimus, tensor fascia lata, medial hamstrings, extensor digitorum longus, and peroneus tertius. The muscles innervated by the sacral segments are paralyzed, whereas the muscles innervated by the lumbar nerve roots are functioning. There is a dynamic imbalance between functioning medial hamstrings and paralyzed biceps femoris; with skeletal growth medial rotation deformity of the leg develops. Coxa valga occurs in one third of the patients, but hips do not dislocate. The feet and ankles are in severe progressive calcaneus deformity.

When *S1 is the lowest neurosegmental level* functioning, the muscles acting in addition to L5 neurosegmental level are gluteus maximus, biceps femoris, triceps surae, extensor digitorum longus and brevis, and flexor digitorum longus and brevis. The deep tendon patellar and ankle reflexes are present. The gluteus maximus in relation to the hip flexor is weak; therefore, a mild flexion deformity of the hip is ordinarily present. In the foot, clawing of the toes is a common deformity.

In myelomeningocele, severe lordosis, scoliosis, and kyphosis are common spinal deformities and often most disabling. It is imperative that the spine of MM patients be examined at each clinic visit and that AP and lateral radiograms of the entire spine be made periodically. The vertebral column and neural arches are the primary sites of involvement in MM.

Scoliosis in MM is usually evident after the age of 6 years. It may be due to (1) *congenital anomalies* of the vertebral column such as hemivertebrae, unilateral segmental bar, or failure of segmentation, (2) *local instability* of the spine because of absence of posterior elements and intervening ligaments, (3) *paralysis* of spinal musculature, (4) *neurologic dysfunction* due to hydromyelia, and (5) *tethering of the cord* at the site of sac closure.

The paralytic curves are long and associated with pelvic obliquity. The trunk is decompensated, and sitting is uneven. Decubitus ulcers because of abnormal pressure commonly occur. Distinguish the congenital and paralytic scoliosis in MM. Perform dermatomal sensory evoked potentials, high-resolution CT scanning, and MRI studies.

Kyphosis is evident at birth in MM. It presents as a rigid posterior angulation of the spine limited at the site of the osseous defect (Fig 6–35). The pedicles in the lesional area are spread widely apart, projecting posterolaterally and tenting the skin. The pelvic inclination is markedly increased, giving an appearance of severe flexion deformity of the hips. Turn the patient prone from lateral or supine position and hyperextend the spine by elevating the knees off the table. The kyphosis does not decrease; it is rigid. In sitting and standing posture, the degree of kyphosis increases due to static forces of body weight. A compensatory thoracic and lumbar lordosis develops above and below the kyphosis.

The kyphotic deformity increases with growth. The spinal cord is stretched over the apex of the kyphos; the neural tissues are stretched, and progressive neurologic deficit develops. Pressure on the skin by the bony prominences causes skin necrosis and ulcers.

Radiograms of the spine show the kyphos, anterior wedging of the vertebrae, the absence of laminae and spinous processes, and the marked widening of the interpedicular spaces.

Hyperlordosis is the most common spinal deformity in MM. It develops later on in childhood. The level of paralysis determines the location and extent of lordosis. The exaggerated anterior angulation of the spine may be below the third lumbar vertebra (distal type of lordosis), or it may be located above the second lumbar vertebra, extending to the thoracic spine, a site where lordosis is normally not present (Fig 6–36).

Lordosis may be caused by (1) posterior osseous defect of the lumbosacral spine, (2) posterior postoperative scarring, (3) congenital spondylolisthesis and flexion contracture of the hip, which increase the pelvic inclination and force the lumbar spine into hyperlordosis. Lordosis may be compensatory in origin for purposes of balance. The MM patient with paralysis of the triceps surae and hip extensor muscles, but strong hip flexors and knee extensor muscles, stands with a calcaneus crouch posture. The lumbar spine is tilted into severe lordosis to compensate the forward inclination of the trunk (Fig 6–37).

Bone fragility due to paralysis and atrophy of the lower limbs is common in MM. Pathologic fractures occur in about 30 percent of the cases, especially following postoperative immobilization in a hip spica or above-knee cast.

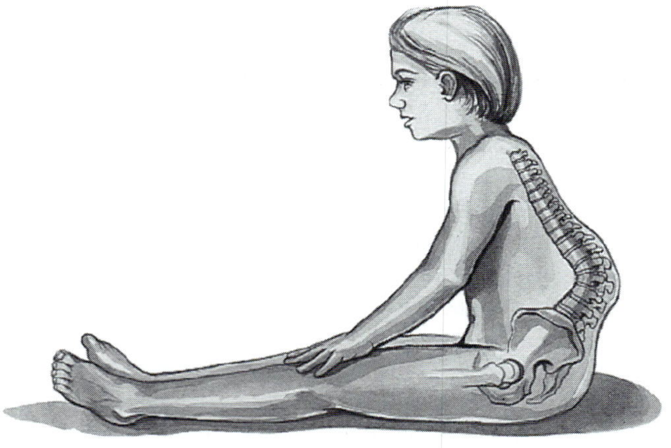

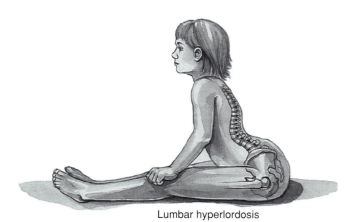

Lumbosacral kyphosis

Figure 6–35. Lumbosacral kyphosis in myelomeningocele.

Lumbar hyperlordosis

Figure 6–36. Lumbar hyperlordosis in myelomeningocele (distal type).

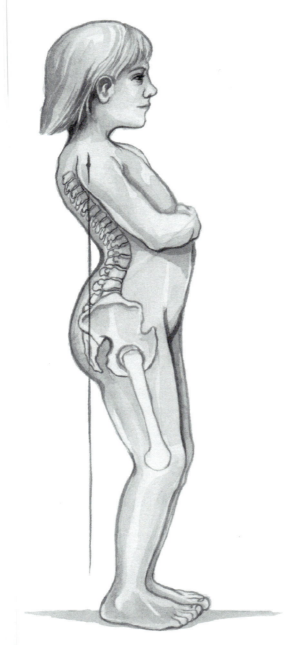

Figure 6–37. Compensatory hyperlordosis in myelomeningocele. Trunk inclined forward due to paralysis of the gluteus maximus and triceps surae. Balance is provided by posterior tilting of the trunk and lumbar hyperlordosis.

Physeal injuries and epiphyseal displacement are frequent. The fractures heal with hypoplastic callus.

Skin anesthesia and deformity of the limbs, especially equinovarus feet, predispose the MM patient to pressure sores, infected decubitus ulcers, and sometimes osteomyelitis of superficial bones. There is no pain sensation to warn the patient, parents, or surgeon. Correction of deformities and careful padding of orthoses are crucial. Frostbite due to poor circulation is another problem in MM children. Warn the parents and patient that these children should avoid extremes of temperature.

Management. An infant born with MM requires total care. A neurosurgeon, urologic surgeon, pediatric surgeon, orthopedic surgeon, neurologist-pediatrician, plastic surgeon, orthotist, physical therapist, administrative coordinator, social worker, psychologist, vocational counselor, special educator, occupational therapist, and the parents need to be involved.

The meningocele is closed as an emergency measure by the neurosurgeon. With immediate repair, there is maximal preservation of innervation, and with successful control of hydrocephalus by shunting, the mortality rate of MM has markedly decreased. A selective approach is not recommended. All children with MM should be treated with realistic goals. It is best that the MM child be managed in a major institution in a multidisciplinary care clinic. The orthopedic surgeon is only a member of the team of medical and surgical specialists.

The objectives of orthopedic management are (1) to provide a stable standing posture with the center of gravity over plantigrade feet and the knees and hips in complete extension or preferably slight hyperextension, and (2) to enable these children to walk.

The quality of walking is subdivided into the following diminishing grades: (1) Community walker. (2) Household walker. (3) Nonfunctional walkers who are essentially wheelchair bound and walk during physiotherapy sessions with orthoses and crutches or walkers. Most nonfunctional walkers regress in adolescence or adult life to nonwalkers. (4) Nonwalkers who are sitters and use the wheelchair to get around, transferring themselves in and out of their wheelchair to their beds.

Factors affecting the ability to walk are (1) the extent and severity of musculoskeletal deformity, (2) motor strength of the muscles functioning within a neurosegmental level, (3) obesity (overweight children with MM have difficulty in ambulating because of increased demand for energy expenditure, (4) intelligence, age, and motivation of patient. Patients with mental retardation and gross spasticity have a poor prognosis for ambulation, (5) the presence of brain damage, (6) the design and effectiveness of orthoses, and (7) a multitude of shunt revisions adversely affecting walking ability.

In sacral level lesions, over half of the patients are community ambulators; in lower lumbar level lesions, a third; in upper lumbar lesions, a tenth; and in thoracic level lesions, none.[290] Ordinarily, patients with upper lumbar and thoracic neurosegmental level lesions are not functional ambulators.[274]

The principles of orthopedic management of MM patients are as follows: (1) Assume in the beginning that all children have the potential to walk, unless they have some

CNS damage with marked spasticity, hydrocephalus, and brain damage; (2) perform simple surgery in those who will be nonfunctional walkers; the objective of care of these children with high level lesions is to provide a stable standing and sitting posture. Upright posture gives new vistas to life to these paralyzed children. (3) Functional walkers who will continue to walk in adult life require more extensive surgery to provide them the function to meet the greater demands of society later on in their lives. (4) Perform surgery in both limbs and at several levels under one anesthesia. (5) The period of cast immobilization should be as short as possible; prolonged immobilization of the limbs in cast causes osteoporosis and results in stress fractures. (6) Always correct muscle imbalance to prevent recurrence of deformity. (7) Resect rather than section fibrotic muscle tendons. (8) Employ operative correction of rigid deformities (such as rigid clubfoot, vertical talus, or hyperextensor contracture of knees) and not "conservative" cast methods. (9) Do not accept undercorrection because the deformity will recur and further surgery will be required.

Orthopedic management varies according to stage of development, age of the patient, neurosegmental level of the lesion, and the deformities present.

The *first year of life* is essentially a neurosurgical year—excision of sac and shunting. At birth the orthopedists evaluate the neuromusculoskeletal system, the neurosegmental level of paralysis, and the associated deformities. The physical therapist instructs the parents to place the newborn in physiologic posture in order to prevent deformity due to malposture. Developmental therapy is employed to enhance motor development of the head, neck, trunk, and limbs. Foot deformities such as talipes equinovarus or vertical talus are treated by passive stretching exercises, splinting, and serial casting. When the patient develops head and neck control, encourage sitting balance. When prone mobility and sitting balance develop, encourage the patient to develop hand skills, coordinated hand function, and strength of the upper limb muscles. Sitting aids are provided as necessary.

In the *second year of life,* when the child attempts to pull himself up to upright position, orthotic devices are provided to assist the child in standing. The type of brace given depends upon the neurosegmental level of the lesion, trunk balance, and upper limb function. The child with thoracic and upper lumbar level lesions is placed initially in a total body splint—a posterior thoracolumbosacral hip-knee-ankle-foot orthosis and later on in an A-frame. These devices support the hips in neutral extension and 10 to 15 degrees of abduction and the knees, ankles, and feet in neutral position. The child is placed in these standing devices for several hours a day. Upright posture stimulates the child to be interested in his or her environment and opens new vistas. Later on the child is fitted with a parapodium that enables him or her to stand without crutches and allows some degree of mobility.

Children with lower lumbar level lesions are fitted with a KAFO or AFO. The younger child begins with more extensive bracing; as he develops greater motor control and balance, the components of the brace are removed cephalocaudally. Rotational malalignment is controlled with cable twisters. Children with sacral level lesions are supported initially with AFO and later on have no braces. Wheelchairs and other mobility aids are provided as necessary to meet individual requirements.

Foot deformities require correction between 6 and 18 months of age. Ninety percent of children with MM have some type of significant foot deformity. Rigid equinovarus (clubfoot) deformity is the most troublesome. Weight-bearing on a small lateral area of the sole and forefoot results in abnormal pressure, ulcers, cellulitis, and osteomyelitis, which, if untreated, eventually results in amputation. It is vital to provide flexible, normally aligned plantigrade feet with persistent and diligent care. Muscle imbalance, fibrosis, and contracture of denervated muscles present difficult problems. The recurrence rate is high. Radical posteromedial, lateral, and plantar release is necessary to provide plantigrade feet. Excise the tendons of fibrotic muscles. Perform capsulectomy and not capsulotomy. The anterior tibial tendon is released to prevent recurrent varus deformity. Tendon transfers do not ordinarily succeed in MM feet. In the older child with recurrent deformity, perform osteotomy to preserve some motion. Avoid arthrodesis. Hindfoot varus is corrected by lateral closing wedge osteotomy of the calcaneus. Midfoot varus is treated by lateral column shortening or double osteotomy (closing cuboid and open-up medial cuneiform).

Congenital convex pes valgus (rigid vertical talus) equinus and severe cavus deformity require surgical correction between 1 and 2 years of age.

Calcaneus deformity of the feet is very common in low lumbar lesions because of muscle imbalance between strong anterior tibial and paralyzed triceps surae muscles; functionally, it is very disabling. Treat it by anterolateral release to provide a plantigrade, flexible foot that can be braced in an AFO.

Valgus feet remain flexible and can be controlled by an appropriate AFO; however, as the child gets older, lateral torsion deformity of the tibia and ankle valgus develop. The fibula shortens and the distal tibial epiphysis becomes wedged laterally. It causes bracing problems with pressure sores on the medial malleolus. In the young child, tenodesis of the Achilles tendon to the fibula is performed. In the older child, medial hemiepiphyseodesis of the distal tibia corrects the ankle valgus by asymmetric growth of the distal tibia. In the child over 10 to 12 years of age, supramalleolar varus osteotomy of the tibia is indicated.

Hindfoot valgus may be associated with ankle valgus. It is treated by medial sliding osteotomy of the calcaneus in the older child.

In the *third and fourth year of life,* the MM child improves upright mobility and walking ability. Aggressive physical therapy is carried out to achieve maximal function, and part-time splints are used to prevent development of deformities of the limbs and spine.

In this age group and in older patients, progressive deformities of the hip, leg, and knee develop; they are presented briefly.

HIP DEFORMITIES

Paralytic Hip Subluxation and Dislocation

Determine the cause. Hip dislocation has several causes: (1) *Muscle imbalance* between hip flexors-adductors and paralyzed hip extensors-abductors. In L3–L4 neurosegmental level lesions, 60 to 80 percent of the hips dislocate, whereas in L2 level when the hip adductors are weak and at L5 level when the hip abductors get stronger the hip only subluxates. (2) *Bone deformity*—namely, coxa valga, excessive femoral antetorsion, and posterior and superolateral deficiency of the acetabulum. Wear of the acetabulum is posterior as the hips are flexed at night and the patient sits most of the day. (3) *Capsular laxity* due to stretching. (4) *Pelvic obliquity.*

The second factor to consider in management of hip dislocation in MM is the *potential for walking.* The presence of a strong quadriceps femoris muscle is a reliable prognostic sign for walking—household or community. The most important factor in walking is muscle strength and not whether the hips are located or dislocated. An MM child who walks does so by 6 years of age. If a patient is 8 years of age and still not walking, the odds are very strong that he will not be a household or community walker. In a child who requires above-knee orthoses and crutches for walking, there is no difference in gait and posture between those with hips dislocated and those with hips located. In these patients, the presence or absence of fixed flexion deformity of the hip and knee is the determining factor in standing posture and gait. Correction of fixed deformity is vital. Ability to flex the hip is important in walking.

The third factor to consider is whether dislocation of the hip is unilateral or bilateral. When only one hip dislocates, it causes significant lower limb length disparity, pelvic obliquity, and contractural deformities of the dislocated side.

In the infant and young child, the subluxated hips or reducible dislocated hips are splinted with the hips in extension and abduction. The flexion braces such as Pavlik or Ilfeld should not be used, as they cause flexion deformity of the hip and aggravate the posterior deficiency of the acetabulum. Muscle-tendon transfers do not function adequately and are not effective. Posterolateral transfer of the iliopsoas removes a deforming force but does not function as a hip abductor in gait; it causes lateral rotation deformity of the hip and takes away hip flexion power, which is very

important in gait. An operation commonly performed in the 1960s and 1970s, it is rarely performed at present. The iliopsoas transfer is considered only in unilateral dislocation of the hip.

Posterior transfer of a hip adductor to the ischium does not function as a hip extensor. External oblique transfer to the greater trochanter does not function effectively as a hip abductor and does not decrease or eliminate gluteus medius limp or lurch.

In the older MM child with subluxation or dislocation of the hip, bony procedures are performed consisting of varus derotation intertrochanteric osteotomy of the proximal femur to correct coxa valga and femoral antetorsion. The markedly subluxated hip is treated by open reduction and capsular plication and posterior coverage of the femoral head by either Staheli shelf or Chiari medial displacement osteotomy. Do not perform a Salter or Pemberton innominate osteotomy; they provide anterior coverage. In MM hip the deficiency is posterior.

Hip flexion deformity is a common deformity in L3 and higher level lesions, and often it is accompanied by knee flexion contracture. It is caused by muscle imbalance between strong hip flexors and paralyzed hip extensors and from static forces of malposture because most of these patients are primarily sitters. There is a direct relationship between the time spent sitting and the degree of severity of hip flexion deformity. Hip flexion deformity increases anterior pelvis tilt and causes compensatory excessive lumbar lordosis.

In T12 and higher level lesions, flexion deformity of the hip is associated with abduction-lateral rotation contracture of the hip. When it is unilateral or asymmetric, it causes pelvic obliquity.

Treatment of hip flexion deformity initially should be conservative, consisting of passive stretching exercises of the hip flexors, prone posturing, and splinting of the hips and knees in extension. When the child gets older and the hip flexion deformity progressively increases and exceeds 25 to 30 degrees, soft tissue release is performed. In the older patient, when flexion deformity of the hip is 50 degrees or greater, extension osteotomy of the proximal femur at the intertrochanteric level is indicated.

Abduction-lateral rotation contracture of the hip is corrected by soft-tissue release (Ober-Yount procedure). Postoperatively, the hips are postured properly to prevent recurrence of deformity.

Hip adduction deformity, if severe, is treated by surgical release of adductor longus and brevis.

KNEE DEFORMITIES

Knee flexion deformity is treated early by splinting of the knee in extension and by encouraging standing in a KAFO with the knee in extension. Knee flexion contracture that exceeds 25 to 30 degrees requires surgical correction by soft tissue release. It is important to completely correct the flexion deformity and hyperextend the knee 10 to 15 degrees on the operating table. Often knee flexion and hip flexion deformity coexist; both are corrected at the same time.

Extension contracture and recurvatum of the knee are usually bilateral. The degree of deformity varies; it is usually rigid and associated with varying degrees of anterior subluxation of the knee joint. Pathogenic factors are fibrosis of the quadriceps muscle (seen in T12–L1 and higher level lesions) or dynamic imbalance between strong quadriceps and paralyzed hamstrings (seen in lesions at neurosegmental L3 or L4 levels or distal to it). Sometimes a malunited distal femoral or proximal tibial fracture is the cause because of anterior tilting of the distal femoral condyle or posterior tilting of proximal tibial metaphysis.

Extension contracture of the knee impedes walking and makes fitting orthoses difficult. Treatment consists of soft tissue release or lengthening of the quadriceps mechanism.

Rotational Deformities of the Lower Limb

Medial tibiofibular torsion causes toeing-in gait. It occurs commonly at L4–L5 neurosegmental level because of muscle imbalance between strong medial hamstrings and paralyzed biceps femoris. The muscle imbalance causes progressive structural medial tibiofibular torsion. MM patients with clubfoot have excessive medial tibiofibular torsion.

Lateral tibiofibular torsion is often associated with ankle valgus. Contracture of the iliotibial band aggravates the deformity. It causes the child to toe out in gait. The anteriorly displaced prominent medial malleolus creates problems with fitting of orthoses and pressure sores.

Initially treat torsional problems of the leg with cable twisters and braces (KAFO). Often the deformity increases with skeletal growth and impedes gait. At about 6 to 7 years of age, the excessive medial tibial torsion is treated with lateral derotation osteotomy of the tibia and lateral tibiofibular torsion with medial rotation and varization osteotomy of the distal tibia at the supramalleolar level. Use internal fixation with AO compression plate and above-knee cast. The child should not bear weight until adequate healing has taken place. Nonunion, delayed union, wound slough, and infection are common complications.

■ TUMORS AND TUMOROUS CONDITIONS OF BONE

A bone tumor is suspected when a patient presents with a mass, pain, altered function, or a pathologic fracture resulting from a trivial injury. Occasionally a bone tumor is detected incidentally in a radiogram made for some other reason.

A specific diagnosis of tumor cannot be made from the clinical features; however, a detailed history and thorough physical examination assist the surgeon in localizing the region to be imaged. In the medical history, the *age* of the patient is relevant because most bone tumors develop in certain age groups; for example, a destructive bone lesion in a patient 5 years or younger is most commonly due to histiocytosis, whereas giant cell tumor occurs at 18 years and older. The race of the patient is of some consideration; for example, Ewing's sarcoma is very rare in blacks. A rapidly growing mass suggests an aggressive lesion—more likely to be malignant than benign. A benign bone tumor, unless it is an osteoid osteoma, osteoblastoma, or aneurysmal bone cyst, is ordinarily not painful. A deep aching pain relieved by salicylates or other analgesics is suggestive of osteoid osteoma. The pain is often worse at night. Inquire about the onset of pain; an insidious onset of pain that is transient suggests a benign lesion, whereas rapid onset of pain that is persistent, increases in severity, and keeps the patient awake at night is a feature of malignant tumors. Ask about the duration of the pain. Determine the site of pain and its distribution. A sudden increase in pain suggests a pathologic fracture.

In the medical history, ask about previous fractures and any kidney or gastrointestinal disorders or recent infections. In the present history, ask about fever, chills, or weight loss.

On examination, a *mass* may be palpable, particularly if it is an osteochondroma, expansile cyst, osteoid oseoma, or malignant bone tumor such as osteogenic sarcoma or Ewing's sarcoma. Determine the size of the mass and its consistency. Is it soft and cystic or hard and bony? Are its margins distinct and smooth, or infiltrating to surrounding tissues? Is it mobile? A fixed mass that does not alter on muscle contraction indicates a bony lesion. Muscle tumors are usually mobile, and they move with relaxation and contraction of the muscle. Transilluminate superficial masses with a flashlight to see if they are cystic, such as a ganglion. Is the mass locally tender? Feel the mass with the dorsum of your proximal phalanges for temperature differences from surrounding tissues. A warm mass indicates either a malignant lesion or an inflammatory condition. Are there any café-au-lait spots? Are there any hemangiomas or pulsation in the mass to indicate a vascular tumor? A blood vessel lesion decreases in size on elevation of the limb and with steady, firm pressure. Is there any erythema, dilatation of superficial veins, or edema? Is there any lymphadenopathy?

Assess the neurologic picture. Is there any sensory loss or motor weakness? Neurologic deficit is uncommon except when the expanding bone tumor is in an anatomic site, such as the sciatic notch or the sacrum, where nerves cannot move freely. Determine range of motion of the joint. Is there any stiffness? Any effusion in the adjacent joints?

Imaging.   When a bone tumor is suspected, the initial assessment is made by plain radiogram. These should include an AP and lateral projection of the involved area. Always rule out the possibility of referred pain, especially when a radiogram of the painful area is normal. Pain in the antero-medial aspect of the thigh may be referred from the hip, whereas pain in the posterolateral aspect of the thigh may be referred from lumbosacral pathology and pain in the anterior aspect of the hip region and lower abdomen from the lumbar region. Imaging the proper area is crucial. Conventional radiography often makes the correct diagnosis; it is an excellent, cost-effective diagnostic tool in orthopedic oncology.

In assessing the radiographic appearance, first determine the *anatomic location* of the tumor, as often it has diagnostic importance. In a long bone, is it in the epiphysis, metaphysis, or diaphysis? Tumors that involve the *epiphysis* are eosinophilic granuloma, chondroblastoma, and enchondroma when the physis is open, and most probably a giant cell tumor when the growth plate is closed. A lesion in the *metaphysis* is quite common to many benign tumors such as unicameral bone cyst. This is also a common site for osteogenic sarcoma. The metaphyseal site is not diagnostically discriminating. Is the lesion in the *diaphysis* of a long bone? This is a common site for fibrous dysplasia, histiocytosis X, osteoblastoma, adamantinoma, and Ewing's sarcoma. When a lesion affects the ribs, in children and adolescents, it most probably is fibrous dysplasia or Ewing's sarcoma. In the adult, chondrosarcoma may occur in the ribs. In the skeletally mature patient, common sites for multiple myeloma and metastatic tumors are the ribs, pelvis, and spine. In the vertebral column, when the site of the lesion is the posterior element, that is, spinous process, lamina, or pedicles, one should consider the possibility of aneurysmal bone cyst, osteoblastoma, or osteoid osteoma. When the vertebral body is involved, consider histiocytosis X (eosinophilic granuloma) or hemangioma. The scapula and pelvis are common sites of fibrous dysplasia, aneurysmal bone cyst, and Ewing's sarcoma. When multiple bones are affected, suspect multiple hereditary exostosis, fibrous dysplasia, enchondromatosis (Ollier's disease), histiocytosis X, or metastatic tumors. When metaphyseal transverse areas of translucence are present, rule out leukemia.

Second, determine *the effect on the local bone.* Assess the internal radiographic characteristics of the lesion. Use a magnifying lens to see detail. Are the bone trabeculae destroyed? Is there new bone formation? Don't mistake ossification for calcification. In ossification, the matrix is ossified, depicting an appearance of organization and structure. In calcification, mineralization is unstructured, haphazard, and dense. Tumor bone formation suggests osteogenic sarcoma, whereas calcification suggests cartilaginous lesions such as enchondroma or chondrosarcoma.

Third, assess the *reaction of surrounding tissues in the zone of transition* between the lesion and the host bone. Clear demarcation with a narrow zone of transition and an area of surrounding sclerosis is suggestive of a benign lesion, whereas a poorly demarcated, wide, irregular zone of transition with jagged outlines and no clear boundaries in-

dicates an aggressive, rapidly growing lesion; it may be due to a malignant tumor, locally aggressive lesion, or infection. Is the cortex thinned and expanded? This is seen in unicameral bone cysts, aneurysmal bone cysts, fibrous dysplasia, and enchondroma.

Codman's triangle is reactive bone under the elevated periosteum at the margin of the tumor. It is seen in aggressive tumors. A sunburst pattern is seen in rapidly growing tumors such as osteosarcoma, which produces radially directed bone spicules along Sharpey's fibers and blood vessels. Onion skin and sunburst appearance, however, are not sufficiently specific to be of diagnostic value. Inspect the plain radiograms carefully for any extraosseous extension of the tumor; when it is present, suspect malignancy. Is there any associated soft tissue mass? It may be visible in the plain radiogram. A tumor located on the surface of a bone is termed parosteal or juxtacortical.

CT is indicated to depict bone detail in anatomic areas where visualization is difficult by simple plain radiography, such as the subscapular region, spine, pelvis, and sacrum.[363,369,384] CT assesses the composition of the abnormal osseous matrix. It clearly shows punctate calcification in cartilaginous tumors and intraosseous as well as extraosseous extension of the lesion. CT also shows mineralization and detects subtle cortical distraction and fracture. In aneurysmal bone cyst it visualizes the thin rim of reactive bone around the expanded and destroyed cortex.

MRI can make axial, coronal, and sagittal images. It shows nerves, vessels, ligaments, articular cartilage, and physes. T1 weighting or stir sequences are used in marrow involvement, and T2 weighting or gradient-echo sequences are used for soft tissue extension.[364,365] In aneurysmal bone cyst, fluid levels are shown clearly by MRI and are diagnostically helpful.[377,378,392] In lipoma, the fat content is depicted. MRI is superior to CT in delineating the margins of the lesion and extraosseous extension of the tumor and its relationship with the surrounding neurovascular structures. The disadvantage of MRI is that it provides poor bone detail, and subtle changes in bone structure can be missed. MRI shows an abnormal signal when edema is present. MRI does not accurately distinguish between benign and malignant bone tumor.

Isotope scanning is a very sensitive but nonspecific imaging tool. Technetium-99m shows increased uptake when the lesion is osteoid osteoma, osteoblastoma, aneurysmal bone cyst, fibrous dysplasia, osteogenic sarcoma, Ewing's sarcoma, and neuroblastoma.[375,380,390]

Laboratory Tests. CBC and differential, ESR or C-reactive proteins, and calcium phosphate and alkaline phosphatase levels are indicated when metabolic bone disease is suspected. In bone tumors, this is not useful.[391]

In the *differential diagnosis* of bone tumors, consider first the following non-neoplastic conditions: (1) osteomyelitis, (2) stress fracture, (3) metabolic bone disease, such as brown tumor of hyperparathyroidism, (4) circulatory diseases of bone such as infection, (5) synovial disease such as pigmented villonodular synovitis or synovial chondromatosis, and (6) myositis ossificans.

Then consider these major categories of bone tumor: (1) benign primary bone tumor, (2) malignant primary bone tumor, and (3) a metastatic bone tumor. Table 6–2 is a listing of tumors of bone. Using such a classification as a general framework, the common tumors of bone occurring in children and adolescents are briefly discussed.

BENIGN RADIOLUCENT BONE LESIONS

Often in the literature, these are referred to as cystic lesions, but this is a misnomer because the radiolucent lesion in bone may contain fluid, fibrous tissue, cartilage, or cells without calcification or ossification. A lytic bone lesion is not an accurate term either, because the area of radiolucency may be caused by failure of bone formation and not bone destruction.

Unicameral Bone Cyst (UBC)[393–407]

In this benign lesion of the growing skeleton there is a true bone cyst which consists of a single cavity—hence the

TABLE 6–2. CLASSIFICATION OF TUMORS AND TUMOROUS LESIONS OF BONES

  I. Benign—primary
  A. Fibrous-cystic
    1. Unicameral bone cyst
    2. Aneurysmal bone cyst
    3. Fibrous dysplasia
    4. Fibrous cortical defect
    5. Nonossifying fibroma
  B. Cartilaginous
    1. Enchondroma
    2. Multiple enchondromatosis
    3. Osteochondroma
    4. Multiple cartilaginous extoses
    5. Periosteal chondroma
    6. Benign chondroblastoma (Codman's tumor)
    7. Chondromyxoid fibroma
  C. Osseous
    1. Osteoid osteoma
    2. Osteoblastoma
    3. Osteofibrous dysplasia (Campanacci syndrome)
  D. Marrow cell tumors
    1. Histiocytosis
  II. Malignant primary tumors
  A. Osteosarcoma
  B. Ewing's sarcoma
  C. Chondrosarcoma
  D. Adamantinoma
  E. Fibrosarcoma
  F. Malignant fibrous histiocytoma
  G. Chordoma
  III. Metastatic tumors in children
  A. Neuroblastoma
  B. Nephroblastoma (Wilms' tumor)

name unicameral. It is the most common rarefied cystic lesion in bone. The proximal metaphyses of the humerus and femur are the most common sites, occurring in 75 percent of all cases. The upper and lower ends of the fibula are the next most frequent sites.

It can occur in any bone. The exact cause of the cyst is unknown. It is due to blockage of the circulation and drainage of the interstitial fluid. The fluid of the cyst has characteristics similar to those of serum plasma.[397] Lysosomes may have a role in the pathogenesis of UBC.[401]

Clinical Features. UBCs are asymptomatic. They may be incidentally found in a radiogram made for some other reason. Often they are discovered after a pathologic fracture sustained by trivial injury. When complicated by a fracture, the presenting complaints are local pain and swelling; when the femur or tibia is the site of the lesion, the child limps.

Imaging. The radiolucent lesion is concentric and juxtaphyseal, occupying the entire metaphysis with varying degrees of thinning and expansion of the cortex. The cyst has a clear radiolucency because of its fluid content (Fig 6–38). Ordinarily the regional cortex does not expand more than the width of the physis. UBCs are in the active phase when they are located in the metaphysis and extend to the growth plate. With bone growth, the cyst grows away from the growth plate and involves the diaphysis; at this stage, the UBC is considered to be inactive. Very rarely, a UBC may extend through the physis into the epiphysis.[404] Following a fracture, fragments of bone may fall into the bottom of the cyst; this is referred to as a fallen fragment sign.[406] Twenty-five percent of UBCs heal following a fracture.[400]

Treatment. The fracture is treated by immobilization of the part. In the case of the proximal humerus, a Velpeau splint is used. After healing of the fracture and persistence of the UBC, treatment consists of aspiration of the cyst and injection with 80 to 120 mg of methyl prednisone acetate. Perform the procedure under general anesthesia under radiographic control using the two-needle technique. The fluid in the cyst is clear and straw-colored except following a recent fracture, when it may be serosanguineous. A cystogram is performed to ensure that the cavity is unicameral and not partitioned by bone septa following a fracture. Corticosteroid injection is repeated in 2 to 3 months if there is no healing of the lesion. It is the method of choice in initial treatment of UBC; it is much simpler and equally effective as an open operative procedure. The success rate is 90 percent following two or three repeat injections.[393,399,405,407]

Curettage and bone grafting are indicated in cases where there is no response to injection, particularly in the neck of the femur with a pathologic fracture, especially if it involves the inferior cortex of the femoral neck and results in coxa vara; involvement of the capital physis causes

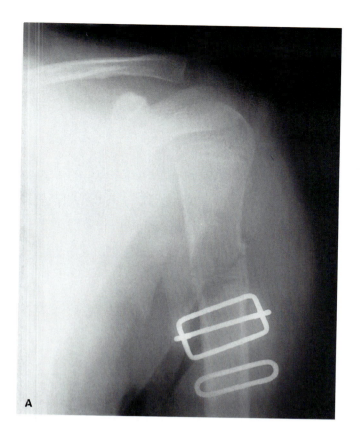

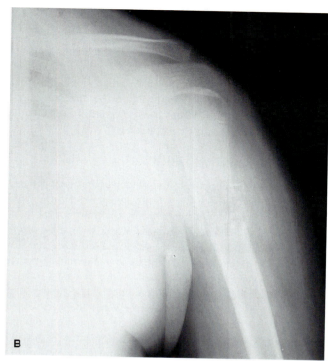

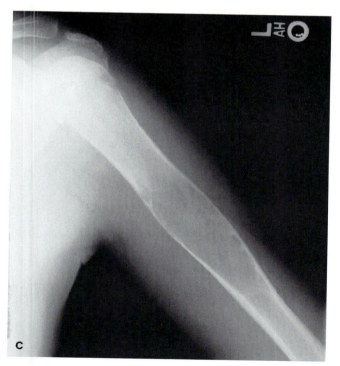

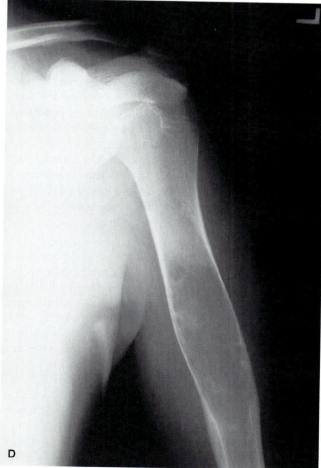

Figure 6–38. Unicameral bone cyst of the left proximal humerus in a 12-year-old boy. **A, B.** AP and lateral projections showing pathologic fracture through the radiolucent lesion. Note the thinning and expansion of the regional cortex. This was treated in a hanging cast. **C, D.** AP and lateral radiograms of the left humerus. The fracture has healed and the radiolucent lesion has grown away from the proximal humeral physis. The cyst is persistent and is larger. The transverse diameter of the cyst is not greater than the transverse diameter of the proximal humeral metaphysis.

coxa breva.[393,398,402] At present, I recommend packing the cavity of the cyst with collograft and Grafton. In the proximal femur, it is best to support the hip in a single hip spica cast or with crutches, depending upon the age and cooperation of the patient. When internal fixation is used, the growth plate should not be violated.

Aneurysmal Bone Cyst (ABC)[409–417]

This benign, non-neoplastic radiolucent bone lesion has a characteristic expansile, blown-out appearance in the radiogram. The lesion is characterized by the presence of channels and spaces that usually contain blood, with some of the locules containing blood-tinged or clear fluid. On gross inspection, it is characterized by the honeycomb mesh appearance with a surrounding thin shell of subperiosteal bone.

ABC occurs in older children, adolescents, and young adults, with 80 percent occurring between the ages of 10 and 20 years. About 50 percent occur in the long tubular bones, usually the humerus, femur, or tibia, and 30 percent in the vertebral column involving the posterior elements.

Clinically, the patient presents with local pain of several weeks or months' duration. If the site of affection is a superficial bone, local tenderness and swelling are present on palpation. In the vertebral column, compression of the spinal cord and nerve roots may occur.

Imaging. In the long bones the area of radiolucency is metaphyseal in its location and eccentric (in contrast to UBC, which is concentric). There is expansion and thinning of the regional cortex with the extent of expansion wider than the physis (Fig 6–39). The radiographic appearance is aggressive. The ABC can cross the physis and cause growth arrest. Telangiectatic osteosarcoma may give the radiographic appearance of ABC. Obtain an adequate biopsy and examine the tissue by frozen and permanent sections to confirm the diagnosis of ABC. Do not miss a telangiectatic sarcoma. The bone scan shows increased uptake. The MRI shows a multitude of fluid levels.

Treatment. Treatment consists of curettage and bone grafting. Angiostatic agents such as oral dexamethasone may induce healing.[412] One should be cautious not to disturb the growth of the physis. The periosteum should be preserved. Make a wide surgical exposure and large hole in the cortex to remove the tumor. There is a high rate of recurrence. When the ABC recurs following the curettage, grows rapidly, and involves the soft tissues, review the original pathology to reconfirm that the original lesion is an ABC and not a telangiectatic osteosarcoma. Wide resection with use of an external fixator to maintain length is indicated in recurrent cases. The bone regenerates if the periosteum is preserved. Vascular occlusion with embolization is indicated when the lesion is very large and located in a surgically inaccessible site such as the vertebral column.

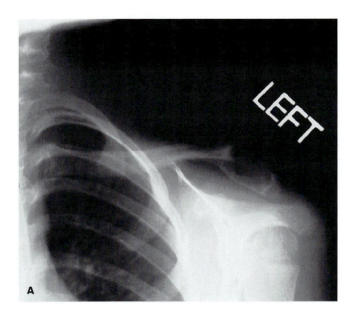

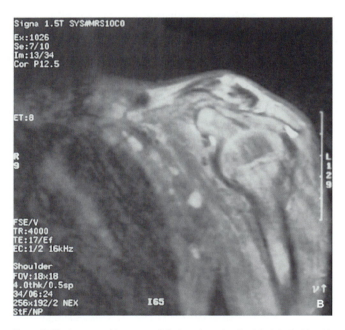

Figure 6–39. Aneurysmal bone cyst of the lateral one fourth of the left clavicle with a healed pathologic fracture. **A.** AP radiogram. Note that the cystic rarefaction is larger than the diameter of the shaft of the clavicle. **B.** MRI showing the radiolucent lesion.

FIBROUS DEFECTS OF BONE AND NONOSSIFYING FIBROMA[418–426]

These radiolucent lesions, commonly found in the metaphyseal region of long bone, consist of spindle-shaped connective tissue cells with an occasional multinucleated giant cell. They should be considered as sites of developmental defect of bone maturation; they tend to disappear spontaneously with skeletal growth. They occur in children and adolescents and are noted on radiograms taken for some other reason.

Fibrous cortical defects are ovoid or circular in shape and are eccentrically located in the metaphyses of long bones with a geographic border and sclerotic rim (Fig 6–40). *Nonossifying fibroma* is medullary in location, tends to persist, or sometimes increases in size, and occasionally nonossifying fibroma may present with a pathologic fracture (Fig 6–41).

Treatment.   Fibrous metaphyseal cortical defects are simply observed; they ossify and disappear within 3 to 5 years. Nonossifying fibromas are observed unless they increase in size and sustain recurrent pathologic fractures. Surgical treatment consists of curettage and autogenous bone grafting or grafting with collograft and Grafton.

FIBROUS DYSPLASIA

This lesion, involving primarily the growing skeleton, is characterized by expanding fibro-osseous tissue in the interior of the bone. There are two principal forms of fibrous dysplasia; monostotic and polyostotic.

In the *monostotic type,* the femur, tibia, and humerus are common sites, although a rib, facial bone, or calvarium is not infrequently involved. Almost any bone may be affected by fibrous dysplasia. Fibrous dysplasia may be localized to the metaphysis or diaphysis of a long bone, or it may involve the full length of the bone.

Most monostotic lesions are asymptomatic and the lesion is discovered incidentally in a radiogram made for some other reason, such as a chest radiogram or intravenous pyelogram. When the proximal femur is involved, progressive varus angulation occurs and the child presents with a short-leg, gluteus medius limp. When the tibia is involved, anterolateral bowing with local swelling develops. When the maxilla or mandible is affected, asymmetry and deformity of the face due to enlargement of the affected bone are obvious on inspection. Local pain develops when there is a stress fracture or when the lesion is rapidly expanding.

The *polyostotic form* of fibrous dysplasia can be associated with a variety of endocrine disorders; for example, in McCune-Albright syndrome, polyostotic fibrous dysplasia occurs with precocious puberty and café-au-lait pigmentation of the skin.[427,428,430] McCune-Albright syndrome is due to mutation of the gene encoding the alpha subunit of the stimulatory G protein of adenyl cyclase. Prior to surgical intervention, it behooves the surgeon to request a

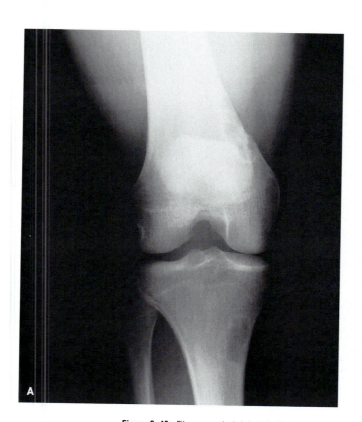

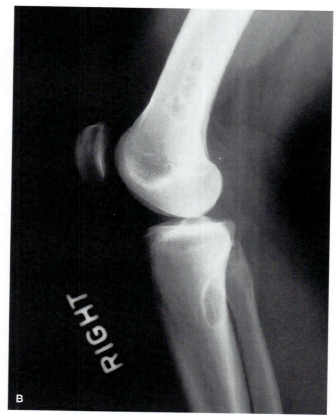

Figure 6–40. Fibrous cortical defect. **A, B.** AP and lateral radiograms of the distal femur and proximal tibial metaphyses.

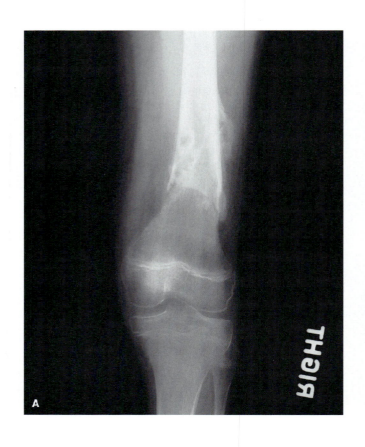

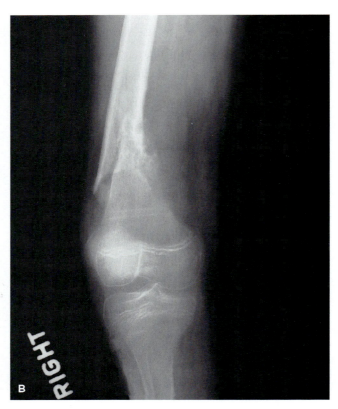

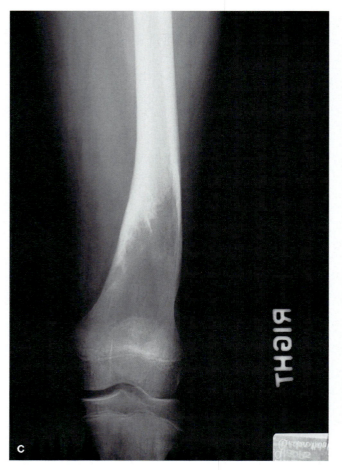

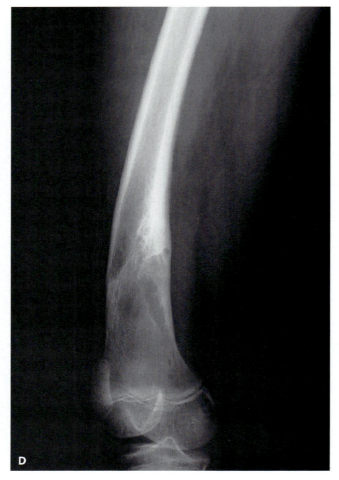

Figure 6–41. Pathologic fracture through a nonossifying fibroma of the distal femoral metaphyseal-diaphyseal region. **A, B.** AP and lateral radiograms showing the healing fracture through the area of irregular rarefaction. **C, D.** Radiograms of the distal femur 1 year later showing that the fracture and the lesion are healed.

thorough endocrine assessment to rule out other endocrinopathies such as hyperparathyroidism, Cushing's syndrome, and hypophosphatemic rickets. In polyostotic fibrous dysplasia, bone changes are more extensive than in the monostotic form; bowing of long bones, pathologic fractures, pain, and limping are common.

Imaging Findings. In the long bones fibrous dysplasia involves the metaphysis and diaphysis; the epiphysis is rarely involved. Fibrous dysplasia gives a radiolucent shadow in the interior of the involved bone. The area of radiolucency has a ground glass appearance due to the mixture of fibrous tissue and thin calcified trabeculae. The regional cortical bone is thinned with a scalloped, undulating pattern due to endosteal erosion (Figs 6–42 and 6–43). The bony ridges on the inner surface of the affected bone cast a "multiloc-

ular" appearance. There may be expansion of the bone. There is no periosteal reaction, except in the presence of a pathologic fracture.

CT clearly shows the ground glass appearance of fibrous dysplasia. Bone scan with technetium-99m depicts moderately increased uptake.

Treatment. Asymptomatic fibrous dysplasia does not require treatment. It is simply observed at periodic intervals. Significant angular deformities such as severe genu varum or valgum or coxa vara and "shepherd's crook" deformity of the proximal femur or pathologic fractures require surgical intervention.[423] Refrain from thorough curettage and massive bone grafting, especially in polyostotic fibrous dysplasia, as the recurrence rate is high. An exception to this conservative approach is an expanding fibrous dysplasia in

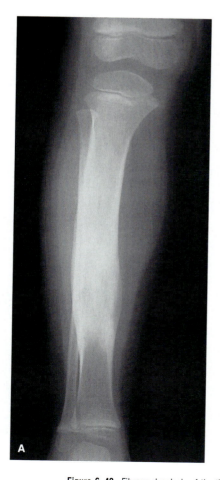
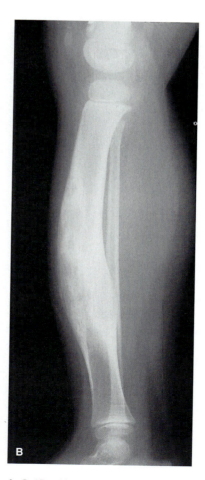

Figure 6–42. Fibrous dysplasia of the tibia. **A., B.** AP and lateral of the tibia.

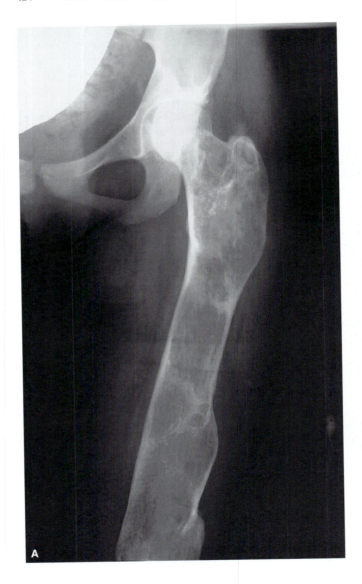

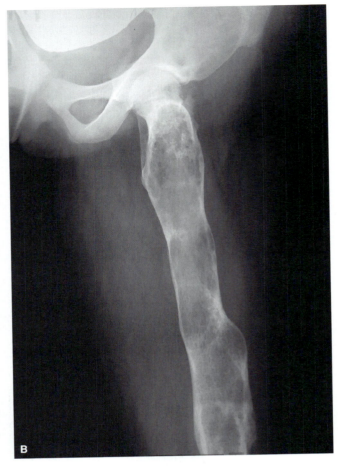

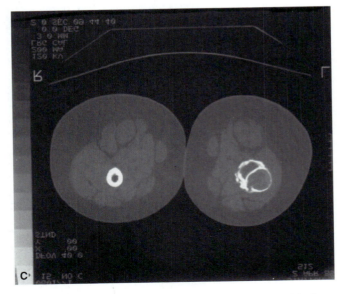

the neck or subtrochanteric region of the femur with a thin cortex and a pathologic stress fracture. In such an instance, aggressive measures are indicated in the form of thorough curettage, cortical and cancellous bone grafting, and internal fixation. When coxa vara is present, it is corrected by intertrochanteric valgus osteotomy and fixed internally with an intramedullary rod with screws extending into the neck and head of the femur.

Sarcomatous transformation occurs very rarely in fibrous dysplasia; be suspicious of such change when persisting pain and rapid expansion of the radiolucent area develop in the radiogram.[435] The types of secondary sarcomas developing in fibrous dysplasia are osteogenic sarcoma, chondrosarcoma, and fibrosarcoma. Most cases occur in the adult. A definitive diagnosis is made by biopsy following appropriate staging by scintigraphy, CT, and/or MRI.

Figure 6–43. Fibrous dysplasia. **A. & B.** AP and lateral radiogram of the femur showing the areas of rarefaction with the ground glass appearance and thinning of the cortices. **C.** CT scan of the normal right and affected left femur.

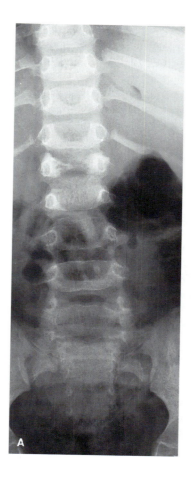

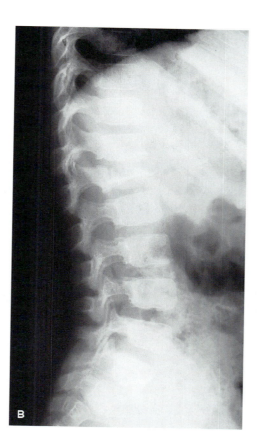

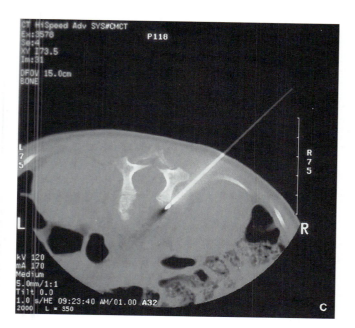

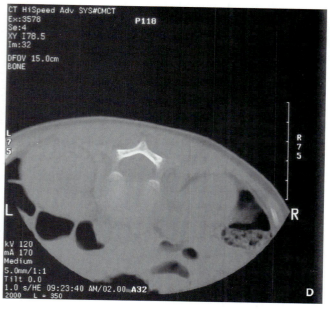

Figure 6–53. Eosinophilic granuloma of the right ilium. **A.** Note the punched out area of rarefaction in the superior roof of the acetabulum extending proximally for a distance of 3.5 cms. **B.** AP and lateral radiograms of the thoracolumbar spine, showing the decreased height and collapse of the first lumbar vertebral body. **C, D.** CT scans showing localization of the lesion and injection by hydrocortisone. *(Continues)*

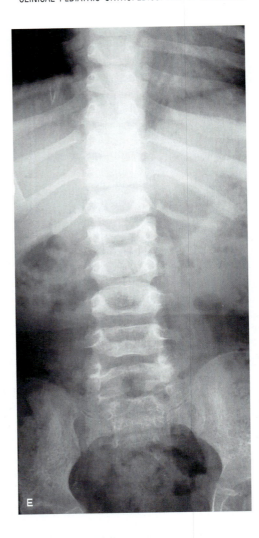

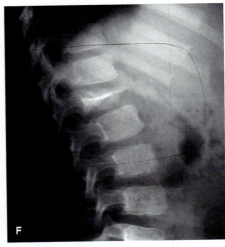

Figure 6–53 *(Continued).* **E, F.** AP and lateral radiograms of the thoracolumbar region 1 year later, showing healing of the lesion but persisting collapse of the body of L1.

there is increased local heat. The range of motion of the adjacent joint is restricted, and progressive disuse atrophy develops. Occasionally a pathologic fracture is the presenting complaint.

The usual site of osteogenic sarcoma is the metaphysis of a long bone; in 50 percent of cases, the distal end of the femur and the proximal end of the tibia are involved. Next in frequency are the proximal metaphyses, the humerus, and the femur. Occasionally osteogenic sarcoma is located in the fibula, innominate bone, or vertebral column.

There is no sex predilection; it occurs equally in males and females. The usual age is 10 to 20 years, although it can occur in the young child and older adult.

Osteogenic sarcoma develops from cells of the mesenchymal series and forms tumor osteoid and osseous tissue. The *classic osteogenic sarcoma* develops in the interior of bone. *Juxtacortical or parosteal osteogenic sarcoma* develops on the surface of bone in relation to the periosteum and immediate parosteal connective tissue. *Telangiectatic osteogenic sarcoma* grows rapidly and undergoes cystic and necrotic changes with evidence of neoplastic osseous tissue formation; it is highly malignant. In telangiectatic osteogenic sarcoma, the bone is weakened by the rapid destructive osteolytic process and pathologic fracture is not uncommon. Classification of osteogenic sarcoma is given in Table 6–3.

Etiology. The exact cause of osteogenic sarcoma remains obscure. Cytogenetic studies have shown that in some cases of osteosarcoma, an anti-oncogene, a specific retinoblastoma gene, is absent. The absence of the same gene leads to retinoblastoma. Patients with hereditary retinoblastoma are 1000 times more prone to develop osteogenic sarcoma than are normal individuals. The male to female ratio is 1.6 to 1.

TABLE 6–3. CLASSIFICATION OF OSTEOSARCOMA

Primary
    Intramedullary—central
        Classic-conventional
        Telangiectatic
        Small cell
        Fibrohistiocytic
        Low-grade intraosseous
        Multicentric
    Surface—juxtacortical
        Parosteal
        Periosteal
        High-grade surface
        Undifferentiated parosteal
Secondary
    Radiation induced
    Developing in benign presenting conditions (such as fibrodysplasia)
    Paget's disease (in adults)

Imaging.   In the radiograms, destructive and osteoblastic changes are the characteristic findings of osteogenic sarcoma. Bone destruction is depicted by ill-defined, irregular, ragged radiolucent defects and tumor bone formation by irregular areas of increased radiopacity (Fig 6–54).

The growing intramedullary tumor mass involves and destroys the regional cortex, raises the periosteum, and produces a "sunburst" image on the radiogram; spicules of new bone are formed and lie perpendicular to the shaft along the vessels passing from the periosteum to the cortex. Codman's triangle is formed, which represents subperiosteal new bone with its base perpendicular to the shaft. Both the "sunburst" appearance and Codman's triangle are not diagnostic of osteogenic sarcoma; they may be seen in Ewing's sarcoma and osteomyelitis.

In the differential diagnosis of osteogenic sarcoma, one should consider subacute osteomyelitis, exuberant callus of stress fracture, eosinophilic granuloma, aneurysmal bone cyst, active myositis ossificans, fibrosarcoma, Ewing's sarcoma, and metastatic carcinoma. Prior to definitive treatment, it is crucial to confirm the diagnosis of osteogenic sarcoma by pathologic examination of the lesion.

When osteogenic sarcoma is suspected in the plain radiogram, the following imaging investigations are carried out (1) *CT,* which demonstrates the bone destruction, tumor bone formation, and the degree of local extension in detail; (2) *MRI* of the entire bone, which delineates the intramedullary extent of the tumor, extension and exact involvement of soft tissues, including vessels and nerves, and rules out skip lesions; (3) *bone scan with technetium-99m,* which shows marked increased uptake as well as other bony and soft tissue sites[549,552,565]; (4) *chest x-ray* and *chest CT,* which demonstrate absence or presence of pulmonary metastases; and (5) *biplanar peripheral angiography,* which delineates the extent of soft tissue extension and its relationship to adjacent vessels and nerves; it is performed preoperatively to assist in decision-making in limb salvage versus amputation.

Laboratory Tests.   In osteogenic sarcoma the serum level of alkaline phosphatase is elevated because of osteogenesis in the tumor tissue. Following ablation of the tumor, levels of alkaline phosphatase fall to normal values; with recurrence and metastases they elevate. There is disagreement as to the prognostic value of monitoring the course of osteogenic sarcoma by serial determination of serum alkaline phosphatase levels.

The presence of anti-osteosarcoma antibody in the serum can be determined by hemagglutinins or by precipitins against extracts of osteosarcoma. The level of antibodies against extract of osteosarcoma increases following excision of the tumor and decreases following recurrence or development of metastases.

Staging.   Definitive diagnosis of osteogenic sarcoma is made by histologic examination of tissue from the lesion by open biopsy. The tumor should be surgically staged prior to biopsy.[555] Both the staging and open biopsy should be performed by the surgeon who will carry out the definitive treatment.

Tumors are separated into (1) *two histologic grades* (low grade [G_1] and high grade [G_2], (2) *two anatomic sites* (intracompartmental [T_1] and extracompartmental [T_2]), and (3) *two categories as to metastases* (none [M_0] and with metastases [M_1]).

Patients with low-grade histologic lesions are graded as stage I, those with high grade as stage II, and those with metastases (either in regional lymph nodes or distal sites) as stage III (Table 6–4). Each *bone* is considered to have its own separate anatomic compartment. A soft tissue anatomic compartment is defined as a muscle group separated by fascial boundaries that act as barriers to tumor extension (Table 6–5).

Biopsy.   Prior to biopsy, obtain a consultation with the radiologist, pathologist, and oncologist (who may perform a bone marrow aspiration when the child is anesthetized prior to beginning chemotherapy). Osteogenic sarcoma demands interdisciplinary coordination and management.

There are three *types of biopsy:* (1) needle, (2) incisional, and (3) excisional. When the lesion is surgically accessible,

TABLE 6–4. SURGICAL STAGING

Stage	Grade	Site	Metastases
IA	Low (G_1)	Intracompartmental (T_1)	None (M_0)
IB	Low (G_1)	Extracompartmental (T_2)	None (M_0)
IIA	High (G_2)	Intracompartmental (T_1)	None (M_0)
IIB	High (G_2)	Extracompartmental (T_2)	None (M_0)
III	Any (G)	Any (T)	With regional or distant metastasis (M_1)

TABLE 6–5. SURGICAL SITES

Intracompartmental (T_1)	Extracompartmental (T_2)
Intraosseous	Soft tissue extension
Intra-articular	Soft tissue extension
Superficial to deep fascia	Deep fascial extension
Paraosseous	Intraosseous or extrafascial extension
Intrafascial compartments	Extrafascial planes or spaces
Ray of hand or foot	Mid- and hindfoot
Posterior calf	Popliteal space
Anterolateral leg	Groin–femoral triangle
Anterolateral thigh	Intrapelvic
Medial thigh	Midhand

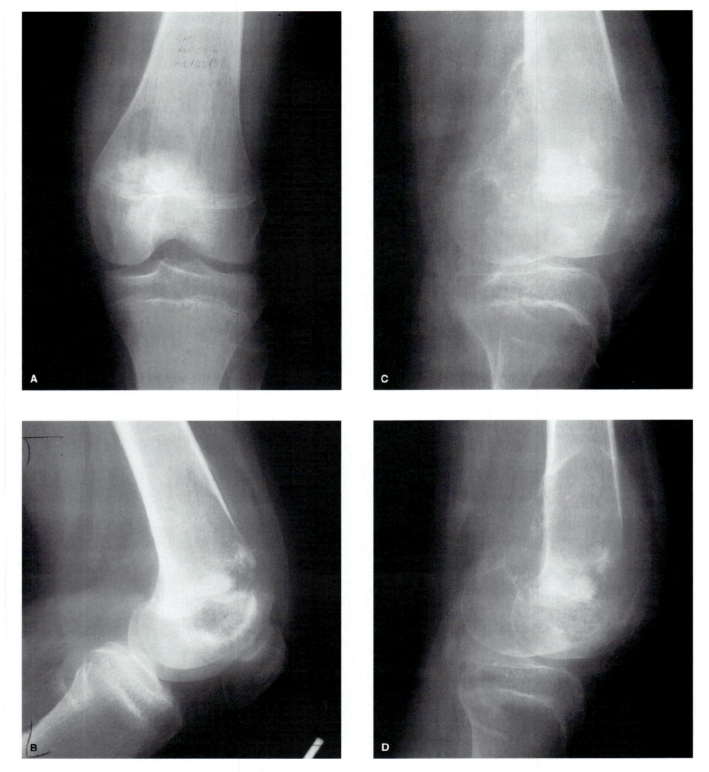

Figure 6–54. Osteogenic sarcoma involving the left distal femur in a 14-year-old boy. The patient complained of pain, which was diagnosed as internal derangement of the right knee. **A, B.** AP and lateral radiograms. Note the bone destruction and tumor bone formation. Diagnosis of osteogenic sarcoma was not suspected from these initial radiograms. **C, D.** AP and lateral radiograms of the distal femur showing the marked increase in the extent of destruction and tumor bone formation. The patient presented with an increasing, painful mass on the medial aspect of the distal thigh. *(Continues)*

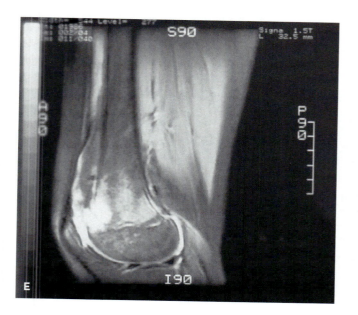

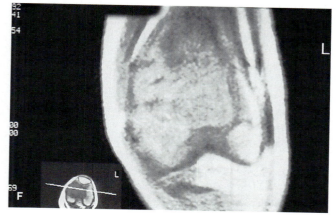

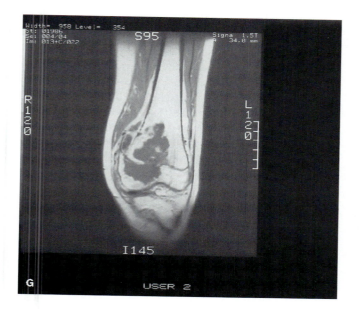

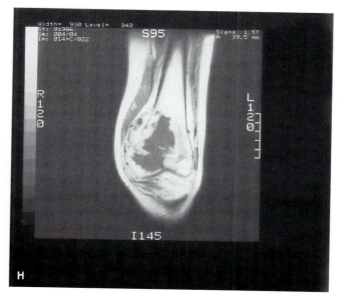

Figure 6–54 *(Continued).* **E–H.** MRI of the distal femur showing the bone destruction and tumor bone formation.

open biopsy should be performed because it enables the surgeon to visualize the tumor tissue and obtain adequate representative tissue. Mistakes are often made by needle biopsy. The disadvantage of open biopsy is tumor spillage.

Incisional biopsy is performed in malignant and aggressive lesions involving soft tissues. Excisional biopsy is performed when the lesion is small and easily removed with a safe margin and in benign bone tumors.

Exercise the following technique during biopsy: (1) Always verify the anatomic site of biopsy by biplanar radiography in the operating room. (2) Perform frozen section, if possible, to ensure that adequate tissue has been obtained for diagnosis. (3) Perform culture studies routinely. (4) Use a tourniquet and elevate the limb (do not exsanguinate with bandage) prior to inflation. (5) Use longitudinal and not transverse incisions. (5) Do not develop wound flaps. (6) Consider the possibility of limb salvage during surgical exposure; incision and deep dissection must be resectable. (7) Go straight through muscle to tumor. (8) Avoid and do not expose neurovascular structures. (9) Use sharp dissection and a coagulation diathermy knife in order to prevent spillage of neoplastic cells into vascular channels. (10) When soft tissue extension is present and adequate tissue is available for pathologic diagnosis, do not biopsy bone. If you have to violate the cortex, make round and oblong apertures to diminish the risk of fracture. Plug the hole with thrombin-soaked Gelfoam and collograft. (11) Achieve complete hemostasis and drain the wound with the suction tubes in line with the excision. (12) Close the wound tautly in layers.

Treatment. The current treatment of osteosarcoma consists of surgical resection of the tumor and adjuvant chemotherapy. The treatment plan is as follows: First, *open biopsy* to make the diagnosis, and second, adjuvant chemotherapy for 4 to 6 weeks. The principal chemotherapeutic drug is methotrexate. Other neoadjuvant chemotherapeutic agents given in combination are cyclophosphamide, actinomycin D, doxorubicin, cisplatin, and blecomycin.

Preoperative chemotherapy reduces edema and decreases the size of the tumor, making limb salvage surgery possible. It also determines the efficacy of the chemotherapeutic agents being used, thereby allowing the administration of the most effective drug postoperatively. The drugs are changed following ablation of the tumor if there is no response to the preoperative chemotherapeutic agent.

The third phase is *definitive surgery.* Total removal of the tumor with clear margins is top priority. If possible, function is preserved by limb salvage; if not feasible, the limb is amputated. The *fourth phase* is post–definitive surgery adjuvant chemotherapy for an additional 12 months. The choice of the chemotherapeutic agent is individualized, depending upon the response of the tumor tissue to the drug used preoperatively; there should be greater than 90 percent tumor necrosis. With effective neoadjuvant chemotherapy and surgical resection of the tumor, the 5-year survival rate of osteogenic sarcoma is 70 percent. Of the various prognostic factors, the histologic response to preoperative chemotherapy is the most important. The worst prognosis is in patients with pulmonary metastases and skip lesions.

When resecting the tumor, localize the exact site and extent of the lesion on the MRI (longitudinal cuts) which involve the entire bone. Determine the extent of the resection on the MRI performed when the tumor mass was at its largest, usually on the first MRI. Always excise the biopsy wound and site.

Limb salvage has the disadvantages of risk of local recurrence, the possible presence of skip lesions, the extensive operative procedure and its possible complications, quality of life during recovery, and the disfiguring aspects of the procedure. Limb salvage entails excision of the segment of bone involved with the tumor and replacement and reconstruction of the intercalary segment with autograft—usually vascularized fibula. Chemotherapy does not delay union of the graft, and with the stress loading of weight-bearing, the fibula hypertrophies in time. A problem is fracture of the graft because these children want to lead a normal life. The fractures heal normally, with the hypertrophic callus increasing the diameter of the autograft. The use of allografts, particularly osteoarticular replacements for the lower limb and pelvis, is controversial. Some surgeons utilize allografts in reconstruction of the proximal humerus and femur in combination with prostheses (allograft prosthetic composites). Expandable prostheses are used occasionally, but they are associated with numerous problems and complications such as infection, loss of length, and loosening, requiring reoperations.

Large lesions of the distal femur, proximal tibia, and proximal femur with extensive soft tissue involvement are best managed by rotationplasty and a modified below-knee prosthesis. When the distal femur is resected, the ankle joint becomes the knee and the triceps surae functions as the quadriceps. When the proximal tibia is resected, the ankle joint becomes the knee and the quadriceps is preserved to function as the knee extensor. On the rare occasion when the proximal femur is resected, the knee joint is converted to become the hip, the ankle to become the knee, and the triceps surae to function as the "quadriceps." Functionally the children with rotationplasty have an efficient gait and walk with greater efficiency because they are provided with a "motorized knee"; that is, the ankle is converted to function as a knee and provides swing phase control.

In the upper limb when the scapula is involved, limb salvage consists of excision of the scapula and resection of the lateral clavicle. It preserves satisfactory function. When the proximal humerus, radius, or ulna is involved, the involved segments of the long bones are resected and replaced with vascularized fibula. Limb salvage combined with neoadjuvant and adjuvant chemotherapy has increased the 5-year disease-free survival rate to about 65 percent.[551,563,573]

Amputation is indicated in (1) patients with excessively large tumors with extension of the tumor into soft tissues and involvement of major vessels and nerves, rendering limb salvage impossible, (2) those who have pulmonary metastases, and (3) those in whom the disease cannot be controlled by chemotherapy. With aggressive surgery and chemotherapy, the survival rate of these children is improved.

When pulmonary metastases develop, the lobe involved with tumor is resected.

SURFACE OSTEOSARCOMAS[545,548,556,572,574]

These tumors develop on the surface, the periosteal aspect of bone. They comprise the following biologically heterogeneous group of neoplasms: (1) parosteal osteosarcoma, (2) periosteal osteosarcoma, (3) high-grade surface osteosarcoma, and (4) dedifferentiated parosteal osteosarcoma.

Both parosteal and periosteal osteosarcomas occur exclusively on the appendicular skeleton, with the distal femur and proximal tibia being the most common sites. Parosteal osteosarcoma occurs in the third to fifth decades of life, whereas periosteal osteosarcoma occurs in the second or third decade of life. They are slow-growing tumors and usually not painful. The presenting complaint is a progressively enlarging mass and interference with joint function such as inability to fully extend the knee. The treatment of both parosteal and periosteal osteosarcomas is wide surgical excision; they do not respond to chemotherapy. The prognosis is good.

High-grade surface osteosarcoma and dedifferentiated parosteal osteosarcoma are life-threatening. They are treated with a combination of chemotherapy and surgery.

EWING'S SARCOMA[578–590]

This primary malignant tumor of bone arises from the non-mesenchymal cells of the bone marrow; it is second in prevalence to osteogenic sarcoma, which is twice as common as Ewing's sarcoma in white children. Ewing's sarcoma is very rare in the Black race. There is a definite predilection for the 10 to 15 year age group. Cytogenetic studies have demonstrated that the majority of the tumor cells in Ewing's sarcoma have a translocation between chromosomes 11 and 22.

Common sites of Ewing's sarcoma are the femur, tibia, humerus, fibula, innominate bone, rib, scapula, and vertebrae. In the long bones, the sarcomatous lesion is located in the diaphysis rather than the metaphysis. The hands and feet are very rarely affected by Ewing's sarcoma.

Clinical Features. The presenting complaint is local pain. In the long bones, varying degrees of stiffness of the adjacent joints is common. When the femur, tibia, or fibula is affected, the child has an antalgic limp. When the lumbar vertebrae are the site of the lesion, back pain with sciatica is the presenting complaint. When the ilium, ischium, or pelvis is affected, impingement of the pelvic organs such as the bladder may occur. Pleural effusion may be noted when the ribs are affected.

On examination, a tumor mass can often be palpated and is tender on pressure. With penetration of the cortex and extraosseous spread of the neoplasm, the mass rapidly increases in size. When the ilium is the site of the lesion, the painful tumor mass is palpable in the lower quadrant of the abdomen or in the buttocks. When the ischium or pelvis is involved, the mass is palpable on rectal examination.

The child or adolescent with Ewing's sarcoma has a low-grade fever, is anemic, and lethargic, and has no appetite. Progressive weight loss is commonly found. The leukocytes shift to the left and the ESR is elevated.

Imaging. Plain radiograms show mottled rarefaction with permeation of the overlying cortex. The affected bone displays some expansion and periosteal new bone formation in the form of laminated "onion peel" appearance (Fig 6–55). These radiographic findings are not specific to Ewing's sarcoma; they can occur in osteomyelitis, eosinophilic granuloma, metastatic neuroblastoma, reticulum cell sarcoma, malignant lymphoma, and "osteolytic" osteogenic sarcoma.

Soft tissue mass overlying the area of bone is often present. MRI clearly demonstrates the soft tissue mass and extent of the tumor. CT shows the extent of intraosseous involvement and the extraosseous soft tissue spread. Scintigraphy with technetium-99m discloses markedly increased uptake at the site of the lesion. All of these imaging modalities are used to stage Ewing's sarcoma.

At the time of presentation, Ewing's sarcoma may be staged as follows: *stage I*—solitary and intraosseous; *stage II*—solitary and extraosseous; *stage III*—metastatic but confined to the affected bone; and *stage IV*—distinct metastases.

Treatment. Historically, when surgery was the only option for treatment of Ewing's sarcoma, the 5-year survival rate was less than 10 percent. The tumor is radiosensitive, and irradiation controlled the tumor initially and markedly reduced the size of the tumor. Irradiation, however, does not completely eradicate the tumor; there is a substantial local recurrence rate of 30 percent. Radiation therapy also has definite drawbacks and complications; it interferes with normal bone growth and causes limb length disparity, scoliosis and kyphosis, osseous necrosis, soft tissue

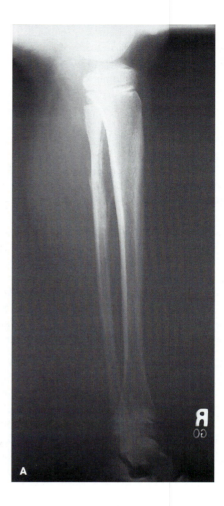

and articular changes, osteitis, and pathologic fracture. The most serious complication is radiation-induced osteosarcoma.

At present, the treatment recommended for Ewing's sarcoma is chemotherapy combined with wide excision of the tumor. Radiation therapy is added when the margins of the resected tumor are questionably narrow and not wide. The chemotherapy is of the neoadjuvant type, consisting of vincristine, cyclophosphamide, doxorubicin, and etoposide. With such a protocol of management, the survival rate of Ewing's sarcoma has markedly improved. Approximately 20 percent of patients with Ewing's sarcoma have metastases at the time of diagnosis. The survival rate of children with metastasis is poor. Early diagnosis is crucial to improve survival.

CHONDROSARCOMA

Chondrosarcoma occurs rarely in the adolescent and is extremely rare in childhood. Most of the chondrosarcomas are secondary, developing in benign cartilaginous lesions such as solitary enchondroma, multiple enchondromatosis, osteochondroma, and multiple hereditary exostosis. Primary chondrosarcoma almost never occurs in a child.

Malignant transformation arises in the metaphysis of long bones in enchondroma and multiple enchondromatosis, whereas in exostosis and multiple hereditary exostoses it occurs in the region of the shoulder girdle, vertebral column, and pelvis (Fig 6–56).

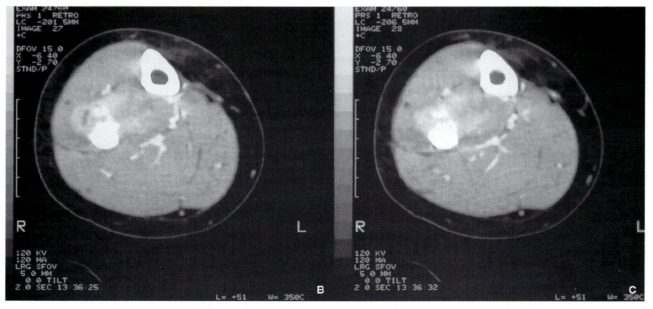

Figure 6–55. Ewing's sarcoma of the proximal fibula. **A.** Lateral view of the tibia and fibula. **B, C.** MRI showing the destruction of the fibula with soft tissue extension.

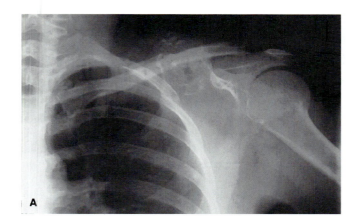

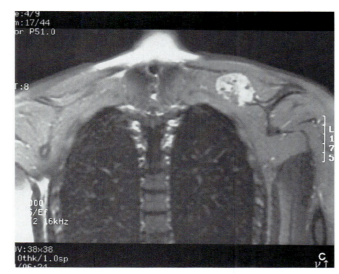

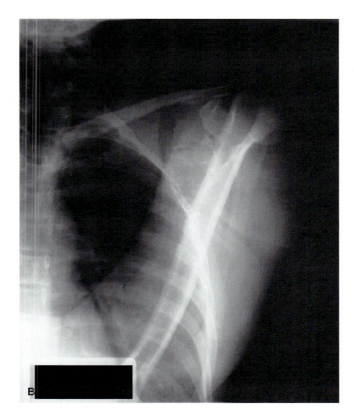

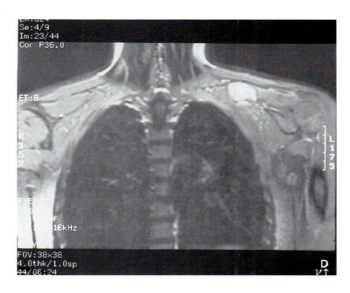

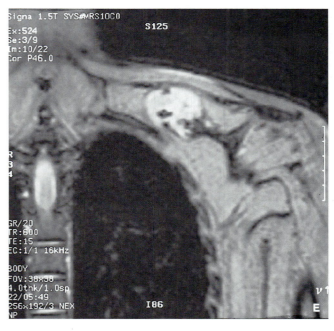

Figure 6–56. Chondrosarcoma of the left scapula. **A, B.** AP and lateral radiograms showing the calcification of the tumor mass. **C–E.** MRI clearly showing the calcified tumor.

The presenting complaint varies with the location of the chondrosarcoma. When it is centrally located, the patient complains of steady, dull aching pains; in peripheral chondrosarcoma, the patient presents with a deformity of the limb or slowing enlarging mass.

MRI delineates the thickness, irregularity, and calcification of the cartilaginous cap of secondary chondrosarcoma of an exostosis and also the internal structure of chondrosarcoma developing secondary to enchondroma.

Chondrosarcomas are slow-growing malignant tumors that do not metastasize early. Treatment consists of resection of an expendable bone. Limb salvage is possible in almost all cases. The ablated part is replaced by autograft or vascularized autograft. Occasionally in advanced cases, limb salvage by rotationplasty is performed. The prognosis for survival is excellent.

ADAMANTINOMA[591–594]

A tumor of unknown origin, adamantinoma occurs most commonly in the tibia, involving the anterior cortex of the diaphysis.

The presenting complaint is local pain. The onset is insidious; when there is a pathologic fracture, the onset of pain is acute. Anterior bowing of the tibia is common. Palpation reveals a localized mass that is warm and tender.

In plain radiograms, the lesion demonstrates a "soap bubble" appearance. On bone scan with technetium-99m the tumor shows markedly increased uptake. CT clearly demonstrates the area of bone destruction.

Treatment consists of excision with a wide surgical margin. When the medullary canal is penetrated, segmented resection with a wide margin and reconstruction of the limb with allograft are performed. When attempted segmental resection fails, a below-knee or knee disarticulation is indicated.

Malignant fibrous histiocytosis and fibrosarcoma of bone are very rare tumors in childhood.

METASTATIC TUMORS OF BONE[595–601]

In the radiogram the metastatic bone tumors are characterized by "punched-out" osteolytic areas with minimal or no reactive new bone formation. A solitary metastatic bone lesion may be mistaken for primary tumor. In children, neuroblastoma and nephroblastoma (Wilms' tumor) are the two malignant tumors that frequently metastasize to bone.

Neuroblastoma

This tumor occurs in infants and children under 5 years of age. It is a malignant round cell tumor that usually originates from the medulla of the adrenal gland, but it can arise from any part of the sympathetic nervous system. It metas-

tasizes to bone, liver, and lymph nodes via the hematogenous and lymphatic routes. The skeletal lesions usually are multiple.

The presenting complaint is pain in the affected bone and discomfort at the site of origin of the neuroblastoma, usually the abdomen. Ultrasonography, CT, and MRI studies disclose the primary location of the neuroblastoma. Scintigraphy with fluorine-18 and technetium-99m show increased uptake in the osseous and extraosseous lesions.

Diagnosis is made by the presence of neoplastic cells in bone marrow smears or histologic examination of the metastatic lesion in bone. In the urine, 3-methoxy-4-hydroxymandelic acid and homovanillic acid levels are elevated.

Treatment consists of chemotherapy and irradiation. The prognosis is very poor when neuroblastoma has metastasized to bone.

Wilms' Tumor

This usually occurs in infants and children under 3 years of age. It presents as an abdominal mass. Lower limb length disparity and hemihypertrophy may be the first signs of Wilms' tumor. Don't miss it! Order an ultrasonogram of the abdomen. In late diagnosed cases, metastasis to the skeleton may have occurred and back pain may be the presenting complaint.

Treatment consists of immediate nephrectomy. Function of the opposite kidney should be assessed prior to surgery. Metabolic bone lesions are treated by chemotherapy and irradiation.

SOFT TISSUE TUMORS[607–621]

When a child presents with a soft tissue mass in the limbs, it may be due to (1) an inflammatory process, (2) trauma such as myositis ossificans or false aneurysm, (3) a benign soft tissue tumor, or (4) malignant soft tissue tumor.

History and Examination. Ask when the soft tissue mass was first noted and whether it is increasing in size. Is there any history of injury or infection? Most soft tissue tumors, benign or malignant, do not cause pain or limb dysfunction. Inflammatory and traumatic masses may be painful and tender on palpation. Feel the consistency of the mass; is it soft or hard? Does it pulsate? On auscultation, is there a bruit? Is there a Tinel sign (on percussion of the tumor involving a nerve, a tingling sensation in the distal end of the limb)? A positive Tinel sign suggests a nerve sheath tumor. What is the exact location of the soft tissue mass? Is it subcutaneous or deep? Try to measure its size. As a rule, soft tissue masses that are deep and larger than 5 cm are more likely to be malignant than smaller subcutaneous masses. What is the mobility of the soft tissue mass? Is it fixed to surrounding tissues or loose? Does it move when the adjacent joint is flexed and extended? Does it transilluminate? Clinical assessment of soft tissue masses is ordinarily unreliable.

Imaging Findings. In evaluation of soft tissue masses, *plain radiograms* are of no diagnostic value. Soft tissue masses usually have the same radiographic density as muscle. A lipoma shows a homogeneous fat density. Calcification may be present due to deposition of calcium in necrotic tissue; it occurs in malignant soft tissue tumors such as synovial sarcoma. Calcification is also visualized in the rounded phlebolith of hemangioma. Plain radiograms show areas of ossification in soft tissue masses such as in myositis ossificans. Plain radiograms also demonstrate extrinsic pressure on bone.

Ultrasound imaging determines the depth and size of a soft tissue mass and whether it is cystic or solid.[613] A soft tissue mass that is superficial in location, less than 5 cm in size, and entirely cystic is most probably benign, especially if located around a joint such as the knee. If it is deep, greater than 5 cm in size, and not entirely cystic, it is likely to be malignant, such as a rhabdomyosarcoma (especially in the thigh). It must be pointed out, however, that benign tumors such as intramuscular lipoma, desmoid tumor, hemangioma, and nerve sheath tumors can be deep in their location and that one third of all soft tissue sarcomas are subcutaneous. A biopsy is vital in making the definitive diagnosis.

Staging studies are carried out when malignancy is suspected. *CT* shows that the soft tissue mass is often isodense, similar to muscle. Exceptions to this are the homogeneous fat density of lipoma and heterogeneous fat density of liposarcoma. CT demonstrates extrinsic cortical invasion and calcification or ossification in the soft tissue mass. CT does not assist in differentiation between a benign and malignant soft tissue tumor.

Scintigraphy with gallium is of diagnostic value; malignant soft tissue sarcomas show increased uptake, whereas benign soft tissue tumors show normal uptake.[611] MRI is performed in the sagittal and coronal planes; it shows the location of the soft tissue mass, its size, extent, and relationship to bone, and its neurovascular status. It distinguishes masses that are composed of fat from those that are not. On the T1- and T2-weighted images, fat produces a higher signal than muscle. MRI is preferable to CT in assessment of soft tissue tumors.[612,620] *Angiography* to delineate the vascular relations is indicated only when limb salvage is considered.

Next, only a few of the benign and malignant soft tissue tumors are presented.

Lipoma. This common soft tissue tumor in infants and children may be subcutaneous or intramuscular. The instep of the foot is a common site. It presents as a soft, flabby mass with indistinct boundaries. On palpation, a suggestion of fluctuation is felt. It does not transilluminate. Lipomas cast a soft tissue shadow of "fat density" in the radiogram and a cystic appearance in the ultrasonogram. Treatment consists of surgical excision. Lipomas are surrounded by a definite capsule.

Ganglions. These thin-walled cysts contain clear, colorless, gelatinous fluid. They seem to arise from tendon sheaths or from within the connective tissue of the subjacent joint capsule. They usually are located around the wrist, foot and ankle, or knee. The presenting complaint is a soft tissue mass that may feel hard when distended and tense with fluid. The mass transilluminates. Radiograms are made to rule out the presence of a bony spur or osteochondroma that is irritating the tendon and causing the ganglions. Ultrasonography shows a fluid consistency in the mass. It is indicated only in deep lesions.

Treatment is indicated when the ganglion enlarges and causes pain. In the foot, a ganglion may be painful on weight-bearing. Aspiration and prednisone injection are ordinarily not successful; the ganglion recurs. Complete excision of the ganglion results in a cure.

Hemangiomas. These comprise 7 percent of benign soft tissue tumors. They may be congenital in origin, presenting at birth, or they may develop in childhood or adolescence. *Solitary hemangiomas* are of two types: (1) *capillary hemangioma*, which occurs in 1 in every 200 live births; ordinarily treatment is not indicated, as 95 percent involute by 7 years of age; and (2) *cavernous hemangioma*, which may be *superficial*, involving the skin, or *deep*. Cavernous hemangiomas usually do not regress. Deep lesions may involve muscle, nerves, or bone and become painful. Thrombophlebitic areas develop in cavernous hemangiomas. Superficial cavernous hemangiomas are treated by laser surgery; the deep lesions may be excised or embolized. Cavernous hemangioma does not undergo malignant transformation.

Diffuse hemangioma or angiomatosis may involve a segment or an entire limb. Diagnosis is obvious. Increased circulation to the part causes hypertrophy and increased length of the limb. Treatment is by embolization or surgical excision, best performed by vascular and plastic surgeons.

Benign tumors of *nerve* origin are *neurilemoma* and *neurofibroma*. Neurilemomas develop from the Schwann cells of the nerve sheath.[615] The presenting complaint is a soft tissue mass that is firm in consistency. Often asymptomatic, it may become painful when located in weight-bearing areas of the foot. A neurilemoma does not cause neurologic deficit. When painful, it is treated by marginal excision.

Neurofibromas may be solitary or multiple (von Recklinghausen's disease). Nerves may become affected. (See section on neurofibromatosis.)

Rhabdomyosarcoma. This malignant muscle tumor comprises 3.5 percent of all childhood malignancies. In the United States there are 350 new cases each year.

The *embryonal type* of rhabdomyosarcoma is the most common, occurring in the child under 10 years of age. Common sites are the retroperitoneum, genitourinary tract, and head and neck; it does occur in the limbs. Metastasis is to local lymph nodes. The *alveolar type* of rhabdomyosarcoma is seen in older children. Treatment consists of wide surgical excision and chemotherapy.

Synovial Cell Sarcoma.[607–610,614,621] This malignant tumor accounts for 10 percent of all soft tissue sarcomas and is very rare in children. Half of the lesions occur in the limbs, with 10 percent involving the hands and feet. The tumor arises from the primitive synovial cells but rarely invades the joint.

The presenting complaint is a soft tissue mass that is often superficial in location and fixed to surrounding soft tissues. The mass grows slowly in size and may become painful. Often the diagnosis is delayed for months or longer. Radiograms may show spotty radiopacity representing focal calcifications in the necrotic tissue of the malignant soft tissue mass. CT is of value in depicting the soft tissue mass and finite areas of calcification which may not be visualized in the plain radiograms. Scintigraphy with technetium-99m shows increased uptake. The tumor metastasizes to local lymph nodes. Treatment consists of surgical resection.

TUMORAL CALCINOSIS[622–627]

The presenting complaint is a mass, which may be of varying sizes, fixed deeply to the periarticular tissues. Stiffness of involved joints is minimal. The usual site is the extensor aspect of the shoulder, hip, or elbow. Occasionally small joints are involved.[624]

Treatment. Excision of the tumor is ordinarily not indicated because the condition is asymptomatic. Successful treatment with an oral suspension of dihydroxyaluminum-sodium carbonate and limiting the dietary intake of calcium and phosphorus are reported by Gregosiewicz et al.[622] Surgery is performed when the tumor enlarges, becomes unsightly, interferes with joint motion, or ulcerates and develops secondary infection. The recurrence rate is high.

NEUROFIBROMATOSIS (NF)[628–705]

In this neural crest disorder, cells derived from the neural crest invade the pigmented cells of the skin, parts of the central and peripheral nervous systems, adrenals, and skeleton. The exact pathogenesis and pathobiology are unknown.

NF is a genetic disorder, autosomal dominant in inheritance, with 100 percent penetrance. About half of the cases are fresh mutations. Neurofibromatosis affects 1 in 3000 newborns. The prevalence increases with increasing paternal age.

Classification. NF manifests in two types: (1) NF1 or peripheral type; this is the classic disease as described by von Recklinghausen and accounts for 85 percent of all cases; and (2) NF2 or the central type, which is characterized by bilateral acoustic neuromas and only a few peripheral manifestations.[654] The gene for NF1 is mapped to the long arm of chromosome 17; it is a very large gene, the intron containing three smaller genes, one of which encodes for a protein neurofibrin similar to the glutamyl transpeptidase–activating proteins. NF2 is very rare, occurring in 1 in 35,000 live births. It is autosomal dominant in inheritance. The gene of NF2 is localized on the long arm of chromosome 22 and has been cloned. In this section only NF1 is discussed.

Diagnosis. The clinical manifestations of NF1 vary widely. This marked diversity of physical findings and the fact that a child with NF may appear to be normal at birth make its clinical diagnosis difficult. In order to make the diagnosis of NF1, the patient should have two or more of the following findings: (1) Six or more café-au-lait spots, which should be 5 mm or more in diameter in a child and 15 mm or more in an adult. The café-au-lait spots are the hallmark of NF; they are tan-colored and smooth-edged, they may take 12 months to appear, and their size and number increase with increasing age. Do not mistake the dark brown hyperpigmented nevi for café-au-lait spots. (2) Axillary and inguinal freckling, a common skin marking in NF1. It is very rare in persons who do not have NF1. (3) Neurofibromas, at least two cutaneous or a single plexiform. The *cutaneous neurofibromas* are ordinarily found immediately underneath the skin; they consist of benign Schwann cells and fibrous connective tissue. Cutaneous neurofibromas are not associated with neurologic deficit. Clinically they are not evident in the first decade of life. At puberty the cutaneous neurofibromas increase in number. The term *fibroma molluscum* denotes a number of neurofibromas conglomerating on the skin. *Plexiform neurofibromas* are highly vascular, infiltrate the adjacent tissues, and produce gigantism of the involved limb. They may be painful to touch and pressure. The overlying skin is usually darkly pigmented. (4) One or more of the following skeletal lesions, which are distinctive to NF1, such as pseudarthrosis of long bones (commonly of the tibia or fibula), dystrophic kyphoscoliosis, scalloping of the posterior surface of the vertebral bodies, enlargement of neural foramina, and local or generalized overgrowth of a limb. This is sometimes associated with verrucous hyperplasia, in which there is a tremendous overgrowth of the skin, which is thickened with a soft papillary feel and with crevices that tend to break down easily. There may be some oozing between the skin folds. A foul odor may emanate from the superficial infection. Large soft tissue masses with rough, raised villous skin are the characteristic finding of elephantiasis, which is a very unsightly manifestation of the disease. (5) At least two Lisch nodules, which are melanocystic hamartomas protruding from the surface of the iris; these are easily detected by slit-lamp examination. (6) A first-degree relative with NF1.

Other clinical features of NF1 are hypertension (which is due to stenosis of the renal artery), pheochromocytoma, short stature with an enlarged head, and mental retardation. Malignancy may develop in 2 to 5 percent of patients with NF1. It is usually an astrocytoma of the CNS or a glioma of the optic nerve. Neurofibromas may undergo sarcomatous changes.[632,657]

Orthopedic Implications.

The three most serious problems are pseudarthrosis of the long bones, kyphoscoliosis, and overgrowth of the limbs, both bony and soft tissue. Often the tibia and fibula are the sites of pseudarthrosis of the long bones. Management of this complex problem is discussed in Chapter 2. Occasionally the clavicle, radius, ulna, or femur is involved. Their management follows the same principles as that of the tibia and fibula.

Dystrophic scoliosis in NF1 is characterized by a sharp and short (four to six vertebrae) curvature with marked rotation of the apical vertebra and distortion of the ribs. The site of scoliosis is usually thoracic.[628,630,636,639,640,644] The natural history is relentless progression with marked deformity. This dystrophic kyphoscoliosis does not respond to orthotic management. It requires early surgical intervention. In NF1, curves resembling idiopathic scoliosis may occur. Other vertebral abnormalities are the following: (1) Enlargement of the neural foramina (in such an instance, rule out a dumbell neurofibroma in the spinal canal which protrudes through the neural foramina). MRI of the spinal canal makes the diagnosis. (2) Pedicle defects occasionally occur and a vertebra may become completely displaced. This is treated by spinal fusion and instrumentation. (3) Anterolateral meningoceles have been demonstrated by MRI. They may erode the pedicles and require combined neurosurgical and orthopedic management for excision of the meningocele and stabilization of the spine with fusion and internal fixation.

Overgrowth of soft tissue and bone in NF is a difficult problem to manage. Limb length disparity is managed by epiphyseodesis. A multidisciplinary approach combining plastic and orthopedic surgery is required to debulk the grotesque soft tissue enlargement in stages.

PROTEUS SYNDROME[662–665]

Proteus syndrome is characterized by grotesque overgrowth of limbs and soft tissues, marked disfigurement of the facies, angular deformities of the limbs, and severe kypho-

scoliosis. The Elephant Man, John Merrick, who in the past was thought to have NF, has now been diagnosed with Proteus syndrome.[664] The condition was first described in detail by Wiedemann et al.[665] They named the syndrome after the ancient Greek demigod Proteus, who could change his appearance at will to avoid enemies. Proteus syndrome is a congenital hamartomatous affection of unknown cause. It should be differentiated from other hamartomatous diseases such as Klippel-Trenaunay-Weber syndrome, NF, Mafucci syndrome, and Banayan-Zonana syndrome. *Treatment* should be individualized. Leg length disparity, angular deformities, and macrodactyly are treated appropriately.

ARTHROGRYPOSIS MULTIPLEX CONGENITA[666–705]

Arthrogryposis, a term derived from the Greek, means literally curved or hooked joint. It encompasses a heterogeneous group of congenital disorders characterized by multiple joint contractural deformities. In the literature it is referred to by a number of other names, such as amyoplasia congenita and multiple congenital articular rigidity. Multiple congenital contracture (MCC), which was first used by Schanz and endorsed by Swinyard and Bleck, is the English translation of arthrogryposis multiplex congenita.[693,701] Arthrogryposis multiplex congenita (AMC) is a distinctive sign and not a diagnosis.

Multiple joint contractures are classified into three broad categories by Hall: (1) those primarily involving the limbs with no other abnormalities; (2) those with multiple congenital joint contractures plus anomalies in some other areas of the body such as the craniofacies or viscera; and (3) those with multiple congenital contractures of the limbs and severe CNS dysfunction.[676–678] The presenting clinical picture varies widely according to the type of MCC.

Multiple Congenital Contracture Primarily Involving the Limbs.

This category is divided into two subtypes: amyodysplasia congenita and distal arthrogryposis.

Amyodysplasia congenita is the most common type, comprising about half of the cases of MCC; the infant presents with the classic picture of arthrogryposis. This type of MCC is not hereditary, with no recurrence risk in the family. Despite the bizarre appearance of the child at birth, the disease is nonprogressive; however, joint deformities do increase with growth if not treated. The term *amyodysplasia,* however, is not correct; in the embryo the muscles are formed normally, but they undergo fibrosis and fibrofatty changes. The contractural deformity of the joints is caused by lack of motion and failure of normal development. The joint deformities represent in utero posture of the limbs when akinesia of the fetus takes place.

The distinctive clinical features of *classic AMC* are present at birth. They include (1) rigidity of multiple joints with some degree of free passive and painless motion between the extremes of range; the contractural deformity of the joints may be flexion and extension, and all four limbs may be affected or only the upper or only the lower; (2) dislocation of joints, most frequently the hips, knees, radial heads; talipes equinovarus deformity or congenital convex pes valgus deformity of the feet is common; (3) absence of normal creases and presence of deep dimples, usually at the elbows and patellae, (4) hypoplasia and fibrosis of muscles which, with a diminished mass of subcutaneous tissue, give the limbs a cylindrical shape and a "wooden doll" appearance; deep tendon reflexes may be absent or diminished, (5) normal intelligence and no CNS deficit (Fig 6–57).

Distal Arthrogryposis. In this form only the hands and feet are involved. The thumb is flexed and adducted across the palm; the fingers are flexed in the palm, overlapping each other; and the feet are clubbed or in severe calcaneo-

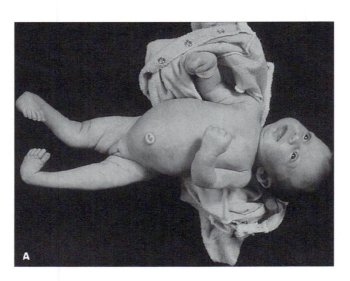

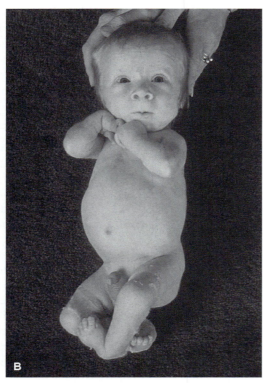

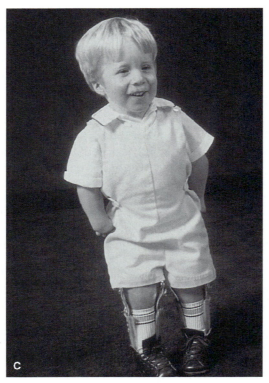

Figure 6–57. Clinical appearance of arthrogryposis multiplex congenita. **A.** Note the talipes equinovarus deformities of the feet, extension contractures of the knees, and flexion contractures of both elbows. **B.** An infant with arthrogyposis multiplex congenita with severe flexion deformity of the knees, hips and elbows. **C.** The same patient two years later following surgical correction of his deformities. *(Courtesy of Dr. John Sarwark.)*

valgus. The toes are contracted into hyperflexion. Distal arthrogryposis is inherited as an autosomal dominant trait.[678]

Multiple congenital joint contractures with involvement in other body parts are a very heterogeneous group of conditions, some of which are specific entities and syndromes such as diastrophic dwarfism and Freeman-Sheldon syndrome. Multiple congenital joint contractures with CNS dysfunction include many chromosomal abnormalities. Prognosis in this group is poor; the infants fail to thrive, and about 50 percent die during infancy or early childhood.

Etiology. Amyodysplasia is due to fetal akinesia.[683] The exact cause of lack of motion of the fetus in utero is unknown. Experimentally in the chick embryo, arthrogryposis has been produced by the Newcastle disease virus and Coxsackie virus.[691] In cattle, infection by the Akabane virus during early pregnancy has caused arthrogryposis. The survey by Wynne-Davies has demonstrated that arthrogryposis multiplex congenita is a nongenetic disease of early pregnancy, associated with a variety of unfavorable intrauterine factors and possibly caused by a viral environmental agent.[704]

Management. The deformities vary widely in extent, and the care of a child with arthrogryposis should be individualized depending upon the joints and limbs involved and the severity of the deformities. It is imperative that the surgeon explain to the parents what is involved in the overall care of the child and discuss the natural history. Children with amyodysplasia have normal intelligence and are able to walk and develop adequate function of the upper limbs for activities of daily living such as dressing, toilet needs, and self-feeding.

The joints are restricted in range of motion because of contracture of extra-articular tissues—the capsules, ligaments, and fibrosed muscles. These should be released surgically, as plaster casts and splints cause further rigidity of the joints. Following release of contractural deformities, physical therapy is performed to maintain range of motion and splints are used at night to prevent recurrence of deformities.

Surgery in the lower limbs is performed first. For example, a newborn child with arthrogryposis presents with congenital dislocation of both hips and knees and severe talipes equinovarus of both feet. The order of management is to reduce the knee subluxation first at 2 to 3 months of age by appropriate soft tissue release, followed at 4 to 5 months of age by surgical release and correction of clubfoot deformity and at 9 to 12 months of age by open reduction of both hips with femoral shortening. During this period of reconstruction of the lower limbs, upper limb deformities are splinted part-time and range of motion exercises are taught to the family. Upper limb surgery is postponed until

the child is 3 to 4 years of age, when adequate cooperation with postoperative care is possible. Lack of elbow flexion is a serious problem. Muscle tendon transfers are performed to provide elbow flexion so that the child can get his or her hand to the mouth.

BONE DYSPLASIAS[706–727]

Bone dysplasia is an intrinsic disturbance of the formation, growth, and remodeling of bone and cartilage due to genetic and inborn biochemical errors. In the long bones, the developmental affection may involve the epiphysis, physis, metaphysis, or diaphysis.

The presenting complaint varies according to the type of bone dysplasia. The diagnosis is readily made at birth in some of the bone dysplasias such as achondroplasia and diastrophic dysplasia, whereas in others the possibility of a developmental affection of the skeletal system is not suspected until later in childhood.

Bone dysplasia is suspected when an infant or child presents with short stature (proportionate or disproportionate) or very tall stature with slender and long fingers and feet (such as in Marfan's syndrome); angular deformation of the limbs, such as genu varum or valgum (particularly if asymmetric); lower limb length inequality; enlargement of the epiphysis; joint deformity, such as flexion contracture; or abnormal appearance of the head and face or deformities of the ear such as cauliflower ears. Pain is ordinarily not a feature of bone dysplasia unless a stress fracture develops in osteoporotic bones, such as in osteogenesis imperfecta.

History and Examination. First obtain a detailed family history, as most of the bone dysplasias are heritable disorders. Next, measure the child's standing and sitting height. Is there any disproportion between the length of the trunk and the length of the lower limbs? The lower segment is measured from the superior border of the symphysis pubis to the plantar surface of the feet with the ankles in neutral dorsiflexion. The upper segment is measured from the top of the head to the top of the symphysis pubis. In whites, the ratio between the upper and lower segments is 1.7:1 in the infant; then it gradually decreases to 1:1 in the older child. In blacks the lower segment is normally longer than the upper segment, whereas in the Chinese this proportion is reversed.

Determine the span of the upper limbs by measuring the distance between the tips of the long fingers with the shoulders abducted 90 degrees and the elbows, wrists, and fingers in neutral extension. In the normal child, the stature is approximately equal to the span of the upper limbs. In proportionate short stature, such as in pituitary dwarfism, the proportions between the limbs and the upper segment of the body are normal, whereas in disproportionate short stature such as in achondroplasia, the limbs in relation to the upper segment are disproportionately short. In the upper limb, measure the length of the arms (humeri) from the posterior tip of the acromion to the tip of the olecranon and that of the forearms from the tip of the olecranon to the tip of the radial and ulnar styloids (radius and ulna). In the lower limb, measure the length of the thighs (femurs) from the inferior surface of the anterior superior iliac spine to the medial knee joint line, and the length of the legs from the knee joint line to the distal tip of the medial malleolus (tibia) and that of the lateral malleolus (fibula). The shortness of the limbs is *rhizomelic* when the humeri and femora are relatively short, such as in achondroplasia; whereas the shortness is *centrifugal* when the limbs become progressively shorter toward the fingers and toes, as in Ellis–van Creveld syndrome. In Marfan's syndrome, the limbs are relatively long.

Inspect the face and head. Fine and sparse hair on the head, a large pear-shaped nose, and a long philtrum are findings in trichorhinophalangeal syndrome. Is the hair coarse, as in cretinism? A low hairline, bushy eyebrows meeting in the midline, small nose with anteverted nostrils, in-turned upper lip, and microcephaly are the distinctive features of *Cornelia de Lange syndrome* (a very rare disorder characterized also by short stature, mental retardation, congenital longitudinal deficiency of long bones, primarily on the ulnar or fibular side, and failure to thrive). The whistling face with a long philtrum, small nose, pursed mouth, deeply sunken eyes, and U- or H-shaped scarlike contractures that extend from the middle of the lower lip to the chin is distinctive of *craniocarpotarsal dysplasia (Freeman-Sheldon syndrome)*.

In *achondroplasia,* the bridge of the nose is depressed and flattened, the forehead bulges, the face is broad with a small maxillary region, the mandible is prognathous, the head appears disproportionately enlarged, and the skull is brachycephalic with decrease of its AP diameter. In *Hurler's syndrome* (mucopolysaccharidosis I), the facies is grotesque and heavy, resembling a gargoyle; the head is enlarged with a scaphocephalic (boat-shaped) skull; the forehead is low; the eyes are set wide (hypertelorism); the nose is saddle-shaped with a depressed bridge and wide nostrils; the lips are patulous, broad, and everted; the tongue is enlarged and thick; and the ears are set low. In *osteogenesis imperfecta,* the face is elfin-shaped and the forehead is broad, with prominent parietal and temporal bones and an overhanging occiput, resembling a soldier's helmet. In *Larsen's syndrome,* the facies is flat with a depressed nasal bridge, bulging forehead, and widely spaced eyes (hypertelorism). In *congenital contractural arachnodactyly,* the head is oval with retrognathia and a small mouth. In Down's syndrome, the eyes are slanted with prominent epicanthal folds. In osteogenesis imperfecta, the sclerae may be blue. In Marfan's syndrome, the lenses may be dislocated.

Next, inspect the *ears.* Are they abnormal? The cauliflower ears of diastrophic dysplasia and the crumpled ears of congenital contractural arachnodactyly are distinctive. Are the ears set low? How is the child's hearing? These examples illustrate the diagnostic importance of inspection of the skull, face, and eyes in bone dysplasia.

Inspect the *teeth!* Are they late in developing or abnormal? In *osteogenesis imperfecta,* the teeth are affected because of deficiency of dentition; they are discolored, yellowish brown or bluish gray, break easily, and are prone to caries. In *Hurler's syndrome* the teeth are poorly formed, small, and widely spaced. Examine the *palate;* is there a cleft palate or is it normal and high-arched?

Examine the *skin!* Is it hypermobile and hyperextensible, as in Ehlers-Danlos syndrome? In the hypogonadic male, the skin is smooth and the hairline is low. In hypopituitarism, the skin is wrinkled and the face is rounded. In cretinism, the skin is dry and the hair is coarse and scarce. Are there any subcutaneous calcifications as in hypoparathyroidism? Are there any abnormal scars with poor healing to suggest collagen disorders? Are there any café-au-lait spots as in NF? Are there any hemangiomas to suggest Maffuci's syndrome?

Is there any ligamentous or joint capsule hyperlaxity? Does the wrist hyperflex so that the thumb touches the volar surface of the forearm (Fig 6–58A)? Does the thumb protrude beyond the ulnar border of the clenched fist (Steinberg sign) (Fig 6–58B)? Does the wrist hyperextend so that the dorsa of the fingers are parallel to the dorsum of the forearm (Fig 6–58C)? Do the elbows and knees hyperextend (Fig 6–58D, F)? Does the ankle dorsiflex excessively (Fig 6–58E)?

Is the neck short as in Hurler's syndrome? Is there webbing of the neck as in Turner's syndrome? Are the neck muscles in spasm? Determine range of motion of the cervical spine; in Klippel-Feil syndrome, the neck is short, the hairline low, and the neck restricted in motion, especially lateral flexion. Atlantoaxial instability is a common problem in bone dysplasia; for example, in Morquio's disease, it occurs in almost 100 percent of cases, caused by a combination of ligamentous hyperlaxity and odontoid aplasia. In spondyloepiphyseal dysplasia, it is present in about one third of the cases; it is due to dysplasia of the odontoid (hypoplasia, aplasia, or separation). Always examine the neck and limbs to rule out cervical myelopathy and neurologic deficit.

Next, inspect the thoracic cage. Is there pectus excavatum or carinatum? In Jeune's disease (asphyxiating thoracic dysplasia), the long, narrow, cylindrical chest with marked decrease in both the AP and lateral diameters is distinctive. In Ellis–van Creveld syndrome, the ribs are short and the thoracic cage is long and narrow. In rickets the pull of the diaphragm on the rib cage produces a horizontal depression that is called "Harrison's groove"; also in rickets, the sternum projects forward,

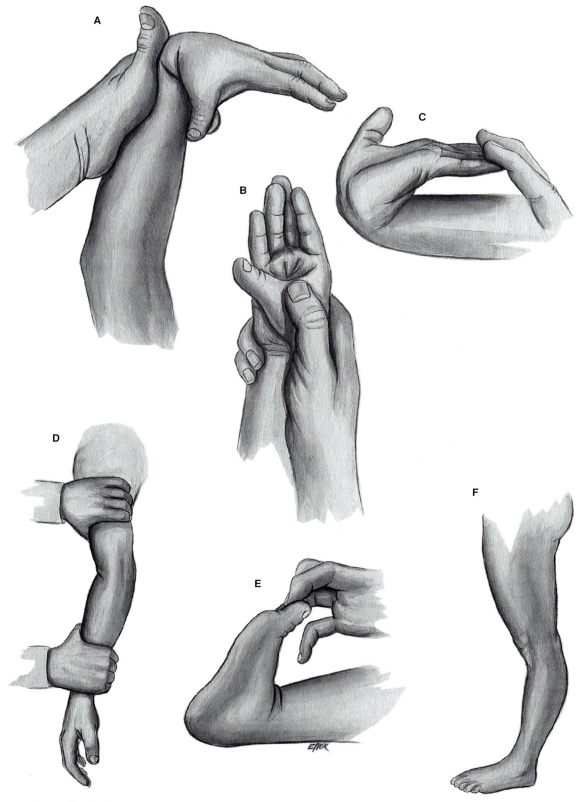

Figure 6–58. Physical findings in ligamentous hyperlaxity. **A.** On hyperflexion of the wrist, the thumb touches the volar surface of the forearm. **B.** The thumb protrudes beyond the ulnar border of the hand. **C.** On dorsiflexion of the wrist and fingers, the dorsa of the fingers are parallel with the dorsum of the forearm. **D.** Hyperextension of the elbow. **E.** Hyperextension of the ankle. **F.** Hyperextension of the knees (genu recurvatum).

giving the appearance of a pigeon breast (pectus carinatum).

Palpate the clavicles. Are they deficient centrally as in cleidocranial dysplasia, or are they hypoplastic and deficient laterally as in pycnodysostosis? In mucopolysaccharidosis, the medial ends of the clavicles are broad.

Next, examine the spine. Is there scoliosis or exaggerated thoracic kyphosis? A thoracolumbar gibbus suggests mucopolysaccharidosis. In achondroplasia there is severe lumbar lordosis.

Examine the hands. In achondroplasia, the hand is short and broad, with all the fingers of equal length ("starfish hand") and the long and ring fingers spread apart, forming a V-shaped space ("main en trident"). Long, thin fingers suggest Marfan's syndrome. In congenital contractural arachnodactyly, the fingers are long and gracile, with flexion contractures of the PIP joint. Ask the patient to make a fist, and inspect the length of the metacarpals. In pseudohypoparathyroidism, the third and fourth metacarpals are short. In multiple hereditary exostoses, the third, fourth, and fifth metacarpals may be short; palpate for the presence of exostoses. Inspect the palm; in Down's syndrome there is a single palmar crease (simian palmar crease), and the hands are short and stubby with incurving of the little finger. Is there polydactyly? In Ellis–Van Creveld syndrome the extra digits are often on the ulnar side, the fingers are short, and there is hypoplasia or absence of the ossification centers of the distal phalanges. In diastrophic dysplasia, the first metacarpal is very short, giving the appearance of a "hitchhiker's thumb."

Inspect the feet. Are they long and narrow with slender toes, with the big toe protruding beyond the second toe, suggesting Marfan's syndrome? The big toe and thumb are very short in fibrodysplasia ossificans progressiva. Inspect the plantar surface of the feet. In melorheostosis, the plantar skin is thickened, firm, and woody, with contracture of the plantar fascia and flexion contracture of the toes.

Radiographic Examination.   This should include the following projections: (1) AP view of the pelvis, which should include both hips and the symphysis pubis; (2) AP view of one knee; (3) AP view of one forearm to include the elbow and wrist; (4) PA view of one hand (preferably the left) to include all metacarpals and digits; (5) AP view of the entire spine; (6) lateral view of the entire spine; (7) AP view of the thoracic cage, which should show the shoulders and clavicles; and (8) lateral view of the skull.

Laboratory Studies.   The following diagnostic determinations of the blood are made as necessary: calcium, phosphates, alkaline phosphatase, and urine examinations.

Bone biopsy, skin biopsy, hair examination, and cytogenetic studies are guided by the abnormal radiographic findings.

MULTIPLE EPIPHYSEAL DYSPLASIA[728–737]

In multiple epiphyseal dysplasia (MED), the development of the epiphyseal ossification center is disturbed and disorganized. The ossification centers appear late and are mottled. Initially the articular cartilage is normal, but in time with stress loading it becomes flattened and misshapen, particularly in the weight-bearing joints. The degree and extent of involvement vary from severe and extensive (Fairbanks' dysplasia multiplex) to minimal and limited.[728,729,734] The femoral and humeral heads, short tubular bones of the hands and feet, distal epiphysis of the femur, and proximal epiphysis of the tibia are common sites. The vertebral column is normal, but the ring apophysis of the vertebrae may ossify late and is irregular in appearance. The facial bones, skull, and pelvis are not affected. Funnelization, diaphyseal cylindricization, and modeling are normal.

MED is inherited as an autosomal dominant trait. There is no sex predilection; it occurs equally in males and females. The prevalence is about 11 per million index patients.[737]

The presenting complaint is stiffness of joints and a waddling gait in a child between 4 and 8 years of age. Diagnosis is not made in infancy or early childhood, and occasionally not until adolescence. The fingers and toes are short and stubby. The affected joints are restricted in range of motion to a varying degree. Flexion contracture of the elbows and knees is commonly present. Determine range of extension and flexion; ordinarily there is no limitation of elbow or knee flexion, that is, no extension deformity. There is no effusion, synovial thickening, or increased warmth of the affected joints; absence of such inflammatory findings assists in distinguishing the stiff joint of MED from that of rheumatoid arthritis.

Angular malalignment of the knees in the form of genu varum or valgum may be present.

The stature of patients with MED is somewhat short. The height of the trunk is normal; the decreased stature is of the short limb type.

Pain is not a clinical feature in childhood. Occasionally epiphyseal dysplasia of the femoral heads is complicated by avascular necrosis; in such a case an antalgic limp may develop in childhood (Fig 6–59).

In late adolescence or early adult life, degenerative arthritis of the weight-bearing joints develops because of the irregularity and deformity of the joints. Pain in the hip with restriction of motion is a common complaint. Knee and ankle pain are not uncommon.

Imaging Findings.   The principal finding in the early stages is the delay of appearance of the ossification centers of the epiphyses. Once the ossification centers of the epiphyses develop, they are mottled and fragmented and later on become flattened (Fig 6–60). Metacarpals and phalanges are short.

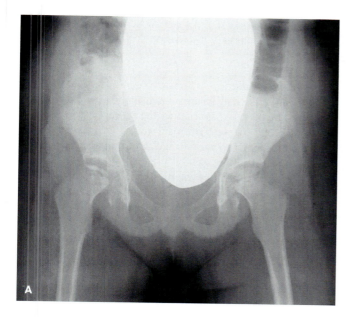

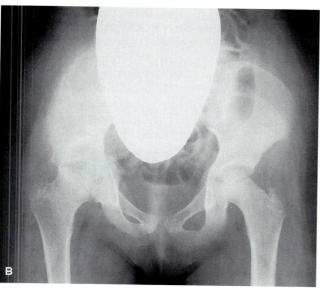

Figure 6–59. Multiple epiphyseal dysplasia in a 4-year-old girl. **A.** AP radiogram of the hips. Note the flattening of the femoral heads. The right hip is complicated by avascular necrosis. **B.** Postoperative radiogram of the hips following Salter innominate osteotomy to contain the femoral head.

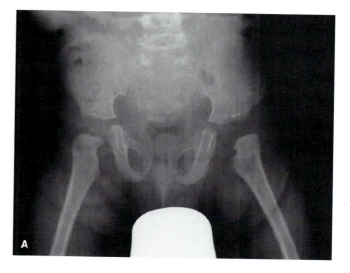

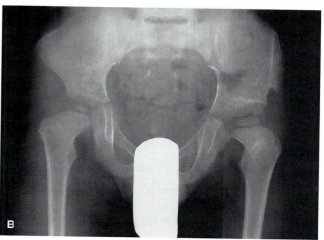

Figure 6–60. Multiple epiphyseal dysplasia. **A.** AP of both hips showing marked delay in ossification of the ossific nuclei and subluxation of the left hip. The child is 2 years old. **B.** At 3 years of age, there is still delayed ossification of the right hip. The left hip was treated by innominate osteotomy. Note the ossification of the femoral head, which is flat.

Differential Diagnosis. Distinguish MED of the hips from Legg-Perthes disease. In uncomplicated MED there is no avascular necrosis, and the progressive radiographic stages of Legg-Perthes disease (necrosis, fragmentation, regeneration) are not seen. In bilateral Perthes' disease the degree of involvement and stages of the disease vary from one side to the other. Bone imaging with technetium-99m shows lack of uptake in Perthes' disease. MRI shows the avascularity of the femoral ossification center and articular pathology in Perthes' disease.

On occasion, MED of the hips is complicated by avascular necrosis of the femoral heads. The vertebral column in spondyloepiphyseal dysplasia is abnormal (see below), whereas in MED it is normal.

In cretinism, ossification centers of the epiphyses are delayed in appearance and irregular; cretinism is differentiated from MED by its characteristic clinical features and thyroid function tests.

Treatment. There is no specific therapy. Innominate osteotomy is indicated to contain the flattened, extruded femoral heads. Restore concentric mobility of the hip by the use of a continuous passive motion machine and aggressive physical therapy.

DYSPLASIA EPIPHYSEALIS HEMIMELICA[738–740]

The presenting complaint is limitation of motion of the affected joint, an angular deformity such as valgus of the knee, or a localized enlargement of the affected epiphysis. It is recognizable at birth. Involvement is usually unilateral, affecting one limb. The most common sites are the distal femur, proximal tibia, or tarsus. It is limited to the medial or lateral half of the epiphysis. It is caused by abnormal cartilage proliferation and associated enchondral ossification in the epiphysis of a tarsal, carpal, or flat bone.

Imaging Findings. Plain radiograms show irregular and often multicentric areas of radiopacity adjacent to the involved epiphysis. In the mature bone, the lesion appears as an irregular bony mass similar to an exostosis. In dysplasia epiphysealis hemimelica, the lesion is in the epiphysis, whereas in exostosis, the lesion is in the metaphysis or diaphysis.

Treatment. This consists of excision of the exostosis when it produces deformity or interferes with joint motion. Recurrence is common.

ACHONDROPLASIA[741–757]

Achondroplasia is the most common form of dwarfism, with a prevalence of 1 per 26,000 live births. The mode of inheritance is autosomal dominant; 80 percent of the cases, however, are spontaneous mutations. Familial cases in siblings are rare. In achondroplasia, enchondral bone formation is defective but intramembranous bone formation is normal.

The *clinical features* are distinctive: (1) The dwarfism is disproportionate, with rhizomelic short limbs and a relatively long trunk. (2) The head is disproportionately large with a prominent forehead, broad face, depressed and flattened bridge of the nose, and projecting lower jaw. (3) Exaggerated thoracolumbar kyphosis (gibbus) in the infant is flexible, disappearing in prone posture and decreasing in severity when the child begins to walk. The posture is distinctive and is characterized by marked lumbar hyperlordosis, protruding abdomen, prominent buttocks, and a flat chest with flaring of the costal margins. (4) Short and broad hands with fingers of equal length (due to a short middle finger) give the appearance of "starfish hand"; also, the long and ring fingers are spread apart with a V-shaped space between them and are referred to as *trident* hand. (5) Bowing of the lower limbs is due primarily to tibia vara with relative overgrowth of the fibula; in the older patient, ligamentous laxity on the lateral side of the knee causes genu varum. The hindfoot is in varus. Peroneal nerve stretching at the level of the neck of the fibulae may cause paresthesia and drop foot. (6) A robust general appearance is seen, with above-average muscular development and overabundance of skin and soft tissues. Mentation is normal or above average.

Radiographic Features. (1) The skull is large with a relatively short base and a narrow and funnel-shaped foramen magnum (Fig 6–61A, B). (2) In the vertebral column, the interpediculate distance from L1 to L5 progressively decreases, in contrast to the normal spine, in which this distance becomes progressively greater (Fig 6–61C). This cephalocaudal tapering of the lumbar spinal canal is due to premature synostosis between the vertebral body and its arch. The pedicles are short and thick, and the posterior surfaces of the vertebral bodies are concave. The ossification centers of the vertebral bodies are smaller than normal, giving a bullet shape to the vertebral bodies in early life. (3) The inner contour of the *pelvis* has a typical, classic "champagne glass" appearance because the width of the pelvic inlet is greater than its depth (Fig 6–61D). The iliac wings are squared off (elephant ears), with a short narrow sciatic notch and flat acetabular roof. The sacrum is narrow, articulating low on the ilia with exaggeration of its tilt.

The long and short tubular bones are short and thick, with apparent increased diameter. The epiphyses are normal, but the metaphyses are flared and splayed. The physes are notched or V-shaped. The two flared limbs of the metaphyses seem to embrace the epiphyses, giving a ball-and-socket appearance to the epiphyseal-metaphyseal junction. This is best depicted in the distal femur and proximal tibia (Fig 6–61E, F). The diaphyses are of normal diameter. All of the long tubular bones are affected. The micromelia is rhizomelic, with the proximal segments of the limbs (the femurs and humeri) more shortened than the distal segments. The fibula is less affected than the tibia; consequently, the fibula is longer than the tibia. At the knee the head of the fibula is more proximal than normal, and at the ankle the lateral malleolus is more distal than normal. The relative overgrowth of the fibula causes medial bowing of the leg and varus of the hindfoot. Radiograms of the chest disclose short ribs with deep concave rib ends and a stubby sternum.

Prenatal diagnosis of achondroplasia can be made; homozygous cases can be diagnosed in the second trimester and heterozygous achondroplasia during the third trimester of pregnancy.[746] This poses an ethical dilemma.

Natural History and Treatment. The general health of achondroplasts is good. The prognosis is excellent for normal longevity. The epiphyses are normal, and osteoarthritis of the knee or hip is not a problem.

Avoid the pitfall of mistaking the large skull for hydrocephalus, resulting in unnecessary shunting. CT makes the definitive diagnosis.

In the older patient with achondroplasia, spinal stenosis and intervertebral disc protrusion or rupture cause

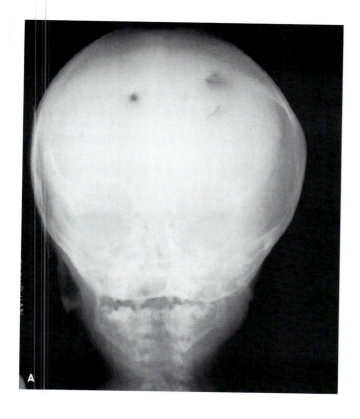

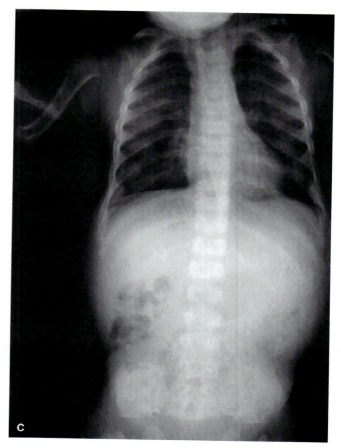

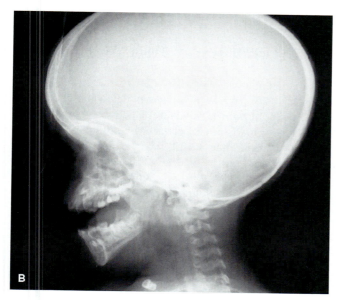

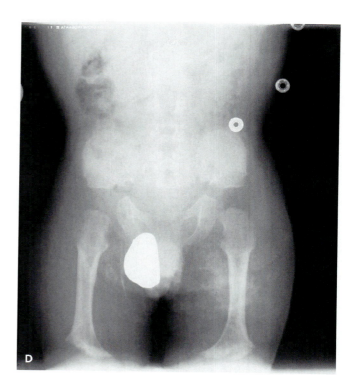

Figure 6–61. Radiographic findings in achondroplasia. **A, B.** AP and lateral views of the skull. Note the large skull with a short base. **C.** AP view of the spine. Note the cephalocaudal tapering of the spinal canal in the lumbar region. **D.** AP view of the pelvis. Note that the center of the pelvic inlet is greater than its depth, giving the appearance of a champagne glass. Also note the short sciatic notches and flat roofs of the acetabuli. *(Continues)*

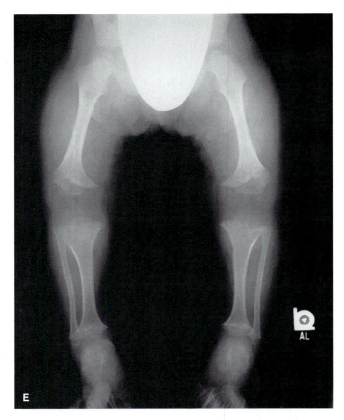

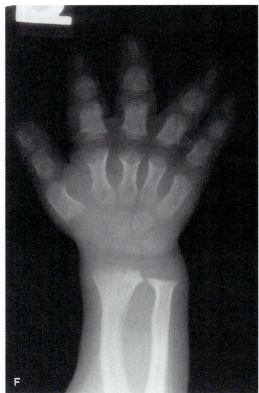

Figure 6–61 (Continued). E. AP view of both lower limbs. Note the short femurs and tibias and relatively long fibulas. Also note the flaring and splaying of the metaphyses and the V-shaped physes. **F.** AP view of the hand. Note the short and thick phalanges and metacarpals and the V space between the long and ring fingers. The equal length of the digits gives the appearance of a starfish hand.

backache, sciatica, paresthesia, and occasionally paraplegia. Lumbar hyperlordosis and spurring of the facet joints aggravate the condition. Often the patient squats to correct the hyperlordosis and alleviate the back pain and paresthesia. Laminectomy and disc excision are performed when disability is great.

Occasionally, kyphosis may become unstable and painful, requiring spinal fusion with internal fixation. Spinal orthotics are not tolerated.

Severe varus deformity of the tibiae is corrected by realignment osteotomy; it improves the mechanism of gait and provides normal foot alignment. Relative overgrowth of the fibula can be corrected by epiphyseodesis of the proximal and distal fibula. Limb lengthening to increase upper limb length and stature is controversial. It is performed when there is marked disability from the short limbs and not to improve appearance.

HYPOCHONDROPLASIA[758,759]

The clinical and radiographic features of hypochondroplasia are similar to those of achondroplasia, but much less severe; they probably are allelic developmental affections. The manifestations are mild in infancy; hypochondroplasia is not detected at birth. The height at skeletal maturity is between 4 feet, 5 inches and 5 feet. There are no disabling symptoms. Orthopedic treatment is not indicated. Growth hormone therapy has minimal or no effect.

SPONDYLOEPIPHYSEAL DYSPLASIA[760–765]

Spondyloepiphyseal dysplasia (SED) manifests in two types: (1) *SED congenita,* which can be diagnosed at birth, and (2) *SED tarda,* which manifests later in childhood. The inheritance of SED congenita is autosomal dominant, linked to chromosome 12q13; whereas the mode of inheritance of SED tarda is heterogeneous; most cases are X-linked recessive and linked to Xp22, and some cases are autosomal dominant. Sporadic cases do occur. The prevalence of SED congenita is 1 to 2 per million, whereas that of SED tarda is 3 to 4 per million population.

The presenting feature of SED is disproportionate dwarfism with marked shortening of the trunk and progressive involvement of the epiphyses of the long bones, particularly those of the proximal and distal femur and proximal tibia.

SED congenita is subdivided into two types: (1) that with severe coxa vara, and (2) that with mild coxa vara. These two types can be differentiated by 3 to 4 years of age, when the degree of coxa vara and shortness of stature becomes apparent. At birth the severe dwarfism with short trunk is apparent. There is increased thoracic kyphosis and marked lumbar lordosis. The vertebrae are flattened (platyspondyly), and the odontoid process is hypoplastic, with atlantoaxial instability. The thorax is barrel-shaped with pectus excavatum. The epiphyses of long bones are markedly delayed in ossification and irregular in development. The ossification centers of the femoral heads do not appear until 5 years of age. The pubic bone is late to ossify. The gait is waddling. Not infrequently the radiographic appearance is mistaken for congenital hip dislocation. Ultrasonography and MRI demonstrate that the femoral heads are contained in the acetabuli and are irregular. The epiphyses of other long bones, such as the distal femur and proximal tibia, show marked delay in ossification and incongruity of development. The metaphyses are normal. The diaphyses appear normal. Other associated anomalies are cleft palate, myopia, and retinal detachment. In young adult life, severe degenerative arthritis of the hip develops.

Treatment consists of upper cervical fusion for atlantoaxial subluxation and abduction osteotomy of the proximal femur to correct coxa vara. In the adult, degenerative osteoarthritis of the hip and knee are managed by total joint replacement.

In SED the presenting complaint is back pain and stiffness in an adolescent. The vertebrae are flattened (platyspondyly), and the disc spaces are narrowed. There is a hump-shaped mound of bone in the central and posterior portion of the superior and inferior end plates; the ossification centers of the upper and lower anterior margins of the vertebral bodies are absent. The proximal epiphyses of the femora-humeri are minimally involved. The distal epiphyses of the long bones and the epiphyses of the hands and feet are not affected.

Management of back pain is symptomatic. Joint deformities are usually not severe enough to warrant operative treatment.

DIASTROPHIC DYSPLASIA[766–772]

The term *diastrophic* is derived from the Greek; it means crooked or twisted. The mode of inheritance of diastrophic dysplasia is autosomal recessive, and the abnormal gene is located on the distal long arm of chromosome 5 (5q31.3). The defect lies in abnormal collagen organization of cartilage.

The clinical picture of this severe micromelic dwarfism is distinctive, and the diagnosis is readily made at birth. The typical deformities are the following: (1) Cauliflower ears. (2) Cleft or high-arched palate. (3) "Hitchhiker's thumb" due to excessive shortness of the first metacarpal, which is triangular in shape. The MP joint of the thumb is subluxated medially and the thumb is recessed proximally and almost perpendicular to the other digits. (4) Flexion deformities of the knees and hips which are present at birth and progressively increase in severity to a degree that impedes standing and walking. The contractural deformity of the joints is due to shortness of soft tissue and deformation of osteocartilaginous components of the joints. (5) The trunk appears normal at birth, but as the infant starts walk-

ing, he or she develops progressive scoliosis and kyphosis, which become fixed and severe in the preadolescent. (6) Equinovarus deformity of the feet and ankles; other mild deformities of the feet are symphalangism, short first metatarsals, and deformed great toes. (7) The stature of patients with diastrophic dysplasia is very short; height at skeletal maturity is 80 to 140 cm. The dwarfism is disproportionate; the limbs are very short, and flexion contractures of the knees and hips accentuate the lower limb shortening. Intelligence is normal.

Treatment. Soft tissue release is performed to correct equinovarus deformity of the feet and flexion contracture of the knees and hips. Orthoses are ineffective to control the severe kyphoscoliosis; early surgical intervention is recommended. The hip dislocation is rigid and high and best left alone. Cervical kyphosis can cause canal compression. It is treated by anterior cervical fusion.

CHONDROECTODERMAL DYSPLASIA (ELLIS–VAN CREVELD SYNDROME)[773–776]

In this disproportionate short limb dwarfism, the shortening is centrifugal, that is, greater in the lower legs and forearms than in the thighs and upper arms. The femora and humeri are often bowed. Genu valgum is common; it is due to hypoplasia of the lateral side of the upper tibial epiphysis and disproportionately short fibulae in relation to the tibia. The patellae subluxate and dislocate laterally. The spine is normal. Other manifestations of Ellis–van Creveld syndrome are the following: (1) *Polydactyly,* which is invariably present; often the digits on the ulnar side are duplicated. Often there is fusion of the carpal and tarsal bones. (2) *Ectodermal dysplasia,* with nails that are small, hypoplastic, dystrophic, and spoon-shaped; *teeth* that are late in eruption, absent, irregular, or pointed; denture defects and dental caries are commonly present; sparse hair; and fusion between the upper lip and gums. (3) *Congenital heart disease* is present in 60 percent of the cases; atrial or ventricular septal defect is the most common anomaly.

Treatment of heart anomalies is top priority; they are managed by the cardiologist and cardiac surgeon. The extra digits of the hands and feet are ablated between 1 and 2 years of life. Severe valgum deformity of the knee is corrected by varus osteotomy at the appropriate age.

■ OSTEOGENESIS IMPERFECTA[777–838]

The presenting complaint of osteogenesis imperfecta (OI) is fracture (one, several, or multiple) due to fragility of bone. It is genetically heterogeneous, some types inherited as autosomal dominant, others as recessive traits, and some occurring as mutations. OI comprises a number of distinct entities with wide variation in severity of involvement. In

TABLE 6–6. CLASSIFICATION OF OSTEOGENESIS IMPERFECTA (SILLENCE)

| | Type I | | Type II | |
	A	B	A	B
Inheritance	Autosomal dominant	Autosomal dominant	Autosomal dominant	Autosomal dominant
Incidence	1/30,000	1/30,000	1/62,000	
Bone fragility	Variable—slight to moderately severe. Frequency of fractures markedly decreases after puberty.	Variable—slight to moderately severe	Very severe	Very severe
Deformity of long bones	Moderate—less severe than other types	Moderate—less severe than other types	Broad, crumpled accordion-like, especially femurs and humerus; beaded ribs	Broad, crumpled; beaded ribs; rib fractures
Hypermobility of joints—ligamentous laxity	Marked genu recurvatum. Pes planovalgus. Dislocated hip may develop.	Marked genu recurvatum. Pes planovalgus. Dislocated hip may develop.	Unknown because of perinatal death	Unknown because of perinatal death
Spine deformity	Kyphoscoliosis—20%	Kyphoscoliosis—20%	?	?
Skull	Wormian bones; marked osteoporosis of membranous bones	Wormian bones; marked osteoporosis of membranous bones	Wormian bones with severe demineralization	Wormian bones with severe demineralization
Teeth	Normal	Dentinogenesis imperfecta	Unknown because of perinatal death	Unknown because of perinatal death
Sclerae	Blue—persists through life	Blue—persists through life	Blue	Blue
Deafness	Present—40%	Present—40%		
Other	Eyes—premature arcus senilis; easy bruising; bleeding tendency	Eyes—premature arcus senilis; easy bruising	Flattened acetabuli; nonimmune hydrops; microscopic calcification of aorta and endocardium	Same —
Prognosis	Fair—ambulatory with or without support	Fair—ambulatory with or without support	Perinatal lethal respiratory disease	Survival possible; respiratory disease
Chondro-osseous and biochemical defect	Collagen normal; quantitative defect—50% of normal production	Collagen normal	Collagen produced structurally abnormal	

the most severe form, the infant is stillborn with multiple fractures or dies in the early neonatal period. In the mildest form, the diagnosis is made in the young adult when osteoporosis is detected.

The classification of OI proposed by Sillence is most useful clinically; it is based on the genetic types, age of onset, frequency of fractures, color of sclerae, teeth, presence or absence of wormian bones, and progression. This classification is given in Table 6–6.[824]

OI is a connective tissue disorder caused by biochemical defects in the genes for collagen A1 and collagen A2. The gene mutations result in either quantitative defects or qualitative defects. In type I OI, the collagen is normal, but only 50 percent of the normal amount is produced, whereas in types II, III, and IV, the collagen produced is structurally abnormal with molecular defects.

The incidence of the various types of OI varies. The birth incidence and population frequency of type I is 1 in 30,000, whereas that of type II is 1 in 62,000. At present, the exact incidence of types III and IV is unknown.

Clinical Features. These vary according to the type of OI. Repeated and multiple fractures, occurring after the slightest injury, are the hallmark of OI. Diagnosis is readily made in the very severe type II (Sillence) form. There are a multitude of fractures of the long bones and ribs sustained by minimal trauma, either in utero or during delivery. On gentle palpation of the deformed short limbs, you feel crepitation. The skull is soft and membranous. The sclerae are blue. Inheritance of type II OI is autosomal dominant. The prognosis is very poor; perinatal death occurs because of intracranial hemorrhage.

In type III OI, bone fragility and deformities of the long bones are severe. The patient is born with fractures or sustains them with minimal or no trauma in early infancy.

| Type II | Type III | Type IV | |
C		*A*	*B*
Autosomal recessive Extremely rare Very severe	Autosomal recessive Very rare Severe numerous fractures by 2 yrs of age	Autosomal dominant Unknown Moderate—newborn fracture—25%	Autosomal dominant Unknown
Thin, fractured long bones; ribs slightly beaded	Fractures at birth; severe deformities of long bones	Moderate	Moderate
Unknown because of perinatal death	Marked	Moderate	Moderate
?	Severe kyphoscoliosis; cod fish vertebrae	Kyphoscoliosis	Kyphoscoliosis
Wormian bones with severe demineralization	Membranous bone; severe deossification; wormian bones; occiput, facial bones fairly well ossified; triangular facies	Moderate deossification; wormian bones	Same
Unknown because of perinatal death	Dentinogenesis imperfecta	Normal	Dentinogenesis imperfecta
Blue	Blue at birth and infancy, but become normal later	Normal	Normal
		Deafness less severe—otosclerosis or nerve	
Same —	"Popcorn" calcification	No bleeding tendency	Same
Perinatal lethal respiratory disease	Wheelchair bound; utmost household ambulator Collagen produced structurally abnormal	Fair	Fair

In general, the earlier the fractures occur, the more severe the disease. The femora, humeri, and tibiae are frequently affected. Fractures heal normally with normal-appearing callus, but remodeling into mature lamellar bone does not occur, making the long bone susceptible to refracture. Nonunion can occur if the fracture is markedly displaced with soft tissue interposition and not reduced. Occasionally the fracture heals with hyperplastic callus. Malignant degeneration of the hyperplastic callus into osteosarcoma has been reported.[807]

Anterior, posterior, medial, or lateral bowing of the long bones is a common sequela. Deformity is caused by malunion of the fracture, multiple microscopic stress fractures on the tension side, and the pull of strong muscles. Deformities that result are anterolateral angulation in the distal half of the femur, coxa vara in the proximal femur, anterolateral bowing of the tibia, and lateral angulation in the humerus. Angular and rotational deformities of the radius and ulna restrict range of rotation of the forearm. Genu recurvatum and flexion deformity of the elbow occur commonly. Fortunately, the incidence of fractures declines after adolescence.

In type I and type IV (Sillence) OI, bone fragility is moderate to mild. The number of fractures varies; in general they occur later in life and less often.

Blue sclerae are caused by thinness of the scleral collagen layer. A well-known manifestation of OI, blue sclerae are not present in all of its types. In type IV, the color of the sclerae is normal; in type III, they are bluish at birth and become less blue in time and white in the adult. In type I, the sclerae are distinctly blue throughout life. In type II, they are blue.

Hyperlaxity of ligaments, a manifestation of collagen abnormality, occurs almost universally in OI. It causes hypermobility of joints, such as genu recurvatum, elbow hyperextension, severe pes valgus, atlantoaxial subluxation, knee and patellofemoral joint instability (which predisposes the patient to fall, causing fractures), and occasionally hip or radial head dislocation.

The *teeth* are abnormal because of deficiency of dentin (dentinogenesis imperfecta). The teeth are late to erupt; both deciduous and permanent teeth are affected. They are small, yellowish brown or translucent blue in color, break easily, and are prone to caries. In type IA and type IVA, the teeth are normal; in type IB and type IVB, dentinogenesis imperfecta is present; and in type III it may be present. In type II, it is unknown because of perinatal death.

Kyphoscoliosis develops in about one third of the patients with OI (Fig 6–62A, B). Causative factors are severe osteoporosis, compression fractures of vertebrae, and ligamentous hyperlaxity. The more severe the osteoporosis, the greater the spinal deformity.

Pathologic spondylolisthesis develops due to elongation of the pars interarticularis and sometimes due to stress fracture.

Deafness develops in adult life due either to otosclerosis (conduction type) or to pressure on the auditory nerve. It is present in 40 percent of type I and about 15 percent of type IV.

Deformities of the limbs (due to angulation and overriding of fractures), growth disturbance, and kyphoscoliosis cause short stature in OI.

Children with OI are intelligent, bright, and usually outgoing; occasionally they become fearful and withdrawn because of the multiplicity of fractures.

Imaging. The findings in the plain radiogram depend upon the type and severity of OI. The hallmark of OI is

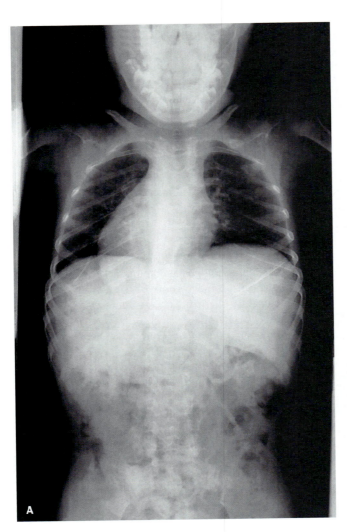
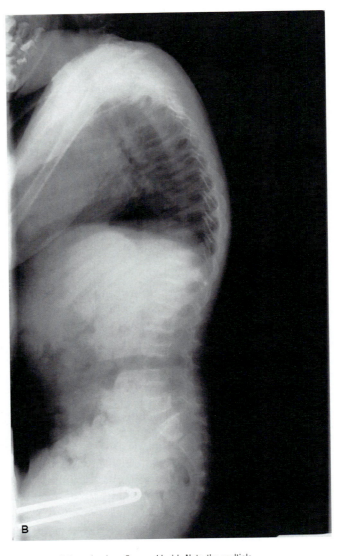

Figure 6–62. The spine in osteogenesis imperfecta. **A, B.** AP and lateral views of the spine in a 5-year-old girl. Note the multiple compression fractures and exaggerated thoracic kyphosis.

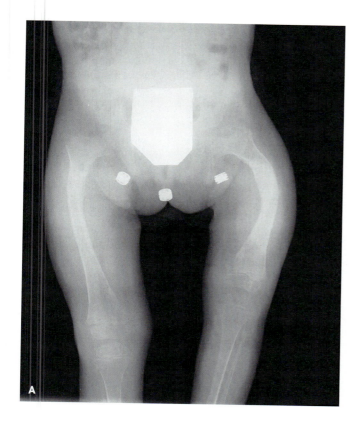

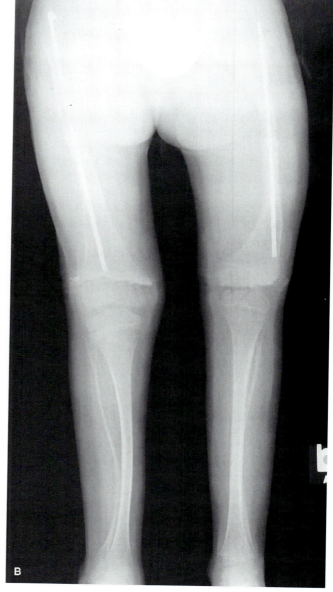

Figure 6–63. Radiographic findings in osteogenesis imperfecta. **A.** AP view of both femurs and proximal tibias. Note the severe osteoporosis and the bowing of the femurs due to multiple fractures. The left femur is congenitally short. **B.** AP view of both lower limbs showing postoperative fragmentation and rodding of the femurs. Note the very thin fibulas and the lateral angulation of the tibias at their middle one third.

osteoporosis, which is always present in varying degrees. In severe OI, the osteoporosis is very marked, with diffuse demineralization of the skeleton. The radiographic manifestations are striking at birth. The skull shows almost no ossification. The ribs are beaded, with multiple fractures. The severe atrophy of the thoracic cage simulates asphyxiating thoracic dysplasia. The long bones are short, crumpled (accordion-like), and wide with thin cortices. The diaphysis is as wide as the metaphysis. The long bones are angulated, with malunion of fractures in different stages of repair (Fig 6–63A, B). Popcorn calcifications may develop.

Wormian bone appears radiographically as islands of ossification in the skull in nonossified membranous bone. To be of diagnostic value, the wormian bones should be 4 mm by 6 mm in size, 10 in number, and arranged in a mosaic pattern. Wormian bones are not present in normal skulls, but they may be present in other bone dysplasias such as cleidocranial dysplasia.[792]

Hyperplastic callus formation may develop following a fracture; it should not be mistaken for osteogenic sarcoma.

Laboratory Findings. The alkaline phosphatase level may be elevated; the serum calcium and phosphorus levels are normal.

Type I collagen is found in skin, bone, and ligament. In quantitative OI (type I), there is no structural abnormality of collagen, but there is a 50 percent underproduction of structurally normal type I collagen (COL IA gene linked to chromosome 7q21). In qualitative OI (types II, III, and IV), there are structurally normal and abnormal collagen molecules, either COL 1A or COL 1A2 gene—chromosome 7q21. Skin biopsy and study of collagen fibers distinguish quantitative from qualitative forms of OI.

Differential Diagnosis. In the newborn type II OI with multiple fractures, short limbs, and an enlarged head, clinically it may be mistaken for camptomelic dwarfism, achondroplasia, or congenital hypophosphatasia. Radiograms and laboratory studies establish the diagnosis.

In the milder forms of OI, proclivity for fractures and radiologic evidence of the presence of multiple fractures in various stages of healing may arouse suspicion for battered child syndrome. Sometimes it is difficult to definitively separate OI from battered child syndrome. Bruising can occur in OI because of capillary fragility; external bruises on the battered child appear when assaulted and disappear when in a protected environment.

Fractures in the battered child are more metaphyseal in location than in osteogenesis imperfecta. In OI, the sclerae may be white and the teeth normal. In cystinosis and pycnodysostosis, multiple fractures do occur and the possibility of OI may be suggested. In the early stages of leukemia, diffuse osteoporosis similar to that seen in OI may be present.

Management. There is no specific treatment. Various medications (fluorides, magnesium oxide, calcitonin, and ascorbic acid) have been tried, but they have been unable to correct the basic defect. Claims of decrease in the fracture rate have not been supported by further studies.

The objective of orthopedic treatment is to prevent fractures or to decrease the frequency of fractures, prevent and correct musculoskeletal deformity, and provide the maximal possible function.

Problems vary with the severity of the disease and the age of the child. When a baby is born with severe OI, it is necessary to explain the nature of the disease to the parents in detail, outline a course of treatment, and inform them as to the likely future of the child. Relate these facts in simple terms; don't go into surgical details such as long bone rodding and treatment of kyphoscoliosis.

The pressing problems are the pulmonary insufficiency due to multiple rib fractures, which is managed by the neonatologist, and the subdural hematoma due to skull fracture, which is treated by the neurosurgeon. The multiple long bone fractures present a problem of nursing care and handling of the baby. The displaced fractures are splinted in simple, well-padded posterior plastic shells; often, however, the fractures are stable and actual splinting is not needed. The fractures heal in 14 days. Prolonged immobilization causes increased osteoporosis and initiates a vicious circle. Instruct the parents in the delicate technique of handling the fragile baby. Provide the parents with publications by the Osteogenesis Imperfecta Foundation; put them in touch with the parents of other OI patients. Inspire confidence in the fearful parents. The basic principles of care are gentleness and patience.

Hypotonia is a problem in OI. Developmental therapy by the physical therapist promotes head and neck control and use of the upper limbs. In severe OI, the occurrence of multiple fractures impairs functional development. In the care of fractures, maintain adequate alignment and splint for as short a time as possible to prevent exaggeration of osteopenia and progressive muscular atrophy.

An active but gentle exercise program increases muscle strength. External support by light plastic orthoses promotes stance and walking. The extent of orthotic support is diminished, for example from HKAFO to KAFO to AFO, as the child develops greater motor and bone strength.

Surgical intervention in the form of fragmentation by multiple osteotomies, realignment, and intramedullary rod fixation corrects deformity of the long bones and provides internal support, enhancing the potential for stance and assisted or independent walking in severe OI. The indications for fragmentation and rodding are the multiplicity of fractures and increasing moderate to severe deformity of long bones, interfering with the fitting of orthotic support and impairing function. The surgical procedure of rodding these fragile, thin bones requires experience and technical skill. Rodding should not be performed in the infant and young child. The 3 year old or older child, who is beginning to pull himself up to standing, is at the optimal age. The operative procedure has problems and complications and does not alter the basic pathobiology of bone fragility. Patients with OI are at risk for malignant hyperthermia; it behooves the anesthesiologist to be aware of the potential complication of anesthesia. Blood loss is a problem due to capillary fragility.

■ BATTERED CHILD (SILVERMAN'S) SYNDROME[839–854]

A battered child is one who has sustained injury, not by accident but because of deliberate assault by a person or persons responsible for the child's care. Silverman first described the battered child syndrome, and sometimes it is referred to by his name.[852] It occurs in the young child, about two thirds of them under 3 years of age and one third under 6 months of age. The abused child is ordinarily malnourished, underweight, and in poor general health. The socioeconomic condition is often poor, with overcrowded and deplorable environmental conditions; however, a child from a middle or upper class family can be willfully and criminally assaulted by an emotionally maladjusted person.

The assault may be inflicted by a parent, an older sibling in the same family, or a neighbor. The mechanism of assault is a direct blow, throwing the infant on the floor, vigorous pulling and twisting of the limbs, or vigorous shaking.[843,847]

The possibility of battered child syndrome should be suspected when there are (1) multiple fractures, inflicted at different times, (2) bruises and lacerations in different areas of the body, (3) subdural hematoma, and/or (4) visceral trauma in the thorax or abdomen such as rupture of the intestines, laceration or contusion of the liver, subpleural hemorrhage, and injury to the lung.[841,842]

On initial presentation of the child, the history of injury given by the parents is unsatisfactory; they don't know how it happened, and the questions are answered evasively. A radiogram cannot distinguish between assault and accident; the following features of the bone lesions are very suggestive: (1) in battered child syndrome, the fractures are multiple in various stages of healing, (2) they have a predilection for the metaphysis, and (3) there is exaggerated periosteal new bone formation (Fig 6–64).[841,844] The latter are explained by vascularity and thickness of the periosteum and the relative softness of the metaphysis in the long bones of infants and young children. The metaphysis displaces where the periosteum is attached to the physis, and subperiosteal hematoma elevates the periosteum. Initially this may not be visible in the plain radiogram. Physeal injuries are common, with minimal or marked separation and displacement of the epiphysis. In 2 to 3 weeks after injury, abundant subperiosteal calcification and ossification occur, and later the cortex of the long bone becomes relatively thick.

Diagnosis. Radiograms of suspect areas are vital, and bone scan with technetium-99m should be performed. When subdural hematoma is suspected, CT of the head is made. Chest radiograms and ultrasonograms of the abdomen depict the presence and extent of visceral injuries. Make ultrasonograms of the abdomen and determine serum amylase and lipase levels to rule out injury to the pancreas when abdominal pain and tenderness are present.

The differential diagnosis between osteogenesis imperfecta and battered child syndrome is always a problem. During delivery a newborn with osteogenesis imperfecta may sustain multiple fractures; other clinical features of OI assist in making the proper diagnosis. Scurvy, congenital syphilis, and infantile cortical hyperostosis should be considered in the differential diagnosis, as they show excessive new subperiosteal bone formation in the plain radiograms.

Children with congenital insensitivity to pain may have multiple fractures, but they are not in pain.

Management. The problem is complex, with sociologic, psychopathologic, and legal implications. In North America, the physician reports his suspicion to the appropriate committee in the hospital, who in turn report to the appropriate legal authorities in the child welfare department. The law grants immunity to the reporter. The welfare department is required to investigate, and, if there is adequate evidence of willful assault, brings the case to the attention of the juvenile court and removes the child from the dangerous environment and places him in a foster home. Repeated assault can cause death of the abused child; be mindful of the mortality of battered child syndrome.

■ INFANTILE CORTICAL HYPEROSTOSIS (CAFFEY DISEASE)[855–862]

This self-limited disease of early infancy has its onset usually at 2 months of age and rarely occurs after the fifth month of postnatal life. The child presents with a soft tissue swelling over the affected bone; the local mass is deep, firm, and somewhat tender, but there is no increased local heat or redness. The infant is irritable with moderate fever.

The mandible is the most common site of involvement; the next most frequent sites are the tibiae, clavicles, scapulae, ribs, and ulnas.

Imaging. In the plain radiogram, massive subperiosteal new bone formation with cortical hyperostosis (the width and density of the cortex is increased) is the characteristic finding (Fig 6–65). The hyperostosis is confined to the di-

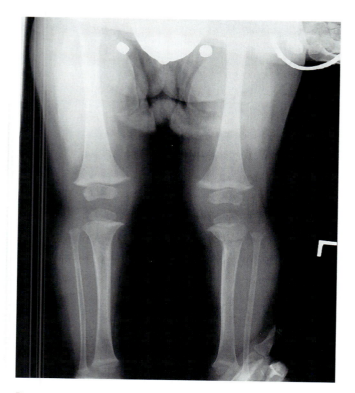

Figure 6–64. A metaphyseal fracture of the proximal tibia in battered child syndrome.

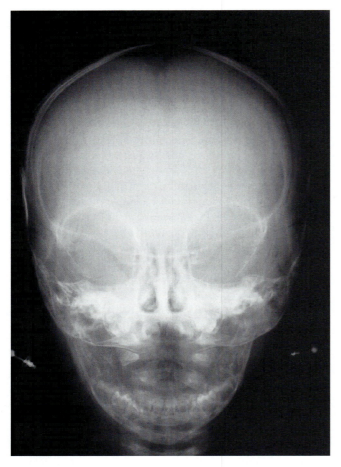

Figure 6–65. Infantile cortical hyperostosis of the mandible.

aphysis; the epiphysis and metaphysis are spared. Early in the course of the disease, the newly formed osseous tissue is coarse and the underlying cortex is visible, but later on the new bone increases in density and becomes homogeneous with the cortex. Bone scan with technetium-99m shows increased uptake, before changes on plain radiograms are visible.

Laboratory Studies. The white blood cell count and ESR are elevated, and there is also increase in immunoglobulin concentration (IgA and IgM), C-reactive protein, and serum alkaline phosphatase levels.

A diagnosis of infantile cortical hyperostosis is readily made by its distinctive features of (1) narrow age group of birth to 5 months; (2) mandibular involvement, and (3) the findings of irritability and fever, local swelling, and cortical hyperostosis. In the differential diagnosis, rule out osteomyelitis, congenital syphilis, scurvy, hypervitaminosis A, trauma (especially in osteogenesis imperfecta), and Ewing's sarcoma.

Treatment. Corticosteroids or other nonsteroidal anti-inflammatory medications are given when the systemic manifestations are acute and the infant is very uncomfortable. Antibiotics and surgical drainage are not indicated. Complete recovery takes place in 6 to 9 months; the disease is self-limiting.

■ TRICHORHINOPHALANGEAL DYSPLASIA (GIEDION SYNDROME)[863–866]

Clinically this disease is characterized by (1) sparse and slowly growing hair on the head, (2) pear-shaped nose, (3) brachyphalangy with thin nails, and (4) short stature, below the third percentile. In the plain radiogram, the epiphyses of the phalanges are cone-shaped, and the femoral heads are flattened and fragmented, with "Perthes"-like changes; involvement of hips is usually bilateral. The inheritance is autosomal dominant, with the abnormal gene located on 8q24.12.

■ LARSEN'S SYNDROME[867–870]

The presenting complaint is multiple congenital dislocation of the hips, knees, and radial heads, and occasionally rigid club feet. The facial appearance is distinctive—flat with a depressed nasal bridge, bulging forehead, and widely spaced eyes (hypertelorism). The joints are very lax. In the feet, a juxtacalcaneal accessory bone (or bifid calcaneus) is present. The fingers are long and cylindrical, with short and broad fingertips. The thumbs have a spatulate distal phalanx. Other abnormalities are failure of segmentation of vertebrae, scoliosis, hypoplasia of the cervical vertebrae with dislocation of the upper cervical spine, and cervico-thoracic lordosis. Cardiovascular anomalies and malacia of the trachea may occur.

The inheritance of Larsen's syndrome is autosomal dominant in most cases; on occasion it is autosomal recessive or sporadic.

■ EHLERS-DANLOS SYNDROME[871–881]

This heterogeneous group of connective tissue disorders is characterized by (1) excessive ligamentous hyperlaxity and hyperextensibility of the joint, (2) abnormal stretchability (hyperelasticity) of the skin, and (3) excessive bruisability and fragility of blood vessels.[876,877]

The orthopedic surgeon should rule out Ehlers-Danlos syndrome whenever he encounters a child with severe flat feet, genu recurvatum, recurrent subluxation or dislocation of the patellofemoral joint, hip dislocation, scoliosis, thoracic hypokyphosis or lordosis, poor posture with thoracolumbar kyphosis, recurrent subluxation or dislocation of the shoulder joint, instability and subluxation of the sternoclavicular joint, and atlantoaxial subluxation or dislocation.

History. Ask about the presence of skin hyperextensibility, bruising, and joint hypermobility in other members of the family. The mode of inheritance in Ehlers-Danlos syndrome is autosomal dominant or recessive. Inquire in detail about the gastrointestinal, cardiovascular, genitourinary, venous, and respiratory systems. Ehlers-Danlos syndrome is a generalized connective tissue disorder that affects multiple systems. Is there any bleeding from the gastrointestinal or urinary tract? Rupture and hemorrhage from the bowel may occur. Is the patient constipated? Is there any rectal prolapse?

Examination. Gently pull on the *skin*. Is it hyperextensible (Fig 6–66A, B)? Does it bruise easily? The skin on the dorsum of the hands and feet is redundant. On the subcutaneous bones such as the anterior aspect of the tibia and the dorsum of the ulna, the skin is thin (cigarette paper–like) and often hyperpigmented.

The *joints* are hypermobile. The elbows and knees hyperextend markedly. The thumb protrudes way beyond the ulnar border of the hand, and on dorsiflexion of the hand, the fingers are parallel to the forearm. On longitudinal distraction, the bones can be pulled apart to an abnormal degree. Joint instability may cause traumatic effusion and hemarthrosis. Test for dislocation of the hips, the patellae, the radial heads, the shoulders, and the temporomandibular joints. Is there any atlantoaxial instability with stiffness of the neck due to pain and any neurologic deficit in the upper and lower limbs? Examine the *spine* for scoliosis, spondylolisthesis, and hyperlordosis.

Inspect the teeth—are they malformed? Do the gums bleed easily? Is there gingivitis? The retina may detach and the sclerae may perforate. Check the heart for signs of aortic and/or mitral valve insufficiency. Cardiac consultation and echocardiogram should be obtained as necessary. Varicose veins are common. Resorptive osteolysis may occur. Diaphragmatic hernia, rectal prolapse, dilation of the alimentary tract, hydronephrosis, polycystic kidney, bladder diverticuli, spontaneous pneumothorax, and pulmonary hypertension are some of the other systemic findings in Ehlers-Danlos syndrome. It is vital to examine the entire child in this generalized connective tissue disorder.

Classification. Eleven different types of Ehlers-Danlos syndrome have been described. However, type IX is now reclassified as a disorder of copper metabolism and type XI as a simple joint instability disorder, and both have been removed as types of the syndrome.

Type 1 is the gravis or severe form; the marked skin hyperextensibility and joint hyperlaxity are associated with

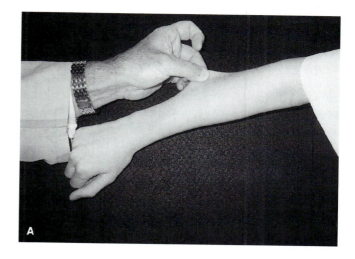

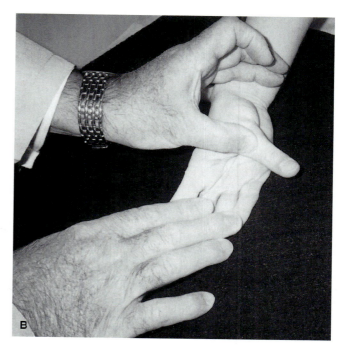

Figure 6–66. Ehlers-Danlos syndrome. **A.** Hyperextensibility of the skin. **B.** Note the hypermobility of the MCP joint of the thumb.

friability of the tissues, recurrent bruising of the skin, "cigarette paper" scars, and pigmentation of the skin. Subcutaneous calcified nodules may be present. It is inherited as an autosomal dominant trait with complete penetrance. In *type II* (mutis), the clinical picture is similar to type I, but much milder; its inheritance is autosomal dominant. In *type III*, both the large and small joints are hypermobile, but the skin hyperextensibility is minimal and scar formation is normal. Inheritance is autosomal dominant. *Type IV* is the vascular or ecchymotic form. It is caused by a defect in type III collagen. The production and secretion of pro-alpha 2 is diminished. It is inherited either as an autosomal dominant or autosomal recessive trait. Clinically it is characterized by thin, pale, and translucent skin that is minimally hyperextensible. Skin bruising and pigmented scars are common. The hypermobility of the joints is restricted to the IP and MCP joints of the hand. Rupture of vessels and bowel does occur. Life expectancy is short.

Type V, inherited as X-linked recessive, is characterized by marked hyperextensibility and bruising of the skin; hypermobility of the joints is minimal or absent.

Type VI is the oculoscoliotic form, which is inherited as an autosomal recessive trait. It is caused by deficiency of lysine hydroxylase; the concentration of hydroxylysine in the collagen is low. The collagen fibers are loose. Ocular manifestations are retinal detachment, perforation of the sclerae, and microcornea. Scoliosis is common. Joint hypermobility and skin hyperextensibility are mild to moderate.

Type VII is subdivided into two subtypes: *type VIIA* due to structural defect of pro-alpha 1 collagen and *type VIIB,* which is due to a structural defect of pro-alpha 2 collagen. Inheritance is either autosomal dominant or autosomal recessive. Clinically it is characterized by extreme hypermobility of the joints, and the name *arthrochalasis multiplex congenita* is given to this type of Ehlers-Danlos syndrome. The skin is soft with mild hyperextensibility. The stature is short. Micrognathia may be present.

Type VIII is characterized by progressive periodontal disease with gingival recession and loss of teeth between 10 and 30 years of age. The skin is fragile, with easy bruising and abundant scarring. Its inheritance is autosomal dominant.

Management. There is no specific treatment for the collagen disorder. Orthopedic manifestations are treated symptomatically. Patellofemoral joint and hip dislocation and severe hallux valgus require operative intervention. Wound healing is a problem; obtain a plastic surgery consultation.

■ MUCOPOLYSACCHARIDOSIS (MPS)[882–899]

In this storage disease, the lysosomal enzymes are deficient and the degradation of micromolecular components into smaller component units is blocked, resulting in abnormal intracellular accumulation of semidegraded compounds. Heparan sulfate, dermatan sulfate, and chondroitin sulfate are the mucopolysaccharides that accumulate in abnormal quantities. The chemical and radiographic manifestations vary according to the type of enzyme deficiency. The mucopolysaccharides are excreted in the urine, and the various mucopolysaccharidoses can be diagnosed by biochemical analysis of the urine. The specific enzyme defect can also be detected in the cultured skin fibroblasts.

Bone growth and development are affected in MPS. Common radiographic features include (1) enlarged sella turcica and thickening of the skull, (2) broad medial ends of the clavicles, (3) ribs that are narrowed and attenuated posteriorly and widened anteriorly, (4) platyspondyly or ovoid vertebral bodies with underdevelopment of the AP portion, giving the appearance of a broad hook, (5) flaring of the iliac wings with oblique acetabular roofs and coxa valga, (6) lack of diaphyseal modeling, with the diaphysis thicker than the metaphysis, and (7) changes in the hand consisting of delayed ossification of the carpal bones, second to fifth metacarpals that are pointed proximally, and phalanges that are bullet-shaped. The term *dysostosis multiplex* has been proposed by Spranger to embrace these skeletal changes in MPS.[898]

The classification of MPS is given in Table 6–7. For the sake of brevity, only Morquio's disease is described in the text; for a description of the clinical manifestations and radiographic features of MPS, the reader is referred to the references.

MORQUIO'S DISEASE[900–909]

This MPS occurs in 1 in 100,000 births. It is inherited as an autosomal recessive trait. The enzyme deficiency of Morquio-A disease is *N*-acetylgalactosamine-6-sulfatase, with its gene mapped to 16q24.3. The enzyme deficiency of Morquio-B disease is β-galactosidase; it is demonstrated in the fibroblasts. Excess keratan sulfate is secreted in the urine. The clinical features of Morquio-A disease and Morquio-B disease are similar. Morquio-A disease presents in grades of clinical involvement: severe, intermediate, and mild.

Clinically the newborn and infant appear normal; ordinarily Morquio's disease is not detected at birth. Between the first and second years of life, the following characteristic findings become evident: (1) kyphosis (gibbus) at the thoracolumbar juncture, with a short lordotic curve below, prominent buttocks, and prominent abdomen. The spleen and liver are not enlarged. (2) Pectus carinatum; the sternum projects forward with a manubrial-sternal angle of 90 degrees. Premature fusion of the sternal segments restricts chest excursion and decreases vital capacity. Thoracic cage immobility and deformity cause microatelectasis and recurrent or chronic pneumonia. (3) Marked shortness of stature (under 4 feet). The dwarfism is due to the short trunk; the limbs are relatively long. (4) Extreme ligamentous joint laxity causes hyperextensibility of the elbows, wrists, and ankles, severe genu valgum, flexible flat feet, and valgus ankles. This generalized joint hyperlaxity is a feature of Morquio's disease and is dissimilar to other MPS, in which joints may be stiff. The valgus deformity of the ankles and knees gradually increases in severity and becomes disabling

TABLE 6–7. CLASSIFICATION OF THE MUCOPOLYSACCARIDOSES

Type	Eponym	Enzyme Deficiency	MPS Stored-Excretion in Urine	Inheritance	Salient Manifestation
IH	Hurler	α-L-iduronidase	DS ++, HS +	Autosomal recessive	Grotesque gargoyle facies; organomegaly; mental retardation; corneal clouding
IS	Scheie	α-L-iduronidase	HS +, DS ++	Autosomal recessive	Normal intelligence; no hepatosplenomegaly; corneal clouding; stature normal
II	Hunter	Iduronate sulfatase	HS ++, DS +	Sex-linked recessive; all patients male	Gargoyle facies, but less severe; organomegaly; mental retardation; no corneal clouding; flesh-colored papules
IIIA	Sanfilippo	Heparan sulfate sulfaminidase	HS ++	Autosomal recessive	Severe mental retardation; severe neurologic degeneration; no corneal clouding; normal stature
IIIB	Sanfilippo	α-N-acetyl-D glucosaminidase	HS	Autosomal recessive	Same as above
IIIC	Sanfilippo	Glucosamine-N-acetyl transferase	HS	Autosomal recessive	Same as above
IIID	Sanfilippo	N-acetyl glucosamine-6-sulfatase	HS	Autosomal recessive	Same as above
IVA	Morquio	N-acetyl galactosamine-6-sulfatase	KS	Autosomal recessive	Dysostosis multiplex bone changes; odontoid hypoplasia; corneal clouding; short stature
IVB	Morquio	β-Galactosidase	KS	Autosomal recessive	Similar to above
VI	Maroteaux-Lamy	Arylsulfatase B (N-acetyl galactosamine)	DS	Autosomal recessive	Dysostosis multiplex; corneal clouding; hepatosplenomegaly; normal intelligence
VIII	Sly	β-Glucuronidase	CS, DS, HS	Autosomal recessive— gene mapped to 7q11, 23-714	Dysostosis multiplex; heptosplenomegaly

DS = Dermatan sulfate; KS = keratan sulfate; HS = heparan sulfate; CS = chondroitin sulfate; MPS = mucopolysaccharidosis.

by the age of 10 years. Developmental osseous deformity aggravates the knock knees. (5) The hands and feet are short, with broad digits. (6) Symptoms due to *atlantoaxial instability,* which is due to hypoplasia of the odontoid process and ligamentous hyperlaxity. This occurs in almost 100 percent of the cases. Spinal cord compression causes myelopathy. Hypertrophy of the longitudinal ligament, which develops gradually, causes further cord compression. The signs of myelopathy develop insidiously at about 5 years of age. The child complains of progressive decrease of endurance and ability to run. Pyramidal signs gradually develop in the form of spasticity, hyperreflexia, clonus, and a positive Babinski reflex. Sphincter tone disturbance is rare. (7) Normal level of intelligence. (8) Mild corneal clouding, progressive deafness, and dental abnormalities in the form of thin enamel layers and pointed cusps of the permanent teeth.

Imaging Findings. These are distinctive. The lumbar and thoracic vertebrae are flattened (platyspondyly) and beaked anteriorly. The 12th thoracic vertebra is hypoplastic and displaced posteriorly on L1, accentuating the thoracolumbar kyphosis (Fig 6–67A). The odontoid process is almost always hypoplastic or absent in Morquio's disease; this is best depicted by MRI. Atlantoaxial instability and subluxation are demonstrated on flexion-extension lateral views of the cervical spine (Fig 6–67B, C).

Ossification of the long bones, particularly of the femoral heads, is delayed and irregular. The femoral necks are widened and flared. The acetabula are very dysplastic because the lateral acetabular epiphyses do not develop properly and fail to ossify. The hips progressively subluxate. The pelvis becomes narrower with growth, with the width and length of the inner pelvic contour of equal length, resembling the shape of a wine glass (Fig 6–67E, F). The shafts of the long bones are short and thick but otherwise normal. The ulna is relatively short in relation to the radius, and the carpus subluxates ulnarward (Fig 6–67D).

Management. Atlantoaxial instability is treated by C1–C2 fusion. The severe genu valgum is treated by varization osteotomy; braces are not effective in correcting or controlling progression. Ulnar deviation of the wrists is treated by elongation of the ulna.

The prognosis is guarded. Rigidity of the rib cage and decrease in vital capacity may compromise pulmonary function and result in respiratory failure. The disease is rarely fatal.

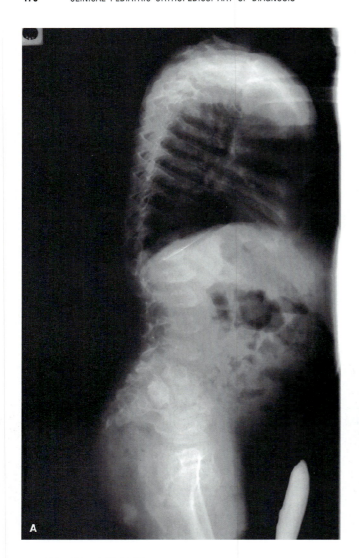

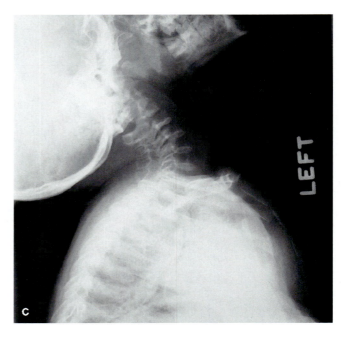

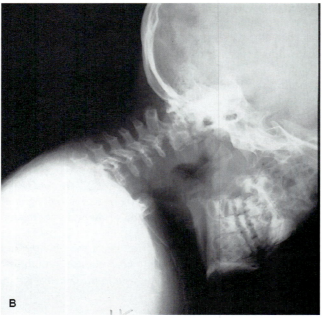

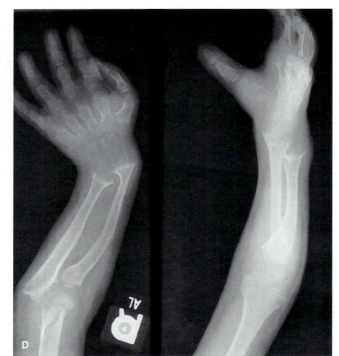

Figure 6–67. Radiographic findings in Morquio disease. **A.** Lateral view of the spine. Note the platyspondyly and anterior beaking of the lumbar and lower thoracic vertebrae. **B, C.** Flexion-extension views of the cervical spine showing excessive mobility between C1 and C2. **D.** AP and lateral views of the forearm. Note the delay in ossification of the distal ulnar and radial epiphyses and the short ulna and ulnar subluxation of the wrist. *(Continues)*

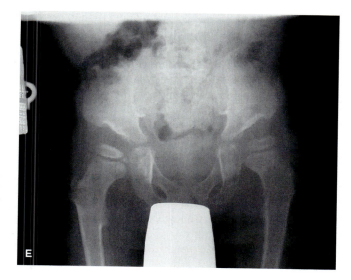

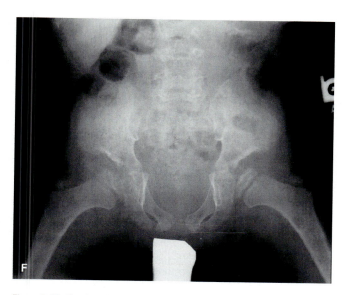

Figure 6–67 *(Continued).* **E, F.** AP and lateral views of the pelvis. Note the delay and irregularity of ossification of the femoral heads, with subluxation of the hips and failure of ossification of the lateral acetabular epiphysis. Note the wine glass appearance of the pelvic inlet.

TABLE 6–8. CONDITIONS THAT CAUSE JOINT PAIN AND SIMULATE ARTHRITIS

I. Tumors and tumorous lesions
  A. Malignant
    Leukemia, neuroblastoma, lymphoma, Hodgkin's disease, synovial sarcoma
  B. Benign
    Bone
      Histiocytosis X, eosinophilic granuloma, osteoid osteoma, osteoblastoma, enchondroma, benign chondroblastoma
    Joint
      Synovial hemangioma, intra-articular lipoma, synovial chondromatosis, pigmented villonodular synovitis

II. Infectious diseases
  Septic arthritis, gonococcal arthritis
  Subacute osteomyelitis involving epiphyses with sympathetic effusion in adjacent joint
  Lyme disease
  Tubercular arthritis
  Viral arthritis (such as postrubella, varicella, or mumps)
  Reactive arthritis

III. Inflammatory and other collagen affections
  Toxic synovitis, nonspecific synovitis
  Rheumatic fever
  Henoch-Schönlein purpura
  Inflammatory bowel disease
  Reiter's syndrome
  Foreign body synovitis
  Psoriatic arthritis
  Polyarteritis nodusa
  Collagen disorder with vasculitis
  Systemic lupus erythematosus
  Dermatomyositis and polymyositis
  Mediterranean fever

IV. Hemophilia and other disorders of coagulation

V. Structural-anatomic conditions
  Legg-Perthes disease
  Slipped capital femoral epiphysis
  Osteochondritis dissecans
  Chondromalacia of the patella—recurrent subluxation of the patellofemoral joint
  Occult stress fracture
  Tarsal coalition
  Ligamentous hyperlaxity such as Ehler-Danlos syndrome, Down's syndrome

VI. Referred pain
  Lumbosacral spine to hip and lower limbs
  Cervical spine to upper limbs

VII. Endocrine-metabolic affections
  Gout
  Thyroid disease
  Mucopolysaccharidosis, Hurler syndrome

■ DIFFERENTIAL DIAGNOSIS OF JOINT PAIN

Pain in and around a joint is a very common complaint. Many conditions can cause and simulate acute or chronic arthritis (Table 6–8). In order to make the correct diagnosis, it is important to be thorough in history taking, to be diligent in physical examination, and to perform the appropriate imaging studies and laboratory tests.

History. Which joint or joints are involved—the knees, ankles, hips, wrists, elbows, and/or fingers? Is the arthritis monoarticular, pauciarticular (four or fewer large joints), or polyarticular? Any history of enlargement (tumefaction) of a finger or toe? Was there any swelling of the joint? Was it warm and painful on movement? Any limp when joints of the lower limbs are involved? What is the severity of the joint pain—mild, moderate, or severe? Is it constant or intermittent? How long does the pain last? Are the joint pains fleeting? Are they increasing in severity?

Inquire as to the *onset* of the joint disease; was it acute or insidious? Did it follow an injury or was it present to a mild degree before and has become aggravated by trauma? Is there any history of antecedent joint disease? Is there any history of recent illness, such as diarrhea or upper respiratory infection, as predisposing factors for infectious arthritis? Any history of rubella, mumps, chickenpox, or glandular fever to suggest a viral basis to the arthritis?

Did the child have a *rash* to suggest exanthem? Ask about the appearance and distribution of the rash. In juvenile rheumatoid arthritis (JRA), the rash is salmon pink, discrete, maculopapular, and circular; it develops over the arms, thighs, axilla, and trunk; and it does not itch. Rheumatic fever rash is recurrent and fleeting, disappearing within a few hours. In Henoch-Schönlein purpura the rash is maculopapular and purpuric. In Lyme arthritis, the rash (erythema chronicum migrans) is characteristic. Is there any history of tick bite?

An *antecedent infection* such as otitis media or a boil or other skin infection suggests the possibility of septic arthritis. Any history of fever? Is there chronic cutaneous moniliasis or other fungal infection to suggest the possibility of fungus infection in the joints? Did the child have a puncture wound from a fall on the knee to indicate foreign body arthritis? Is there a history of easy bruising or bleeding to suggest a bleeding disorder or hemophilic arthropathy?

Is there any contact with a patient with active tuberculosis? The incidence of tuberculosis has greatly declined in civilized countries, but it still occurs, especially in an immunocompromised host. What is the immunologic status of the child? Ask whether the child has been on medications (such as steroids for asthma or methotrexate for vasculitis) that cause suppression of the immune system. Any possibility of AIDS or hypogammaglobulinemia? What is the hematologic status? Is there neutropenia or sickle cell disease?

Inquire as to bowel symptoms such as diarrhea and abdominal pain. Is there any previous history of ulcerative colitis or regional enteritis? Arthritis of inflammatory bowel disease is often transient and involves a few large joints; it may precede intestinal complaints. Consider its possibility when arthritis in a child is associated with weight loss, recurrent fevers, failure to thrive, anemia, and erythema nodosum.

In *reactive arthritis,* one or several large joints are affected; it is characterized by sterile synovitis and joint fluid and association with bacterial infection of the gastrointestinal tract such as shigellosis or salmonellosis.

Are there any symptoms of urethritis or sexual exposure to gonococcal infection to suggest gonorrheal arthritis? Any history of conjunctivitis? The triad of Reiter's syndrome consists of urethritis, conjunctivitis, and arthritis.

Inquire as to previous treatment (medications, physical therapy, splinting) and the response to it. Do the symptoms increase with activity and subside with rest?

Take a detailed family history as to the incidence of rheumatoid arthritis and other joint disease, immunologic disorders, and collagen disease.

Examination. The physical examination should be thorough, assessing the whole child. Does the child appear ill, listless, irritable, malnourished, and underweight? Weigh the patient and measure the standing and sitting heights. Take the patient's blood pressure; when the blood pressure is elevated, consider the possibility of collagen disease with vasculitis. Take the temperature; in systemic rheumatoid arthritis with polyarthritis, the child has a fever, which may be low grade and sustained or quotidian with one or two daily rises from normal to 104°F. When the child is feverish, ask the parents about its duration (days or weeks) and whether acetaminophen (Tylenol), salicylates, or antibiotics were given and the response of the fever to medication.

Look for skin rashes; they are an important diagnostic clue to the nature of arthritis. Gluteal and/or foot rash is indicative of Henoch-Schönlein disease; whereas in systemic rheumatoid disease with polyarthritis, the rashes are salmon pink, discrete, and circular or circinate. The rash of Lyme arthritis is characteristic. It apppears as a "bull's eye" on the thighs, arms, axilla, and trunk. In rheumatic fever the rash is fleeting and recurrent, disappearing within a few hours.

Inspect the eyes. Is there any asymmetry of the pupils? How is the vision? Is it diminished? The acute iritis associated with HLA-B27 is usually painful, and the red conjunctivitis is clinically obvious; whereas iridocyclitis of pauciarticular JRA requires slit-lamp examination by an ophthalmologist to detect it. Palpate the abdomen. Is there any abnormal enlargement of the liver or spleen? Is there any lymphadenopathy in the axilla, groin, posterior triangle of the neck, or supraclavicular region? Although hepatosplenomegaly and generalized lymphadenopathy are frequently present in systemic rheumatoid disease with polyarthritis, the possibility of malignancy should always be entertained with such physical findings.

Palpate near the olecranon process of the elbows, along the anterolateral surface of the tibia, and over the extensor tendon of the wrist and fingers. Are there any *subcutaneous* nodules? When present, JRA is a probability.

Auscultate the heart. Any cardiac murmur to indicate rheumatic fever? Pericarditis and myocarditis with enlargement of the heart do occur in systemic rheumatoid polyarthritis.

Next, examine the musculoskeletal system. First, inspect the standing patient. Is there any muscle atrophy around the painful joint? What is the position of the joint? Is it held in flexion? Is there any lower limb disparity because of overgrowth of the long bone due to increased circulation from the arthritis? Is there scoliosis? Ask the patient to walk. Is there any antalgic limp?

Then examine the joints for effusion, swelling, synovial thickening, and increased local heat. Test range of motion of the joint. Examine all of the large and small joints, beginning with the normal and then proceeding to the painful ones.

Investigations. The clinical presentation determines the extent of imaging and other laboratory examinations.

Imaging. Always obtain (1) *plain radiograms* of the affected joint; (2) *ultrasonograms* of the joint to demonstrate the presence of fluid and other soft tissue changes; (3) *bone scan* with technetium-99m in some cases, especially when the diagnosis is not certain; it shows increased uptake in both sides of the joint; (4) *CT and MRI* studies, performed when internal derangement of the joint or tumor is suspected.

Laboratory Studies. The following laboratory tests are made as indicated: (1) CBC, (2) routine urinalysis, (3) ESR and C-reactive protein, (4) bleeding and clotting time, (5) blood cultures, (6) agglutination test for IgM, (7) rheumatoid factor test, (8) antinuclear antibody tests, (9) identification of antibodies to *Brucella, Salmonella, Ixodes dammini* (Lyme disease), and the like, (10) synovial fluid analysis and culture, and (11) tuberculosis test.

JUVENILE RHEUMATOID ARTHRITIS

Rheumatoid disease in children and adolescents may manifest in three patterns: (1) pauciarticular (four or fewer joints), (2) polyarticular (five or more joints) with minimal systemic manifestation, and (3) systemic disease with polyarthritis. The onset, course, and prognosis of rheumatoid disease vary greatly according to its clinical pattern.[912,913,922,925,957]

Pauciarticular Arthritis

This is characterized by involvement of a few large joints with minimal or no systemic involvement and is sometimes associated with tumefaction of a finger or toe. The prefix *pauci* is derived from the Latin *paucus,* which means "few."[921,934]

The diagnostic criteria for a joint to be rheumatoid are inflammation (swelling, tenderness, effusion), pain on motion, and heat in one or more joints for 6 weeks or longer.

The *age* of onset is usually between 2 and 4 years, with 50 percent of the cases occurring before 4 years of age; however, it may begin at any time between 4 months and 15 years of age. There is definite sex predilection for the female, with a female to male ratio of 7:3.

The knee and ankle are the two most common joints involved; next in order of frequency are the subtalar joint, elbow, wrist, and hip. Digits are involved in some children. In about one half of the cases, one joint is involved; in one quarter, two joints; and in one fifth, three joints. Ordinarily when only one joint is involved initially, the pauciarticular pattern develops within weeks or months. Often large joint involvement is asymmetric.

The presenting complaint may be an antalgic limp when the joints of the lower limbs are involved. The onset is insidious. In-toeing due to inversion of the heel is the initial manifestation when the subtalar joint is affected.

On examination, the inflamed joint is swollen. A palpable effusion is present in the acute stage. The inflamed synovium is thickened and boggy, and it remains thickened as long as the disease is active. Palpate the joint with the dorsum of the proximal phalanges of your hand; the inflamed joint is slightly warm. Local tenderness is minimal. Range of motion of the affected joints is restricted. Flexion deformity of the knee, hip, and elbow is always present. The hip is also limited in abduction and medial rotation. The subtalar joint is inverted, with a varus deformity of the hindfoot and midfoot. Muscle atrophy is always present, its degree dependent upon the severity and duration of the arthritis. Increased blood supply to the physis due to chronic synovitis causes overgrowth of the affected lower limb and results in lower limb length disparity and functional scoliosis.

The eyes of children with pauciarticular arthritis should be examined every 4 to 6 months. Iridocyclitis is a serious complication, which, if left untreated, results in loss of eyesight in 20 percent of the cases.[939,964] Refer the patient to an ophthalmologist.

Systemic manifestations are none or minimal; fever, hepatosplenomegaly, rash, and subcutaneous nodules are absent.

Laboratory Studies. Complete blood count is normal. The ESR may be slightly or moderately elevated. The rheumatoid factor is negative. Antinuclear antibodies may be positive (homogeneous or speckled pattern). Bone scan with technetium-99m shows increased uptake in the affected joints, but its routine use is not recommended.

In the diagnostic work-up of pauciarticular JRA, always perform serologic tests to rule out Lyme arthritis, in which the titers of IgM and IgG antibodies against *Ixodes dammini* are elevated. Lyme disease characteristically develops in the summer and autumn—periods when ticks are very active. Inquire as to a history of tick bite and whether the child had a rash or prodromal systemic signs such as a low-grade fever, headache, or stiff neck.

The *clinical course* of pauciarticular JRA is benign. Occasionally it may evolve into polyarticular JRA; often, however, it resolves in 2 years with periods of remission and exacerbation.

Treatment. This consists of nonsteroidal anti-inflammatory medications. It is essential to provide local care to the affected joint in the form of rest, relief of muscle spasm, prevention of deformity by part-time use of splints and counterpoised traction (if necessary), and restoration and maintenance of motion by active and passive exercises. The prognosis is good.

Polyarthritis with Minimal Systemic Manifestations

In this polyarticular form of JRA, five or more joints are affected. The onset is usually insidious, although on occasion it may be acute. Any joint may be affected—the wrists, PIP joints of the fingers, subtalar and midtarsal joints of the feet, knees, elbows, hips, shoulders, temporomandibular joints, and cervical spine are frequent sites.

The age of onset has two peaks; 1 to 3 years and 8 to 10 years. In the younger age group, there is no sex predilection, whereas in the juvenile age group, females are more commonly affected.

The involved joints in the polyarticular form of JRA are more severely inflamed than those of pauciarticular JRA. The child is apprehensive, guarding the affected limb against movement. The involved joint is painful, locally tender on palpation, swollen with effusion and synovial thickening, and warm. Range of motion of the affected joint is restricted. When the cervical spine is involved, neck motion is limited and torticollis may develop. A receding chin is commonly present when the temporomandibular joint is affected. Subcutaneous nodules may develop over bony prominences such as the elbows and heels or in the flexor tendons of the hands and feet.

Systemic manifestations are minimal; many of these children have low-grade fever, malaise, slight hepatosplenomegaly, and mild anemia.

Laboratory and Imaging Findings.   Often the CBC shows mild anemia with hemoglobin below 10, the ESR is elevated, and the rheumatoid factor may be positive or negative. The osteocalcin is decreased. Plain radiograms demonstrate regional osteoporosis with cortical thinning. MRI with gadolinium discloses moderate to extreme cartilage destruction; the intercarpal distance is decreased.

The *clinical course* is chronic and protracted, lasting many years with periods of partial remission with minimal joint involvement interspersed with acute exacerbation. Polyarticular JRA with a negative rheumatoid factor may digress to pauciarticular disease and eventually resolve. Those cases of polyarticular JRA with the rheumatoid factor positive, however, have a poorer prognosis, resulting in marked destruction of the affected joints. The rheumatoid factor–positive polyarticular JRA is similar to adult rheumatoid arthritis; the only difference is its age of onset, developing in late childhood.

Management.   Polyarticular JRA with minimal systemic involvement is treated with nonsteroidal anti-inflammatory medications such as naproxen sodium, tolmetin sodium, or ibuprofen.[914,916,917,919,922,943] When there is no adequate response to nonsteroidal anti-inflammatory drugs and inflammation and pain are severe, a short period of steroid therapy, such as prednisone, should be considered. During medical treatment, monitor adverse reactions of the bone marrow and liver to the drugs every 3 months (or more often if abnormal) by the following tests: CBC, white blood cell count and differential, platelet count, and serum glutamic-oxaloacetic transaminase. When steroids are given, bone mineral metabolism is checked by determination of serum osteocalcin. The diet should be adequate for calcium intake. The eyes should be examined for iridocyclitis, uveitis, glaucoma, vasculitis, and hemorrhage; these are rare complications.[939]

Local care of joints, physical therapy, and occupational therapy are given as outlined for pauciarticular JRA.

Systemic Rheumatoid Disease with Polyarthritis

The onset of this type of JRA is acute with high fever. The sick child is usually consulted by the pediatrician and pediatric rheumatologist. The orthopedic surgeon is asked to assess the patient when there is difficulty in the differential diagnosis between acute onset of systemic JRA and septic arthritis with septicemia. Hepatosplenomegaly and generalized lymphadenopathy are common. Rheumatoid rash occurs in 50 to 75 percent of the cases. Subcutaneous nodules over the olecranon process and along the subcutaneous surface of the tibia are commonly present. Pericarditis with enlargement of the heart develops in 10 percent of cases. Ocular inflammation, iridocyclitis, and amyloidosis are serious problems.[954]

Laboratory Findings.   CBC and hemoglobin disclose moderate anemia with leukocytosis. ESR is elevated. Antinuclear antibody and rheumatoid factor tests are often negative.

When septicemia and septic arthritis are considered in the differential diagnosis, blood cultures should be made.

Imaging.   The initial findings in the plain radiogram are soft tissue swelling, capsular distention, and regional osteoporosis. These are nonspecific changes, reflecting the acute synovitis and response to the inflammatory hyperemia.

Juxta-articular new bone formation may occur in the phalanges. With progression of the disease, the articular cartilage space narrows due to destruction of hyaline cartilage by the inflammatory process. In the late stages, when fibrous ankylosis occurs, the articular cartilage space is obliterated.

In the cervical spine, atlantoaxial instability and subluxation develop due to erosion of the odontoid process.

Ultrasonography shows the fluid and soft tissue changes in the affected joints. *Bone scan with technetium-99m* shows minimal increased uptake on both sides of the joint. MRI with gadolinium shows the extent of destruction of articular cartilage.

The *clinical course* is chronic and protracted with periods of partial remission. Growth and development are retarded. The affected children are chronically ill, in pain, and lose too much time from school. Despite aggressive therapy, some of the patients with systemic rheumatoid polyarticular arthritis become wheelchair bound or household ambulators because of deformity of the joints, hypotonia, and pain.

Management. It is crucial to provide multidisciplinary care with involvement by the pediatrician, pediatric rheumatologist, immunologist, physical and occupational therapists, psychologist, and social worker.

Nonsteroidal anti-inflammatory drugs are tried first. Often steroids are required to control the progression of the disease process. Immunosuppressive agents are given on occasion.

Death can occur in severe systemic rheumatoid disease from complications of amyloidosis or complications of drug therapy.

Juvenile Spondyloarthropathy[918,953]

This form of JRA usually has its onset in older children (usually 9 years or older), and it is more common in boys. A positive family history can often be obtained in the form of rheumatoid arthritis or psoriasis and bowel disease. The arthritis begins in a few of the large joints of the lower limbs, with the knees, ankles, and hips most commonly involved. The joints of the upper limbs, with the exception of the elbow, are rarely affected. The small joints are occasionally involved, suggesting psoriasis. The patient complains of intermittent pain, which is aggravated by rest and relieved by motion. After a few years, the patient complains of a painful and stiff low back. Occasionally atlantoaxial subluxation is the presenting complaint. Iridocyclitis develops in 25 percent of the cases; obtain ophthalmologic consultation.

The plain *radiograms* are normal in the beginning, but a *bone scan* with technetium-99m shows increased uptake in the sacroiliac joints and the affected large joint.

Laboratory Findings. CBC and ESR are often normal. HLA-B27 is positive. The antinuclear antibodies may be positive.

Treatment. Nonsteroidal anti-inflammatory medications are given to control inflammation of the joints. Early in the disease, a course of sulfasalazine may be tried (40 to 60 mg/kg/day) in three to six divided doses with milk or food; after 6 weeks decrease the dosage to 30 mg/kg/day. NSAIDs are given as necessary depending upon the activity of the arthritis. Liver function should be monitored at three-month intervals.

In 2 to 3 percent of the cases of juvenile spondyloarthropathy, the arthritis persists into adult life.

Operative treatment may be indicated when an adequate trial of aggressive nonsurgical treatment fails to control progression of the synovitis and when deformity needs correction.[917] Operative measures consist of (1) *soft tissue procedures*—muscle-tendon lengthening, synovectomy, capsulotomy, and capsulectomy, and (2) *bone and joint procedures*—osteotomy, arthroplasty and arthrodesis, and epiphyseodesis to equalize limb lengths.

Synovectomy is indicated in the early stages of JRA when 1 to 2 years of aggressive medical and non-surgical orthopedic treatment fails to suppress the active synovitis and the joint undergoes progressive deformity.[910,930,938,946,948,950] Synovectomy is effective when the hyaline articular cartilage appears normal or when there is mild cartilage erosion with yellow areas and flaking. Synovectomy is contraindicated when there are large, deep erosions of articular cartilage. Synovectomy is best performed through the arthroscope.

Soft tissue release is performed to correct fixed contractural deformity of joints. Musculotendinous lengthening of contracted muscles corrects deformity, decompresses the joint, relieves muscle spasm and pain, and provides greater range of joint motion. Capsulotomy or capsulectomy is indicated when flexion deformity of the knee or hip or equinus deformity of the ankle is rigid and severe.

Lower limb disparity is corrected by epiphyseodesis of the distal femur and/or proximal tibia of the long limb. Mobility of completely destroyed hip and knee joints is restored by total joint replacement of the hip and/or knee.[917,941,951,952,961,963]

Atlantoaxial subluxation with neurologic deficit may require cervical fusion.[911,927,931] This is especially true when JRA develops in children with Down syndrome or Ehlers-Danlos syndrome with marked ligamentous hyperlaxity. In other conditions, a simple cervical orthosis may stabilize the neck and prevent progressive subluxation.

RHEUMATIC FEVER

Rheumatic fever follows beta-hemolytic streptococcal infection. The arthritis is acutely painful, migratory (persisting in one joint only a few days), and involves large joints, predominantly the knees, ankles, and wrists. Carditis, skin rash (erythema marginatum), subcutaneous nodules, and occasionally chorea are other associated findings. Joint symptoms are immediately controlled by an adequate dose of salicylates. The antistreptococcal titer is elevated. Appropriate antibiotic therapy prevents recurrence and cures the streptococcal infection.

REITER'S SYNDROME

Following *Shigella* infections, a child occasionally develops Reiter's syndrome, which consists of the triad of urethritis, conjunctivitis, and arthritis. Only a few large joints are affected and ordinarily the arthritis is transient, responding to nonsteroidal anti-inflammatory medication.

HENOCH-SCHÖNLEIN PURPURA

The diagnosis of this rare form of vasculitis is readily made when the typical clinical picture is fully developed, with abdominal pain, nephritis, and patchy angioneurotic edema of the hands, feet, and genital area. The orthopedic surgeon, however, is not consulted at this stage of the disease; he sees the patient with one or more swollen and painful joints prior to the appearance of the skin manifestations. Consider the possibility of Henoch-Schönlein purpura when a painful swollen joint has relatively normal range of motion despite the discomfort. The diagnosis is probable when a maculopurpural and purpuric rash develops over the ankles and gluteal regions.

INFECTIOUS ARTHRITIS

Diagnosis and management of septic arthritis and subacute osteomyelitis of the epiphysis with sympathetic effusion in adjacent joints are discussed in Chapters 2 and 3.

GONOCOCCAL ARTHRITIS[967–970]

Gonococcal arthritis is rare in children; it occurs in the sexually active, careless adolescent or is transmitted to an infant by maternal infection. Do not hesitate to ask about urethral discharge! Arthritis usually develops 2 to 4 weeks following the initial infection. One or several joints may be affected; common sites are the knees, ankles, wrists, and sternoclavicular joints. Caution! When the sternoclavicular joint is inflamed and swollen, gonococcal arthritis is the most likely diagnosis.

The affected joints are swollen, hot, tender, and tense, with marked restriction of motion. Destruction of articular cartilage occurs rapidly in gonococcal arthritis. Immediate treatment with penicillin is effective; it prevents damage to the joint.

In infants, gonococcal arthritis is in the form of erythematous papules surrounded by hemorrhagic or vesiculopustulous lesions. The joint-skin combination is referred to as gonococcal arthritis dermatitis.[970]

TUBERCULOUS ARTHRITIS

This form is rare, but it still occurs and should be considered in the differential diagnosis of arthritis. It is blood-borne and caused by *Mycobacterium tuberculosis*. Radiograms of the chest are made to rule out pulmonary infection. Examine the abdomen for mesenteric lymphadenopathy and the neck for enlarged infected lymph nodes. The infection may be the human or bovine type.

Tuberculous arthritis is often monoarticular. The hip and knee are common sites of involvement; next in order of frequency are the ankle, sacroiliac joint, shoulder, and wrist. The vertebral column is a common site; tuberculous arthritis should always be considered in the differential diagnosis of spondyloarthropathy.

The onset of tuberculous arthritis is insidious. The child is ill, has evident weight loss, and is easily fatigued. When a weight-bearing joint is involved, the presenting complaint is slight local discomfort and an antalgic limp. On palpation of superficial joints, such as the knee, ankle, or elbow, the soft tissues are boggy due to synovial thickening and effusion. Absence of local heat and redness are distinctive of tuberculosis. Muscle atrophy is marked. The range of joint motion is limited.

Imaging Findings. In the plain radiogram, initial findings consist of regional osteoporosis, capsular distention, and soft tissue swelling; these changes are nonspecific. With progression of the disease, the tuberculous granulomatous tissue destroys the hyaline cartilage and the articular cartilage space narrows; this is especially evident in the hips, where there is a congruous fit of the opposing articular surfaces. Areas of radiolucency in the epiphysis soon develop due to bone destruction. Reactive bone formation is characteristically absent. CT detects bone and soft tissue changes in detail. Chest radiogram, intravenous pyelogram, and flat plate and ultrasonogram of the abdomen are other imaging studies that are performed.

Laboratory tests should include CBC, sedimentation rate, and skin test for tuberculosis. Synovial fluid analysis and culture and histologic examination of tissue obtained by biopsy make the diagnosis.

Treatment consists of antitubercular drugs and rest to the part. Synovectomy and curettage of the bone lesion are indicated when diagnosis is not made early. The prognosis is good.

FOREIGN BODY ARTHRITIS

Following a fall on the knee or walking barefoot on the playground or beach, a piece of wood, broken glass, or stone may penetrate a superficial joint. The child complains of pain and swelling of the joint. There may be a low-grade fever, suggesting infectious arthritis. Inspect the skin for scars of a puncture wound. There is effusion and synovial thickening. Point tenderness suggests the diagnosis. Plain radiograms are normal unless the foreign body is radiopaque. An ultrasonogram may detect the foreign body; if it is not helpful, an MRI should be performed.

Treatment consists of removal of the foreign body and irrigation of the wound, either through the arthroscope or with open surgery. It is important to place the incision over the likely site of the foreign body.

ARTHRITIS AND JOINT SYMPTOMS RELATED TO MALIGNANT TUMORS AND TUMOROUS LESIONS

Joint pain and stiffness can be caused by leukemia, neuroblastoma, lymphoma, Hodgkin's disease, sarcoma, and osteogenic and Ewing's sarcoma, simulating arthritis. Always consider and rule out malignancy when a painful joint does not respond to nonsteroidal anti-inflammatory medication. Leukemic and neuroblastoma cells can infiltrate articular ends of long bones and involve periarticular tissues. In malignancies, the patient complains of pain at rest. In the beginning, the pain is mild to moderate; then it persists and increases to become very severe, keeping the patient awake at night.

The child with malignancy is pale and ill, with a fever that cannot be explained. Rule out lymphadenopathy. Palpate the abdomen for masses and hepatosplenomegaly. CBC demonstrates anemia and other leukocyte abnormalities. The sedimentation rate is often elevated. Next perform an appropriate diagnostic oncology work-up consisting of plain radiograms, bone scan with technetium-99m, CT, MRI, ultrasonography, and bone marrow biopsy. Remember that the most common presenting complaint of a child with leukemia is bone and joint pain.

Benign tumors and tumorous lesions can involve the epiphyses of long bones and cause joint pain. Some of the tumors are osteoid osteoma, osteoblastoma, eosinophilic granuloma (histiocytosis X), enchondroma, and benign chondroblastoma. (See section on tumors and tumorous conditions of bone.)

SYNOVIAL HEMANGIOMA[971–975]

The presenting complaint is a swollen, boggy joint that is painful on motion and warm to touch. The pain and swelling are intermittent with recurrent effusion.

A rare cause of joint pain, it is often misdiagnosed as rheumatoid arthritis. It is usually seen in adolescents and young adults, although on careful inquiry, the joint complaints date back to childhood. The knee is the most common site of involvement; the elbow, ankle, and shoulder are occasional sites. When the hemangioma is pedunculated, there may be a history of locking of the knee, suggesting a loose body.

On examination, one can palpate a soft and doughy mass that is exquisitely tender. Elevate and exsanguinate the limb; the mass decreases in size. On dependency, the mass becomes larger. Measure the circumference of the limbs; there is marked muscle atrophy about the joint. Look for the presence of subcutaneous hemangiomas. Is there any lower limb length disparity?

Imaging. Plain radiograms are usually normal; phleboliths, however, when present, are a diagnostic clue. Varying degrees of local osteoporosis are present. Ultrasonograms disclose effusion of the joint and may detect the hemangiomatous mass. MRI is often necessary to delineate the pathology.

Treatment. This consists of excision of the hemangioma through the arthroscope. Diffuse cavernous hemangiomas require synovectomy. Postoperative joint stiffness is a problem.

INTRA-ARTICULAR LIPOMA

The presenting complaint is swelling of varying degrees in the joint. The mass consists of mesenchymal fat cells. Intra-articular lipomas are usually asymptomatic and do not cause any dysfunction. The plain radiogram discloses the mass, which is radiolucent. Surgical treatment is not indicated.

SYNOVIAL CHONDROMATOSIS[976–981]

In this very rare condition, metaplastic and multiple foci of cartilage form in the intimal layer of a large joint. The knee is the most common site. The hip, ankle, elbow, or wrist may be involved.

The presenting complaints are pain, swelling, and stiffness of the involved joint. When loose bodies form, the joint may lock. Physical findings are joint crepitus, synovial thickening, and limitation of joint motion.

Plain radiograms disclose the stippled calcification in and around the joint. MRI clearly depicts the synovial chondromata.

Treatment consists of synovectomy.

PIGMENTED VILLONODULAR SYNOVITIS[982–987]

The presenting complaint is pain and swelling of the involved joint, the knee being the most common site. It may affect the fingers, ankles, hips, wrists, and shoulders. Range of joint motion is limited; there may be a history of locking. The synovium proliferates and becomes nodular, villous, and brownish in color.

Plain radiograms disclose irregular synovial thickening and erosion of the articular ends of the bones. CT and MRI depict the lesion in detail.

On aspiration of the joint, a dark brown or serosanguineous fluid is obtained.

In the differential diagnosis, rule out juvenile rheumatoid arthritis, synovial hemangiomatosis, and low-grade infectious arthritis. The diagnosis is made by histologic examination of the proliferated synovium.

Treatment consists of total synovectomy, which is best performed through the arthroscope.

Structural-anatomic conditions that cause joint pain are discussed in Chapters 1 through 3.

Referred pain and endocrine-metabolic affections should always be considered in the differential diagnosis of joint pain.

■ HEMOPHILIA

In this genetically determined disorder, the coagulation mechanism is deranged due to functional deficiency of a specific factor, namely Factor VIII or IX. The hallmarks of hemophilia are repeated episodes of bleeding and uncontrolled hemorrhage. There are three types of hemophilia: (1) *Hemophilia A* is the most common type, comprising 80 percent of the cases. It is due to Factor VIII deficiency. The gene responsible for hemophilia A is carried on the X-chromosome. Transmitted by an asymptomatic female carrier, it occurs in the male. (2) *Hemophilia B* is due to Factor IX deficiency and is also called "Christmas disease." Comprising 15 percent of the cases, it is transmitted by an X-linked recessive gene. Clinical manifestations of hemophilia A and hemophilia B are quite similar. (3) *Hemophilia C* (von Willebrand's disease) is caused by both Factor VIII deficiency and platelet abnormality. Its inheritance is autosomal dominant, occurring in both sexes. The hemorrhage disorder is relatively mild.

The orthopedic implications of hemophilia are the following: (1) hemarthrosis and hemophilic arthropathy, (2) soft tissue hematoma, (3) nerve palsy, (4) hemophilic pseudotumor, (5) fractures, (6) dislocations, and (7) myositis ossificans.

Hemarthrosis and Hemophilic Arthropathy. Bleeding into the joint occurs most commonly in the knee; next, in descending order, are the ankle, elbow, wrist, shoulder, and hip. *Acute bleeding* causes considerable pain, muscle spasm, and swelling. There may or may not be a history of injury. The posture of the joint is one of minimal discomfort; the knees and elbows are held in flexion, the ankle in equinus, and the hip in moderate flexion and some abduction and lateral rotation. On palpation, there is increased warmth and local tenderness. The overlying skin is tense. Passive and active motion of the affected joint is restricted and painful, eliciting further muscle spasm.

Ordinarily, the parents and patient are instructed to immediately administer Factor VIII or XI, which is followed by rapid subsidence of the intense pain and acute bleeding.

Following several episodes of bleeding into the joint, subacute hemarthrosis develops. Clinically the pain is minimal and restriction of joint motion moderate. Progressive flexion deformity of the joint develops. The following pathophysiologic changes occur consequent to multiple bleeds into the joint. The synovium hypertrophies and undergoes fibrosis due to uptake of iron and leukocyte and platelet enzymes. The diseased synovium bleeds easily, setting up a vicious circle. The proliferating synovium forms pannus, which erodes articular cartilage peripherally. The action of proteolytic enzymes degrades articular cartilage. Compression of opposing cartilaginous surfaces results in progressive degeneration and destruction of the joint with fibrosis and loss of motion. Hemorrhage into the subchondral bone causes necrosis of overlying cartilage. Progressive destruction of the joint leads to disabling arthritis in adult life.

Plain radiograms demonstrate the progressive destruction of the joint. (1) Initially only soft tissues are swollen, and there is no osseous deformity (stage I). (2) Then there is osteoporosis and overgrowth of the epiphysis, with the integrity of the joint maintained (stage II). (3) With recurrent bleeding, destruction of the articular cartilage is then mild to moderate, narrowing the articular cartilage space. Subchondral cysts develop. In the knee, the intercondylar notch widens and in the elbow the trochlear notch increases in diameter (stage III). (4) The osseous changes become pronounced, and the articular cartilage space becomes severely narrowed (stage IV). (5) Finally, fibrous ankylosis of the joint occurs, with total loss of articular cartilage space, marked incongruity of the joint, and irregular hypertrophy of the epiphysis (stage V).[989]

Soft Tissue Bleeding and Nerve Palsy. Minor intramuscular and intermuscular bleeding occurs frequently. Bleeding becomes serious when it is severe and produces pressure on neuromuscular structures. Muscle necrosis and fibrosis result in contractural deformity. The quadriceps femoris, triceps surae, iliopsoas, and forearm muscles are common sites of hemorrhage into muscle. Bleeding into the iliacus sheaths causes femoral nerve palsy. Hemorrhage into the volar compartment of the forearm causes ischemic necrosis and fibrosis of forearm muscles and Volkmann's contracture.

The presenting complaint is pain on motion of the part or at rest. The site of hemorrhage is swollen and tender on palpation.

Diagnosis of hemorrhage into superficial muscles and soft tissues is readily made by physical examination. Bleeding into deep soft tissues such as the retroperitoneum, iliopsoas, and hip is readily detected by ultrasonography.[1015] Occasionally MRI is performed, especially when nerve palsy is present.

Neuropraxia is caused by compression of the nerve from the hematoma. The femoral nerve is commonly involved in its course in the closed, rigid compartment within the iliacus fascia.[1003] Next in frequency is median nerve palsy; occasionally the ulnar, radial, peroneal, and lateral femoral cutaneous nerves are involved. A history of strenuous physical activity or injury such as twisting of the limb or a fall may be obtained. The patient complains of pain and weakness of the affected muscles. When the femoral nerve is involved, the posture of the hip is one of flexion and lateral rotation. On range-of-motion testing, extension and medial rotation are restricted and painful. A tender mass may be palpable in the iliac fossa. The patient is unable to extend the knee and there is anesthesia of cutaneous sensory nerve distribution of the femoral nerve.[995,1017]

Hemophilic Pseudotumors. These are cystic swellings in soft tissue produced either by recurrent uncontrolled bleeding into muscles which is confined within a compartment or by subperiosteal hemorrhage which progressively strips the periosteum from the cortex. Erosion of subjacent bone by compression may occur. Occasionally, pseudotumors result from hemorrhage into bone.[988,989,991,1009,1012,1029,1034] The overlying muscle is raised and undergoes necrosis.

The most common site of pseudotumor is in the thigh; next, in decreasing order, are the abdomen, pelvis, tibia, hand, and calcaneus. Pathologic fracture of an affected bone may occur. Do not mistake a hemophilic pseudotumor for a malignant lesion.

Dislocation of the Hip. This may develop from intraarticular bleeding into the hip and stretching of the capsule. A serious complication is avascular necrosis of the femoral head due to tamponade of its blood supply.[993,998,1001,1028,1031]

Fractures. In hemophilia fractures occur commonly in the lower limbs, especially in children with stiff knees and osteoporotic bones who sustain supracondylar fracture of the distal femur.[997] Pathologic fracture may also occur after trivial injury to a bone weakened by pseudotumor. The problem is uncontrolled bleeding into a closed fascial compartment, muscle necrosis, and Volkmann's ischemic contracture.[993,994,1000,1014]

Myositis Ossificans. This develops because of intramuscular or intermuscular bleeding. It occurs in 15 percent of patients with hemophilia. It causes some restriction of adjacent joints, but otherwise disability is minimal.[1010,1018]

***Management.*[999]** The care of a child with hemophilia should be provided at a hemophilia clinic in a children's hospital by a multidisciplinary team of medical specialists consisting of a hematologist, orthopedic surgeon, physical therapist, nurse clinician, psychologist, and social worker.

Prevention of injury is crucial. Provide the family with a list of instructions as to the appropriate toys, games, and physical activities. The child with hemophilia should avoid contact sports; he or she should be involved in physical activities that are not likely to cause injury, such as swimming and golf.

Medical Management. The goal is to control bleeding by hemostasis achieved by administration of freeze-dried Factor VIII or IX concentrates, which are commercially available. *Home treatment* consists of training the family or the mature patient to administer Factor VIII or IX at home; such home programs do function effectively, provided that the child and parents are compliant and thoroughly instructed as to dosage schedules and appropriate sterile technique and handling of the materials.[1008,1020] Parents may be apprehensive about causing AIDS or hepatitis B by infusion of infected blood products. They should understand that delay in early treatment is the primary cause of crippling joint deformity.

The indication for Factor VIII or IX replacement is immediate control of soft tissue and joint hemorrhage. Prevention of sizeable hemarthrosis checkreins the secondary changes in synovial tissue that result from exposure to blood for prolonged periods. Factor VIII or IX replacement is administered as soon as the joint bleed is diagnosed. Pain and swelling are the hallmark of hemarthrosis. External compression with one or two elastic bandages over the site of hemorrhage minimizes bleeding and swelling. If the bleed is severe, the affected joint is temporarily immobilized in a soft, padded splint. Do not apply a circular cast or taut constricting bandages! There should be adequate follow-up and proper communication between the parents and the physician and nurse clinician.

Analgesics to allay pain should be avoided as much as possible. The severity of pain decreases after cessation of bleeding. If absolutely necessary, only acetaminophen—plain or with codeine—is given. Avoid potent analgesics, as they are likely to lead to drug addiction. Do not give analgesic drugs that contain salicylates (aspirin) or antihistamine because they inhibit platelet aggregation and prolong bleeding time.

Aspiration of Hemarthrosis. This is performed less and less due to the efficacy of early diagnosis and early effective treatment by factor replacement. The indication for aspiration is severe *progressive* hemarthrosis with marked distention of the joint capsule and excruciating pain that cannot be controlled by factor replacement. The acute bleeding episode should be of less than 24 hours' duration. The knee is the joint most commonly requiring aspiration. What is the previous history of bleeding in the involved and other joints and the response to treatment? Are there antibodies to Factor VIII or IX?

Arthrocentesis should be performed under strict aseptic conditions and under local anesthesia. Factor VIII or IX replacement should be given immediately before (20 to 30 minutes) aspiration and 12 hours later. When aspiration is delayed after factor replacement, thickening and clotting of the blood make aspiration unsuccessful. Avoid multiple punctures. In severe bleeds, factor replacement is continued for 3 to 5 days following cessation of hemorrhage.

Local care of the joint is crucial to prevent deformity. Following aspiration, the part is immobilized in a posterior splint for 2 to 3 days. The patient is instructed to perform isometric exercises in the splints. Two to three days after aspiration, the splint is removed and active knee flexion-extension exercises are performed several times a day. Support in the posterior splint is continued for 2 weeks; then it is gradually discontinued. The importance of habilitation of the joint cannot be overemphasized.

Surgical Treatment. Wounds, soft tissues, and bone heal normally in the hemophilic patient. If the clotting mechanism is restored to normal by administration of Factor VIII or IX, open surgery is relatively safe. Antihemophilic factor is given the day before surgery and continued for 3 weeks postoperatively; the sutures are removed the 14th day after surgery. Deformities that are severe, interfere with function, and cannot be corrected by closed nonoperative methods are treated by open surgery. Rigid equinus deformity is corrected by Achilles tendon lengthening and fixed flexion contracture of the knee by fractional lengthening of the hamstrings, and if necessary, by posterior capsulotomy of the knee. Extension contracture of the knee is treated by V-Y lengthening of the rectus femoris and quadriceps mechanism. Compartment syndrome due to a soft tissue bleed is treated by fasciotomy and epimysiotomy.

Synovectomy, particularly of the knee, is indicated in patients with recurrent hemarthrosis (two or three major bleeds into the joint per month) and those who fail to respond to aggressive, persistent medical management, physical therapy, crutch protection, and orthotic support for a period of 6 to 12 months. The radiographic stage of hemophilic arthropathy should be II or III; synovectomy is contraindicated in stages IV and V arthropathy because it is ineffective.

Joints, particularly the knee or hip, that are destroyed and stiff with severe disabling pain are treated by total joint replacement, whereas in the ankle or subtalar and midfoot joints, ankle or triple arthrodesis is performed.

Pseudotumors, if disabling, are excised following careful preoperative planning by MRI.

Fractures heal normally in hemophilics. On the first to the third day of the fracture, administer Factor VIII or IX to raise the blood levels to 40 to 60 percent of normal. Subsequently, it should be 20 to 30 percent of normal for a period of 7 to 14 days, depending upon the severity of associated soft tissue surgery.

Crippling deformities of the musculoskeletal system can be prevented and corrected by collaboration between the hematologist and orthopedic surgeon and appropriate *early* treatment.

References

Spinal Muscular Atrophy

1. Beevor CE: A case of congenital spinal muscular atrophy (family type), and a case of haemorrhage into the spinal cord at birth, giving similar symptoms. *Brain* 25:85, 1902
2. Benady SG: Spinal muscular atrophy in childhood: Review of 50 cases. *Dev Med Child Neurol* 20:746, 1978
3. Brandt S: *Werdnig-Hoffmann's Infantile Progressive Muscular Atrophy.* Copenhagen, E Munksgaard, 1950
4. Burke SW, Jameson VP, Roberts JM, Johnston CE, Willis J: Birth fractures in spinal muscular atrophy. *J Pediatr Orthop* 6:34, 1986
5. Byers RK, Banker BQ: Infantile muscular atrophy. *Arch Neurol* 5:140, 1961
6. Daher YH, Lonstein JE, Winter RB, Bradford DS: Spinal surgery in spinal muscular atrophy. *J Pediatr Orthop* 5:391, 1985
7. Dubowitz V: Benign infantile spinal muscular atrophy. *Dev Med Child Neurol* 16:672, 1974
8. Dubowitz V: *The Floppy Infant.* London, William Heineman, 1969
9. Evans GA, Drennan JC, Russman BS: Functional classification and orthopaedic management of spinal muscular atrophy. *J Bone Joint Surg* 73B:516, 1981
10. Hoffmann J: Ueber chronische spinale Muskelatrophi im Kindsalter, auf familiarer Basis. *Dtsch Z Nervenheilk* 3:427, 1893
11. Kugelberg E, Welander L: Heredo-familial juvenile muscular atrophy simulating muscular dystrophy. *AMA Arch Neurol Psychiatry* 75:500, 1956
12. Pearn J: Autosomal dominant spinal muscle atrophy. A clinical and genetic study. *J Neurol Sci* 38:263, 1978
13. Schwentker EP, Gibson DA: The orthopedic aspects of spinal muscular atrophy. *J Bone Joint Surg* 58A:32, 1976
14. Shapiro F, Bresnan MJ: Orthopaedic management of childhood neuromuscular disease. Part I: Spinal muscular atrophy. *J Bone Joint Surg* 64A:785, 1982
15. Welander L: Myopathia distalis tarda hereditaria. *Acta Med Scand* (Suppl) 265:1, 1951
16. Werdnig G: Zwei fruhim famile hereditare fall von progressiver muskelatrophie unter dem bild der dystrophie, aber auf neurotishcer grundlage. *Arch Psychiatr Nervenkr* 22:237, 1891
17. Wohlfart G, Fex J, Eliasson S: Hereditary proximal muscle atrophy: A clinical entity simulating progressive muscular dystrophy. *Acta Psychiatr Scand* 39:395, 1955
18. Zellweger H, Simpson J, McCormick WF, Ionasescu V: Spinal muscular atrophy with autosomal dominant inheritance. *Neurology* 22:957, 1972

Cerebral Palsy

19. Bagg MR, Farber J, Miller F: Long-term follow-up of hip subluxation in cerebral palsy patients. *J Pediatr Orthop* 13:32, 1993
20. Baker LD, Dodelin R, Bassett FH III: Pathological changes in the hip in cerebral palsy: Incidence, pathogenesis and

treatment. A preliminary report. *J Bone Joint Surg* 44A: 133, 1962

21. Banks HH, Green WT: Adductor myotomy and obturator neurectomy for the correction of adduction of the hip in cerebral palsy. *J Bone Joint Surg* 42A:111, 1960

22. Banks HH, Green WT: The correction of equinus deformity in cerebral palsy. *J Bone Joint Surg* 40:1359, 1958

23. Bleck EE: *Orthopaedic Management in Cerebral Palsy.* Philadelphia, MacKeith Press, 1987

24. Bleck EE: I. Cerebral palsy hip deformities: Is there a consensus? II. Botulinum toxin A: A clinical experiment. *J Pediatr Orthop* 14:281, 1994

25. Boscarino LF, Oonpuu S, Davis RB III, Gage JR, DeLuca PA: Effects of selective dorsal rhizotomy in gait in children with cerebral palsy. *J Pediatr Orthop* 13:174, 1993

26. Brunner R, Baumann JU: Clinical benefit of reconstruction of dislocated or subluxated hip joints in patients with spastic cerebral palsy. *J Pediatr Orthop* 14:290, 1994

27. Cassidy C, Craig CL, Perry A, Karlin LI, Goldberg MJ: A reassessment of spinal stabilization in severe cerebral palsy. *J Pediatr Orthop* 14:731, 1994

28. Chong KC, Vojnic CD, Quanbury AO, Letts RM: The assessment of the internal rotation gait in cerebral palsy. *Clin Orthop* 132:145, 1978

29. Cooke PH, Cole WG, Carey RPL: Dislocation of the hip in cerebral palsy. Natural history and predictability. *J Bone Joint Surg* 71B:441, 1989

30. Crawford AH, Kucharzyk D, Roy DR, Bilbo J: Subtalar stabilization of the planovalgus foot by staple arthroereisis in young children who have neuromuscular problems. *J Bone Joint Surg* 72A:840, 1990

31. Damron TA, Breed AL, Cook T: Diminished knee flexion after hamstring surgery in cerebral palsy patients: Prevalence and severity. *J Pediatr Orthop* 13:188, 1993

32. Davids JR, Holland WC, Sutherland DH: Significance of the confusion test in cerebral palsy. *J Pediatr Orthop* 13:717, 1993

33. DeLuca PA: Gait analysis in the treatment of the ambulatory child with cerebral palsy. *Clin Orthop* 264:65, 1991

34. Dhawlikar SH, Root L, Mann RL: Distal lengthening of the hamstrings in patients who have cerebral palsy. *J Bone Joint Surg* 74A:1385, 1992

35. Elmer EB, Wenger DR, Mubarak SJ, Sutherland DH: Proximal hamstring lengthening in the sitting cerebral palsy patient. *J Pediatr Orthop* 12:329, 1992

36. Filler BC, Stark IT: Capsulodesis of the MDH of the thumb in cerebral palsy. *J Bone Joint Surg* 58A:667, 1976

37. Gage JR: *Gait Analysis in Cerebral Palsy.* London, MacKeith Press, 1991, pp 143–149

38. Gage JR: Surgical treatment of knee dysfunction in cerebral palsy. *Clin Orthop* 253:45, 1990

39. Gage JR: The clinical use of kinetics for evaluation of pathological gait in cerebral palsy. *J Bone Joint Surg* 76A:622, 1994

40. Gage JR: The role of gait analysis in the treatment of cerebral palsy. *J Pediatr Orthop* 14:701, 1994

41. Gage JR, Fabian D, Hicks R, Tashman S: Pre- and postoperative gait analysis in patients with spastic diplegia: A preliminary report. *J Pediatr Orthop* 4:715, 1984

42. Gage JR, Perry J, Hicks RR, Koop S, Werntz JR: Rectus femoris transfer to improve knee function of children with cerebral palsy. *Dev Med Child Neurol* 29:159, 1987

43. Goldner JL: Reconstructive surgery in the hand in cerebral palsy. *J Bone Joint Surg* 37A:1141, 1955

44. Goldner JL: Upper extremity surgical procedures for patient with cerebral palsy. *AAOS Instr Course Lect* 28:37, 1979

45. Green NE, Griffin PP, Shiavi R: Split posterior tibial tendon transfer in spastic cerebral palsy. *J Bone Joint Surg* 65A: 748, 1983

46. Green WB, Dietz FR, Goldberg MJ, Gross RH, Miller F, Sussman MD: Rapid progression of hip subluxation in cerebral palsy after selective posterior rhizotomy. *J Pediatr Orthop* 11:494, 1991

47. Green WT: Tendon transplantation of the flexor carpi ulnaris for pronator flexor deformity of the wrist. *Surg Gynecol Obstet* 75:337, 1942

48. Green WT, Banks H: Flexor carpi ulnaris transplant. *J Bone Joint Surg* 44A:1343, 1962

49. Hoffer MM: Management of the hip in cerebral palsy. Current concepts review. *J Bone Joint Surg* 68:629, 1986

50. Hoffer MM, Abraham E, Nickel V: Salvage surgery at the hip to improve sitting posture of mentally retarded, severely disabled children with cerebral palsy. *J Bone Joint Surg* 67A:1229, 1985

51. Hoffer MM, Perry J, Melkonian G: Electromyographic analysis of grasp and release in cerebral palsied children. *J Hand Surg* 4:424, 1979

52. Hoffer MM, Stein GA, Koffman M, Prietto M: Femoral varus-derotation osteotomy in spastic cerebral palsy. *J Bone Joint Surg* 67A:1229, 1985

53. Hoffinger SA, Rab GT, Abou-Ghaida H: Hamstrings in cerebral palsy crouch gait. *J Pediatr Orthop* 13:722, 1993

54. House JH, Gwathney FW, Fidler MO: A dynamic approach to the thumb-in-palm deformity in cerebral palsy. *J Bone Joint Surg* 63A:216, 1981

55. Hsu LCS, Li HSY: Distal hamstring elongation in the management of spastic cerebral palsy. *J Pediatr Orthop* 10:378, 1990

56. Ireland ML, Hoffer M: Triple arthrodesis for children with spastic cerebral palsy. *Dev Med Child Neurol* 27:623, 1985

57. Kalen V, Bleck EE: Prevention of spastic paralytic dislocation of the hip. *Dev Med Child Neurol* 27:17, 1985

58. Koman LA, Mooney JF III, Goodman A: Management of valgus hindfoot deformity in pediatric cerebral palsy patients by medial displacement osteotomy. *J Pediatr Orthop* 13:180, 1993

59. Koman LA, Mooney JF III, Smith BP, Goodman A, Mulvaney T: Management of cerebral palsy with botulinum A toxin: Report of a preliminary randomized, double-blind trial. *J Pediatr Orthop* 14:299, 1994

60. Krum SD, Miller F: Heterotopic ossification after hip and spine surgery in children with cerebral palsy. *J Pediatr Orthop* 13:739, 1993

61. Laplaza FJ, Root L: Femoral anteversion and neck-shaft angles in hip instability in cerebral palsy. *J Pediatr Orthop* 14:719, 1994

62. Marty GR, Dias LS, Gaebler-Spira D: Selective posterior rhizotomy and soft-tissue procedures for the treatment of cerebral diplegia. *J Bone Joint Surg* 77A:713, 1995

63. Matev IB: Surgical treatment of "thumb in palm." *J Bone Joint Surg* 45B:703, 1963

64. Matev IB: Surgical treatment of flexion adduction contracture of the thumbs in cerebral palsy. *Acta Orthop Scand* 41:439, 1970

65. McCue FC, Honner R, Chapman WC: Transfer of the brachioradialis for hand deformed by cerebral palsy. *J Bone Joint Surg* 52:1171, 1970

66. Minear WL: A classification of cerebral palsy. *Pediatrics* 18:841, 1956

67. Mubarak SJ, Valencia FG, Wenger DR: One-stage correction of the spastic dislocated hip. Use of pericapsular acetabuloplasty to improve coverage. *J Bone Joint Surg* 74A:1347, 1992

68. Nene AV, Evans GA, Patrick JH: Simultaneous multiple operations for spastic diplegia. *J Bone Joint Surg* 75B:488, 1993

69. Ounpuu S, Muik E, Davis RB, Gage JR, DeLuca PA: Rectus femoris surgery in children with cerebral palsy. Part II: A comparison between the effect of transfer and release of the distal rectus femoris in knee motion. *J Pediatr Orthop* 13:331, 1993

70. Ounpuu S, Muik E, DeLuca PA, Gage JR: Rectus femoris surgery in children with cerebral palsy. Part I: The effect of rectus femoris transfer location on knee motion. *J Pediatr Orthop* 13:325, 1993

71. Osterkamp J, Caillouette JT, Hoffer MM: Chiari osteotomy in cerebral palsy. *J Pediatr Orthop* 8:274, 1988

72. Payne LZ, DeLuca PA: Heterotopic ossification after rhizotomy and femoral osteotomy. *J Pediatr Orthop* 13:733, 1993

73. Peacock WJ, Arens LJ: Selective posterior rhizotomy for the relief of spasticity in cerebral palsy. *South Afr Med J* 62:119, 1982

74. Perry J: Distal rectus femoris transfer. *Dev Med Child Neurol* 29:153, 1987

75. Perry J: *"Phases of Gait" Gait Analysis: Normal and Pathological Function.* Thorofare, NJ, Slack, 1992, pp 9–16

76. Perry J, Hoffer MM: Preoperative and postoperative dynamic electromyography as an aid in planning tendon transfers in children with cerebral palsy. *J Bone Joint Surg* 59A:531, 1977

77. Perry J, Hoffer MM, Giovan P, Antonelli D, Greenberg R: Gait analysis of the triceps surae in cerebral palsy. A preoperative and postoperative clinical and electromyographic study. *J Bone Joint Surg* 56:511, 1974

78. Phelps WP: Prevention of acquired dislocation of the hip in cerebral palsy. *J Bone Joint Surg* 41A:440, 1959

79. Pope DF, Bueff HU, DeLuca PA: Pelvic osteotomies for subluxation of the hip in cerebral palsy. *J Pediatr Orthop* 14:724, 1994

80. Rab GT: Determination of muscle length in patients with cerebral palsy. *Dev Med Child Neurol* 55(Suppl):34, 1987

81. Rang M, Douglas G, Bennet GC, Koreska J: Seating for children with cerebral palsy. *J Pediatr Orthop* 1:279, 1981

82. Rattey TE, Leahey L, Hyndman J, Brown DCS, Gross M: Recurrence after Achilles tendon lengthening in cerebral palsy. *J Pediatr Orthop* 13:184, 1993

83. Reimers J: A scoring system for the evaluation of ambulation in cerebral palsied patients. *Dev Med Child Neurol* 14:332, 1972

84. Reimers J: Contracture of the hamstrings in spastic cerebral palsy. *J Bone Joint Surg* 56B:102, 1974

85. Reimers J: Functional changes in the antagonists after lengthening the agonists in cerebral palsy. I. Triceps surae lengthening. *Clin Orthop* 253:30, 1990

86. Reimers J: Functional changes in the antagonists after lengthening the agonists in cerebral palsy. II. Quadriceps strength before and after distal hamstring lengthening. *Clin Orthop* 253:35, 1990

87. Reimers J: The stability of the hip in children: A radiological study of the results of muscle surgery in cerebral palsy. *Acta Orthop Scand* (Suppl) 184:1, 1972

88. Reimers J: Static and dynamic problems in spastic cerebral palsy. *J Bone Joint Surg* 55B:822, 1973

89. Roberts WM, Adams JP: The patellar-advancement operation in cerebral palsy. *J Bone Joint Surg* 35A:958, 1953

90. Root L, Goss JR, Mendes J: The treatment of the painful hip in cerebral palsy by total hip replacement or hip arthrodesis. *J Bone Joint Surg* 68:590, 1986

91. Root L, LaPlaza FJ, Brourman SN, Angel DH: The severely unstable hip in cerebral palsy. *J Bone Joint Surg* 77A:703, 1995

92. Rose SA, DeLuca PA, Davis RB III, Ounpuu S, Gage JR: Kinematic and kinetic evaluation of the ankle after lengthening of the gastrocnemius fascia in children with cerebral palsy. *J Pediatr Orthop* 13:727, 1993

93. Rosenthal RK, Deutsch SD, Miller W, Schumann W, Hall JE: A fixed ankle, below-the-knee orthosis for the management of genu recurvatum in spastic cerebral palsy. *J Bone Joint Surg* 57A:545, 1975

94. Rosenthal RK, Levine DB: Fragmentation of the distal pole of the patella in spastic cerebral palsy. *J Bone Joint Surg* 59A:934, 1977

95. Samilson RL: *Orthopaedic Aspects of Cerebral Palsy.* Clinics in Developmental Medicine No. 52/53. London, William Heinemann Medical Books, 1975

96. Samilson RL, Tsou P, Aamoth G, Green WT: Dislocation and subluxation of the hip in cerebral palsy. Pathogenesis, natural history, and management. *J Bone Joint Surg* 54A:863, 1967

97. Segal L, Thomas SE, Mazur JM, Mauterer M: Calcaneal gait in spastic diplegia after heelcord lengthening: A study with gait analysis. *J Pediatr Orthop* 9:697, 1989

98. Silfverskiöld N: Reduction of the uncrossed two joint muscles of the leg to one joint muscles in spastic conditions. *Acta Chir Scand* 56:315, 1923

99. Simon SR, Deutsch SD, Nuzzo RM, Mansour MJ, Jackson JL, Koskinen M, Rosenthal RK: Genu recurvatum in spastic cerebral palsy. *J Bone Joint Surg* 60A:882, 1978

100. Smith JT, Stevens PM: Combined adductor transfer, iliopsoas release, and proximal hamstring release in cerebral palsy. *J Pediatr Orthop* 9:1, 1989

101. Staheli LT, Chew DE: Slotted acetabular augmentation in childhood and adolescence. *J Pediatr Orthop* 12:569, 1992

102. Steel HH: Gluteus medius and minimus insertion advancement for correction of internal rotation gait in spastic cerebral palsy. *J Bone Joint Surg* 62A:919, 1980

103. Sussman MD: Casting as an adjunct to neurodevelopmental therapy for cerebral palsy. *Dev Med Child Neurol* 25:804, 1983

104. Sutherland DH: *Gait Disorders in Childhood and Adolescents.* Baltimore, Williams & Wilkins, 1984
105. Sutherland DH, Cooper L: The pathomechanics of progressive crouch gait in spastic diplegia. *Orthop Clin North Am* 9:143, 1978
106. Sutherland DH, Davids JR: Common gait abnormalities of the knee in cerebral palsy. *Clin Orthop* 288:139, 1993
107. Sutherland DH, Olshen R, Cooper L, Wood SL-Y: The development of mature gait. *J Bone Joint Surg* 62A:336, 1980
108. Sutherland DH, Santi M, Abel MD: Treatment of stiff knee gait in cerebral palsy: A comparison by gait analysis of the distal rectus femoris transfer versus proximal rectus release. *J Pediatr Orthop* 10:433, 1990
109. Sutherland DH, Schottstaedt ER, Larsen LJ, Ashley RK, Callander JM, James PM: Clinical and electromyographic study of seven spastic children with internal rotation gait. *J Bone Joint Surg* 51A:1070, 1969
110. Swanson AB: Treatment of swan-neck deformity in cerebral palsied hand. *Clin Orthop* 48:167, 1966
111. Tachdjian MO, Minear WL: Sensory disturbances in the hands of children with cerebral palsy. *J Bone Joint Surg* 40A:85, 1958
112. Tenuta J, Shelton YA, Miller F: Long-term follow-up of triple arthrodesis in patients with cerebral palsy. *J Pediatr Orthop* 13:713, 1993
113. Thometz J, Simons S, Rosenthal R: The effect on gait of lengthening of the medial hamstrings in cerebral palsy. *J Bone Joint Surg* 71A:345, 1989
114. Tylkowski CM, Howell-Garvey V, Miller G: The influence of hamstring and hip flexor musculature on crouch gait in spastic cerebral palsy as determined by gait analysis. *Dev Med Child Neurol* 30(Suppl 57):14, 1988
115. Tylkowski CM, Rosenthal RK, Simon SR: Proximal femoral osteotomy in cerebral palsy. *Clin Orthop* 151:183, 1980
116. Waters RL, Garland DE, Perry J, Habig T, Slabaugh P: Stiff-legged gait in hemiplegia: Surgical correction. *J Bone Joint Surg* 61A:927, 1976
117. Watts HG: Gait laboratory analysis for preoperative decision making in spastic cerebral palsy: Is it all it's cracked up to be? *J Pediatr Orthop* 14:703, 1994
118. White WF: Flexor slide in spastic hand. *J Bone Joint Surg* 54B:453, 1972
119. Winter DA: *The Biomechanics and Motor Control of Human Gait.* Waterloo, Ontario, Canada: University of Waterloo Press, 1987, pp 29–43
120. Winters T, Hicks R, Gage JR: Gait patterns in spastic hemiplegia in children and young adults. *J Bone Joint Surg* 69A:437, 1987
121. Woods G: *Cerebral Palsy in Childhood.* Bristol, John Wright & Sons, 1957
122. Zuckerman JD, Staheli LT, McLaughlin JF: Acetabular augmentation for progressive hip subluxation in cerebral palsy. *J Pediatr Orthop* 4:436, 1984

Progressive Muscular Dystrophy

123. Arikawa E, Hoffman EP, Kaido M, Nonaka I, Sugita H, Arahata MD: The frequency of patients with dystrophin abnormalities in a limb-girdle patient population. *Neurology* 41:1491, 1991
124. Bach JR, McKeon J: Orthopedic surgery and rehabilitation for the prolongation of brace-free ambulation of patients with Duchenne muscular dystrophy. *Am J Phys Med Rehab* 70:323, 1991
125. Banker BQ: Congenital muscular dystrophy, in *Myology, Basic and Clinical,* Vol 2. New York, McGraw-Hill, 1986, pp 1367–1377
126. Becker PE, Kiener F: Eine neve x-chromasomale Muskeldystrophie. *Arch Psychiatr Nerven* 193:427, 1955
127. Beggs AH, Hoffman EP, Snyder JR, Arahata K, Specht L, Shapiro F, Angelini C, Sugita H, Kunkel LM: Exploring the molecular basis for variability among patients with Becker muscular dystrophy: Dystrophy gene and protein studies. *Am J Hum Genet* 49:54, 1991
128. Bradley WG, Jones MZ, Mussini JM, Fawcett PRW: Becker-type muscular dystrophy. *Muscle Nerve* 1:111, 1978
129. Bunch WH, Siegel IM: Scapulothoracic arthrodesis in facioscapulohumeral muscular dystrophy. Review of seventeen procedures with three to twenty-one-year follow-up. *J Bone Joint Surg* 75A:372, 1993
130. Cambridge W, Drennan JC: Scoliosis associated with Duchenne muscular dystrophy. *J Pediatr Orthop* 7:436, 1987
131. Castillo J, Pumar JM, Rodriguez JR, Prieto JM, Arrojo L, Martinez F, Noya M: Magnetic resonance imaging of muscles in myotonic dystrophy. *Europ J Radiol* 17:141, 1993
132. Consalez GG, Thomas NST, Stayton CL, Knight SJL, Johnson M, Hopkins LC, Harper PS, Elsas LJ, Warren ST: Assignment of Emery-Dreifuss muscular dystrophy to the distal region of Xq28: The results of a collaborative study. *Am J Human Genet* 48:468, 1991
133. Dubowitz V: *Muscle Biopsy,* 2nd ed. London, Bailliere Tindall, 1985
134. Emery AEH: *Duchenne Muscular Dystrophy,* 2nd ed. New York, Oxford University Press, 1988
135. Fenton-May J, Bradley DM, Sibert JR, Smith R, Parsons EP, Harper PS, Clarke A: Screening for Duchenne muscular dystrophy. *Arch Dis Child* 70:551, 1994
136. Galasko CS, Delaney C, Morris P: Spinal stabilisation in Duchenne muscular dystrophy. *J Bone Joint Surg* 74B:210, 1992
137. Gerschwind N, Simpson JA: Procaine amide in the treatment of myotonia. *Brain* 78:81, 1955
138. Goebel HH: Congenital myopathies, in Adachi M, Sher JH (eds): *Neuromuscular Disease.* New York, Igaku-Schoin, 1990, pp 197–244
139. Gowers WR: A lecture on myopathy of a distal form. *Br Med J* 2:89, 1902
140. Gowers WR: *Pseudohypertrophic Muscular Paralysis.* London, Churchill Livingstone, 1879
141. Granata C, Giannini S, Ballestrazzi A, Merlini L: Early surgery in Duchenne muscular dystrophy. Experience at Istituto Ortopedico Rizzoli, Bologna, Italy. *Neuromusc Dis* 4:87, 1994
142. Greene WB: Transfer versus lengthening of the posterior tibial tendon in Duchenne's muscular dystrophy. *Foot Ankle* 13:526, 1992

143. Heckmatt JZ, Dubowitz V, Hyde SA, Florence J, Gabain AC, Thompson N: Prolongation of walking in Duchenne muscular dystrophy with lightweight orthoses: Review of 57 cases. *Devel Med Child Neurol* 27:149, 1985

144. Hoffman EP, Kunkel LM: Dystrophin abnormalities in Duchenne/Becker muscular dystrophy. *Neuron* 2:1019, 1989

145. Hoffman EP, Kunkel LM, Angelini C, Clarke A, Johnson M, Harris JB: Improved diagnosis of Becker muscular dystrophy by dystrophin testing. *Neurology* 39:1011, 1989

146. Hsu JD: The natural history of spine curvature progression in the nonambulatory Duchenne muscular dystrophy patient. *Spine* 8:771, 1983

147. Jakab E, Gledhill RB: Simplified technique for scapulocostal fusion in facioscapulohumeral dystrophy. *J Pediatr Orthop* 13:749, 1993

148. Jennekens FG, ten Kate LP, deVisser M, Wintzen AR: Diagnostic criteria for Duchenne and Becker muscular dystrophy and myotonic dystrophy. *Neuromusc Dis* 1:389, 1991

149. Johnson J: Thomsen and myotonia congenita. *Med Hist* 12:190, 1968

150. Kazakov VM, Bogorodinsky DK, Znoyko ZV, Skorometz AA: The facio-scapulo-limb (or the facioscapulohumeral) type of muscular dystrophy. Clinical and genetic study. *Eur Neurol* 11:236, 1974

151. Ketenjian AY: Scapulocostal stabilization for scapula winging in facioscapulohumeral muscular dystrophy. *J Bone Joint Surg* 60A:476, 1978

152. Korf BR, Bresnan MJ, Shapiro F, Sotrel A, Abroms IF: Facioscapulohumeral dystrophy presenting in infancy with facial diplegia and sensorineural deafness. *Ann Neurol* 17:513, 1985

153. Landouzy L, Déjérine J: De la myopathie atrophique progressive (myopathie héréditaire, débutant dans l'enfance par la face, sans alteration de système nerveaux). *CR Acad Sci* 98:53, 1984

154. Letournel E, Fardeau M, Lytle JO, Serrault M, Gosselin RA: Scapulothoracic arthrodesis for patients who have facioscapulohumeral muscular dystrophy. *J Bone Joint Surg* 72A:78, 1990

155. Leyden E: *Klinik der Ruckenmarks-Krankheiten.* Berlin, Hirschwald 2:531, 1876

156. Meryon E: On granular or fatty degeneration of the voluntary muscles. *Trans Med Chir Sco Edinb* 35:72, 1852

157. Mubarak SJ, Morin WD, Leach J: Spinal fusion in Duchenne muscular dystrophy—fixation and fusion to the sacropelvis? *J Pediatr Orthop* 13:752, 1993

158. Munsat TL, Baloh R, Pearson CM, Fowler W Jr: Serum enzyme alterations in neuromuscular disorders. *JAMA* 226:1536, 1973

159. Nicholson LV: Advances in Duchenne and myotonic dystrophy. *Rev Curr Opinion Rheum* 5:706, 1993

160. Oda T, Shimizu N, Yonenobu K, Ono K, Nabeshima T, Kyoh S: Longitudinal study of spinal deformity in Duchenne muscular dystrophy. *J Pediatr Orthop* 13:478, 1993

161. Padberg G: *Facioscapulohumeral Disease.* Thesis, University of Leiden, 1982

162. Partridge TA: Invited review. Myoblast transfer: A possible therapy for inherited myopathies? *Muscle Nerve* 14:197, 1991

163. Partridge TA, Morgan JE, Coulton GR, Hoffman EP, Kunkel LM: Conversion of mdx myofibres from dystrophin-negative to-positive by injection of normal myoblasts. *Nature* 337:176, 1989

164. Personius KE, Pandya S, King WM, Tawil R, McDermott MP: Facioscapulohumeral dystrophy natural history study: Standardization of testing procedures and reliability of measurements. The FSH DY Group. *Phys Ther* 74:253, 1994

165. Ramsey PL, Hensinger RN: Congenital dislocation of the hip associated with central core disease. *J Bone Joint Surg* 57A:648, 1975

166. Rodillo EB, Fernandez-Bermejo E, Heckmatt JZ, Dubowitz V: Prevention of rapidly progressive scoliosis in Duchenne muscular dystrophy by prolongation of walking with orthoses. *J Child Neurol* 3:269, 1988

167. Schonk D, Coerwinkel-Driessen M, van Dalen I, Oerlemans F, Smeets B, Schepens J, Hulsebos T, Cockburn D, Boyd Y, Davis M, Rettig W, Shaw D, Roses A, Ropers H, Wieringa B: Definition of subchromosomal intervals around the myotonic dystrophy gene region at 19q. *Genomics* 4:384, 1989

168. Schwentker EP, Gibson DA: The orthopedic aspects of spinal muscular atrophy. *J Bone Joint Surg* 58A:32, 1976

169. Shapiro F, Bresnan MJ: Current concepts review. Orthopaedic management of childhood neuromuscular disease. Part III: Diseases of muscle. *J Bone Joint Surg* 64A:1102, 1982

170. Shapiro F, Specht L: Orthopedic deformities in Emery-Dreifuss muscular dystrophy. *J Pediatr Orthop* 11:336, 1991

171. Shapiro F, Specht L: The diagnosis and orthopaedic treatment of inherited muscular diseases of childhood. *J Bone Joint Surg* 75A:439, 1993

172. Shapiro F, Specht L, Korf BR: Locomotor problems in infantile facioscapulohumeral muscular dystrophy. Retrospective study of 9 patients. *Acta Orthop Scand* 62:367, 1991

173. Siegel IM: Diagnosis and management in orthopedic treatment of muscle dystrophy. *AAOS Instr Course Lect* 30:3, 1981

174. Smith RA, Newcombe RG, Sibert JR, Harper PS: Assessment of locomotor function in young boys with Duchenne muscular dystrophy. *Muscle Nerve* 14:462, 1991

175. Smith SE, Green NE, Cole RJ, Robison JD, Fenichel GM: Prolongation of ambulation in children with Duchenne muscular dystrophy by subcutaneous lower limb tenotomy. *J Pediatr Orthop* 13:336, 1993

176. Specht LA: Molecular basis and clinical applications of neuromuscular disease in children. *Curr Opin Pediatr* 3:966, 1991

177. Specht LA, Kunkel LM: Duchenne and Becker muscular dystrophies, in Rosenberg RN, Prusiner SB, DiMauro S, Barchi RL, Kunkel LM (eds): *The Molecular and Genetic Basis of Neurological Disease.* Boston, Butterworth-Heinemann, 1993, pp 613–631

178. Speer MC, Pericak-Vance MA, Yamaoka L, Hung W-Y, Ashley A, Stajich JM, Roses AD: Presymptomatic and prenatal diagnosis in myotonic dystrophy by genetic linkage studies. *Neurology* 40:671, 1990

179. Spencer GE Jr, Vignos PJ Jr: Bracing for ambulation in childhood progressive muscular dystrophy. *J Bone Joint Surg* 44A:234, 1962

180. Sussman MD: Advantage of early spinal stabilization and fusion in patients with Duchenne muscular dystrophy. *J Pediatr Orthop* 4:532, 1984

181. Suput D, Zupan A, Sepe A, Demsar F: Discrimination between neuropathy and myopathy by use of magnetic resonance imaging. *Acta Neurol Scand* 87:118, 1993

182. Thomsen J: Tonische Kranfe in willkurlich beweglichen Muskein in Folge von erebier psychischer Disposition. *Arch Psychiat Nervenkr* 6:706, 1876

183. Vignos PJ Jr, Wagner MB, Kaplan JS, Spencer GE Jr: Predicting the success of reambulation in patients with Duchenne muscular dystrophy. *J Bone Joint Surg* 65A:719, 1983

184. Wagner MB, Vignos PJ Jr, Carlozzi C, Hull AL: Assessment of hand function in Duchenne muscular dystrophy. *Arch Phys Med Rehabil* 74:801, 1993

185. Walton JN, Gardner-Medwig D: Progressive muscular dystrophy and the myotonic disorders, in Walton JN (ed): *Disorders of Voluntary Muscle,* 4th ed. Edinburgh, Churchill Livingstone, 1980, pp 205–237

186. Walton JN, Natrass FJ: On the classification, natural history and treatment of the myopathies. *Brain* 77:169, 1954

187. Weimann RL, Gibson DA, Moseley CF, Jones DC: Surgical stabilization of the spine in Duchenne muscular dystrophy. *Spine* 8:776, 1983

188. Welander L: Myopathia distalis tarda hereditaria. *Acta Med Scand* (Suppl) 265:1, 1951

189. Wijmenga C, Frants RR, Brouwer OE, Moerer P, Weber JL, Padberg GW: Location of facioscapulohumeral muscular dystrophy gene on chromosome 4. *Lancet* 336:651, 1990

190. Williams EA, Read L, Ellis A, Morris P, Galasko CSB: The management of equinus deformity in Duchenne muscular dystrophy. *J Bone Joint Surg* 66B:546, 1984

191. Winters JL, McLaughlin LA: Myotonia congenita. *J Bone Joint Surg* 52A:1345, 1970

192. Zellweger H, Afifi A, McCormick WF, Mergner W: Severe congenital muscular dystrophy. *Am J Dis Child* 114:591, 1967

193. Zellweger H, Antonik A: Newborn screening for Duchenne muscular dystrophy. *Pediatrics* 5:30, 1975

Hereditary Motor and Sensory Neuropathies

194. Aramideh M, Hoogendijk JE, Aalfs CM, Meyjes FE, DeVisser M, Ongerboer de Visser BW: Somatosensory evoked potentials, sensory nerve potentials and sensory nerve conduction in hereditary motor and sensory neuropathy type I. *J Neurol* 239:277, 1992

195. Charcot JM, Marie P: Progressive muscular atrophy. Often familial, starting in the feet and legs and later reaching the hands. *Arch Neurol* 17:553, 1967

196. Charcot JM, Marie P: Sur une forme particulaire d'atrophie musculaire progressive, souvent familiale, débutant par les pieds et les jambes et atteignant plus tard les mains. *Rev Med (Paris)* 6:97, 1886

197. Christie BG: Electrodiagnostic features of Charcot-Marie-Tooth disease. *Proc R Soc Med* 54:321, 1961

198. Daher YH, Lonstein JE, Winter RB, Bradford DS: Spinal deformities in patients with Charcot-Marie-Tooth disease. A review of 12 patients. *Clin Orthop* 202:219, 1986

199. Déjérine J, Sottas J: Sur la nevrite interstitielle, hypertrophique et progressive de l'enfance. *CR Soc Biol* 5:63, 1893

200. Drummond RP: A twenty-one year review of a case of congenital indifference to pain. *J Bone Joint Surg* 57B:241, 1975

201. Dyck PJ: Histologic measurements and fine structure of biopsied sural nerve: Normal, and in peroneal muscular atrophy, hypertrophic neuropathy, and congenital sensory neuropathy. *Mayo Clin Proc* 41:742, 1966

202. Dyck PJ, Ott J, Moore SB, Swanson CJ, Lambert EH: Linkage evidence for genetic heterogeneity among kinships with hereditary motor and sensory neuropathy, type I. *Mayo Clin Proc* 58:430, 1983

203. Dyck PJ, Lambert EH: Lower motor and primary sensory neural disease with peroneal muscular atrophy. I. Neurologic, genetic and electrophysiologic findings in hereditary polyneuropathies. *Arch Neurol* 18:603, 1968

204. Dyck PJ, Lambert EH: Lower motor and primary sensory neural disease with peroneal muscular atrophy. II. Neurologic, genetic and electrophysiologic findings in various neuronal degenerations. *Arch Neurol* 18:619, 1968

205. Dyck PJ, Lambert EH, Mulder DW: Charcot-Marie-Tooth disease. Nerve conduction and clinical studies of a large kinship. *Neurology* 13:1, 1963

206. Gibberd FB, Billimoria JD, Goldman JM, Clemens ME, Evans R, Whitelaw MN, Retsas S, Sherratt RM: Heredopathia atactica polyneuritiformis: Refsum's disease. *Acta Neurol Scand* 72:1, 1985

207. Goldman JM, Clemens ME, Gibberd FB, Billimoria JD: Screening of patients with retinitis pigmentosa for hereditary actactica polyneuritiformis (Refsum's disease). *Br Med J* 290:1109, 1985.

208. Heimans JJ, Lindhout D: Charcot-Marie-Tooth disease. *J Med Genet* 20:77, 1983

209. Hensinger RN, MacEwen GD: Spinal deformity associated with heritable neurologic conditions: Spinal muscular atrophy, Friedreich's ataxia, familial dysautonomia and Charcot-Marie-Tooth disease. *J Bone Joint Surg* 58A:13, 1976

210. Homberg BH: Charcot-Marie-Tooth disease in northern Sweden: An epidemiological and clinical study. *Acta Neurol Scand* 87:416, 1993

211. Jacobs JE, Carr CR: Progressive muscular atrophy of the peroneal type (Charcot-Marie-Tooth disease). Orthopedic management and end-result study. *J Bone Joint Surg* 32A:27, 1950

212. Jones SJ, Carroll WM, Halliday AM: Peripheral and central sensory nerve conduction in Charcot-Marie-Tooth disease and comparison with Friedreich's ataxia. *J Neurol Sci* 61:135, 1983

213. Kaku DA, Parry GJ, Malamut R, Lupski JR, Garcia CA: Nerve conduction studies in Charcot-Marie-Tooth polyneuropathy associated with a segmental duplication of chromosome 17. *Neurology* 43:1806, 1993

214. Karlholm S, Nilsonne U: Operative treatment of the foot deformity in Charcot-Marie-Tooth disease. *Acta Orthop Scand* 39:101, 1968

215. Krishna Rao CVG, Fits CR, Harwood-Nash DC: Déjérine-Sottas syndrome in children (hypertrophic interstitial polyneuritis). *AJR* 122:70, 1974

216. Levitt RL, Canale ST, Cooke AJ, Gartland JJ: The role of foot surgery in progressive neuromuscular disorders in children. *J Bone Joint Surg* 55A:1396, 1973

217. Lidge RT, Chandler FA: Charcot-Marie-Tooth disease. *J Pediatr* 43:152, 1953

218. MacEwen GD, Floyd GC: Congenital insensitivity to pain and its orthopaedic implications. *Clin Orthop* 68:100, 1970

219. Mann DC, Hsu JD: Triple arthrodesis in the treatment of fixed cavovarus deformity in adolescent patients with Charcot-Marie-Tooth disease. *Foot Ankle* 13:1, 1992

220. Miller MJ, Williams LL, Slack SL, Nappi JF: The hand in Charcot-Marie-Tooth disease. *J Hand Surg* 16B:191, 1991

221. Nielsen VK, Pilgaard S: On the pathogenesis of Charcot-Marie-Tooth disease. A study of the sensory and motor conduction velocity in the median nerve. *Acta Orthop Scand* 43:4, 1972

222. Refsum S: Heredopathia atactica polyneuritiformis: A familial syndrome not hitherto described. *Acta Psychiatr Neurol* (Suppl) 38, 1946

223. Roussy G, Levy G: A propos de la dystasie aréflexique héréditaire. *Rev Neurol* (*Paris*) 62:763, 1934

224. Roussy G, Levy G: Sept cas d'une maladie familiale particulaire: Troubles de la marche, pieds, bots, et aréflexie tendineuse généralisée avec accessoirement légère maladresse des mains. *Rev Neurol* (*Paris*) 45:427, 1926

225. Sabir M, Lyttle D: Pathogenesis of pes cavus in Charcot-Marie-Tooth disease. *Clin Orthop* 175:173, 1983

226. Saunders JT: Etiology and treatment of clawfoot. *Arch Surg* 30:179, 1935

227. Shapiro F, Specht L: The diagnosis and orthopaedic treatment of inherited muscular diseases of childhood. *J Bone Joint Surg* 75A:439, 1993

228. Shapiro F, Specht L: The diagnosis and orthopaedic treatment of childhood spinal muscular atrophy, peripheral neuropathy, Friedreich ataxia, and arthrogryposis. *J Bone Joint Surg* 75A:1699, 1993

229. Skre H: Genetic and clinical aspects of Charcot-Marie-Tooth's disease. *Clin Genet* 6:98, 1974

230. Symonds SCP, Shaw ME: Familial claw-foot with absent tendon-jerks. A "forme fruste" of the Charcot-Marie-Tooth disease. *Brain* 49:387, 1926

231. Tooth HH: *The Peroneal Type of Progressive Muscular Atrophy.* London, HK Lewis, 1886

232. Tynan MC, Klenerman L, Helliwell TR, Edwards RH, Hayward M: Investigation of muscle imbalance in the leg in symptomatic forefoot pes cavus: A multidisciplinary study. *Foot Ankle* 13:489, 1992

233. Walker JL, Nelson KR, Stevens DB, Lubicky JP, Ogden JA, VandenBrink KD: Spinal deformity in Charcot-Marie-Tooth disease. *Spine* 19:1044, 1994

Friedreich's Ataxia

234. Aronsson DD, Stokes IA, Ronchetti PJ, Labelle HB: Comparison of curve shape between children with cerebral palsy, Friedreich's ataxia, and adolescent idiopathic scoliosis. *Dev Med Child Neurol* 36:412, 1994

235. Boyer SH, Chisholm AW, McKusick VA: Cardiac aspects of Friedreich's ataxia. *Circulation* 25:493, 1962

236. Child JS, Perloff JK, Bach PM, Wolfe AD, Perlman S, Kark RA: Cardiac involvement in Friedreich's ataxia: A clinical study of 75 patients. *J Am Coll Cardiol* 7:1370, 1986

237. Cocozza S, Antonelli A, Campanella G, Cavalcanti F, DeMichele G, Di Donato S, Filla A, Monticelli A, Pianese L, Piccinelli A, et al: Evidence of a genetic marker associated with early onset in Friedreich's ataxia. *J Neurol* 240:254, 1993

238. Friedreich N: Uber degenerative Atrophie der spinalen Hinterstrange. *Virchow Arch Pathol Anat* 26:391; 27:1, 1863

239. Hensinger RN, MacEwen GD: Spinal deformity associated with heritable neurological conditions: Spinal muscular atrophy, Friedreich's ataxia, familial dysautonomia and Charcot-Marie-Tooth disease. *J Bone Joint Surg* 58A:13, 1976

240. Hewer RL: Study of fatal cases of Friedreich's ataxia. *Br Med J* 3:649, 1968

241. Labelle H, Tohme S, Suhaime M, Allard P: Natural history of scoliosis in Friedreich's ataxia. *J Bone Joint Surg* 68A:564, 1986

242. Makin M: The surgical treatment of Friedreich's ataxia. *J Bone Joint Surg* 35A:425, 1953

243. Melancon SB, Cloutier R, Potier M, Dallaire L, Vanasse M, Geoffroy G, Barbeau A: Friedreich's ataxia: Malic enzyme activity in cellular fractions of cultured skin fibroblasts. *Can J Neurol Sci* 11:637, 1984

244. Ormerod IE, Harding AE, Miller DH, Johnson G, MacManus D, du Boulay EP, Kendall BE, Moseley IF, McDonald WI: Magnetic resonance imaging in degenerative ataxic disorders. *J Neurol Neurosurg Psychiatry* 57:51, 1994

245. Palau F, Monros E, Prieto F, Vilchez JJ, Lopez-Arlandis JM: Genetic diagnosis of Friedreich's ataxia. *Lancet* 338:1087, 1991

246. Pelosi L, Fels A, Petrillo A, Senatore R, Russo G, Lonegren K, Calace P, Caruso G: Friedreich's ataxia: Clinical involvement and evoked potentials. *Acta Neurol Scand* 70:360, 1984

247. Quebec Cooperative Study on Friedreich's Ataxia. *Can J Neurol Sci* 11:501, 1984

248. Roussy G, Levy G: Sept cas d'une maladie familiale particulaire; Troubles de la marche, pieds, bots et aréflexie tendineuse généralisée, avec accessoirement, légère maladresse des mains. *Rev Neurol* (*Paris*) 45:427, 1926

249. Salisachs P, Findley LJ, Codina M, La Torre P, Martinez-Lage JM: A case of Charcot-Marie-Tooth disease mimicking Friedreich's ataxia: Is there any association between Friedreich's ataxia and Charcot-Marie-Tooth disease? *Can J Neurol Sci* 9:99, 1982

250. Saunders JT: Etiology and treatment of clawfoot. *Arch Surg* 30:179, 1935

251. Spillane JD: Familial pes cavus and absent tendon jerks. Its relationship with Friedreich's disease and peroneal muscular atrophy. *Brain* 63:275, 1940

252. Subramony SH: Degenerative ataxias. *Curr Opinion Neurol* 7:316, 1994

253. Symonds CP, Shaw ME: Familial claw-foot with absent tendon jerks. *Brain* 49:387, 1926

254. Thilenius OG, Grossman BJ: Friedreich's ataxia with heart disease in children. *Pediatrics* 27:246, 1961

Dermatomyositis and Polymyositis

255. Banker BQ: Dermatomyositis of childhood. Ultrastructural alterations of muscle and intramuscular blood vessels. *J Neuropathol Exp Neurol* 34:46, 1975
256. Bohan A, Peter JB: Polymyositis and dermatomyositis. *N Engl J Med* 292:344, 1975
257. Bohan A, Peter JB, Bowman RL, Person CM: A computer-assisted analysis of 153 patients with polymyositis and dermatomyositis. *Medicine* 56:255, 1977
258. Brown M, Swift TR, Spies SM: Radioisotope scanning in inflammatory muscle disease. *Neurology* 26:517, 1976
259. Cassidy JT, Petty RE: *Juvenile Dermatomyositis, Textbook of Pediatric Rheumatology.* Philadelphia, WB Saunders, 1995, pp 323–364
260. Lian JB, Pachman LM, Gundberg CM, Partridge REH, Maryjowski ML: Gamma-carboxyglutamate excretion and calcinosis in juvenile dermatomyositis. *Arthritis Rheum* 25: 1094–1100, 1982
261. Mechler F: Changing electromyographic findings during chronic course of polymyositis. *J Neurol Sci* 23:237, 1974
262. Miller M, Carton FX: Vasculitis in children's dermatomyositis (author's transl.). *Ann Dermatol Venereol* 107: 841, 1980
263. Miller G, Heckmatt JZ, Dubowitz V: Drug treatment of juvenile dermatomyositis. *Arch Dis Child* 58:445, 1983
264. Pachman LM: Juvenile dermatomyositis: A clinical overview. *Pediatr Rev* 12:117, 1990
265. Pachman LM: Juvenile dermatomyositis (JDMS): New clues to diagnosis and pathogenesis. *Clin Exp Rheumatol* 12:S69, 1994
266. Pachman LM: Polymyositis and dermatomyositis in children, in Maddison PJ, Isenberg DA, Woo P, Glass DN (eds): *Oxford Textbook of Rheumatology.* Oxford, Oxford University Press, 1993, pp 821–830
267. Pachman LM, Litt DL: An adapted nailfold capillary (NFC) photographic technique for children with juvenile dermatomyositis (JDMS). *Arthritis Rheum* 35:S257, 1993 (abstract)
268. Sarrat P: Periungual capillaroscopy in children with scleroderma and dermatomyositis. *J Med Vasc* 8:175, 1983
269. Walton JN, Adams RD: *Polymyositis.* Baltimore, Williams & Wilkins, 1958
270. Winkelmann RK: Dermatomyositis in childhood. *Clin Rheum Dis* 8:353, 1982

Myelomeningocele

271. Abraham E, Verinder DGR, Sharrard WJW: The treatment of flexion contracture of the knee in myelomeningocele. *J Bone Joint Surg* 59B:433, 1977
272. Allen BL Jr, Ferguson RL: The operative treatment of myelomeningocele spinal deformity—1979. *Orthop Clin North Am* 10:845, 1979
273. Aprin H, Kilfoye RM: Extension contracture of the knee in patients with myelomeningocele. *Clin Orthop* 144:260, 1979

274. Asher M, Olson J: Factors affecting the ambulatory status of patients with spina bifida cystica. *J Bone Joint Surg* 65A:350, 1983
275. Bazih J, Gross RH: Hip surgery in the lumbar level myelomeningocele patient. *J Pediatr Orthop* 1:405, 1981
276. Birch R: Surgery of the knee in children with spina bifida. *Dev Med Child Neurol* (Suppl 37) 18:111, 1976
277. Boytim MJ, Davidson RS, Charney E, Melchionni JB: Neonatal fractures in myelomeningocele patients. *J Pediatr Orthop* 11:28, 1991
278. Brock DJ, Sutcliffe RG: Alphafetoprotein in the antenatal diagnosis of anencephaly and spina bifida. *Lancet* 2:197, 1972
279. Bunch WM, Cas AS, Bensman AS, Long DM (eds): *Modern Management of Meningomyelocele.* St. Louis, Warren H. Green, 1972
280. Bunch WM, Hakala MW: Iliopsoas transfers in children with myelomeningocele. *J Bone Joint Surg* 66:224, 1984
281. Burkus JK, Moore DW, Raycroft JF: Valgus deformity of the ankle in myelodysplastic patients. Correction by stapling of the medial part of the distal tibial physis. *J Bone Joint Surg* 65A:1157, 1983
282. Canale ST, Hammond NL, Cotler JM, Sneddon HE: Pelvic displacement osteotomy for chronic hip dislocation in myelodysplasia. *J Bone Joint Surg* 57A:177, 1975
283. Carroll NC: The orthotic management of spina bifida children. Present status—future goals. *Prosthet Orthot Int* 1: 39, 1977
284. Carroll NC, Sharrard WJ: Long-term follow-up of posterior iliopsoas transplantation for paralytic dislocation of the hip. *J Bone Joint Surg* 54A:551, 1972
285. Carstens C, Paul K, Niethard FU, Pfeil J: Effect of scoliosis surgery on pulmonary function in patients with myelomeningocele. *J Pediatr Orthop* 11:459, 1991
286. Carter CO, Evans K: Children of adult survivors with spina bifida cystica. *Lancet* 2:924, 1973
287. Charney EB, Melchionni JB, Smith DR: Community ambulation by children with myelomeningocele and high-level paralysis. *J Pediatr Orthop* 11:579, 1991
288. Childs V: Physiotherapy for spina bifida. *Physiotherapy* 63: 281, 1977
289. Clarkson JD: Self-catheterization training of a child with myelomeningocele (toileting independence, incontinent children). *Am J Occup Ther* 36:95, 1982
290. DeSouza LJ, Carroll NC: Paralysis of hip abductor muscles in spina bifida: Results of treatment by the Mustard procedure. *J Bone Joint Surg* 52:1364, 1970
291. Dias LS: Ankle valgus in children with myelomeningocele. *Dev Med Child Neurol* 20:627, 1978
292. Dias LS, Jasty MJ, Collins P: Rotational deformities of the lower limbs in myelomeningocele. *J Bone Joint Surg* 66A: 215, 1984
293. Dirschl DR, Greene WB: Pseudotumor of the distal part of the femur in a patient who had myelomeningocele. A case report. *J Bone Joint Surg* 74:935, 1992
294. Drabu J, Walker G: Stiffness after fractures around the knee in spina bifida. *J Bone Joint Surg* 67B:266, 1985
295. Drennan JC: Management of neonatal myelomeningocele. *AAOS Instr Course Lect* 25:65, 1976

296. Drummond DS, Moreau M, Cruess RL: The results and complications of surgery for the paralytic hip and spine in myelomeningocele. *J Bone Joint Surg* 62B:49, 1980

297. Duncan JW, Lovell WW, Bailey SC, Ransom D: Surgical treatment of kyphosis in myelomeningocele. *J Bone Joint Surg* 58A:155, 1976

298. Feiwell E: Paralytic calcaneus in myelomeningocele, in McLaurin RL (ed): *Myelomeningocele.* New York, Grune & Stratton, 1977, pp 447–460

299. Fraser RK, Hoffman EB, Sparks LT, Buccimazza SS: The unstable hip and mid-lumbar myelomeningocele. *J Bone Joint Surg* 74B:143, 1992

300. Freeman JM: *Practical Management of Meningomyelocele.* Baltimore, University Park Press, 1974

301. Goessens H, Parsch K: Surgical treatment of knee and foot deformities in spina bifida. *Acta Orthop Belg* 37:216, 1971

302. Golding C: Spina bifida and epiphyseal displacement. *J Bone Joint Surg* 42B:387, 1960

303. Golski A, Menelaus MB: The treatment of intoed gait in spina bifida patients by lateral transfer of the medial hamstrings. *Aust NZ J Surg* 46:157, 1976

304. Hall PV, Lindseth RE, Campbell RK, Kalsbeck JE: Myelodysplasia and developmental scoliosis: A manifestation of syringomyelia. *Spine* 1:50, 1976

305. Hannigan KF: Teaching intermittent self-catheterization to young children with myelodysplasia. *Dev Med Child Neurol* 21:365, 1979

306. Heydemann JS, Gillespie R: Management of myelomeningocele kyphosis in the older child by kyphectomy and segmental spinal instrumentation. *Spine* 12:37, 1987

307. Hobbins JC: Diagnosis and management of neural-tube defects today (Editorial). *N Engl J Med* 7:690, 1991

308. Hoffer MM, Feiwell E, Perry J, Bonnett C: Functional ambulation in patients with myelomeningocele. *J Bone Joint Surg* 55A:137, 1973

309. Hollingsworth RP: An x-ray study of valgus ankles in spina bifida children with valgus flat foot deformity. *Proc R Soc Med* 68:481, 1975

310. Hull W, Moe JH, Winter RB: Spinal deformity in myelomeningocele: Natural history, evaluation and treatment. *J Bone Joint Surg* 56A:1767, 1974

311. James CCM: Fractures of the lower limb in spina bifida cystica: A survey of 44 fractures in 122 children. *Dev Med Child Neurol* 22:88, 1970

312. Kumar SJ, Cowell HR, Townsend P: Physeal, metaphyseal, and diaphyseal injuries of the lower extremities in children with myelomeningocele. *J Pediatr Orthop* 4:25, 1984

313. Lee EH, Carroll NC: Hip stability and ambulatory status in myelomeningocele. *J Pediatr Orthop* 5:522, 1985

314. Lindseth RE, Dias LS, Drennan JC: Myelomeningocele. *AAOS Instr Course Lect* 40:271, 1991

315. Lindseth RE, Glancy J: Polypropylene lower-extremity braces for paraplegia due to myelomeningocele. *J Bone Joint Surg* 56A:556, 1974

316. Lindseth RE, Stelzer L Jr: Vertebral excision for kyphosis in children with myelomeningocele. *J Bone Joint Surg* 61A:699, 1979

317. Lintner SA: Kyphotic deformity in patients who have a myelomeningocele. Open treatment and long-term follow-up. *J Bone Joint Surg* 76:1301, 1994

318. Lorber J: Incidence and epidemiology of myelomeningocele. *Clin Orthop* 45:81, 1966

319. Lorber J: Selective treatment of myelomeningocele. To treat or not to treat. *Pediatrics* 53:307, 1974

320. Lorber J, Salfiedl S: Results of selective treatment of spina bifida cystica. *Arch Dis Child* 56:822, 1981

321. Lowe GP, Menelaus MB: The surgical management of kyphosis in older children with myelomeningocele. *J Bone Joint Surg* 60B:40, 1978

322. Mackel JC, Lindseth RE: Scoliosis in myelodysplasia. *J Bone Joint Surg* 57A:1031, 1975

323. Martin J Jr, Kumar SJ, Guille JT, Ger D, Gibbs M: Congenital kyphosis in myelomeningocele: Results following operative and nonoperative treatment. *J Pediatr Orthop* 14:232, 1994

324. Maynard MJ, Weiner LS, Burke SW: Neuropathic foot ulceration in patients with myelodysplasia. *J Pediatr Orthop* 12:786, 1992

325. Mazur JM, Stillwell A, Menelaus M: The significance of spasticity in the upper and lower limbs in myelomeningocele. *J Bone Joint Surg* 68B:211, 1986

326. McKibbin B: Conservative management of paralytic dislocations of the hip in myelomeningocele. *J Bone Joint Surg* 53B:758, 1971

327. McKibbin B: The use of splintage in the management of paralytic dislocation of the hip in spina bifida cystica. *J Bone Joint Surg* 55B:163, 1973

328. McMaster JJ: The long-term results of kyphectomy and spinal stabilization in children with myelomeningocele. *Spine* 13:417, 1988

329. Menelaus MB: Dislocation and deformity of the hip in children with spina bifida cystica. *J Bone Joint Surg* 51B:238, 1969

330. Menelaus MB: Orthopaedic management of children with myelomeningocele. A plea for realistic goals. *Dev Med Child Neurol* (Suppl) 37:18, 1976

331. Menelaus MB: *The Orthopedic Management of Spina Bifida Cystica,* 2nd ed. Edinburgh, Churchill-Livingstone, 1980

332. Middleton RWD: Ankle valgus due to fibular growth abnormality. *J Bone Joint Surg* 57B:118, 1975

333. Mintz L, Sarwark JF, Dias L, Schafer MF: The natural history of congenital kyphosis in myelomeningocele. *Spine* 16:S348, 1991

334. Muller EB, Norwall A: Brace treatment of scoliosis in children with myelomeningocele. *Spine* 19:151, 1994

335. Muller EB, Nordwall A, Oden A: Progression of scoliosis in children with myelomeningocele. *Spine* 19:147, 1994

336. Parsch K, Manner G: Prevention and treatment of knee problems in children with spina bifida. *Dev Med Child Neurol* (Suppl 37) 18:114, 1976

337. Parsch K, Rossak K, Schultz KP: *Spina-Bifida-Kind, Klinik und Rehabilitation.* Stuttgart, Thieme, 1972

338. Passo SD: Positioning infants with myelomeningocele. *Am J Nurs* 74:1658, 1974

339. Reigel DH, Scarff TB, Woodford JE: Surgery for tethered spinal cord in myelomeningocele patients. American Association of Neurological Surgeons, April 1976. *Dev Med Child Neurol* (Suppl 37) 18:165, 1977

340. Rose GK, Sankarankutty M, Stallard J: A clinical review of the orthotic treatment of myelomeningocele patients. *J Bone Joint Surg* 65A:242, 1983

341. Schafer MF, Dias LS: *Myelomeningocele. Orthopaedic Treatment.* Baltimore, Williams & Wilkins, 1983

342. Sharrard WJW: The mechanism of paralytic deformity in spina bifida. *Dev Med Child Neurol* 4:319, 1962

343. Sharrard WJW: Neuromotor evaluation of the newborn, in *AAOS Symposium on Myelomeningocele.* St. Louis, CV Mosby, 1972

344. Sharrard WJW: Posterior iliopsoas transplantation in the treatment of paralytic dislocation of the hip. *J Bone Joint Surg* 46B:426, 1964

345. Sharrard WJW, Carroll NC: Long-term follow-up of posterior iliopsoas transplant for paralytic dislocation of the hip. *J Bone Joint Surg* 52B:779, 1970

346. Sharrard WJW, Grosfield I: The management of deformity and paralysis of the foot in myelomeningocele. *J Bone Joint Surg* 50B:456, 1968

347. Sherk HH, Ames MD: Functional results of iliopsoas transfer in myelomeningocele hip dislocation. *Clin Orthop Rel Res* 137:181, 1978

348. Stanitski CL, Stanitski DF, LaMont RL: Spondylolisthesis in myelomeningocele. *J Pediatr Orthop* 14:586, 1994

349. Stillwell A, Menelaus MB: Walking ability in mature patients with spina bifida. *J Pediatr Orthop* 3:184, 1983

350. Taylor LJ: Excision of the proximal end of the femur for hip stiffness in myelomeningocele. *J Bone Joint Surg* 68B: 75, 1986

351. Thomas LI, Thompson TC, Straub LR: Transplantation of the external oblique muscle for abductor paralysis. *J Bone Joint Surg* 32A:207, 1950

352. Townsend PF, Cowell HR, Steg NL: Lower extremity fractures simulating infection in spina bifida. *Clin Orthop Rel Res* 144:255, 1979

353. Turner A: Hand function in children with myelomeningocele. *J Bone Joint Surg* 67B:268, 1985

354. Walker G, Cheong-Leen P: Surgical management of paralytic vertical talus in myelomeningocele. *Dev Med Child Neurol* (Suppl 29) 15:112, 1973

355. Walker JH, Thomas M, Russell IT: Spina bifida—the parents. *Dev Med Child Neurol* 13:462, 1971

356. Wallace SJ: The effect of upper-limb function on mobility of children with myelomeningocele. *Dev Med Child Neurol* (Suppl) 29:84, 1973

357. Westin GW, DiFore RJ: Tenodesis of the tendo Achillis to the fibula for paralytic calcaneus deformity. *J Bone Joint Surg* 56A:1541, 1974

358. Wiltse LL: Valgus deformity of the ankle. *J Bone Joint Surg* 54A:595, 1972

359. Wright JG, Menelaus MB, Broughton NS, Shurtleff D: Natural history of knee contractures in myelomeningocele. *J Pediatr Orthop* 11:725, 1991

360. Yngve DA, Douglas R, Roberts JM: The reciprocating gait orthosis in myelomeningocele. *J Pediatr Orthop* 4:304, 1984

361. Ziller R.: Neuropathic osteolysis following arthrodesis of the ankle joint in myelodysplasia. *Beitr Orthop Traumatol* 21:401, 1974

Tumors and Tumorous Conditions of Bone

362. Belliveau RE, Spencer RP: Incidence and sites of bone lesions detected by ^{99m}Tc-polyphosphate scans in patients with tumors. *Cancer* 36:359, 1975

363. Berger PE, Kuhn JP: Computed tomography of tumors of the musculoskeletal system in children. *Radiology* 127:171, 1978

364. Berquist TH: Magnetic resonance imaging of musculoskeletal neoplasms. *Clin Orthop* 244:101, 1989

365. Berquist TH: Magnetic resonance imaging: Preliminary experience in orthopedic radiology. *MRI* 2:41, 1984

366. Bogumil GP, Schwamm HA: *Orthopaedic Pathology—A Synopsis with Clinical and Radiographic Correction.* Philadelphia, WB Saunders Co, 1985

367. Chang AE, Schaner EG, Conkle DM, Flye MW, Doppman JL, Rosenberg SA: Evaluation of computed tomography in the detection of pulmonary metastases. A prospective study. *Cancer* 43:913, 1979

368. Dahlin DC: *Bone Tumors—General Aspects and Data on 6221 Cases,* 3rd ed. Springfield, IL, Charles C Thomas, 1978

369. deSantos LA, Goldstein HM, Murray JA, Wallace S: Computed tomography in the evaluation of musculoskeletal neoplasms. *Radiology* 128:89, 1978

370. Enneking WF: *Musculoskeletal Tumor Surgery.* Edinburgh, Churchill Livingstone, 1983

371. Enneking WF, Chew FS, Springfield DS, Hudson TM, Spanier SS: The role of nuclide bone-scanning in determining the resectability of soft tissue sarcomas. *J Bone Joint Surg* 62A:249, 1981

372. Enneking WF, Spanier SS, Goodman MA: A system for the surgical staging of musculoskeletal sarcoma. *Clin Orthop* 153:106, 1980

373. Ewing J: A review of the classification of bone tumors. *Surg Gynecol Obstet* 68:971, 1939

374. Greenfield GB: *Radiology of Bone Diseases,* 2nd ed. Philadelphia, JB Lippincott, 1975

375. Hudson TM, Chew FS: Radionuclide bone scanning of osteosarcoma: Falsely extended uptake patterns. *AJR* 139:49, 1982

376. Hudson TM, Haas G, Enneking WF, Hawkins IF Jr: Angiography in the management of musculoskeletal tumors. *Surg Gynecol Obstet* 141:11, 1975

377. Hudson TM, Hamlin DJ, Enneking WF, Pettersson H: Magnetic resonance imaging of bone and soft tissue tumors: Early experience in 31 patients compared with computed tomography. *Skeletal Radiol* 13:134, 1985

378. Hudson TM, Hamlin DJ, Fitzsimmons JR: Magnetic resonance imaging of fluid levels in an aneurysmal bone cyst and in anticoagulated human blood. *Skeletal Radiol* 13:267, 1985

379. Jaffe HL: *Tumors and Tumorous Conditions of the Bones and Joints.* Philadelphia, Lea & Febiger, 1958

380. Kirchner PT, Simon MA: Current concepts review. Radioisotopic evaluation of skeletal disease. *J Bone Joint Surg* 63A:673, 1981

381. Lichtenstein L: *Bone Tumors,* 5th ed. St. Louis, CV Mosby, 1979

382. Lodwick GS: A systematic approach to the roentgen diagnosis of bone tumors, in *Tumors of Bone and Soft*

Tissues. Chicago, Year Book Medical Publisher, 1965, pp 49–68

383. Mankin HJ, Lange TA, Spanier SS: The hazards of biopsy in patients with malignant primary bone and soft-tissue tumors. *J Bone Joint Surg* 64A:1121, 1982

384. McLeod RA, Stephens DH: Computed tomography of pelvic musculoskeletal neoplasm. *Contemp Orthop* 1:36, 1979

385. Muhm JR, Brown LR, Crowe JK: Detection of pulmonary nodules by computed tomography. *AJR* 128:267, 1977

386. Ottolenghi CE: Diagnosis of orthopedic lesions by aspiration biopsy: Results of 1,061 punctures. *J Bone Joint Surg* 37A:443, 1955

387. Schajowicz F: *Tumors and Tumor-Like Lesions of Bone and Joints*. New York, Springer-Verlag, 1981

388. Simon MA: Current concepts review. Biopsy of musculoskeletal tumors. *J Bone Joint Surg* 64A:1253, 1982

389. Simon MA: Diagnostic and staging strategy for musculoskeletal tumors, in Evarts CM (ed): *Surgery of the Musculoskeletal System*. Vol. 4. Chap. 11. New York, Churchill-Livingstone, 1983, pp 5–38

390. Simon MA, Kirschner PT: Scintigraphic evaluation of primary bone tumors. Comparison of technetium 99m phosphonate and gallium citrate imaging. *J Bone Joint Surg* 62A:758, 1980

391. Thorpe WP, Reilly JJ, Rosenberg SA: Prognostic significance of alkaline phosphatase measurements in patients with osteogenic sarcoma receiving chemotherapy. *Cancer* 43:2178, 1979

392. Zimmer WD, Berquist TH, McLeod RA, Sim FH, Pritchard DJ, Shives TC, Wold LE, May GR: Bone tumors: Magnetic resonance imaging versus computed tomography. *Radiology* 155:709, 1985

Unicameral Bone Cyst

393. Bensahel H, Baum C: Traitement des kystes osseux solitaires du col du fémur chez l'enfant. *J Chir* 107:61, 1974

394. Burr BA, Resnick D, Syklawer R, Haghighi P: Fluid-fluid levels in a unicameral bone cyst: CT and MR findings. *J Comput Assist Tomogr* 17:134, 1993

395. Capanna R, Dal Monte A, Gitelis S, Campanacci M: The natural history of unicameral bone cyst after steroid injection. *Clin Orthop* 166:204, 1982

396. Chigira M, Maehara S, Arita S, Udagawa E: The aetiology and treatment of simple bone cysts. *J Bone Joint Surg* 65B:633, 1983

397. Cohen J: Etiology of simple bone cysts. *J Bone Joint Surg* 52A:1493, 1970

398. Czitrom AA, Pritzker KPH: Simple bone cyst causing collapse of the articular surface of the femoral head and incongruity of the hip joint. A case report. *J Bone Joint Surg* 62A:842, 1980

399. Fernbach SK, Blumenthal DH, Poznanski AK, Dias LS, Tachdjian MO: Radiographic changes in unicameral bone cysts following direct injection of steroids: A report of 12 cases. *Radiology* 140:689, 1981

400. Galasko CSB: The fate of simple bone cysts with fracture. *Clin Orthop* 101:302, 1974

401. Gerasimov AM, Toporova SM, Furtseva LN, Berezhnoy AP, Vilensky EV, Alekseeva RI: The role of lysosomes in the pathogenesis of unicameral bone cysts. *Clin Orthop* 266:53, 1991

402. Khermosh O, Weissman SL: Coxa vara, avascular necrosis and osteochondritis dissecans complicating solitary bone cysts of the proximal femur. *Clin Orthop* 126:143, 1977

403. Moreau G, Letts M: Unicameral bone cyst of the calcaneus in children. *J Pediatr Orthop* 14:101, 1994

404. Nelson JP, Foster RJ: Solitary bone cyst with epiphyseal involvement. A case report. *Clin Orthop* 118:147, 1976

405. Oppenheim WL, Galleno H: Operative treatment versus steroid injection in the management of unicameral bone cysts. *J Pediatr Orthop* 4:1, 1984

406. Reynolds J: The "fallen fragment sign" in the diagnosis of unicameral bone cysts. *J Radiol* 92:949, 1969

407. Scaglietti O, Marchetti PG, Bartolozzi P: The effects of methylprednisolone acetate in the treatment of bone cysts: Results of three years follow-up. *J Bone Joint Surg* 61B:200, 1979

408. Scaglietti O, Marchetti PG, Bartolozzi P: Final results obtained in the treatment of bone cysts with methylprednisolone acetate (Depo-Medrol) and a discussion of results achieved in other bone lesions. *Clin Orthop* 165:33, 1982

Aneurysmal Bone Cyst

409. Albinana J, Gonzalez-Moran G, Morcuende JA: Femoral head avascular necrosis associated with metaphyseal aneurysmal bone cyst. *J Pediatr Orthop* 4B:110, 1995

410. Capanna R, Albisinni U, Picci P, Calderoni P, Campanacci M, Springfield DS: Aneurysmal bone cyst of the spine. *J Bone Joint Surg* 67A:527, 1985

411. Davies AM, Cassar-Pullicino VN, Grimer RJ: The incidence and significance of fluid-fluid levels on computed tomography of osseous lesions. *Br J Radiol* 65:193, 1992

412. Fraser RK, Coates CJ, Cole WG: An angiostatic agent in treatment of a recurrent aneurysmal bone cyst. *J Pediatr Orthop* 13:668, 1993

413. Hay MC, Paterson D, Taylor TKF: Aneurysmal bone cysts of the spine. *J Bone Joint Surg* 60B:406, 1978

414. Lichtenstein L: Aneurysmal bone cyst. A pathological entity commonly mistaken for giant cell tumor and occasionally for hemangioma and osteogenic sarcoma. *Cancer* 3:279, 1950

415. Lichtenstein L: Aneurysmal bone cyst. Observations on 50 cases. *J Bone Joint Surg* 39A:873, 1957

416. McCarthy SM, Ogden JA: Epiphyseal extension of an aneurysmal bone cyst. *J Pediatr Orthop* 2:171, 1982

417. Ruiter D, Russel TG, Van Der Velde EA: Aneurysmal bone cysts. A clinicopathological study of 105 cases. *Cancer* 39:2231, 1977

Fibrous Defects of Bone and Nonossifying Fibroma

418. Arata MA, Peterson HA, Dahlin DC: Pathologic fractures through non-ossifying fibromas. *J Bone Joint Surg* 63A:980, 1981

419. Brower AC, Culver JE Jr, Keats TE: Histological nature of the cortical irregularity of the medial posterior distal

femoral metaphysis in children. *Radiology* 99:389, 1971

420. Bullough PG, Walley J: Fibrous cortical defect and non-ossifying fibroma. *Postgrad Med J* 41:672, 1965
421. Dietlein M, Benz Bohm C, Widemann D: The fibrous metaphyseal defect in early stage. Differential diagnosis to metaphysitis. *Pediatr Radiol* 22:481, 1992
422. Hatcher CH: The pathogenesis of localized fibrous lesions in the metaphyses of long bones. *Ann Surg* 122:1016, 1945
423. Jaffe HL, Lichtenstein L: Non-osteogenic fibroma of bone. *Am J Pathol* 18:205, 1942
424. Ponseti IV, Friedman B: Evolution of metaphyseal fibrous defects. *J Bone Joint Surg* 31A:582, 1949
425. Sontag IW, Pyle SI: The appearance and nature of cyst-like areas on the distal femoral metaphyses of children. *AJR* 46:185, 1941
426. Wilner D: *Radiology of Bone Tumors and Allied Disorders.* Philadelphia, WB Saunders, 1982, pp 551–611

Fibrous Dysplasia

427. Albright F: Polyostotic fibrous dysplasia: A defense of the entity. *J Clin Endocrinol* 7:307, 1947
428. Albright F, Butler AM, Hampton AO, Smith P: Syndrome characterized by osteitis fibrosa disseminata, areas of pigmentation and endocrine dysfunction with precocious puberty in females. *N Engl J Med* 216:727, 1937
429. Benjamin DR, McRoberts JW: Polyostotic fibrous dysplasia associated with Cushing's syndrome. *Arch Pathol* 96:175, 1973
430. Chung KF, Alaghband-Zadeh J, Guz A: Acromegaly and hyperprolactinemia in McCune-Albright syndrome. Evidence of hypothalmic dysfunction. *Am J Dis Child* 137:134, 1983
431. Daffner RH, Kirks DR, Gehweiler JA Jr, Heaston DK: Computed tomography of fibrous dysplasia. *AJR* 139:943, 1982
432. DePalma A, Almad I: Fibrous dysplasia associated with shepherd's crook deformity of the humerus. *Clin Orthop* 97:38, 1973
433. Harris WH, Dudley HR Jr, Barry RJ: The natural history of fibrous dysplasia. *J Bone Joint Surg* 44A:207, 1962
434. Henry A: Monostotic fibrous dysplasia. *J Bone Joint Surg* 51B:300, 1969
435. Milgram JW: Malignant transformation of polyostotic fibrous dysplasia of bone. *Bull Hosp Joint Dis* 36:137, 1975
436. Rieth KG, Comite F, Shawker TH, Cutler GB: Pituitary and ovarian abnormalities demonstrated by CT and ultrasound in children with features of the McCune-Albright syndrome. *Radiology* 153:389, 1984
437. Savage PE, Stoker DJ: Fibrous dysplasia of the femoral neck. *Skeletal Radiol* 11:119, 1984

Enchondroma

438. Adler CP, Klumper A, Wenz W: Enchondroma—radiology and pathology. *Radiology* 19:341, 1979
439. Campanacci M, Leonessa C, Boni A: Cartilaginous tumors in the hand bones: Report of 112 cases. *Chir Organi Mov* 62:483, 1975
440. Jaffe HL, Lichtenstein L: Solitary benign enchondroma of bone. *Arch Surg* 46:480, 1943
441. Laurence W, Franklin EL: Calcifying enchondroma of long bones. *J Bone Joint Surg* 35B:224, 1953
442. Milgram JW: The origins of osteochondromas and enchondromas. A histopathologic study. *Clin Orthop* 147:264, 1983
443. Remagen W, Nidecker A, Dolanc B: Case report 368: Enchondroma of the tibia with extension degeneration, recurrence with secondary and malignant transformation to highly differentiated chondrosarcoma. *Skeletal Radiol* 15:330, 1986
444. Zimny ML, Redler I: Ultrastructure of solitary enchondromas. *J Hand Surg* 9B:95, 1984

Multiple Enchondromatosis

445. Andren L, Dymling JF, Elner A, et al: Maffucci's syndrome: Report of four cases. *Acta Chir Scand* 126:397, 1963
446. Chen VT, Harrison DA: Maffucci's syndrome. *Hand* 10:292, 1978
447. Fairbank HAT: Dyschondroplasia. Synonyms: Ollier's disease, multiple enchondromata. *J Bone Joint Surg* 30B:689, 1948
448. Lewis RJ, Ketcham AS: Maffucci's syndrome: Functional and neoplastic significance. Case report and review of the literature. *J Bone Joint Surg* 55A:1465, 1973
449. Schnall AM, Genuth SM: Multiple endocrine adenomas in a patient with the Maffucci syndrome. *Am J Med* 61:952, 1976
450. Spranger J, Kemperdieck H, Bakowski H, Opitz JM: Two peculiar types of enchondromatosis. *Pediatr Radiol* 7:215, 1978
451. Sun TC, Swee RG, Shives TC, Unni KK: Chondrosarcoma in Maffucci's syndrome. *J Bone Joint Surg* 67A:1214, 1985

Chondromyxoid Fibroma

452. Dahlin DC: Chondromyxoid fibroma of bone with emphasis on its morphological relationship to benign chondroblastoma. *Cancer* 9:195, 1956
453. Dahlin DC, Wells AH, Henderson ED: Chondromyxoid fibroma of bone; report of two cases. *J Bone Joint Surg* 35A:831, 1953
454. Feldman F, Hecht HL, Johnston AD: Chondromyxoid fibroma of bone. *Radiology* 94:249, 1970
455. Frank MWE, Rockwood CA: Chondromyxoid fibroma: Review of the literature and report of four cases. *South Med J* 62:1248, 1969
456. Jaffe HL, Lichtenstein L: Chondromyxoid fibroma of bone: A distinctive benign tumor likely to be mistaken especially for chondrosarcoma. *Arch Pathol* 45:541, 1948
457. Mayer BS: Chondromyxoid fibroma of lumbar spine. *J Can Assoc Radiol* 29:271, 1978
458. Murphy NB, Price CHG: The radiological aspects of chondromyxoid fibroma. *Clin Radiol* 22:261, 1971
459. Ottolenghi CE, Petracchi LJ: Chondromyxosarcoma of the calcaneus. *J Bone Joint Surg* 35A:211, 1953
460. Prichard RW, Stoy RP, Barwick JTF: Chondromyxoid fibroma of the scapula. *J Bone Joint Surg* 46A:1759, 1964

461. Schajowicz F, Gallardo H: Chondromyxoid fibroma (fibromyxoid chondroma) of bone. *J Bone Joint Surg* 53B:198, 1971

462. Wilson AJ, Kyriakos M, Ackerman LV: Chondromyxoid fibroma: Radiographic appearance in 30 cases and in a review of the literature. *Radiology* 179:513, 1991

Benign Chondroblastoma

463. Bloem JL, Mulder JD: Chondroblastoma: A clinical and radiological study of 104 cases. *Skeletal Radiol* 14:1, 1985

464. Campanacci M, Ginnti A, Martucci E, Trentani C: Epiphyseal chondroblastoma (a study of 39 cases). *Ital J Orthop Traumatol* 3:67, 1977

465. Codman EA: Epiphyseal chondromatous giant cell tumors of the upper end of the humerus. *Surg Gynecol Obstet* 52:543, 1931

466. Fobben ES, Dalinka MK, Schiebler ML: Magnetic resonance imaging: Appearance at 1.5 tesla of cartilaginous tumors involving the epiphysis. *Skeletal Radiol* 16:647, 1987

467. Jaffe HL, Lichtenstein L: Benign chondroblastoma of bone; a reinterpretation of the so-called calcifying or chondromatous giant cell tumor. *Am J Pathol* 18:969, 1942

468. Schajowicz F, Gallardo H: Epiphyseal chondroblastoma of bone. A clinico-pathological study of 69 cases. *J Bone Joint Surg* 52B:205, 1970

Osteoid Osteoma

469. Boriani S, Capanna R, Donati D, Levine A, Picci P, Savini R: Osteoblastoma of the spine. *Clin Orthop* 278:37, 1992

470. Cassar Pullicino VN, McCall IW, Wan S: Intra-articular osteoid osteoma. *Clin Radiol* 45:153, 1992

471. Corbett JM, Wilde AH, McCormack LJ, Evarts CM: Intra-articular osteoid osteoma. A diagnostic problem. *Clin Orthop* 98:225, 1974

472. Cronemeyer RL, Kirchmer NA, DeSmet AA, Neff JR: Intra-articular osteoid-osteoma of the humerus simulating synovitis of the elbow. A case report. *J Bone Joint Surg* 63A:1172, 1981

473. Daunin C, Puget C, Assoun J, Railhac JJ, Cahuzac JP, Clement JL, Sales de Cauzy J: Percutaneous resection of osteoid osteoma under CT guidance in eight children. *Pediatr Radiol* 24:185, 1994

474. Ghelman B, Thompson FM, Arnold WD: Intraoperative radioactive localization of an osteoid osteoma. *J Bone Joint Surg* 63A:826, 1981

475. Goldberg VM, Jacobs B: Osteoid osteoma of the hip in children. *Clin Orthop* 106:41, 1975

476. Greco F, Tamburrelli F, Ciabattoni G: Prostaglandins in osteoid osteoma. *Int Orthop* 15:35, 1991

477. Helms CA, Hattner RS, Vogler JB III: Osteoid osteoma: Radionuclide diagnosis. *Radiology* 151:779, 1984

478. Jaffe HL: Osteoid-osteoma: A benign osteoblastic tumor composed of osteoid and atypical bone. *Arch Surg* 31:709, 1935

479. Jaffe HL, Lichtenstein L: Osteoid-osteoma: Further experience with its benign tumor of bone, with special reference to cases showing the lesion in relation to shaft cortices and commonly misclassified as instances of sclerosing non-suppurative osteomyelitis or cortical-bone abscess. *J Bone Joint Surg* 22:645, 1940

480. Keim HA, Reina EG: Osteoid-osteoma as a cause of scoliosis. *J Bone Joint Surg* 57A:159, 1975

481. Nelson OA, Greer RB: Localization of osteoid osteoma of the spine using computerized tomography. A case report. *J Bone Joint Surg* 65A:263, 1983

482. O'Brien TM, Murray TE, Malone LA, Dervan P, Walsh M, McManus F, Ennis JT: Osteoid osteoma: Excision with scintimetric guidance. *Radiology* 153:543, 1984

483. Ransford AO, Pozo JL, Hutton PAM, Kirwan EOG: The behavior pattern of the scoliosis associated with osteoid osteoma or osteoblastoma of the spine. *J Bone Joint Surg* 66B:16, 1984

484. Rinsky LA, Goris M, Bleck EE, Halpern A, Hirshman P: Intraoperative skeletal scintigraphy for localization of osteoid-osteoma in the spine. Case report. *J Bone Joint Surg* 62A:143, 1980

485. Seitz WH Jr, Dick HM: Intraepiphyseal osteoid osteoma of the distal femur in an 8-year-old girl. *J Pediatr Orthop* 3:505, 1983

486. Simons GW, Sty J: Intraoperative bone imaging in the treatment of osteoid osteoma of the femoral neck. *J Pediatr Orthop* 3:399, 1983

487. Wedge JH, Chang S, MacFadyen DJ: Computed tomography in localization of spinal osteoid osteoma. *Spine* 6:423, 1981

Benign Osteoblastoma

488. Abdelwahab IF, Frankel VH, Klein MJ: Case report 351: Aggressive osteoblastoma of the third lumbar vertebra. *Skeletal Radiol* 15:164, 1986

489. Akbarnia BA, Rooholamini SA: Scoliosis caused by benign osteoblastoma of the thoracic or lumbar spine. *J Bone Joint Surg* 63A:1146, 1981

490. Bertoni F, Unni KK, McLeod RA, Dahlin DC: Osteosarcoma resembling osteoblastoma. *Cancer* 55:416, 1985

491. Capanna RM, Van Horn JR, Ayala A, Picci P, Bettelli G: Osteoid osteoma and osteoblastoma of the talus. A report of 40 cases. *Skeletal Radiol* 15:360, 1986

492. Jackson RO, Reckling FW, Mantz FA: Osteoid osteoma and osteoblastoma: Similar histologic lesions with different natural histories. *Clin Orthop* 128:303, 1977

493. Jaffe HL: Benign osteoblastoma. *Bull Hosp Joint Dis* 17:141, 1956

494. Kirwan EO, Hutton PA, Pozo JL, Ransford AO: Osteoid osteoma and benign osteoblastoma of the spine. Clinical presentation and treatment. *J Bone Joint Surg* 66B:21, 1984

495. Lichtenstein L: Benign osteoblastoma. A category of osteoid and bone-forming tumors other than classical osteoid osteoma, which may be mistaken for giant-cell tumor or osteogenic sarcoma. *Cancer* 9:1044, 1956

496. Lichtenstein L, Sawyer WR: Benign osteoblastoma: Further observations and report of twenty additional cases. *J Bone Joint Surg* 46A:755, 1964

497. Marsh BW, Bonfiglio M, Brady LP, Enneking WF: Benign osteoblastoma: Range of manifestations. *J Bone Joint Surg* 57A:1, 1975

498. Schajowicz F, Lemos C: Osteoid osteoma and osteoblastoma. Closely related entities of osteoblastic derivation. *Acta Orthop Scand* 41:272, 1970

499. Seki T, Fukada H, Ishii Y, Hanaoka H, Yatabe S, Takano M, Koide O: Malignant transformation of benign osteoblastoma. A case report. *J Bone Joint Surg* 57A:424, 1975

500. Weatherly CR, Jaffray D, O'Brien JP: Radical excision of an osteoblastoma of the cervical spine. A combined anterior and posterior approach. *J Bone Joint Surg* 68B:325, 1986

Osteochondroma (Exostosis)

501. D'Ambrosia R, Ferguson ABR: The formation of osteochondroma by epiphyseal cartilage transplantation. *Clin Orthop* 61:103, 1968

502. Garrison RC, Unni KK, McLeod RA, Pritchard DJ, Dahlin DC: Chondrosarcoma arising in osteochondroma. *Cancer* 49:1890, 1982

503. Hudson TM, Chew FS, Manaster BJ: Scintigraphy of benign exostosis and exostotic chondrosarcoma. *AJR* 140:581, 1983

504. Jaffe HL: *Tumors and Tumorous Conditions of Bones and Joints.* Philadelphia, Lea & Febiger, 1958, p 143

505. Keith A: Studies on the anatomical changes which accompany certain growth disorders of the human body. *J Anat* 54:101, 1920

506. Lange RH, Lange TA, Rao BK: Correlative radiographic, scintigraphic, and histological evaluation of exostosis. *J Bone Joint Surg* 66A:1454, 1984

507. Milgram JW: The origins of osteochondromas and enchondromas. A histopathologic study. *Clin Orthop* 174:264, 1983

508. Paling MR: The "disappearing" osteochondroma. *Skeletal Radiol* 10:40, 1983

509. Wilner D: Solitary exostosis, in *Radiology of Bone Tumors and Allied Disorders.* Philadelphia, WB Saunders, 1982, pp 272–355

Multiple Hereditary Exostoses

510. Fogel GR, McElfresh EC, Peterson HA, Wicklund PT: Management of deformities of the forearm in multiple hereditary osteochondromata. *J Bone Joint Surg* 66A:670, 1984

511. Jaffe HL: *Tumors and Tumorous Conditions of the Bones and Joints.* Philadelphia, Lea & Febiger, 1958, p 143

512. Keith A: Studies on the anatomical changes which accompany certain growth-disorders of the human disorder known as multiple exostoses. *J Anat* 54:101, 1920

513. Madigan R, Worrall T, McClain E: Cervical cord compression in hereditary multiple exostosis. Review of the literature and report of a case. *J Bone Joint Surg* 56A:410, 1974

514. McCormack EB: The surgical management of hereditary multiple exostosis. *Orthop Rev* 10:57, 1981

515. Ogden JA: Multiple hereditary osteochondromata: Report of an early case. *Clin Orthop Rel Res* 116:48, 1976

516. Peterson HA: Deformities and problems of the forearm in children with multiple hereditary osteochondromata. *J Pediatr Orthop* 9:427, 1989

517. Peterson HA: Multiple hereditary osteochondromata. *Clin Orthop Rel Res* 239:222, 1989

518. Snearly WN, Peterson HA: Management of ankle deformities in multiple hereditary osteochondromata. *J Pediatr Orthop* 9:427, 1989

519. Shapiro F, Simon S, Glimcher MJ: Hereditary multiple exostoses: Anthropometric, roentgenographic, and clinical aspects. *J Bone Joint Surg* 61A:815, 1979

520. Solomon L: Hereditary multiple exostosis. *Am J Hum Genet* 16:351, 1964

521. Voutsinas S, Wynne-Davies R: The infrequency of malignant disease in diaphyseal aclasis and neurofibromatosis. *J Med Genet* 20:345, 1983

Osteofibrous Dysplasia (Campanacci Syndrome)

522. Campanacci M: Osteofibrous dysplasia of long bones. A new clinical entity. *Ital J Orthop Traumatol* 2:221, 1976

523. Campanacci M, Giunti A, Leonessa C, Pagnani P, Trentani C: Pathological fractures in osteopathies and bony dysplasias. *Ital J Orthop Traumatol* (Suppl 1) 1975

524. Campanacci M, Laus M: Osteofibrous dysplasia of the tibia and fibula. *J Bone Joint Surg* 63A:367, 1981

525. Campanacci M, Leonessa C: Displasia fibrosa dello scheletro. *Chir Organi Mov* 59:195, 1970

526. Fragenheim P: Angeborene Ostitis fibrosa als Ursache einer intrauterinen Unterschenkelfraktur. *Arch Klin Chir,* 117:22, 1921

527. Goergen TG, Dickman PS, Resnick D, Saltzstein SL, O'Dell CW, Akeson SH: Long bone ossifying fibromas. *Cancer* 39:2067, 1977

528. Kempson RL: Ossifying fibroma of the long bones. A light and electron microscopic study. *Arch Pathol* 82:218, 1966

529. McFarland B: "Birth fracture" of the tibia. *Br J Surg* 27:706, 1940

530. Semian DW, Willis JB, Bove KE: Congenital fibrous defect of the tibia mimicking fibrous dysplasia. A case report. *J Bone Joint Surg* 57A:854, 1975

Eosinophilic Granuloma

531. Benz-Bohm G, Georgi P: Scintigraphic and radiographic findings in eosinophilic granuloma. *Radiologe* 21:195, 1981

532. Calvé J: A localized affection of the spine suggesting osteochondritis of the vertebral body, with the clinical aspects of Pott's disease. *J Bone Joint Surg* 7:41, 1925

533. Christian H: Defects in membranous bone, exophthalmos and diabetes insipidus. An unusual syndrome of dyspituitarism. *Med Clin North Am* 3:849, 1920

534. Cohen M, Zornoza J, Cangir A, Murray JA, Wallace S: Direct injection of methylprednisolone sodium succinate in the treatment of solitary eosinophilic granuloma of bone: A report of 9 cases. *Radiology* 136:289, 1980

535. Compere E, Johnson WE, Coventry MB: Vertebra plana (Calvé's disease) due to eosinophilic granuloma. *J Bone Joint Surg* 36A:969, 1954

536. Compere E, Johnson WE, Coventry MB: Vertebra plana (Calvé's disease) due to eosinophilic granuloma. *J Bone Joint Surg* 45A:1322, 1963

537. Farber S, Green WT, Dermott L: The nature of solitary or eosinophilic granuloma of bone. *Am J Pathol* 17:625, 1941

538. Letterer E: Aleukamische Retikulose. (Ein Beitrag zu den proliferativen Erkrankungen des Retikuoendothelialapparates.) *Frankfurt Z Pathol* 30:377, 1924

539. Lichtenstein L: Histiocytosis X. Integration of eosinophilic granuloma of bone. "Letterer-Siwe disease," and Schuller-Christian disease as related manifestations of a single nosologic entity. *Arch Pathol* 56:84, 1953

540. Lichtenstein L: Histiocytosis X (eosinophilic granuloma of bone, Letterer-Siwe disease, and Schuller-Christian disease). *J Bone Joint Surg* 46A:76, 1964

541. McCullough CJ: Eosinophilic granuloma of bone. *Acta Orthop Scand* 51:389, 1980

542. Schajowicz F, Slullitel J: Eosinophilic granuloma of bone and its relationship to Hand-Schuller-Christian and Letterer-Siwe syndromes. *J Bone Joint Surg* 55B:545, 1973

543. Schuller A: Uber eigenartige Schadeldefkte im Jugendalter. *Fortschr Rontgenstr* 23:12, 1915

544. Yabsley RH, Harris WR: Solitary eosinophilic granuloma of a vertebral body causing paraplegia. Report of a case. *J Bone Joint Surg* 48A:1570, 1966

Osteogenic Sarcoma

545. Aliuja SC, Villacin AB, Smith J, Bullough PG, Huvos AG, Marcove RC: Juxtacortical (parosteal) osteogenic sarcoma. *J Bone Joint Surg* 59A:632, 1977

546. Beattie EJ: The management of pulmonary metastasis in children with osteogenic sarcoma with resection combined with chemotherapy. *Cancer* 35:618, 1975

547. Campanacci M, Costa P: Total resection of the distal femur or proximal tibia for bone tumors. *J Bone Joint Surg* 61B:455, 1979

548. Campanacci M, Picci P, Gherlinzoni F, Guerra A, Bertoni F, Neff JR: Parosteal osteosarcoma. *J Bone Joint Surg* 66B:313, 1984

549. Coffre C, Vanel D, Contesso G, Kalifa C, Dubousset J, Genin J, Masselot J: Problems and pitfalls in the use of computed tomography for the local evaluation of long bone osteosarcoma: Report on 30 cases. *Skeletal Radiol* 13:147, 1985

550. Dahlin DC: Pathology of osteosarcoma. *Clin Orthop* 111:23, 1975

551. Dal Monte A: Osteosarcoma of the proximal femur and humerus in children treated by resection, endoprosthesis and complementary chemotherapy. *Ital J Orthop Traumatol* 9:151, 1983

552. De Santos LA, Bernardino ME, Murray JA: Computed tomography in the evaluation of osteosarcoma: Experience with 25 cases. *AJR* 132:535, 1979

553. Dubousset J, Missenard G, Kalifa C: Management of osteogenic sarcoma in children and adolescents. *Clin Orthop* 270:52, 1991

554. Enneking WF, Kagan A: The implications of "skip" metastases in osteosarcoma. *Clin Orthop* 111:33, 1975

555. Enneking WF, Spanier SS, Goodman MA: Surgical staging of musculoskeletal sarcoma. *J Bone Joint Surg* 62A:1039, 1980

556. Farr GH, Huvos AG: Juxtacortical osteogenic sarcoma. An analysis of fourteen cases. *J Bone Joint Surg* 54A:1205, 1972

557. Farr GH, Huvos AG, Marcove BC, Higinbotham NL, Foote FW Jr: Telangiectatic osteogenic sarcoma. *Cancer* 34:1150, 1974

558. Glasser DB, Lane JM: Stage IIB osteogenic sarcoma. *Clin Orthop* 270:29, 1991

559. Glasser DB, Lane JM, Huvos AG, Marcove RC, Rosen G: Survival, prognosis, and therapeutic response in osteogenic sarcoma. The Memorial Hospital experience. *Cancer* 69:698, 1992

560. Hansen MF: Molecular genetic considerations in osteosarcoma. *Clin Orthop* 270:237, 1991

561. Homa DM, Sowers MR, Schwartz AG: Incidence and survival rates of children and young adults with osteogenic sarcoma. *Cancer* 67:2219, 1991

562. Jaffe HL: *Tumors and Tumorous Conditions of the Bones and Joints.* Philadelphia, Lea & Febiger, 1958, p 256

563. Kotz R, Salzer M: Rotation-plasty for childhood osteosarcoma of the distal part of the femur. *J Bone Joint Surg* 64A:959, 1982

564. Lichtenstein L: *Bone Tumors,* 5th ed. St. Louis, CV Mosby, 1977, pp 220–252

565. McKillop JH, Etcubanas E, Goris ML: The indications for and limitations of bone scintigraphy in osteogenic sarcoma: A review of 55 patients. *Cancer* 48:1133, 1981

566. Marcove RC, Martini N, Rosen G: The treatment of pulmonary metastasis in osteogenic sarcoma. *Clin Orthop* 111:65, 1975

567. Marcove RC, Rosen G: "En bloc" resections for osteogenic sarcoma. *Cancer* 45:3040, 1980

568. Matsuno T, Krishman KO, McLeod RA, Unni KK: Telangiectatic osteogenic sarcoma. *Cancer* 38:2538, 1978

569. Patel DV, Hammer RA, Levin B, Fisher MA: Primary osteogenic sarcoma of the spine. *Skeletal Radiol* 12:276, 1984

570. Price CHG, Zhuber K, Salzer-Kunschik M, Salzer M, Willert HG, Immencamp M, Groh P, Matejorsky Z, Keyl W: Osteosarcoma in children. *J Bone Joint Surg* 57B:341, 1975

571. Pritchard DJ, Finkel MP, Reilly CA Jr: The etiology of osteosarcoma. A review of current considerations. *Clin Orthop* 111:14, 1975

572. Raymond AK: Surface osteosarcoma. *Clin Orthop* 270:140, 1991

573. Salzar M, Knahr K, Kotz R: Treatment of osteosarcomata of the distal femur by rotation plasty. *Arch Orthop Trauma Surg* 99:131, 1981

574. Schajowicz F: Juxtacortical chondrosarcoma. *J Bone Joint Surg* 59B:473, 1977

575. Sim FH, Ivins JC, Pritchard D: Osteosarcoma: New developments in diagnosis and treatment. *J Bone Joint Surg* 61B:513, 1979

576. Simon MA: Causes of increased survival of patients with osteosarcoma. Current controversies. *J Bone Joint Surg* 66A:306, 1984

577. Snyder CL, Saltzman DA, Ferrell KL, Thompson RC, Leonard AS: A new approach to the resection of pulmonary

osteosarcoma metastases. Results of aggressive metastasectomy. *Clin Orthop* 270:247, 1991

Ewing's Sarcoma

578. Alman BA, DeBari A, Krajbich JI: Massive allografts in the treatment of osteosarcoma and Ewing sarcoma in children and adolescents. *J Bone Joint Surg* 77A:54, 1995

579. Cara JA, Canadell J: Limb salvage for malignant bone tumors in young children. *J Pediatr Orthop* 14:112, 1994

580. Eckardt JJ, Safran MR, Eilber FR, Rosen G, Kabo JM: Expandable endoprosthetic reconstruction of the skeletally immature after malignant bone tumor resection. *Clin Orthop* 297:188, 1993

581. Ehara S, Kattapuram SV, Egglin TK: Ewing's sarcoma. Radiographic pattern of healing and bony complications in patients with long-term survival. *Cancer* 68:1531, 1991

582. Frassica FJ, Frassica DA, Pritchard DJ, Schomberg PJ, Wold LE, Sim FH: Ewing sarcoma of the pelvis. *J Bone Joint Surg* 75A:1457, 1993

583. Gasparini M, Lombardi F, Ballerini E, Gandola L, Gianni MC, Massimino M, Rottoli L, Fossati-Bellani F: Long-term outcome of patients with monostotic Ewing's sarcoma treated with combined modality. *Med Pediatr Oncol* 23: 406, 1994

584. Glasser DB, Duane K, Lane JM, Healey JH, Caparros-Sison B: The effect of chemotherapy on growth in the skeletally immature individual. *Clin Orthop* 262:93, 1991

585. Hanna SL, Fletcher BD, Kaste SC, Fairclough DL, Parham DM: Increased confidence of diagnosis of Ewing sarcoma using T2-weighted MR images. *MRI* 12:559, 1994

586. Mameghan H, Fisher RJ, O'Orman-Hughes D, Bates EH, Huckstep RL, Mameghan J: Ewing's sarcoma: Long-term follow-up in 49 patients treated from 1967 to 1989. *Int J Radiat Oncol Biol Phys* 25:431, 1993

587. Norman-Taylor FH, Sweetnam DI, Fixsen JA: Distal fibulectomy for Ewing's sarcoma. *J Bone Joint Surg* 76B:559, 1994

588. Toni A, Neff JR, Sudanese A, Ciaroni D, Bacci G, Picci P, Barbieri E, Campanacci M, Giunti A: The role of surgical therapy in patients with nonmetastatic Ewing's sarcoma of the limbs. *Clin Orthop* 286:225, 1993

589. van der Woude HJ, Bloem JL, Holscher HC, Nooy MA, Taminiau AH, Hermans J, Falke TH, Hogendoorn PC: Monitoring the effect of chemotherapy in Ewing's sarcoma of bone with MR imaging. *Skeletal Radiol* 23:493, 1994

590. van der Woude HJ, Bloem JL, Taminiau AH, Nooy MA, Hogendoorn PC: Classification of histopathologic changes following chemotherapy in Ewing's sarcoma of bone. *Skeletal Radiol* 23:501, 1994

Adamantinoma

591. Anderson CE, Saunders JB deCM: Primary adamantinoma of the ulna. *Surg Gynecol Obstet* 75:351, 1942

592. Besemann EF, Perez MA: Malignant angioblastoma, so-called adamantinoma, involving the humerus. A case report. *AJR* 100:538, 1967

593. Campanacci M, Giunti A, Bertoni F, Laus M, Gitelis S: Adamantinoma of the long bones. The experience at the Istituto Ortopedico Rizzoli. *Am J Surg Pathol* 5:533, 1981

594. Unni KK, Dahlin DC, Beabout JW, Ivins JC: Adamantinomas of long bones. *Cancer* 34:1796, 1974

Metastatic Tumors of Bone

595. Anderson OW: Neuroblastoma with skeletal metastases and apparent recovery. *Am J Dis Child* 83:782, 1953

596. Berger PE, Kuh JP, Munschauer RW: Computed tomography and ultrasound in the diagnosis and management of neuroblastoma. *Radiology* 128:663, 1978

597. Evans AE, D'Angio GJ, Randolph J: A proposed staging for children with neuroblastoma. *Cancer* 27:374, 1971

598. Harrison J, Myers M, Rowen M, Vermund H: Results of combination chemotherapy, surgery and radiotherapy in children with neuroblastoma. *Cancer* 34:485, 1974

599. Howman-Giles RB, Gilday DL, Ash JM: Radionuclide skeletal survey in neuroblastoma. *Radiology* 131:497, 1979

600. Kaufman RA, Thrall JH, Keyes JW, Brown ML, Zakem JF: False negative bone scans in neuroblastoma metastatic to the ends of the long bones. *AJR* 130:131, 1978

601. Rosenfield N, Treves S: Osseous and extraosseous uptake of fluorine-18 and technetium 99m polyphosphate in children with neuroblastoma. *Radiology* 111:127, 1974

Wilms' Tumor

602. Aron BS: Wilms' tumor: A clinical study of eighty-one patients. *Cancer* 33:637, 1974

603. Boxer LA, Smith DL: Wilms' tumor prior to onset of hemihypertrophy. *Am J Dis Child* 120:564, 1970

604. Cassaday JR, Jaffe N, Paed D, Filler RM: The increasing importance of radiation therapy in the improved prognosis of children with Wilms' tumor. *Cancer* 39:825, 1977

605. Meadows AT, Litchtenfeld JL, Koop CE: Wilms' tumor in three children of a woman with congenital hemihypertrophy. *N Engl J Med* 291:23, 1974

606. Wara WM, Margolis LW, Smith WB, Kushner J, deLorimier A: Treatment of metastatic Wilms' tumor. *Radiology* 112:695, 1974

Soft Tissue Tumors

607. Buck P, Mickelson MR, Bonfiglio M: Synovial sarcoma: A review of 33 cases. *Clin Orthop* 156:211, 1981

608. Cadman NL, Soule EH, Kelly PJ: Synovial sarcoma: An analysis of 134 tumors. *Cancer* 18:613, 1965

609. Enzinger FM, Weiss S: *Soft Tissue Tumors,* 3rd ed. St. Louis, Mosby–Year Book, 1994

610. Israels SJ, Chan HS, Daneman A, Weitzman SS: Synovial sarcoma in childhood. *AJR* 142:803, 1984

611. Kirchner PT, Simon MA: The clinical value of bone and gallium scintigraphy for soft-tissue sarcomas of the extremities. *J Bone Joint Surg* 66A:319, 1984

612. Kransdorf MJ, Jelinek JS, Moser RP Jr, Utz JA, Brower AC, Hudson TM, Berrey BH: Soft-tissue masses: Diagnosis using MR imaging. *AJR* 153:541, 1989

613. Lange TA, Austin CW, Seibert JJ, Angtuaco TL, Yandow DR: Ultrasound imaging as a screening study for malignant soft-tissue tumors. *J Bone Joint Surg* 69A:100, 1987

614. Mayer DP, Clancy M, Bonakdarpour A, Peterson RO, Steel HH: Case report 152: Synovial sarcoma of the knee. *Skeletal Radiol* 6:221, 1981

615. Murray MR, Stout AP: Schwann cell versus fibroblast as the origin of the specific nerve sheath tumor. *Am J Pathol* 16:41, 1940

616. Myhre-Jensen O: A consecutive 7-year series of 1331 benign soft tissue tumours. Clinicopathologic data. Comparison with sarcomas. *Acta Orthop Scand* 52:287, 1981

617. Petasnick JP, Turner DA, Charters JR, Gitelis S, Sacharias CE: Soft-tissue masses of the locomotor system: Comparison of MR imaging with CT. *Radiology* 160:125, 1986

618. Rydholm A, Berg NO: Size, site and clinical incidence of lipoma. Factors in the differential diagnosis of lipoma and sarcoma. *Acta Orthop Scand* 54:929, 1983

619. Simon MA, Kirschner PT: Scintigraphic evaluation of primary bone tumors. Comparison of technetium-99m phosphonate and gallium citrate imaging. *J Bone Joint Surg* 62A:758, 1980

620. Totty WG, Murphy WA, Lee JKT: Soft-tissue tumors: MR imaging. *Radiology* 160:135, 1986

621. Wright PH, Sim FH, Soule EH, Taylor WF: Synovial sarcoma. *J Bone Joint Surg* 64A:112, 1982

Tumoral Calcinosis

622. Gregosiewicz A, Warda E: Tumoral calcinosis: Successful medical treatment. *J Bone Joint Surg* 71A:1244, 1989

623. Harkess J, Peters H: Tumoral calcinosis: A report of six cases. *J Bone Joint Surg* 49A:721, 1967

624. Malik M, Acharya S: Tumoral calcinosis of the fingers. *Int Orthop* 17:279, 1993

625. Mitnick PD, Goldfarb S, Slatopolsky E, Lemann J Jr, Gray RW, Agus ZS: Calcium and phosphate metabolism in tumoral calcinosis. *Ann Intern Med* 92:482, 1980

626. Viegas J: Tumoral calcinosis: A case report with review of literature. *J Hand Surg* 10A:744, 1985

627. Wilber JF, Slatopolsky E: Hyperphosphatemia and tumoral calcinosis. *Ann Intern Med* 68:1044, 1968

Neurofibromatosis

628. Akbarnia BA, Gabriel KR, Beckman E, Chalk D: Prevalence of scoliosis in neurofibromatosis. *Spine* 17:244, 1992

629. Brill CB: Neurofibromatosis: Clinical overview. *Clin Orthop* 245:10, 1989

630. Calvert PT, Edgar MA, Webb PJ: Scoliosis in neurofibromatosis. The natural history with and without operation. *J Bone Joint Surg* 71B:246, 1989

631. Chee CP: Lateral thoracic meningocele associated with neurofibromatosis: Total excision by posterolateral extradural approach. A case report. *Spine* 14:129, 1989

632. Coleman BG, Arger PH, Dalinka MK, Obringer AC, Raney BR, Meadows AT: CT of sarcomatous degeneration in neurofibromatosis. *AJR* 140:383, 1983

633. Craig JB, Govender S: Neurofibromatosis of the cervical spine. *J Bone Joint Surg* 74B:575, 1992

634. Crawford AH: Neurofibromatosis, in Weinstein SL (ed): *The Pediatric Spine, Principles and Practice,* Vol I. New York, Raven Press, 1994

635. Crawford AH: Neurofibromatosis in children. *Acta Orthop Scand* (Suppl 18) 57, 1986

636. Crawford AH: Pitfalls in the management of spinal deformities associated with neurofibromatosis. *Clin Orthop* 245:29, 1989

637. Crawford AH, Bagamery N: Osseous manifestations of neurofibromatosis in childhood. *J Pediatr Orthop* 6:72, 1986

638. Dolynchuk KN, Teskey J, West M: Intrathoracic meningocele associated with neurofibromatosis: Case report. *Neurosurgery* 27:485, 1990

639. Egelhoff JC, Bates DJ, Ross JS, Rothner AD, Cohen BH: Spinal MR findings in neurofibromatosis types 1 and 2. *AJNR* 13:1071, 1992

640. Funasaki H, Winter RB, Lonstein JB, Denis F: Pathophysiology of spinal deformities in neurofibromatosis. An analysis of 71 patients who had curves associated with dystrophic changes. *J Bone Joint Surg* 76A:692, 1994

641. Graham PW, Oehlschlaeger FH: *Articulating the Elephant Man. Joseph Merrick and His Interpreters.* Baltimore, Johns Hopkins University Press, 1992

642. Gregg PJ, Price BA, Ellis HA, Stevens J: Pseudarthrosis of the radius associated with neurofibromatosis. A case report. *Clin Orthop* 171:175, 1982

643. Gutmann DH, Collins FS: Recent progress toward understanding the molecular biology of von Recklinghausen neurofibromatosis. Brief review. *Ann Neurol* 31:555, 1992

644. Hsu LCS, Lee PC, Leong JCY: Dystrophic spinal deformities in neurofibromatosis. Treatment by anterior and posterior fusion. *J Bone Joint Surg* 66B:495, 1984

645. Huson SM: Recent developments in the diagnosis and management of neurofibromatosis. *Arch Dis Child* 64:745, 1989

646. Huson SM, Compston DAS, Harper PS: A genetic study of von Recklinghausen neurofibromatosis in south east Wales. II. Guidelines for genetic counseling. *J Med Genet* 26:712, 1989

647. Isu T, Miyasaka K, Abe H, et al: Atlantoaxial dislocation associated with neurofibromatosis. Report of three cases. *J Neurosurg* 58:451, 1983

648. Joseph KN, Bowen JR, MacEwen GD: Unusual orthopedic manifestations of neurofibromatosis. *Clin J Orthop* 278:17, 1992

649. Kaempffe FA, Gillespie R: Pseudarthrosis of the radius after fracture through normal bone in a child who had neurofibromatosis. A case report. *J Bone Joint Surg* 71A:1419, 1989

650. Kameyama O, Ogawa R: Pseudarthrosis of the radius associated with neurofibromatosis: Report of a case and review of the literature. *J Pediatr Orthop* 10:128, 1990

651. Lubs ML, Bauer MS, Formas ME, Djokic B: Lisch nodules in neurofibromatosis type 1. *N Engl J Med* 324:1264, 1991

652. Mapstone TB: Neurofibromatosis and central nervous system tumors in childhood. *Neurosurg Clin North Am* 3:771, 1992

653. Neurofibromatosis. Conference Statement. National Institutes of Health Consensus Development Conference. *Arch Neurol* 45:575, 1988

654. von Recklinghausen F: *Ueber die multiplen Fibrome der Haut ihre Beziehung zu den multiplen Neuromen.* August Hirschwald, 1882

655. Rockower S, McKay D, Nason S: Dislocation of the spine in neurofibromatosis. A report of two cases. *J Bone Joint Surg* 64A:1240, 1982

656. Sirois JL III, Drennan JC: Dystrophic spinal deformity in neurofibromatosis. *J Pediatr Orthop* 10:522, 1990

657. Sørensen SA, Mulvihill JJ, Nielsen A: Long-term follow-up of von Recklinghausen neurofibromatosis. Survival and malignant neoplasms. *N Engl J Med* 314:1010, 1986

658. Viskochil D, White R, Cawthon R: The neurofibromatosis type 1 gene. *Ann Rev Neurosci* 16:183, 1993

659. Wanebo JE, Malik JM, VandenBerg SR, Wanego HJ, Driesen N, Persing JA: Malignant peripheral nerve sheath tumors. A clinicopathologic study of 38 cases. *Cancer* 71: 1247, 1993

660. Winter RB: Spontaneous dislocation of a vertebra in a patient who had neurofibromatosis. Report of a case with dural ectasia. *J Bone Joint Surg* 73A:1402, 1991

661. Winter RB, Moe JH, Bradford DS, Lonstein JE, Pedras CV, Weber AH: Spine deformity in neurofibromatosis. A review of one hundred and two patients. *J Bone Joint Surg* 61A: 677, 1979

Proteus Syndrome

662. Demetriades D, Hager J, Nikolaides N, Malamitsi-Puchner A, Bartsocas CS: Proteus syndrome: Musculoskeletal manifestations and management: A report of two cases. *J Pediatr Orthop* 12:106, 1992

663. Stricker S: Musculoskeletal manifestations of Proteus syndrome: Report of two cases with literature review. *J Pediatr Orthop* 12:667, 1992

664. Tibbles JA, Cohen MM: The Proteus syndrome: The Elephant Man diagnosed. *Br Med J* 293:683, 1986

665. Wiedemann HR, Burgio GR, Adenhoff P, Kunze J, Kaufmann HJ, Schirg E: The Proteus syndrome. *Eur J Pediatr* 140:5, 1983

Arthrogryposis Multiplex Congenita

666. Banker BQ: Neuropathologic aspects of arthrogryposis multiplex congenita. *Clin Orthop* 194:30, 1985

667. Bayne LG: Hand assessment and management of arthrogryposis multiplex congenita. *Clin Orthop* 194:68, 1985

668. Bennett JB, Hansen PE, Granberry WM, Cain TE: Surgical management of arthrogryposis in the upper extremity. *J Pediatr Orthop* 5:281, 1985

669. Brown LM, Robson MJ, Sharrard WJ: The pathophysiology of arthrogryposis multiplex congenita neurologica. *J Bone Joint Surg* 62B:291, 1980

670. Carlson WO, Speck GJ, Urcari U, Wenger DR: Arthrogryposis multiplex congenita—a long-term follow-up study. *Clin Orthop* 194:115, 1985

671. Dangles CJ, Bilos ZJ: Surgical correction of thumb deformity in arthrogryposis multiplex congenita. *Hand* 13:55, 1981

672. Drachman DB, Weiner LP, Price DL, Chase J: Experimental arthrogryposis multiplex congenita caused by viral myopathy. *Arch Neurol* 33:362, 1976

673. Drummond DS, Cruess RL: The management of the foot and ankle in arthrogryposis multiplex congenita. *J Bone Joint Surg* 60B:96, 1978

674. Fuller DJ: Immobilisation of foetal joints: A cause of progressive prenatal deformity. *J Bone Joint Surg* 57B:115, 1975

675. Guidera KJ, Kortright L, Berber V, Ogden JA: Radiographic changes in arthrogrypotic knees. *Skeletal Radiol* 20:193, 1991

676. Hall JG: An approach to congenital contracture. *Pediatr Ann* 10:15, 1981

677. Hall JG: Genetic aspects of arthrogryposis. *Clin Orthop* 194:44, 1985

678. Hall JG, Reed SD, Greene G: The distal arthrogryposes: Delineation of new entities—review and nosologic discussion. *Am J Med Genet* 11:185, 1982

679. Herron LD, Westin GW, Dawson EG: Scoliosis in arthrogryposis multiplex congenita. *J Bone Joint Surg* 60A:293, 1978

680. Hoffer MM, Swank S, Eastman R, Clark D, Teige R: Ambulation in severe arthrogryposis. *J Pediatr Orthop* 3:293, 1983

681. Hsu LC, Jaffray D, Leong JCY: Talectomy for clubfoot in arthrogryposis. *J Bone Joint Surg* 66B:694, 1984

682. Huurman WH, Jacobson ST: The hip in arthrogryposis multiplex congenita. *Clin Orthop* 194:81, 1985

683. Inaba Y, Kurogi H, Omori T: Akabane disease: Epizootic abortion, premature birth, stillbirth and congenital arthrogryposis hydranencephaly in cattle, sheep and goats, caused by Akabane virus. *Aust Vet J* 51:584, 1975

684. Lloyd Roberts GC, Lettin AWF: Arthrogryposis multiplex congenita. *J Bone Joint Surg* 52B:494, 1970

685. McCormack MK, Coppola-McCormack PJ, Lee ML: Autosomal-dominant inheritance of distal arthrogryposis. *Am J Med Genet* 6:163, 1980

686. Mead NG, Lithgow WC, Sweeney HJ: Arthrogryposis multiplex congenita. *J Bone Joint Surg* 40A:1285, 1958

687. Mennen U: Early corrective surgery of the wrist and elbow in arthrogryposis multiplex congenita. *J Hand Surg* 18B: 304, 1993

688. Middleton DS: Occurrence of incomplete development of the striated muscle fibre as a cause of certain congenital deformities of the extremities. *Edinburgh Med J* 39:389, 1932

689. Nové-Josserand G, Rendu A: Résultats eloigne et valeur de la méthode de Finck dans le traitement précoce de pieds bots congenitaux. *Lyon Chir* 8:121, 1918

690. Palmer PM, MacEwen GD, Bowen JR, Mathews PA: Passive motion therapy for infants with arthrogryposis. *Clin Orthop* 194:54, 1985

691. Robertson GG, Williamson AP, Blattner RJ: A study of abnormalities in early chick embryos inoculated with Newcastle disease virus. *J Exp Zool* 129:5, 1955

692. Sarwark JF, MacEwen GD, Scott CI: Current concepts review. Amyoplasia (a common form of arthrogryposis). *J Bone Joint Surg* 72A:465, 1990

693. Schanz A: Ein Fall von Multiplen Kongenitalen Kontracturen. *Z Orthop Chir* 5:9, 1898

694. Shapiro F, Specht L: The diagnosis and orthopaedic treatment of childhood spinal muscular atrophy, peripheral neuropathy, Friedreich ataxia, and arthrogryposis. *J Bone Joint Surg* 75A:1699, 1993

695. Sheldon W: Amyoplasia congenita (multiple congenital articular rigidity: Arthrogryposis multiplex congenita). *Arch Dis Child* 7:117, 1932

696. Smith RJ: Hand deformities with arthrogryposis multiplex congenita. *J Bone Joint Surg* 55A:883, 1973

697. Sodergard JM, Jaaskelainen JJ, Ryoppy S: Muscle ultrasonography in arthrogryposis. Comparison with clinical, neuromyographic and histologic findings in 41 cases. *Acta Orthop Scand* 64:357, 1993

698. Sodergard J, Ryoppy S: Foot deformities in arthrogryposis multiplex congenita. *J Pediatr Orthop* 14:768, 1994

699. Solund K, Sonne-Holm S, Kjolbye JE: Talectomy for equinovarus deformity in arthrogryposis. A 13 (2-20) year review of 17 feet. *Acta Orthop Scand* 62:372, 1991

700. Staheli LT, Chew DE, Elliott JS, Mosca VS: Management of hip dislocations in children with arthrogryposis. *J Pediatr Orthop* 7:681, 1987

701. Swinyard CA, Bleck EE: The etiology of arthrogryposis (multiple congenital contractures). *Clin Orthop* 194:15, 1985

702. Williams PF: The elbow in arthrogryposis. *J Bone Joint Surg* 55B:834, 1973

703. Williams PF: Management of upper limb problems in arthrogryposis. *Clin Orthop* 194:60, 1985

704. Wynne-Davies R, Williams PF, O'Connor JC: The 1960's epidemic of arthrogryposis multiplex congenita: A survey from the United Kingdom, Australia and the United States of America. *J Bone Joint Surg* 63B:76, 1981

705. Yonenobu K, Tada K, Swanson AB: Arthrogryposis of the hand. *J Pediatr Orthop* 4:599, 1984

Bone Dysplasias

706. Bailey JA: *Disproportionate Short Stature.* Philadelphia, WB Saunders, 1973

707. Beighton P: *Inherited Disorders of the Skeleton.* New York, Churchill-Livingstone, 1978

708. Beighton P, Cremin BJ: *Sclerosing Bone Dysplasias.* New York, Springer, 1980

709. Brailsford JF: *Radiology of Bones and Joints,* 5th ed. Baltimore, Williams & Wilkins, 1953

710. Carter CO, Fairbank TJ: *The Genetics of Locomotor Disorders.* London, Oxford University Press, 1974

711. Cremin BJ, Beighton P: *Bone Dysplasias of Infancy.* New York, Springer, 1978

712. Fairbank HAT: *An Atlas of General Affections of the Skeleton.* Edinburgh, Livingstone, 1951

713. Haran F, Beighton P: *Orthopaedic Problems in Inherited Skeletal Disorders.* New York, Springer-Verlag, 1982

714. Kaufman HJ (ed): Intrinsic diseases of bones, in *Progress in Pediatric Radiology,* Vol 4. New York, Karger, 1973

715. Lamy M, Maroteaux P: *Les Chondrodystrophies Génotypiques.* Paris, L'Expansion Scientifique Française, 1961

716. McKusick VA: *Heritable Disorders of Connective Tissue.* St. Louis, CV Mosby, 1972

717. McKusick VA: *Mendelian Inheritance in Man.* Baltimore, Johns Hopkins Press, 1978

718. Maroteaux P: *Bone Diseases of Children.* Philadelphia, JB Lippincott, 1979

719. Paterson CR: *Metabolic Disorders of Bone.* Oxford, Blackwell, 1974

720. Rubin P: *Dynamic Classification of Bone Dysplasias.* Chicago, Year Book, 1964

721. Smith DW: *Recognizable Patterns of Human Malformations.* Philadelphia, WB Saunders, 1976

722. Smith R: *Biochemical Disorders of the Skeleton.* London, Butterworth, 1979

723. Spranger JW, Langer LO, Wiedemann HR: *Bone Dysplasia.* Philadelphia, WB Saunders, 1974

724. Taybi H, Lachman RS: *Radiology of Syndromes, Metabolic Disorders, and Skeletal Dysplasias.* St. Louis, CV Mosby, 1996

725. Warkany J: *Congenital Malformations.* Chicago, Year Book, 1971

726. Wynne-Davies R, Fairbank TJ: *Fairbank's Atlas of General Affections of the Skeleton.* Edinburgh, Churchill-Livingstone, 1976

727. Wynne-Davies R, Hall CM, Apley AG: *Atlas of Skeletal Dysplasia.* Edinburgh, Churchill-Livingstone, 1976

Multiple Epiphyseal Dysplasia

728. Fairbank HAT: *An Atlas of General Affections of the Skeleton.* Baltimore, Williams & Wilkins, 1951

729. Fairbank HAT: Generalized diseases of the skeleton. *Proc R Soc Med* 28:1, 611, 1935

730. Herring JA: Rapidly progressive scoliosis in multiple epiphyseal dysplasia. *J Bone Joint Surg* 58A:703, 1976

731. Juberg RC, Holt JF: Inheritance of multiple epiphyseal dysplasia, tarda. *Am J Hum Genet* 20:549, 1968

732. Kozlowski K, Lipska E: Hereditary dysplasia epiphysealis multiplex. *Clin Radiol* 18:330, 1967

733. Maudsley RH: Dysplasia epiphysealis multiplex. A report of fourteen cases in three families. *J Bone Joint Surg* 37B:228, 1955

734. Ribbing S: Hereditare multiple epiphysenstorungen und osteochondrosis dissecans. *Vortag Kongr Nordisch Med Radiol* 6:397, 1951

735. Spranger J: The epiphyseal dysplasias. *Clin Orthop* 114:46, 1975

736. Wenger DR, Ezaki M: Bilateral femoral head collapse in an adolescent with brachydactyly (multiple epiphyseal dysplasia tarda type 1c). *J Pediatr Orthop* 1:267, 1981

737. Wynne-Davies R, Hall CM, Apley AG: *Atlas of Skeletal Dysplasias.* Edinburgh, Churchill-Livingstone, 1985, p 19

Dysplasia Epiphysealis Hemimelica

738. Fairbank TJ: *An Atlas of General Affections of the Skeleton.* Baltimore, Williams & Wilkins, 1951

739. Fasting OJ, Bjerkreim I: Dysplasia epiphysealis hemimelica. *Acta Orthop Scand* 47:217, 1976

740. Trevor D: Tarso-epiphyseal aclasis: A congenital error of epiphysial development. *J Bone Joint Surg* 32B:204, 1950

Achondroplasia

741. Bailey JA: Orthopaedic aspects of achondroplasia. *J Bone Joint Surg* 52:1285, 1970

742. Bergstrom K, Laurent U, Lundbert PO: Neurological symptoms in achondroplasia. *Acta Neurol Scand* 47:59, 1971

743. Epstein JA, Malis LI: Compression of spinal cord and cauda equina in achondroplastic dwarfs. *Neurology* 5:875, 1955

744. Horton WA, Rotter DL, Scott CI, Hall JG: Standard growth curves for achondroplasia. *J Pediatr* 93:435, 1978

745. Kopits SE: Orthopedic implication of dwarfism. *Clin Orthop* 114:153, 1976

746. Lachman RS: Fetal imaging in the skeletal dysplasia: Overview and experience. *Pediatr Radiol* 24:413, 1994

747. Maynard JA, Ippolito EG, Ponseti IV, Mickelson MR: Histochemistry and ultrastructure of the growth plate in achondroplasia. *J Bone Joint Surg* 63A:969, 1981

748. Nehme A-ME, Riseborough EJ, Tredwell SJ: Skeletal growth and development of the achondroplastic dwarf. *Clin Orthop* 116:8, 1976

749. Oberklaid F, Danks DM, Jensen F, Stace L, Rosshandler S: Achondroplasia and hypochondroplasia: Comments on frequency, mutation rate, and radiological features in skull and spine. *J Med Genet* 16:140, 1979

750. Parrot J: Les malformations achondroplastiques. *Soc Anthrop Paris* 1878

751. Ponseti IV: Skeletal growth in achondroplasia. *J Bone Joint Surg* 52A:701, 1970

752. Porter RW, Wicks M, Ottewell D: Measurement of the spinal canal by diagnostic ultrasound. *J Bone Joint Surg* 60B: 481, 1978

753. Rimoin DL: Endochondral ossification in achondroplastic dwarfism. *N Engl J Med* 283:728, 1970

754. Saleh M, Burton M: Leg lengthening: Patient selection and management in achondroplasia. *Orthop Clin North Am* 22: 589, 1991

755. Silverman FN: A differential diagnosis of achondroplasia. *Radiol Clin North Am* 6:223, 1968

756. Vilarrubias JM, Ginebreda I, Jimeno E: Lengthening of the lower limbs and correction of lumbar hyperlordosis in achondroplasia. *Clin Orthop Rel Res* 250:143, 1990

757. Wynne-Davies R, Walsh WK, Gormley J: Achondroplasia and hypochondroplasia. Clinical variation and spinal stenosis. *J Bone Joint Surg* 63B:508, 1981

Hypochondroplasia

758. Beals RK: Hypochondroplasia. *J Bone Joint Surg* 51A:728, 1969

759. Oberklaid F, Danks DM, Jensen F, Stace L, Rosshandler S: Achondroplasia and hypochondroplasia: Comments on frequency, mutation rate, and radiological features in skull and spine. *J Med Genet* 16:140, 1979

Spondyloepiphyseal Dysplasia

760. Fisher RL: Unusual spondyloepiphyseal and spondylometaphyseal dysplasias of childhood. *Clin Orthop* 100:78, 1974

761. Kozlowski K, Bittel-Dobrzynska N, Budsynska A: Spondylo-epiphyseal dysplasia congenita. *Ann Radiol* 11:367, 1958

762. Maroteaux P, Lamy M, Bernard J: La dysplasie spondylo-epiphysaire tardive. Déscription clinique et radiologique. *Presse Med* 65:1205, 1957

763. Sugiura Y, Terashima Y, Furukawa T, Yoneda M: Spondyloepiphyseal dysplasia congenita. *Int Orthop* 2:47, 1978

764. Weinfeld A, Ross MW, Sarasohn SH: Spondyloepiphyseal dysplasia tarda. A cause of premature osteoarthritis. *AJR* 101:851, 1967

765. Wynne-Davies R, Hall C: Two clinical variants of spondylo-epiphysial dysplasia congenita. *J Bone Joint Surg* 64B:435, 1982

Diastrophic Dysplasia

766. Amuso SL: Diastrophic dwarfism. *J Bone Joint Surg* 50A: 113, 1968

767. Hastbacka J, Kaitila I, Sistonen P, de la Chapelle A: Diastrophic dysplasia gene maps to the distal long arm of chromosome 5. *Proc Natl Acad Sci* 87:8056, 1990

768. Herring JA: The spinal disorders in diastrophic dwarfism. *J Bone Joint Surg* 60A:177, 1978

769. Krecak J, Starshak RJ: Cervical kyphosis in diastrophic dwarfism: CT and MR findings. *Pediatr Radiol* 17:321, 1987

770. Lamy M, Maroteaux P: Le nanisme diastrophique. *Presse Med* 52:1977, 1960

771. Poussa M, Merikanto J, Ryoppy S, Marttinen E, Kaitila I: The spine in diastrophic dysplasia. *Spine* 16:881, 1991

772. Ryoppy S, Poussa M, Merikanto J, Marttinen E, Kaitila I: Foot deformities in diastrophic dysplasia. *J Bone Joint Surg* 74B:441, 1992

Chondroectodermal Dysplasia (Ellis–Van Creveld Syndrome)

773. Aird C, McIntosh RA: Shakespeare's Richard III and the Ellis-van Creveld syndrome. *Practitioner* 220:656, 1978

774. Ellis RWB, van Creveld S: Syndrome characterized by ectodermal dysplasia, polydactyly, chondro-dysplasia and congenital morbus cordis: Report of three cases. *Arch Dis Child* 15:65, 1940

775. Mahoney MJ, Hobbins JC: Prenatal diagnosis of chondroectodermal dysplasia (Ellis-van Creveld syndrome) with fetoscopy and ultrasound. *N Engl J Med* 297:258, 1977

776. Milgram JW, Bailey JA II: Orthopaedic aspects of the Ellis-van Creveld syndrome. *Bull Hosp Joint Dis* 36:11, 1975

Osteogenesis Imperfecta

777. Ablin DS, Greenspan A, Reinhart M, Grix A: Differentiation of child abuse from osteogenesis imperfecta. *AJR* 154: 1035, 1990

778. Albright JA: Management overview of osteogenesis imperfecta. *Clin Orthop* 159:80, 1981

779. Albright JA, Grunt JA: Studies of patients with osteogenesis imperfecta. *J Bone Joint Surg* 53A:1415, 1971

780. Astley R: Metaphyseal fracture in osteogenesis imperfecta. *Br J Radiol* 52:441, 1979

781. Bailey RW, Dubow HI: Evolution of the concept of an extensible nail accommodating to normal longitudinal bone growth: Clinical considerations and implications. *Clin Orthop* 159:157, 1981

782. Bauze RJ, Smith R, Francis MJP: A new look at osteogenesis imperfecta. A clinical, radiological and biochemical study of forty-two patients. *J Bone Joint Surg* 57B:2, 1975

783. Beighton P, Spranger J, Versveld G: Skeletal complications in osteogenesis imperfecta. A review of 153 South African patients. *S Afr Med J* 64:565, 1983

784. Benson DR, Donaldson DH, Millar EA: The spine in osteogenesis imperfecta. *J Bone Joint Surg* 60A:925, 1978

785. Bleck EE: Nonoperative treatment of osteogenesis imperfecta: Orthotic and mobility management. *Clin Orthop* 159:111, 1981

786. Bullough PG, Davidson D: The morphology of the growth plate in osteogenesis imperfecta. *Clin Orthop* 116:259, 1976

787. Bullough PG, Davidson DD, Lorenzo JC: The morbid anatomy of the skeleton in osteogenesis imperfecta. *Clin Orthop* 159:42, 1981

788. Carty H: Brittle or battered. *Arch Dis Child* 63:350, 1988

789. Cassis N, Gledhill RB, Dubow H: Osteogenesis imperfecta: Its sociological and surgical implications, with a preliminary report on the use of a telescoping intramedullary nail. *J Bone Joint Surg* 57B:533, 1975

790. Cole WG: Etiology and pathogenesis of heritable connective tissue diseases. *J Pediatr Orthop* 13:392, 1993

791. Cole WG, Jaenisch R, Bateman JF: New insights into the molecular pathology of osteogenesis imperfecta. *QJ Med* 261:1, 1989

792. Cremin B, Goodman H, Spranger J, Beighton P: Wormian bones in osteogenesis imperfecta and other disorders. *Skeletal Radiol* 8:35, 1982

793. Cristofaro RL, Hoek KJ, Bonnett CA, Brown JC: Operative treatment of spine deformity in osteogenesis imperfecta. *Clin Orthop* 139:40, 1979

794. Dent JA, Paterson CR: Fractures in early childhood: Osteogenesis imperfecta or child abuse? *J Pediatr Orthop* 11:184, 1991

795. Epstein DM, Dalinka MK, Kaplan FS, Aronchick JM, Marinelli DL, Kundel HL: Observer variation in the detection of osteopenia. *Skel Radiol* 15:347, 1986

796. Fairbank HAT: Osteogenesis imperfecta and osteogenesis imperfecta cystica. *J Bone Joint Surg* 30B:164, 1948

797. Falvo KA, Bullough PG: Osteogenesis imperfecta: A histometric analysis. *J Bone Joint Surg* 55A:275, 1973

798. Falvo KA, Root L, Bullough PG: Osteogenesis imperfecta: Clinical evaluation and management. *J Bone Joint Surg* 56A:783, 1974

799. Findori G, Rigault JP, Padovari JF, Bensahel H: Expanding intramedullary rods in the treatment of osteogenesis imperfecta. *Rev Chir Orthop* 65:235, 1979

800. Gahagan S, Rimsza ME: Child abuse or osteogenesis imperfecta: How can we tell? *Pediatrics* 88:987, 1991

801. Gamble JG, Strudwick WJ, Rinsky LA, Bleck EE: Complications of intramedullary rods in osteogenesis imperfecta: Bailey-Dubow rods versus nonelongating rods. *J Pediatr Orthop* 8:645, 1988

802. Goldman AB, Davidson D, Pavlov H, Bullough PG: "Popcorn" calcifications: A prognostic sign in osteogenesis imperfecta. *Radiology* 136:351, 1980

803. Hall JG, Rohrt T: The stapes in osteogenesis imperfecta. *Acta Orolaryngol* 65:345, 1968

804. Hanscom DA, Winter RB, Lutter L, Lonstein JE, Bloom B, Bradford DS: Osteogenesis imperfecta. *J Bone Joint Surg* 74A:598, 1992

805. Keats TE: Diffuse thickening of calvarium in osteogenesis imperfecta. Further observations. *Radiology* 86:97, 1966

806. King JD, Bobechko WP: Osteogenesis imperfecta. An orthopaedic description and surgical review. *J Bone Joint Surg* 53B:72, 1971

807. Klenerman L, Ockenden BG, Townsend AC: Osteosarcoma occurring in osteogenesis imperfecta. *J Bone Joint Surg* 49B:314, 1967

808. Lang-Stevenson AL, Sharrard WJW: Intramedullary rodding with Bailey-Dubow extensible rods in osteogenesis imperfecta. An interim report of results and complications. *J Bone Joint Surg* 66B:227, 1984

809. Levin LS: The dentition in the osteogenesis imperfecta syndromes. *Clin Orthop* 159:64, 1981

810. Libman RH: Anesthetic considerations for the patient with osteogenesis imperfecta. *Clin Orthop* 159:123, 1981

811. Marafioti RL, Westin GW: Elongating intramedullary rods in the treatment of osteogenesis imperfecta. *J Bone Joint Surg* 59A:467, 1977

812. McHale KA, Tenuta JJ, Tosi LR, McKay DW: Percutaneous intramedullary fixation of long bone deformity in severe osteogenesis imperfecta. *Clin Orthop* 305:242, 1994

813. Mirbaha M: Multiple osteotomies and intramedullary fixation of the radius and ulna to correct severe deformity and improve function in osteogenesis imperfecta. Report of a case. *J Bone Joint Surg* 48A:523, 1966

814. Nogami H, Ono Y, Katoh R, Oohira A: Microvascular and cellular defects of the periosteum of osteogenesis imperfecta. *Clin Orthop* 292:358, 1993

815. Papagelopoulos PJ, Morrey BF: Hip and knee replacement in osteogenesis imperfecta. *J Bone Joint Surg* 75A:572, 1993

816. Porat S, Heller E, Seidman DS, Meyer S: Functional results of operation in osteogenesis imperfecta: Elongating and nonelongating rods. *J Pediatr Orthop* 11:200, 1991

817. Pozo JL, Crockard HA, Ransford AO: Basilar impression in osteogenesis imperfecta. *J Bone Joint Surg* 66B:233, 1984

818. Roberts JB: Bilateral hyperplastic callus formation in osteogenesis imperfecta. A case report. *J Bone Joint Surg* 58A:1164, 1976

819. Rodriguez RP, Bailey RW: Internal fixation of the femur in patients with osteogenesis imperfecta. *Clin Orthop* 159:126, 1981

820. Root L: Upper limb surgery in osteogenesis imperfecta. *Clin Orthop* 159:141, 1981

821. Ryoppy S, Alberty A, Kaitila I: Early semiclosed intramedullary stabilization in osteogenesis imperfecta. *J Pediatr Orthop* 7:139, 1987

822. Seedorff KS: *Osteogenesis Imperfecta. A Study of Clinical Features and Heredity Based on 55 Danish Families Comprising 180 Affected Persons.* Copenhagen, Munksgaard, 1949

823. Shapiro F: Consequences of an osteogenesis imperfecta diagnosis for survival and ambulation. *J Pediatr Orthop* 5:456, 1985

824. Sillence DO: *Bone Dysplasia. Genetic and Ultrastructural Aspects with Special Reference to Osteogenesis Imperfecta.* M.D. Thesis. University of Melbourne, Australia, 1977

994. Boni M, Ceciliani L: Fractures in haemophilia. *Ital J Orthop Traumatol* 2:301, 1976

995. Brower TD, Wilde AH: Femoral neuropathy in hemophilia. *J Bone Joint Surg* 48A:487, 1966

996. Clark MW: Knee synovectomy in hemophilia. *Orthopaedics* 1:285, 1978

997. Coventry MB, Owen CA Jr, Murphy TR, Mills SD: Survival of patient with hemophilia and fracture of the femur. *J Bone Joint Surg* 41A:1392, 1959

998. Driessen APPM: *Arthropathies in Haemophiliacs.* Groningen, Van-Grocum Company BV-Assen, 1973

999. Duthie RB, Matthews JM, Rizza CR, Steel WM: *The Management of Musculoskeletal Problems in the Haemophilias.* Oxford, Blackwell, 1972

1000. Feil E, Bentley G, Rizza CR: Fracture management in patients with haemophilia. *J Bone Joint Surg* 56B:643, 1974

1001. Floman Y, Niska M: Dislocation of the hip joint complicating repeated hemarthrosis in hemophilia. *J Pediatr Orthop* 3:99, 1983

1002. Gamble JG, Bellah J, Rinsky LA, Glader B: Arthropathy of the ankle in hemophilia. *J Bone Joint Surg* 73A:1008, 1991

1003. Goodfellow JW, Fearn CB d'A, Matthews JM: Iliacus hematoma: A common complication in hemophilia. *J Bone Joint Surg* 49B:748, 1967

1004. Greene WB: Synovectomy of the ankle for hemophilic arthropathy. *J Bone Joint Surg* 76A:812, 1994

1005. Greene WB: Use of continuous passive slow motion in the post-operative rehabilitation of different pediatric knee and elbow problems. *J Pediatr Orthop* 3:419, 1983

1006. Greene WB, McMillan CW: Nonsurgical management of hemophilic arthropathy. *AAOS Instr Course Lect* 38:367, 1989

1007. Greene WB, Yankaskas BC, Guilford WB: Roentgenographic classifications of hemophilic arthropathy. *J Bone Joint Surg* 71A:237, 1989

1008. Hilgartner MW: Home care for hemophilia: Current state of the art. *Scand J Haematol* 30:58, 1977

1009. Horwitz H, Simon N, Bassen FA: Haemophiliac pseudotumor of the pelvis. *Br J Radiol NS* 32:51, 1959

1010. Hutcheson J: Peripelvic new bone formation in hemophilia. *Radiology* 109:529, 1973

1011. Ingram GIC, Brozovic M, Slater NGP: *Bleeding Disorders: Investigation and Management,* 2nd ed. Oxford, Blackwell, 1982

1012. Ivins JC: Bone and joint complications of hemophilia, in Brinkhous KM (ed): *Hemophilia and Hemophilioid Diseases.* International Symposium. Chapel Hill, NC: University of North Carolina Press, 1957, p 225

1013. Katz SG, Nelson IW, Atkins RM, Duthie RB: Peripheral nerve lesions in hemophilia. *J Bone Joint Surg* 73A:1016, 1991

1014. Kemp HS, Matthews JM: The management of fractures in haemophilia and Christmas disease. *J Bone Joint Surg* 50B:351, 1968

1015. Kinnas PA, Woodham CH, MacLarnon JC: Ultrasonic measurements of haematomata of joints and soft tissues in the haemophiliac. *Scand J Haematol* (Suppl) 40:225, 1984

1016. Lachiewicz PF, Inglis JN, Insall JN, Sculco TP, Hilgartner MW, Bussell JB: Total knee arthroplasty in hemophilia. *J Bone Joint Surg* 67A:1361, 1985

1017. Large DF, Ludlam CA, Manicol MF: Common peroneal nerve entrapment in a hemophiliac. *Clin Orthop* 181:165, 1983

1018. Lazerson J, Nagel DH, Becker J: Myositis ossificans as a complication of severe hemophilia A, in *Comprehensive Management of Musculoskeletal Disorders in Hemophilia.* Washington DC, National Academy of Science, 1973

1019. LeBalch T, Ebelin M, Laurian Y, Lambert T, Verroust F, Larrieu M-J: Synovectomy of the elbow in young hemophilic patients. *J Bone Joint Surg* 69A:264, 1987

1020. Levine PH: Efficacy of self-therapy in hemophilia. A study of 72 patients with hemophilia A and B. *N Engl J Med* 291:1381, 1974

1021. Limbird TJ, Dennis SC: Synovectomy and continuous passive motion (cpm) in hemophiliac patients. *Arthroscopy* 3:74, 1987

1022. Madigan RR: Acute compartment syndrome in hemophilia. A case report (letter). *J Bone Joint Surg* 64A:313, 1982

1023. Madigan RR, Hanna WT, Wallace SL: Acute compartment syndrome in hemophilia. A case report. 63A:1327, 1981

1024. McCollough NC III, Enis JE, Lovitt J, Lian ECY, Niemann KMW, Loughlin FC Jr: Synovectomy or total replacement of the knee in hemophilia. *J Bone Joint Surg* 61A:69, 1979

1025. McMillan CW, Greene WB, Blatt PM, White GC II, Roberts HR: The management of musculoskeletal problems in hemophilia. Part I. Principles of medical management of hemophilia. *AAOS Instr Course Lect* 32:210, 1983

1026. Montane I, McCollough NC III, Lian EC-Y: Synovectomy of the knee for hemophilic arthropathy. *J Bone Joint Surg* 68A:210, 1986

1027. Nicol RO, Menelaus MB: Synovectomy of the knee in hemophilia. *J Pediatr Orthop* 6:330, 1986

1028. Serre H, Izran P, Simon L, Rogues JM: Les attients de la hanche au cours de l'hemophilie. *Marseille Med* 106:483, 1969

1029. Starker L: Knochenusur durch ein hamophiles, subperiosteles Hamatom. *Mitt Grenzgeb Med Chir* 31:381, 1918–1919

1030. Stein H, Duthie RB: The pathogenesis of chronic haemophilic arthropathy. *J Bone Joint Surg* 63B:601, 1981

1031. Teitelbaum S: Radiologic evaluation of the hemophilic hip. *Mt Sinai J Med* 44:400, 1977

1032. Triantafyllou SJ, Hanks GA, Handal JA, Greer RB III: Open and arthroscopic synovectomy in hemophilic arthropathy of the knee. *Clin Orthop* 283:196, 1992

1033. Weidel JD: Arthroscopic synovectomy for chronic hemophilic synovitis of the knee. *Arthroscopy* 1:205, 1985

1034. Valderrama JAF de, Natthews JM: The hemophilic pseudotumor or hemophilic subperiosteal hematoma. *J Bone Joint Surg* 47B:256, 1965

INDEX